Manual of Cardio-oncology

Chiara Lestuzzi
Stefano Oliva
Francesco Ferraù
Editors

Manual of Cardio-oncology

Cardiovascular Care in the Cancer Patient

Springer

Editors
Chiara Lestuzzi
Cardiology Unit
IRCCS CRO-National Cancer Institute
Aviano (PN), Italy

Francesco Ferraù
Medical Oncology Unit
Ospedale San Vincenzo
Taormina, Italy

Stefano Oliva
Cardiology Unit
National Cancer Institute "Giovanni Paolo II"
Bari, Italy

ISBN 978-3-319-40234-5 ISBN 978-3-319-40236-9 (eBook)
DOI 10.1007/978-3-319-40236-9

Library of Congress Control Number: 2016961519

Printed on acid-free paper

This Springer imprint is published by Springer Nature
The registered company is Springer International Publishing AG
The registered company address is: Gewerbestrasse 11, 6330 Cham, Switzerland

Foreword

The cancer burden is a worldwide major public health problem. In the developed world, one in three people will develop cancer during their lifetime. As cancer-related survival has improved, an unexpected increase in premature cardiovascular events has occurred. In addition to heart failure, which mainly relates to the fibrosis and apoptosis leading to myocardial dysfunction and arrhythmias, a number of chemotherapeutic agents cause disturbances of microvascular function. In addition, premature coronary artery disease and valvular and pericardial disease are important sequelae of radiotherapy.

Associations have been identified between medications used to treat cancer and cardiovascular events. The agents most commonly associated with cardiovascular injury include the anthracyclines (i.e. doxorubicin), the alkylating agents (i.e. cyclophosphamide), and the tyrosine kinase inhibitors (i.e. trastuzumab). Some of these cancer drugs can cause irreversible and progressive cardiotoxicity, while others can lead only to temporary, stunning-like dysfunction without long-term consequences for the patient.

Long-term cancer survivors now represent one of the largest and fastest growing patient populations at risk for premature cardiovascular disease. In fact, increases in cardiovascular-related morbidity and mortality now threaten to offset some of the advancements in cancer-related survival. However, currently, research initiatives, clinical management, and guidelines addressing the needs of cancer survivors are still lacking.

The definition of what constitutes "cardiotoxicity" is clearly of pivotal importance but remains poorly standardized. The most typical example is heart failure, which can be clinically suspected or only diagnosed during a dedicated cardiac imaging examination. The extent of cardiotoxicity is also variable, depending on the type of drug used, combination with other drugs, prior mediastinal radiotherapy, and the presence of cardiovascular risk factors or history of heart disease. Early detection of the patients prone to developing cardiotoxicity is the key issue to decrease morbidity and mortality.

The Manual of Cardio-oncology coordinated by Chiara Lestuzzi, Stefano Oliva, and Francesco Ferraù provides major clues in the setting of cancer treatment-related cardiotoxicity. The book is very comprehensive covering several major aspects of Cardio-oncology. The book is divided into five main chapters including the current knowledge about epidemiology of the problem, the mechanisms and drugs associated with cardiac toxicity, the diagnostic imaging approaches, the management strategies, and the Cardio-oncology discipline, which is a medical subspecialty concerned with the diagnosis and treatment of heart disease in cancer patients.

With its original approach, the Manual of Cardio-oncology raises awareness of the needs of cancer survivors through a series of recommendations. The book already has an eye to the future and anticipates the priorities for research and management strategies. It should be considered as a reference and will be helpful to Oncologists, Cardiologists, Radiologists, as well as other Clinicians and Students interested in managing patients with cancer.

Patrizio Lancellotti, MD, PhD
Liège, Belgium

Contents

List of Contributors

Adriana Albini
Laboratory of Vascular Biology and Angiogenesis, Scientific and Tecnology Park
IRCCS MultiMedica
Milan, Italy
albini.adriana@gmail.com

Giovanni Donato Aquaro
Fondazione G.Monasterio CNR-Regione Toscana, Via Moruzzi, 1
56124, Pisa, Italy
aquaro@ftgm.it

Riccardo Asteggiano
Cardiology ASL TO 3
Regione Piemonte, Italy
asteggianoricc@hotmail.com

Tanja Baresic
Nuclear Medicine Unit CRO-National Cancer Institute
Aviano, Pordenone, Italy
tbaresic@cro.it

Sandro Barni
The Medical Oncology Hospital Trevigliio
Via Copernico 6, Macherio
Province of Monza and Brianza, Italy
sandro.barni@ospedale.treviglio.bg.it
sandrobarni@alice.it

Barbara Bassani
Laboratory of Vascular Biology and Angiogenesis, Scientific and Tecnology Park
IRCCS MultiMedica
Milan, Italy
babie.bass@gmail.com

Cristina Basso
Department of Cardiac, Thoracic and Vascular Sciences, Pathological Anatomy-Cardiovascular Pathology
Azienda Ospedaliera-University of Padova
Medical School, Via A. Gabelli, 61
35121, Padova, Italy
cristina.basso@unipd.it

Giorgio Battaglia
U.O.C. Nefrologia e Dialisi, Ospedale Santa Marta e Santa Venera
Acireale, Italy
giovanni.giorgio.battaglia@hotmail.it

Massimiliano Berretta
Department of Medical Oncology
National Cancer Institute
Aviano, Pordenone, Italy
mberretta@cro.it

Ettore Bidoli
Unit of Cancer Epidemiology
Centro di Riferimento Oncologico, IRCCS
Aviano, 33081, Italy
bidolie@cro.it

Irma Bisceglia
Cardiovascular Department
S. Camillo Hospital
Rome, Italy
i.bisceglia@libero.it

Sebastiano Bordonaro
Interdisciplinary Unit for Survivors and Chronic Cancer Patients "Lia Buccheri e Nino Tralongo" UO Medical Oncology, RAO Hospital Umberto I
Siracusa, Italy
Bordonaro@raosr.it

Eugenio Borsatti
Nuclear Medicine Unit
CRO-National Cancer Institute
Aviano, Pordenone, Italy
eborsatti@cro.it

Antonino Bruno
Laboratory of Vascular Biology and Angiogenesis, Scientific and Tecnology Park
IRCCS MultiMedica
Milan, Italy
82antonino.bruno@gmail.com

Angela Buonadonna
Department of Medical Oncology
CRO-National Cancer Institute
Aviano, Pordenone, Italy
abuonadonna@cro.it

Maria Agnese Caggegi
Il Gabbiano Hospice and Community
Palliative Care Service, AAS5,
Friuli Occidentale
Pordenone, Italy
agnese.cag@gmail.com

Francesca Cairello
Cardiology Department
Istituto Giannina Gaslini
Genoa, Italy
francesca.cairello@gmail.cpm

Daniela Cardinale
Cardioncology Unit
European Institute of Oncology
Milan, Italy
daniela.cardinale@ieo.it

Annamaria Catino
IRCCS "Giovanni Paolo II"
Clinical Cancer Center
Viale Orazio Flacco 65
70124, Bari, Italy
a.catino@oncologico.bari.it

Anna Clementi
U.O.C. Nefrologia e Dialisi
Ospedale San Giovanni Di Dio
Agrigento, Italy
a.clementi81@virgilio.it

Paola Corradino
Laboratory of Vascular Biology and
Angiogenesis, Scientific and Tecnology Park
IRCCS MultiMedica
Milan, Italy
paolacorradino@yahoo.it

Maria Derchi
Cardiology Department
Istituto Giannina Gaslini
Genoa, Italy
MariaDerchi@ospedale-gaslini.ge.it

Francesco Ferraù
Medical Oncology Unit
Ospedale San Vincenzo
Taormina, Italy
francescoferrau@tin.it

Lucia Fratino
Department of Medical Oncology
National Cancer Institute, IRCCS
Via Franco Gallini 2
Aviano, Pordenone, Italy
lfratino@cro.it

Francesco Furlanello
Arrhythmia and Electrophysiology Center
IRCCS Humanitas Research Hospital
Milan, Italy
ffurlanello@villabiancatrento.it

Domenico Galetta
IRCCS "Giovanni Paolo II"
Clinical Cancer Center
Viale Orazio Flacco 65
70124, Bari, Italy
galetta@oncologico.bari.it

Maurizio Garozzo
U.O.C. Nefrologia e Dialisi, Ospedale Santa
Marta e Santa Venera
Acireale, Italy
maurizio_garozzo@virgilio.it

Laura Ghilardi
Dipartimento Interaziendale
Provinciale Oncologico
Cancer Center OspedalePapa Giovanni XXIII
Bergamo, Italy
lghilardi@hpg23.it

Riccardo Haupt
Epidemiology and Biostatistics Unit
Istituto Giannina Gaslini
Genoa, Italy
riccardohaupt@ospedale-gaslini.ge.it

Cezar Iliescu
Cardiac Catheterization Laboratory, Cardiology
Department MD Anderson Cancer Center
Houston, TX, USA
CIliescu@mdanderson.org

Roberto Labianca
Dipartimento Interaziendale
Provinciale Oncologico
Cancer Center Ospedale Papa Giovanni XXIII
Bergamo, Italy
rlabianca@hpg23.it

Chiara Lestuzzi
Cardiology Unit, IRCCS CRO-National
Cancer Institute
Aviano, Pordenone, Italy
clestuzzi@cro.it

Antonio Logroscino
IRCCS "Giovanni Paolo II"
Clinical Cancer Center
Viale Orazio Flacco 65
70124, Bari, Italy
aflogr@alice.it

Nicoletta Macrì
Laboratory of Vascular Biology and
Angiogenesis, Scientific and Tecnology Park
IRCCS MultiMedica
Milan Italy
nicolettamacri@yahoo.it

Nicola Maurea
Division of Cardiology
National Cancer Institute
Sen. Pascale Foundation
via Mariano Semmola
80131, Naples, Italy
n.maurea@istitutotumori.na.it

Gian Maria Miolo
Department of Medical Oncology
CRO-National Cancer Institute
Aviano, Pordenone, Italy
gmiolo@cro.it

Andrea Misino
IRCCS "Giovanni Paolo II"
Clinical Cancer Center
Viale Orazio Flacco 65
70124, Bari, Italy
dott.misino@oncologico.bari.it

Elisabetta Sara Montagna
IRCCS "Giovanni Paolo II"
Clinical Cancer Center
Viale Orazio Flacco 65
70124, Bari, Italy
es.montagna@libero.it

Ines Monte
Cardio-Thorax-Vascular and Transplant
Department University of Catania
Catania, Italy
inemonte@unict.it

Vera Morsellino
Epidemiology and Biostatistics Unit
Istituto Giannina Gaslini
Genoa, Italy
veramorsellino@gaslini.org

Anju Nohria
Division of Cardiovascular Medicine
Cardio-Oncology Program
Department of Medicine
Dana-Farber Cancer Institute
and Brigham and Women's Hospital
Harvard Medical School
Boston, MA, USA
anohria@partners.org

Douglas M. Noonan
Laboratory of Vascular Biology and
Angiogenesis, Scientific and Tecnology Park
IRCCS MultiMedica
Milan, Italy

Department of Biotechnologies and Life
Sciences, University of Insubria
Varese, Italy
douglas.noonan@gmail.com

Stefano Oliva
Cardiology Unit
National Cancer Institute "Giovanni Paolo II"
Viale Orazio Flacco 65
70124, Bari, Italy
stefano.oliva@alice.it

Antonino De Paoli
Department of Radiation Oncology
CRO-National Cancer Institute
Aviano, Pordenone, Italy
adepaoli@cro.it

Iris Parrini
Department Cardiology, Hospital Mauriziano
Turin, Italy
irisparrini@libero.it

Sara Pessano
Epidemiology and Biostatistics Unit
Istituto Giannina Gaslini
Genoa, Italy
pessara@yahoo.it

Fausto Petrelli
Oncology Unit, Oncology Department
ASST Bergamo Ovest, Ospedale di Treviglio
Piazzale Ospedale 1
24047, Treviglio, BG, Italy
faupe@libero.it

Paolo Pino
Cardiology Unit and Coronary
Intensive Care Unit
Ospedale San Camillo-Forlanini
Rome, Italy
ppino@scamilloforlanini.rm.it

Stefania Rizzo
Department of Cardiac, Thoracic and
Vascular Sciences, Pathological Anatomy-
Cardiovascular Pathology
Azienda Ospedaliera-University of Padova
Medical School, Via A. Gabelli, 61
35121, Padova, Italy
stefania.rizzo-01@sanita.padova.it

Carlos A. Roldan
University of New Mexico School of Medicine
and VA Medical Center
Albuquerque, NM, USA
CRoldan@salud.unm.edu

Antonio Salsano
Division of Cardiac Surgery,
Department of Surgery
University Hospital IRCCS San Martino IST
Largo Rosanna Benzi 10
16132, Genova, Italy
ant.salsano@gmail.com

Loris Salvador
Division of Cardiac Surgery
San Bortolo Hospital, Viale Rodolfi 37
36100, Vicenza, Italy
medloris@yahoo.it

Davide Santeufemia
Oncology Department, Sassari Hospital
Sassari, Italy
davidesanteufemia@gmail.com

Francesco Santini
Division of Cardiac Surgery
Department of Surgery
University Hospital IRCCS San Martino IST
Largo Rosanna Benzi 10
16132, Genova, Italy
francesco.santini@univr.it

Matteo Sarocchi
Clinical Research for
Cardiovascular Diseases
IRCCS San Martino Hospital IST
Genova, Italy
matteosarocchi@gmail.com

Diego Serraino
Unit of Cancer Epidemiology
Centro di Riferimento Oncologico, IRCCS
Aviano, 33081, Italy
serrainod@cro.it

Paolo Spallarossa
Clinic of Cardiovascular Diseases and Coronary
Intensive Care Unit, Department of Internal
Medicine and Medical Specialties
IRCCS San Martino Hospital IST
Genova, Italy
Paolo.spallarossa@unige.it

Brigida Stanzione
Medical Oncology
IRCCS-CRO, National Cancer Institute
Aviano, Pordenone, Italy
brigida.stanzione@cro.it

Gaetano Thiene
Department of Cardiac, Thoracic
and Vascular Sciences, Pathological
Anatomy-Cardiovascular Pathology
Azienda Ospedaliera-University of Padova
Medical School, Via A. Gabelli, 61
35121, Padova, Italy
gaetano.thiene@unipd.it

Olivia Maria Thomas
Il Gabbiano Hospice and Community Palliative
Care Service, AAS5, Friuli Occidentale
Pordenone, Italy
oliviathomas82@gmail.com

Antonino Carmelo Tralongo
Interdisciplinary Unit for Survivors and Chronic
Cancer Patients "Lia Buccheri e Nino Tralongo"
UO Medical Oncology, RAO, Hospital Umberto
I, Siracusa, Italy
tralongolime@hotmail.it

Paolo Tralongo
Interdisciplinary Unit for Survivors and Chronic
Cancer Patients "Lia Buccheri e Nino Tralongo"
UO Medical Oncology, RAO
Hospital Umberto I
Siracusa, Italy
tralongo@raosr.it

Martina Urbani
Radiology Unit
CRO-National Cancer Institute
Aviano, Pordenone, Italy
murbani@cro.it

Marialuisa Valente
Department of Cardiac, Thoracic and Vascular
Sciences, Pathological Anatomy-
Cardiovascular Pathology
Azienda Ospedaliera-University of Padova
Medical School, Via A. Gabelli, 61
35121, Padova, Italy
marialuisa.valente@unipd.it

Paola Vallerio
Cardiology IV Unit, Niguarda
Ca' Granda Hospital
Milan, Italy
valleriopaola@hotmail.com

Gaia Viganò
Division of Cardiac Surgery
Department of Surgery
University Hospital IRCCS San Martino IST
Largo Rosanna Benzi 10
16132, Genova, Italy
gaia_vigano@libero.it

Introductory Aspects

Contents

Epidemiology of Cancer: Prevalence, Incidence of Neoplastic Diseases and Trends in Survival in Europe

Ettore Bidoli and Diego Serraino

C. Lestuzzi et al. (eds.), *Manual of Cardio-oncology*, DOI 10.1007/978-3-319-40236-9_1

1.1 Background

Geographically, Europe consists of 40 countries; some of them are members of the European Union. Estimates of cancer burden in the world or in Europe can be viewed on-line [1–3]. Cancer burden can be measured both as cancer incidence and as cancer mortality, while the 5-year relative cancer survival is a key measure of the effectiveness of health-care systems. Last cancer incidence estimates at country level are updated to year 2012. These estimates are based on the latest incidence data provided by the European Network of Cancer Registries (ENCR), the mortality by the World Health Organization (WHO) mortality database [4] and the population estimates by the United Nations [5].

Herein, we examined the estimates of cancer incidence [6–14], mortality [7, 9, 10, 12, 15] and 5-year survival [2, 16] for the four most frequent cancers representing about 50 % of the cancer burden in European countries.

Moreover, we described the main risk factors likely associated to the geographical pattern observed [14, 17–30], the secondary prevention of specific cancers [31, 32], and lastly the fourth edition of the European Code Against Cancer [17, 20, 24, 25, 31, 33, 34].

1.2 Cancer Distribution

- About 25 % of the worldwide cancers were diagnosed in Europe in 2012. In particular, the estimated total number of cancers (excluding nonmelanoma skin cancers) was 3.4 million. Of them, 1.8 million (53 %) occurred in men and 1.6 million (47 %) in women. The most common cancer sites were breast cancer (464,000 cases, 13.5 % of all cancer cases), followed by colorectal cancer (447,000, 13.0 %), prostate cancer (417,000, 12.1 %) and lung cancer (410,000, 11.9 %). These four cancers represented half (50.5 %) of the estimated overall burden of cancer in Europe in 2012.
- In men, the most common primary sites were prostate (417,000 cases, 22.8 % of the total of the cancers), lung (291,000, 15.9 %) and colon-rectum (242,000, 13.2 %).
- In women, the most frequent primary cancer sites were breast (464,000 cases, 28.8 % of the total), followed by colon-rectum (205,000, 12.7 %) and lung (119,000, 7.4 %).

1.2.1 Incidence of All Cancers Excluding Nonmelanoma Skin Cancers

- The estimated total number of cancer deaths in Europe in 2012 was 1.75 million, of which 56 % (N=976,000) were observed in men and 44 % (N=779,000) in women.
- The most frequent causes of cancer death were due to lung cancer (353,000 deaths, 20 % of the total of cancer deaths), followed by colorectal cancer (215,000 deaths, 12.2 %) and breast cancer (131,000, 7.5 %).
- In men, lung cancer was the leading cause of death from cancer (254,000, 26.1 %) followed by colorectal (113,000, 11.6 %) and prostate (92,000, 9.5 %) cancers.

- In women, breast cancer was the most frequent cause of death in (131,000, 16.8 %), followed by colorectal (102,000, 13.0 %) and lung (nearly 100,000 deaths, 12.7 %) cancers.
- Age-standardised incidence rates were highest in both sexes in Northern and Western European countries (for instance, rates were 550 per 100,000 in men in France and 454 per 100,000 in women in Denmark). In both sexes, the all-cancer incidence rates were lower in the Balkan Peninsula (for instance, in Bosnia and Herzegovina, rates were 254 in men and 195 in women; or in Albania, rates were 263 in men and 234 in women) and in Greece (289 in men and 192 in women).

1.2.2 Mortality of All Cancers Excluding Nonmelanoma Skin Cancers

- Mortality rates, that reflect the frequency and the fatality of cancer, were both high in men in Eastern and Central European countries, i.e. Hungary (306). The high all-cancer mortality rate estimated in Danish women (168) is partially driven by the high incidence and mortality rates of breast cancer.
- The lowest mortality rates in males were estimated for Northern European countries, Finland (163) and Iceland (161) and in females for Southern European countries, Portugal (103) and Spain (99).

1.3 Lung Cancer

1.3.1 Incidence

- In men, incidence rates were highest in Central and Eastern European countries: Hungary (109/100,000), FYR of Macedonia (102), Serbia (99) and Poland (90). Rates were lowest in Northern European countries, for instance, in Finland (45) and Sweden (29).
- In women, the geographical pattern of rates was the opposite of men. Elevated rates were observed in Northern Europe (i.e. Denmark, 55/100,000, and the Netherlands, 44), while low rates were displayed in Eastern Europe (i.e. Ukraine, 9/100,000; Belarus, 9; or Russian Federation, 10).
- Incidence and mortality rates in men are decreasing in many European countries, particularly in Northern and Western areas since the 1980s and the 1990s. These areas were the first in the 1960s where the prevalence of smoking diminished in men.

1.3.2 Mortality

- In both sexes, the geographical pattern of the mortality rates followed generally the geographical pattern of the incidence rates.
- Mortality rates in women, who started smoking later than men, are generally increasing in Europe (particularly in France and Spain) although mortality rates tend to flatten, notably in high-risk countries of Northern Europe.

1.3.3 Risk Factors

- Nearly 90 % of lung cancers are caused by tobacco smoking. Thus, tobacco control is a priority in all European countries, particularly the male populations of Central and Eastern Europe, but also in young women.

1.3.4 Survival

- The European mean age-standardised 5-year survival for lung cancer was the poorest of the ten index cancers (13.0 %) and better for women than for men.
- Geographical differences were small, varying from 9.0 % in the UK and Ireland to 14.8 % in Central Europe.
- Age was a strong determinant of survival, ranging from 24.3 % for patients aged 15–44 years to 7.9 % for patients aged older than 75 years.

1.4 Breast Cancer

1.4.1 Incidence

- Breast cancer was the leading cancer site in women across all Europe in 2012, while a threefold geographical variation in rates was displayed between countries.
- The highest incidence rates were estimated in Western European countries, for instance, Belgium (147), France (137) and the Netherlands (131) and in Northern Europe, in the UK (129) and in the Nordic countries, Denmark (143), Iceland (131) and Finland (121).
- By contrast, incidence rates were much lower in Eastern European countries (i.e. Ukraine rate was 54 and in Moldova rate was 53).
- Moreover, menopausal status should be considered when studying breast cancer:
  - In postmenopausal women, the highest rates of breast cancer women were found in Northern European countries, but in the three Baltic countries, where the incidence rates were similar to those observed in Eastern and Central Europe.
  - Moreover, in Northern, Western and Southern Europe (except for the Baltic countries), incidence rates flatten, with small increases in Slovenia, Germany and the Netherlands. In premenopausal women, the incidence rates of breast cancer were highest in Southern and Western Europe (for instance, above 140/100,000 in Italy, France and the Netherlands).
  - The lowest rates were observed in Central and Eastern Europe and the three Baltic countries (<90/100,000). Finally, rates have flattened in the last 20 years.

1.4.2 Mortality

- Breast cancer was also the first cause of death from cancer in women in Europe. The range of mortality rates varied twofold. Mortality rates were highest in the North (e.g. Belgium, 29, and Denmark, 28) and in the South (i.e. Serbia, 31, and Macedonia, 36).

- Declines in breast cancer mortality rates in most European countries in the 1990s were reported as a consequence of the combined effects of early detection (partly due to screening, partly due to increasing awareness) and a range of advancements in treatment.

1.4.3 Risk Factors

- It is likely that the variation observed in breast cancer incidence across European countries may be linked to a different extent and type of screening activities, a differential prevalence and distribution of known risk factors for breast cancer (e.g. parity, age at first birth), as well as to possible biases in the estimation methods of breast cancer incidence.

1.4.4 Survival

- For most countries, 5-year survival for breast cancer (women only) was fairly close to the European mean (81.8 %). In all countries except Eastern Europe, survival ranged between 76 and 86 %.
  - In all Northern and Central European countries, and also Italy, Spain and Portugal, survival was >80 %.
  - In most Eastern European countries—except the Czech Republic—survival was 10–15 % lower than in the rest of Europe.

1.5 Colorectal Cancer

1.5.1 Incidence

- The incidence rates of colorectal cancer are slightly higher in men than in women, and a nearly fivefold variation in incidence rates was displayed within European countries.
- The higher rates of incidence were observed in Central European countries: Slovakia (92 per 100,000), Hungary (87) and the Czech Republic (81) in men and in Norway (54), Denmark (53) and the Netherlands (50) in women.
- The lower rates were displayed in the Balkan countries of Bosnia and Herzegovina (30 in men and 19 in women), Greece (25 in men and 17 in women) and Albania (13 in men and 11 in women).
- Increasing trends in colon cancer in males were seen in countries in Central, Eastern and Southern Europe.

1.5.2 Mortality

- The geographical patterns of mortality partially followed the pattern of incidence, although mortality was elevated in some countries with relatively low incidence rates (i.e. Moldova, Russia, Montenegro, Poland and Lithuania).

1.5.3 Risk Factors

- Diets low in fruit, vegetables and unrefined plant food, and high in red meat, processed food and fat, have been shown to confer an increased risk of colorectal cancer.
- Avoidance of a sedentary lifestyle and obesity may reduce the risk of colorectal cancer.
- The implementation of an organised population-based colorectal cancer screening, during which precancerous polyps and early-stage cancers can be detected and removed, is underway in higher-resource countries and should remain a high priority as a means of early detection of the disease in Europe.

1.5.4 Survival

- For colon cancer, the European mean age-standardised 5-year survival was 57.0 %, with slight differences between the sexes:
  - Northern, Central and Southern Europe had survival around 60 %.
  - For Eastern Europe, and the UK and Ireland, survival was lower.
  - Several countries had significantly different survival compared with the mean of their respective regions, including Denmark, Croatia, Slovenia and Ireland.
- For patients with rectal cancer, the European mean age-standardised 5-year survival was 55.8 % and was higher for women than for men:
  - Central and Northern Europe had highest the survival, with several countries above 60 %.
  - Southern Europe and the UK and Ireland had intermediate survival.
  - Eastern Europe had much lower survival.

1.6 Prostate Cancer

1.6.1 Incidence

- Incidence rates of prostate cancer vary nearly eightfold across European countries:
  - The highest rates were observed in Northern and Western European countries such as Norway (193) and France (187).
  - The lowest rates were observed in Central and Eastern European countries, such as the Republic of Moldova (30) and Albania (25).
- The incidence rates of prostate cancer increased in all European countries, especially in Northern Europe and in the younger age group (35–64 years), for instance, +28 %/year in Lithuania.

  In some Northern and Western European countries, incidence rates seemed to have flattened or dropped before 2012.

1.6.2 Mortality

- Mortality rates varied much less than incidence rates:
  - The highest rates were displayed in Lithuania (36) and in Denmark (34).
  - The lowest were observed in Malta (14) and Albania (13).

- In most high-resource countries in Northern and Western Europe, the rising trends in incidence are largely attributable to increased detection of latent disease following the widespread availability of PSA tests in the late 1980s and its subsequent and rapid uptake as an inappropriate screening test.

1.6.3 Risk Factors

- The risk factors for prostate cancer are still largely unclear. The strong increase in prostate cancer incidence is mainly due to the introduction of prostate-specific antigen (PSA) testing and consequent biopsy in asymptomatic men and in men with lower urinary tract symptoms.
- The benefit of population screening using PSA testing remains controversial.

1.6.4 Survival

- For prostate cancer, European mean age-standardised 5-year survival was high (83.4 %):
  - In most European countries except those in Eastern Europe, survival was around 80–90 % (exceptions were Croatia, Denmark and Slovenia).
  - Survival was lower in Eastern Europe, except for the Czech Republic and Lithuania.
  - European 5-year relative survival was highest at age 55–64 years and lowest for patients aged 85 years and older.
  - The fall with age was steeper for the UK and Ireland, Central Europe and Southern Europe than for Eastern and Northern Europe.

1.7 Discussion

- The cancer burden and the increasing trends in incidence of the most common cancers in Europe are of concern, in particular those at younger ages, as observed for colorectal cancer.
- The differences in survival of patients with cancer are large for patients diagnosed up to 2002, with high survival in Northern and Central Europe and low survival in the UK and Eastern Europe.
- A large proportion of the studied cancers are potentially avoidable, and primary cancer prevention has achieved some important successes in the past.

  Strategies to reduce the extent of the disease burden on the continent evidently need to be established locally, to reflect the profile of the observed cancer rates in each European country and in comparison with the pattern in the other countries.
- Possible explanations for persistent international differences in survival include differences in cancer biology, use of diagnostic tests and screening, stage at diagnosis and access to high-quality care.

- The differences in survival partly represent differences in resources allocated to health care, so that countries with high total national expenditure on health generally had better survival than did countries that spent less.

  However, differences in cancer survival can be affected by factors other than the provision and organisation of health care, such as socioeconomic status, lifestyle and general health status differences between populations.

  In turn, these factors are likely to lead to differences in health-care-seeking behaviours, patient management decisions and treatment effectiveness that can directly or indirectly affect cancer outcomes. In particular, a poor performance status because of comorbidities can limit the treatment options and their efficacy and thus reduce cancer survival.
- Mass screening and intense diagnostic activity—increasing both incidence and survival—can also contribute to variations in survival.

  Early diagnosis increases detection of early-stage cancers, which might respond well to treatment, but can also result in overdiagnosis and lead time bias, which prolong survival without significantly reducing mortality.
- The increases in survival over time and disparities in cancer survival across Europe suggest that further improvements could be made by application of proven treatment protocols and ensuring that all cancer patients have access to early diagnosis and high-quality treatment.

1.8 European Code Against Cancer

The European Code Against Cancer, 4th edition, was developed as a set of 12 recommendations to give advice on the prevention of cancer and to reduce the risk of dying from cancer (▫ Table 1.1).

The Code follows five main principles:

- Sufficient scientific evidence that following the recommendation to avoid or reduce exposure to a harmful agent, or to adopt a healthy behaviour, or participate in screening or vaccination activities would reduce the individual's risk of developing cancer or dying from cancer.

  Consequently, for the individual, there is a scientifically established benefit, albeit obviously acknowledging the impossibility of totally avoiding cancer.
- The recommendations are suitable for a broad target population.
- The recommendation is something individuals can do to reduce their cancer risk.

  The intention was not to downplay the responsibility of health decision-makers, but to provide a tool for people responding to the question, "what can I do to reduce my cancer risk?"
- The recommendation can be clearly and succinctly communicated to the general population.
- The last principle was to avoid recommendations that would give confusing or mixed messages to people.

1

Table 1.1 European Code Against Cancer: 12 ways to reduce your cancer risk

1	Do not smoke. Do not use any form of tobacco
2	Make your home smoke-free. Support smoke-free policies in your workplace
3	Take action to have a healthy body weight
4	Be physically active in everyday life. Limit the time you spend sitting
5	Have a healthy diet:
	Eat plenty of whole grains, pulses, vegetables and fruits
	Limit high-calorie foods (foods high in sugar or fat) and avoid sugary drinks
	Avoid processed meat; limit red meat and foods high in salt
6	If you drink alcohol of any type, limit your intake. Not drinking alcohol is better for cancer prevention
7	Avoid too much sun, especially for children. Use sun protection. Do not use sunbeds
8	In the workplace, protect yourself against cancer-causing substances by following health and safety instructions
9	Find out if you are exposed to radiation from naturally high radon levels in your home; take action to reduce high radon levels
10	For women:
	Breastfeeding reduces the mother's cancer risk. If you can, breastfeed your baby
	Hormone replacement therapy (HRT) increases the risk of certain cancers. Limit the use of HRT
11	Ensure your children take part in vaccination programmes for:
	Hepatitis B (for newborns)
	Human papillomavirus (HPV) (for girls)
12	Take part in organised cancer screening programmes for:
	Bowel cancer (men and women)
	Breast cancer (women)
	Cervical cancer (women)

Source: International Agency for Research on Cancer/World Health Organization: ▶ http://cancer-code-europe.iarc.fr/index.php/en/ [last access: 29 agust 2016]

Acknowledgements The authors wish to thank Mrs Luigina Mei for editorial assistance.

References

1. European Network of Cancer Registries. ▶ www.encr.eu.
2. Steliarova-Foucher E, O'Callaghan M, Ferlay J, et al. European cancer observatory: cancer incidence, mortality, prevalence and survival in Europe, version 1.0. European Network of Cancer Registries, International Agency for Research on Cancer. 2012. Available at ▶ http://eco.iarc.fr. Accessed 12 Sept 2015.

3. International Agency for Research on Cancer/World Health Organization. GLOBOCAN 2012. Estimated cancer incidence, mortality and prevalence worldwide in 2012. 2012. Available at ► http://globocan.iarc.fr/Default.aspx
4. World Health Organization (WHO) Databank. Geneva, WHO Statistical Information System. 2015. Available at ► http://www.who.int/whosis. Accessed 12 Sept 2015.
5. United Nations, Population Division. World population prospects, the 2010 revision. 2010. Available from ► http://www.un.org/esa/population/unpop.htm. Accessed 12 Sept 2015.
6. Arnold M, Karim-Kos HE, Coebergh JW, et al. Recent trends in incidence of five common cancers in 26 European countries since 1988: analysis of the European cancer observatory. Eur J Cancer. 2015;51(9):1164–87.
7. Bray F, Lortet-Tieulent J, Ferlay J, et al. Prostate cancer incidence and mortality trends in 37 European countries: an overview. Eur J Cancer. 2010;46(17):3040–52.
8. Doll R, Payne P, Waterhouse J. Cancer incidence in five continents: a technical report. Berlin: Springer (for UICC); 1966.
9. Ferlay J, Parkin DM, Steliarova-Foucher E. Estimates of cancer incidence and mortality in Europe in 2008. Eur J Cancer. 2010;46(4):765–81.
10. Ferlay J, Steliarova-Foucher E, Lortet-Tieulent J, et al. Cancer incidence and mortality patterns in Europe: estimates for 40 countries in 2012. Eur J Cancer. 2013;49(6):1374–403.
11. Feuer EJ, Merrill RM, Hankey BF. Cancer surveillance series: interpreting trends in prostate cancer—part II: cause of death misclassification and the recent rise and fall in prostate cancer mortality. J Natl Cancer Inst. 1999;91(12):1025–32.
12. Héry C, Ferlay J, Boniol M, et al. Quantification of changes in breast cancer incidence and mortality since 1990 in 35 countries with Caucasian-majority populations. Ann Oncol. 2008;19(6):1187–94.
13. Torre LA, Bray F, Siegel RL, et al. Global cancer statistics, 2012. CA Cancer J Clin. 2015;65(2):87–108.
14. Lortet-Tieulent J, Soerjomataram I, Ferlay J, et al. International trends in lung cancer incidence by histological subtype: adenocarcinoma stabilizing in men but still increasing in women. Lung Cancer. 2014;84(1):13–22.
15. Malvezzi M, Bertuccio P, Levi F, et al. European cancer mortality predictions for the year 2012. Ann Oncol. 2012;23(4):1044–52.
16. De Angelis R, Sant M, Coleman MP, et al. Cancer survival in Europe 1999–2007 by country and age: results of EUROCARE—5-a population-based study. Lancet Oncol. 2014;15(1):23–34.
17. Anderson AS, Key TJ, Norat T, et al. European code against cancer 4th edition: obesity, body fatness and cancer. Cancer Epidemiol. 2015;39 Suppl 1:S34–45.
18. Arnold M, Pandeya N, Byrnes G, et al. Global burden of cancer attributable to high body-mass index in 2012: a population-based study. Lancet Oncol. 2015;16(1):36–46.
19. Blackadar CB. Historical review of the causes of cancer. World J Clin Oncol. 2016;7(1):54–86.
20. Friis S, Kesminiene A, Espina C, et al. European code against cancer 4th edition: medical exposures, including hormone therapy, and cancer. Cancer Epidemiol. 2015;39 Suppl 1:S107–19.
21. Hakulinen T, Arbyn M, Brewster DH, et al. Harmonization may be counterproductive—at least for parts of Europe where public health research operates effectively. Eur J Public Health. 2011;21(6):686–7.
22. Harris HR, Bergkvist L, Wolk A. Adherence to the world cancer research fund/American institute for cancer research recommendations and breast cancer risk. Int J Cancer. 2016. doi:10.1002/ijc.30015 [Epub ahead of print].
23. International Agency for Research on Cancer (IARC). Monographs on the evaluation of carcinogenic risks to humans, Tobacco smoke and involuntary smoking, vol. 83. Lyon: IARC; 2004.
24. Leitzmann M, Powers H, Anderson AS, et al. European code against cancer 4th edition: physical activity and cancer. Cancer Epidemiol. 2015;39 Suppl 1:S46–55.
25. Leon ME, Peruga A, McNeill A, et al. European code against cancer, 4th edition: tobacco and cancer. Cancer Epidemiol. 2015;39 Suppl 1:S20–33.
26. Nomura SJ, Inoue-Choi M, Lazovich D, et al. WCRF/AICR recommendation adherence and breast cancer incidence among postmenopausal women with and without non-modifiable risk factors. Int J Cancer. 2016. doi:10.1002/ijc.29994 [Epub ahead of print].
27. Soerjomataram I, de Vries E, Pukkala E, et al. Excess of cancers in Europe: a study of eleven major cancers amenable to lifestyle change. Int J Cancer. 2007;120(6):1336–43.
28. Vieira AR, Abar L, Vingeliene S, et al. Fruits, vegetables and lung cancer risk: a systematic review and meta-analysis. Ann Oncol. 2016;27(1):81–96.
29. Wang J, Yang DL, Chen ZZ, et al. Associations of body mass index with cancer incidence among populations, genders, and menopausal status: a systematic review and meta-analysis. Cancer Epidemiol. 2016;42:1–8.

30. World Cancer Research Fund international. Available at ▶ www.wcrf.org. Accessed 09 Mar 2016.
31. Armaroli P, Villain P, Suonio E, et al. European code against cancer, 4th edition: cancer screening. Cancer Epidemiol. 2015;39 Suppl 1:S139–52.
32. Moss SM, Nyström L, Jonsson H, et al. The impact of mammographic screening on breast cancer mortality in Europe: a review of trend studies. J Med Screen. 2012;19 Suppl 1:26–32.
33. Minozzi S, Armaroli P, Espina C, et al. European code against cancer 4th edition: process of reviewing the scientific evidence and revising the recommendations. Cancer Epidemiol. 2015;39 Suppl 1:S11–9.
34. Schüz J, Espina C, Villain P, et al. European code against cancer 4th edition: 12 ways to reduce your cancer risk. Cancer Epidemiol. 2015;39 Suppl 1:S1–10.

Cancer, Heart Diseases, and Common Risk Factors: Smoke

Annamaria Catino, Andrea Misino, Antonio Logroscino, Elisabetta Sara Montagna, and Domenico Galetta

C. Lestuzzi et al. (eds.), *Manual of Cardio-oncology*, DOI 10.1007/978-3-319-40236-9_2

2.1 Key Points

- Cardiovascular disease is the leading cause of death worldwide, with approximately 30 % of deaths. Several studies have demonstrated that both cardiovascular morbidity and mortality are increased by cigarette smoke exposure, and this correlation has been confirmed also for environmental tobacco exposure, such as in the case of passive smoking.
- Cardiovascular disease caused by tobacco use involves multiple mechanisms including thrombosis, endothelial dysfunction, and inflammation.
- Epidemiologic data show that most of the damages produced by smoke exposure reverse quickly after cessation.
- Thus, smoking cessation is a crucial issue of cardiovascular prevention.
- Lung cancer is the leading cause of cancer morbidity and mortality worldwide, and 90 % of the annual cancer deaths worldwide are attributable to cigarette smoke, including passive smoking as a strong risk factor.
- Smoking is directly involved in carcinogenesis; among the over 5000 compounds identified in cigarette smoke, more than 70 substances are carcinogens (both tobacco-specific such as nitrosamines and others derived from tobacco burning such as polycyclic aromatic hydrocarbons) (PAHs).
- In addition, smokers are exposed to other carcinogens including volatile aldehydes, while the addiction of nicotine leads to long-term dependence and cumulative exposure to these substances.
- The relative risk increases with amount smoked, duration, earlier starting age, tar level, and fraction smoked and decreases with time quit.
- Smoking cessation improves risk and mortality from cardiovascular disease and lung cancer; therefore, it is a priority, for the public health system, to reduce smoking prevalence through effective tobacco control policies.

2.2 Epidemiology

Cardiovascular disease is the leading cause of death worldwide, with approximately 30 % of deaths [1]. Several epidemiologic studies have demonstrated that cigarette smoking is associated to higher incidence of myocardial infarction and acute coronary arterial disease, both in men and women [2–6]. This correlation is similar also among low-tar cigarette smokers [7] as well as clearly described for environmental tobacco exposure, such as in the case of passive smoking [8]. The relative risk for cardiovascular events is different by age and is higher in younger smokers, but the absolute excess smoking-related mortality rises with age [9, 10].

> **However, although it is established that cardiovascular morbidity and mortality are both increased by cigarette smoke exposure, the exact role of smoking components is not yet fully clarified as well as the entire and complex pathogenesis.**

The cardiovascular disease caused by tobacco use involves multiple mechanisms including thrombosis, endothelial dysfunction, and inflammation [9, 11]. Another noteworthy issue is the dose–response observation. The correlation between cigarettes daily consumption and ischemic heart disease shows that the risk increases sharply from a scarce tobacco use and reaches a plateau toward heavy smokers [9, 10, 12].

However, epidemiologic data show that most of the detrimental effects produced by smoke exposure reverse quickly after cessation [9].

Thus, smoking cessation is a useful and crucial issue of cardiovascular prevention [8, 10].

2.3 Cigarette Smoke: Chemical–Physical Characteristics

The two phases of cigarette smoke are the tar phase and the gas phase.

- The tar phase is represented by the material remaining after passing through the glass fiber filter, that retains 99.9 % of all particulate material >0.1 μm.
- The gas phase is left after passing through the filter [13].

In these phases a different concentration of free radicals, with a higher rate of long-lived radicals in the tar phase, is contained [13].

The mainstream cigarette smoke, drawn through the tobacco into an active smoker's mouth, consists mainly of gaseous components (92 %), while sidestream smoke, deriving from the burning end of cigarette, contains a relatively higher concentration of the toxic gaseous component than mainstream smoke [14].

Environmental tobacco smoke derives both from sidestream smoke (85 %) and exhaled mainstream smoke (15 %) by smokers [11].

Nicotine, used as additive and present in the tar phase, is involved at multiple levels with smoke-related damages [9, 11].

2.4 Pathophysiology

- Cigarette smoking causes cardiovascular disease by several mechanisms.
  - The correlation between cigarette smoking and different atherosclerotic conditions is the major cause of cardiovascular disease, involving the cardiac vessels as well as big and peripheral vessels, leading to various atherosclerotic clinical syndromes (stable and acute angina, sudden death, stroke, intermittent claudication, and aortic aneurysms) [11].
  - Cigarette smoking interacts with some essential elements of the atherosclerotic process, mainly by the impairment of vasodilatory function, inflammation, and alteration of lipid profile.
  - Several studies have demonstrated that some substances contained in cigarette smoke are related to cardiovascular disease; among them, nicotine, carbon monoxide, and oxidant gases are the most studied.
    - *Nicotine* exposure is very significant in regular smokers, with accumulation patterns persisting high 24 h a day. The effects of nicotine comprise catecholamine release both at the local neurons and from adrenal glands, with persistent sympathetic nervous activation inducing elevated heart rate.

- Cigarette smoking exposes to *carbon monoxide*, that binds to hemoglobin causing persistent high concentrations of carboxyhemoglobin; this significantly reduces the possibility of oxygen carrying and release. As a consequence of carbon monoxide exposure, in cigarette smokers a relative hypoxemia is generally present causing increased red cell mass and blood viscosity, thus favoring a hypercoagulable condition.
- Other oxidizing substances absorbed by smokers are represented by nitrogen oxides as well as several free radicals, all together involved both with the depletion of endogenous antioxidants (such as vitamin C) and also with multiple causes of cardiovascular disease, including inflammation, endothelial injury, dyslipidemia, and platelet activation [15].
- Furthermore, experimental studies reported that polycyclic aromatic hydrocarbons could favor atherosclerosis [16].

Nicotine is primarily correlated with the hemodynamic effects of cigarette smoking; nicotine stimulates the sympathetic nervous system and heart so increasing the myocardial oxygen demand not balanced by the myocardial blood supply. In addition, nicotine induces cutaneous vasoconstriction while other vascular beds become dilated, such as skeletal muscular vessels (Tables 2.1 and 2.2).

Globally, the effects of nicotine encompass higher heart rate and blood pressure as well as myocardial contractility, thus increasing myocardial work and requiring more myocardial blood flow. Moreover, a coronary blood flow impairment is produced by cigarette smoking both by an increase of vascular resistance and also by constriction of epicardial arteries [17]. Indeed, this effect is present even at low dose in humans [18]. Finally, the trend toward stress-induced myocardial ischemia is partially influenced by the carbon monoxide-related effect, which increases the request for coronary blood flow under stress by its induced functional anemia; so, the reduced coronary blood flow vasodilatory reserve could contribute to stress-induced myocardial ischemia in smokers.

Other mechanisms, based on endothelial injury, as well as thrombosis and inflammation, contribute at different levels to cardiovascular smoking-related disease.

The endothelial damage of peripheral and coronary arteries is another mechanism by which cigarette smoking contributes to atherogenesis and acute cardiovascular disease; it is noteworthy that smoking cessation has shown to reverse partially some of these alterations [19].

In this scenario, acute ischemic events are favored by several causes correlated with endothelial injury/dysfunction: a prothrombotic state, a reduced vasodilatory reserve, the inflammation, and an increased adhesion to vessels by neutrophils and monocytes [20]. The oxidative stress is strictly correlated to the development of atherosclerosis and vascular dysfunction, mainly due to the action of free radicals, as reported by some studies [21, 22].

The free radicals could be derived from the gas or tar phase of cigarette smoke, the activation of leucocytes, or other endogenous sources, and one of the consequences is the reduced NO availability [11, 23, 24].

Globally, the enhanced oxidative stress is associated with all cigarette smoking-related alterations, such as endothelial dysfunction, lipid peroxidation, reduced endogenous fibrinolysis, and prothrombotic effects [23, 24]. In fact, the administration of antioxidants or agents reducing the oxidative stress or improving the NO availability could reverse the cigarette smoking-induced mechanisms described above [25–27].

Table 2.1 Smoking harms the whole body, and there are several benefits from smoking cessation, because it is always useful to quit

Organ	Organ damage	Smoking cessation benefits
The brain	Nicotine addiction is similar to drugs as heroin and difficult to eliminate due to some severe brain alterations The brain develops more receptors for nicotine to receive larger amounts This causes the withdrawal syndrome (anxiety, irritability, and a powerful craving for smoking)	To retrieve the brain function to also help stop addiction After smoking cessation, the number of nicotine receptors quickly returns to normal
Hearing/vision	Mild–moderate hearing loss, sometimes permanent (due to the reduced oxygen amount provided to cochlea) It is remarkable that a hearing loss, although mild, could compromise the working activities Vision damage (nicotine affects the production of substances favoring the night vision) Increased risk of blindness caused by cataract and macular degeneration	Hearing improvement Eyesight improvement especially night vision (by contrasting the processes altering the oxygen supply to the retina and optic nerve)
The mouth	Mouth ulcers, early tooth loss, periodontitis, and gingivitis Increased incidence of cancer	Clean mouth and white teeth, brighter smile (less dentist sittings, costs, and free time saving)
The face	The typical "smoker's face" presents dry, dull, and aged skin with many wrinkles	Quitting smoking is a real "antiaging" treatment, with improvement and prevention of wrinkles and dark spots Cost-saving (for beauty centers, medical consulting, other interventions)
Sexuality and fertility	Increased risk and worsening of erectile dysfunction in men Genetic damage of sperm and oocytes and increased incidence of infertility or genetic defects in children	Smoking cessation quickly reduces these harms
Bone and muscles	Muscular damages because of reduced supply of blood and oxygen, with difficult strengthening and easy tiredness as well as myalgias Some substances from cigarette smoke alter the bone composition and physiology, causing osteoporosis and increased risk as well as delayed recovery of fractures *Important:* nowadays, the surgeons consider some orthopedic interventions at higher risk if the patient is a smoker	Smoking cessation quickly improves the bone and muscular health

(continued)

Table 2.1 (continued)

Organ	Organ damage	Smoking cessation benefits
Hormonal status and metabolism	Bigger belly and proportion of fat Increased risk of diabetes as well as worse diabetes control (diabetes involves multiple organs thus disabling them due to several complications: blindness, amputation of limbs caused by severe vasculopathies, etc.) Infertility and earlier menopause in women	Improved control of metabolism, improved dietary efficacy Wellness, fitness, and sexual recovery
Respiratory function	Bronchopulmonary chronic inflammation and emphysema (evolutive and leading to scarred lungs requiring continuous oxygen therapy)	After a short time from smoking cessation, the respiratory symptoms improve as well as the protective function of bronchial cilia The lung emphysema is not curable; hence, it is very important to prevent it by smoking cessation at any time
The heart	Very high risk of cardiovascular diseases (myocardial infarction, ictus cerebri, and Buerger disease frequently causing limb amputation)	Most of these risks are reversible simply by smoking cessation Smoking cessation quickly reduces arterial blood pressure and cardiac frequency The risk of cardiac ischemic disease decreases already by 24 h after smoking cessation The fat level decreases and the blood becomes more fluid by reducing the thromboembolic risk; therefore the heart works easier

The smoking-related endothelial alteration is mediated both by oxidant chemicals and by nicotine.

In addition, smokers present lower levels of antioxidant vitamins, utilized to contrast the increased oxidant stress; consequently, as reported by Heizer [25], the endothelial alteration could be partially improved by the administration of vitamin C. Nicotine affects by itself the endothelium, and an increase of myointimal thickening has been detected in experimental studies [28–31]. Furthermore, in the presence of some comorbidities, such as dyslipidemia, hypertension, and diabetes, the effects of smoking considerably raise the risk of endothelial dysfunction [32].

Cigarette smoking is involved in acute cardiovascular disease by increasing the risk both for myocardial ischemia and also for angina pectoris; the most important pathogenetic mechanism is represented by a hypercoagulable condition [9].

Table 2.2 Main smoking cessation methods. The efficacy of such methods is strongly affected by the reasons and the willingness of smokers. The best choice is represented by an initial approach with a dedicated staff, so the proposed technique will be the single or combined method more suitable according to the personal characteristics of the smoker as well as to the addiction degree

Nicotine-based transdermal plasters and chewing gums	The plasters release the substances contained in the gel, thus reaching the central nervous system and reducing the withdrawal symptoms as well as decreasing the number of smoked cigarettes It is appropriate to use it after medical consultation
Counseling	Groups of smokers guided by an expert (physician, psychologist). Thanks to the communication and the mutual support, it is possible to improve the reasons for quitting smoking, thus increasing the confidence of own possibilities Aside from the comparison of personal experiences, this modality is useful due to the important information provided about the smoking harms as well as a dietary support helpful for detoxification
Pharmacological therapy	Some drugs (e.g., Varenicline) are useful for smoking cessation and are proposed to single patients and also in the context of combined programs developed by Antismoking Centers or by groups belonging to health services/hospitals These therapies are active and appropriate if prescribed by expert physicians
Electronic cigarettes	Several studies and experimental trials are ongoing with the aim of evaluating the safety of the inhaled substances; however, in case of a strong motivation, it could be an option for smoking cessation especially if combined to counseling programs or experimental clinical trials in qualified centers
Other methods	
Acupuncture	The acupuncture technique, belonging to the Chinese culture, is based on the insertion of thin needles in precise points of the body. It is considered a potentially useful method, even in the presence of a strong reason, quite costly
Homeopathy	A medicine "alternative" based on herbal and natural remedies, partially acknowledged also by the "traditional" medicine, could help to quit smoking without drugs and stimulate the natural body defenses There are not yet definitive data about this method that however requires a stronger motivation to quit
Hypnosis	This method is still not much known and validated The technique requires a skilled physician and the strong motivation to quit
To aspirate	Some mouthpieces releasing nicotine are not to be used concurrently with cigarettes. The nicotine mucosal absorption could reduce the smoke craving. Method not validated
The dietary issue	This is a very important factor to consider during smoking cessation It is necessary to avoid overeating (since the ex-smoker could desire food), but the diet could be a very effective support In general, it is recommended to avoid confectionery, fats, alcohol, and fried food; in addition, it is recommended to increase vegetables and fruit intake (rich in vitamins and water). To drink water and herbal teas is useful, because nicotine is water-soluble and is eliminated through urine and sweat Important: the risk of getting fat could be counteracted by the dietary advices provided by the nutritionist, since taking candies or food is often wrongly considered to substitute cigarettes

An enhanced risk of thrombosis relies on multiple factors; among them, the platelet activation as well as endothelial dysfunction and the effects of oxidant substances are closely linked.

Additional causes are represented by the impaired platelet-derived nitric oxide release and a reduced release of tPA from coronary arteries in response to Substance P (endothelium-dependent vasodilator) [33, 34]. It is noteworthy that higher levels of PAI-1 have been detected in smokers as compared in nonsmokers; this finding contributes to impair fibrinolysis [35].

In conclusion, cigarette smoking acts by several mechanisms to thrombosis from atherosclerotic plaques; the activation of platelet aggregation and the high fibrinogen levels as a response to the chronic inflammatory status in smokers are only a part of the complex interaction of multiple factors in the pathogenesis of smoking-related cardiovascular disease.

Indeed, epidemiologic data support this concept, as demonstrated by the rapid reduction of this risk after smoking cessation.

- Smoking-induced cardiovascular disease is correlated with a chronic inflammatory stimulation, as witnessed by increased serum levels of several inflammatory mediators (leukocytes, monocytes, C-reactive protein, and fibrinogen) so favoring atherogenesis [36–39].
- Actually, cigarette smoking favors the vascular inflammation, mostly based on the recruitment and leukocyte adhesion to the blood vessel wall. Oxidant stress is considered the major factor inducing inflammation, while nicotine has been shown to promote inflammation enhancing leukocyte–endothelial links and is also a neutrophil chemotactic agent [9, 40, 41].
- Finally, the insulin resistance associated to cigarette smoking and the hyperinsulinemia-related endothelial alteration represent other interesting elements involved in the smoking-related cardiovascular disease.
- Nicotine could contribute to insulin resistance, so the long-term safety of nicotine medications is to be accurately considered in tobacco cessation programs [9].
- As a concluding remark, smoking is associated with lipid abnormalities, thus favoring atherogenesis.
- Nicotine acts by accelerating lipolysis and inducing insulin resistance, so its role is crucial by increasing the cardiovascular risk in smokers [9].

2.5 Smoke as Risk Factor for Cancer and Other Diseases

Lung cancer is the leading cause of cancer morbidity and mortality worldwide, with almost 1.6 million new cases of lung cancer per year (13 % of total cancer morbidity) and 1.4 million deaths per year (18 % of total cancer mortality) [42]. Globally, lung cancer is the leading cause of cancer deaths in males and the second in females [43]. Tobacco causes almost 6 million people deaths every year, and 90 % of the annual cancer deaths worldwide are attributable to cigarette smoke, although this rate is various across populations, ranging from >80 % in the USA and France to 40 % in sub-Saharan Africa [44].

Besides the pathogenetic processes correlated to the cardiovascular disease and mortality risk, smoking is directly involved in carcinogenesis.

- Among the over 5000 compounds identified in cigarette smoke, more than 70 substances are carcinogens (both tobacco-specific such as nitrosamines and others derived from tobacco burning such as polycyclic aromatic hydrocarbons (PAHs).
- In addition, smokers are exposed to other carcinogens including volatile aldehydes, while the addiction of nicotine leads to long-term dependence as well as cumulative exposure to these substances [45, 46].
- Studies have demonstrated that the higher risk of lung cancer in smokers is dose dependent [47].
- Also passive smoking is considered a strong risk factor for lung cancer [46–49], despite contrasting data about the exact correlation with duration, amount of exposure level, and setting of exposure, respectively [47, 50, 51].
- However, the secondhand tobacco smoke plays a significant role, as reported by Oberg et al. [52], with an estimated 21,400 lung cancer deaths in nonsmokers annually.

The issue regarding the hypothesized higher susceptibility of women to cigarette smoking is not yet fully clarified, as a recent meta-analysis by Yu et al. reports, reaffirming that tobacco control is equally requested in both males and females [53].

A recent systematic meta-analysis has quantitatively demonstrated, by reviewing 287 studies including more than 100 lung cancer cases and published in the last century, the association between lung cancer and smoking [54].

This correlation is strong according to all cancer histotypes and irrespective for sex, although more evident in ever-former and current smokers, as well as for small and squamous subtypes; as expected, the relative risk increases with amount smoked, duration, earlier starting age, tar level, and fraction smoked and decreases with time quit [54].

Furthermore, the covariate adjustment did not affect these findings, thus supporting the causal relationship between smoking and lung cancer.

Notwithstanding the well-known prognostic impact of smoking status on lung cancer patients [55], Okamoto et al. [56] have reported almost partially unforeseen results in a retrospective study evaluating the influence of the amount of tobacco smoking on outcome of patients according to histotype. The prognosis, evaluated in more than 1000 patients submitted to surgery, seems to be better in adenocarcinoma nonsmokers, whereas among squamous subtypes light smokers ($PY \leq 30$) showed a significantly worse prognosis than heavier smokers ($PY > 30$).

These findings support further studies aimed to explore the carcinogenic pathway based on smoking status and histotype, due to the possible different sensitivity to tobacco-related carcinogens irrespective of the extent of DNA damage caused by these smoke components.

As above reported, it is remarkable that most of the pathogenetic mechanisms involved in smoke-related diseases are, at least partially, reversible; hence, the risk reduction of lung cancer incidence and mortality by smoking cessation strongly supports tobacco cessation programs [47, 53, 57].

Furthermore, besides the advantages achievable for smokers who quit, it is important to highlight that, among the former smokers, lung cancer and mortality risk declines progressively with the younger age at smoking cessation [58].

Following previous data about the correlation between the 21 well-known and formally established diseases as caused by smoking [12 types of cancer, 6 categories of cardiovascular disease, diabetes, chronic obstructive pulmonary disease (COPD), and pneumonia including influenza], some studies have suggested that also other causes could contribute to the mortality excess in current smokers [59, 60]. Recently, Carter et al. have reported that approximately 17 % of the excess mortality among current smokers could be associated with some diseases not previously formally attributed to smoking, including renal failure, hypertensive heart disease, infections, respiratory diseases, and breast and prostate cancer [60]. An interesting further finding is the reduction of these risks as the time elapsed since quitting increased [60].

A recent Italian study has estimated the gain in life expectancy with smoking cessation in smokers living in the Mediterranean area [61].

Consistently with previous studies conducted worldwide, Carrozzi et al. have confirmed that quitting smoking improves life expectancy for men and women; in addition, the study presents a tool for estimating the risk reduction associated with quitting smoking for both men and women, by age of quitting, and number of cigarettes smoked per day [61].

Thus, in order to promote and support the fight against tabagism as well as the programs for smoking cessation, it is crucial to accurately estimate the risk. As a consequence, to quantify the gain in health and life expectancy is essential within the National Health System.

- The studies conducted worldwide have showed consistent results about the risk quantification, the improvement of risk by quitting smoking, and the gain in life and health according to the earliness of smoking cessation.
- Despite the improvement in lung cancer therapies, this neoplasm is mostly diagnosed in advanced stage, so efforts have to be made to optimize the screening methods, particularly in high-risk subjects, with the aim of an early detection and a chance of cure. Nevertheless, the rate of lung cancer deaths now preventable by screening is still low, estimated as not more than 8 % in a recent study conducted in the USA [62].
- Tobacco smoke is the major preventable cause of cancer. In the last decade, although the smoking prevalence is decreasing, now representing 28 % in EU-27 (27 Member States) [46], it is still high especially in low-income countries; furthermore, both men and women in European countries show the highest prevalence between 25 and 44 years, with a significant proportion of current heavy smokers [46, 63, 64].

Therefore, it is a priority, for the public health efforts, to prevent cancer deaths and to reduce smoking prevalence as rapidly as possible, through effective tobacco control policies.

Hence, as an important part of the strategy against tobacco smoking and prevalence, according to the WHO's Framework Convention on Tobacco Control (FCTC), the most important measures to be implemented worldwide comprise:

1. Monitoring tobacco use and prevention policies
2. Smoke-free air policies

3. Cessation programs
4. Warnings (health and mass media)
5. Bans on advertising, promotion, and sponsorship
6. Raising tobacco taxes [65]

The reported results about the usefulness of tobacco control policies in the USA with a significant avert of deaths from lung cancer [66] strongly support these programs also in order to decrease the impact on the Health Systems by the multiple smoking-related diseases.

Indeed, a reduction of cardiovascular events has been achieved in many countries by the adoption of smoke-free legislation and smoking ban [46, 67–69], and it is hopeful that these tobacco control policies will protect also the nonsmoker population.

2.6 Conclusions

Smoking cessation has a significant favorable impact on risk and mortality from cardiovascular disease, lung cancer incidence, and mortality as well as on other tobacco-induced cancers and chronic diseases such as chronic obstructive pulmonary disease (COPD).

A global approach, inspired by the WHO-FCTC recommendations, is essential, especially in a Public Health System (as Italian-EU system) aimed to protect the overall population from tobacco; in this scenario, the governmental activities could allow for positive results also within a spending review policy.

References

1. Santulli G. Epidemiology of cardiovascular disease in the 21st century: updated numbers and updated facts. J Cardiovasc Dis. 2013;1(1):1–2.
2. Doll R, Peto R. Mortality in relation to smoking: 20 years' observations on male British doctors. BMJ. 1976;2:1525–36.
3. Doll R, Gray R, Hafner B, Peto R. Mortality in relation to smoking: 22 years' observations on female British doctors. BMJ. 1980;280:967–71.
4. Willett WC, Green A, Stampfer MJ, et al. Relative and absolute excess risks of coronary heart disease among women who smoke cigarettes. N Engl J Med. 1987;317:1303–9.
5. Price JF, Mowbray PI, Lee AJ, Rumley A, Lowe GD, Fowkes FG. Relationship between smoking and cardiovascular risk factors in the development of peripheral arterial disease and coronary artery disease: Edinburgh artery study. Eur Heart J. 1999;20:344–53.
6. Jonas MA, Oates JA, Ockene JK, Hennekens CH. Statement on smoking and cardiovascular disease for health care professionals: American Heart Association. Circulation. 1992;86:1664–9.
7. Negri E, Franzosi MG, La Vecchia C, Santoro L, Nobili A, Tognoni G. Tar yield of cigarettes and risk of acute myocardial infarction: GISSI-EFRIM Investigators. BMJ. 1993;306:1567–70.
8. Law MR, Morris JK, Wald NJ. Environmental tobacco smoke exposure and ischaemic heart disease: an evaluation of the evidence. BMJ. 1997;315:973–80.
9. Benowitz NL. Cigarette smoking and cardiovascular disease: pathophysiology and implications for treatment. Prog Cardiovasc Dis. 2003;1:91–111.
10. Burns DM. Epidemiology of smoking-induced cardiovascular disease. Prog Cardiovasc Dis. 2003;46:11–29.
11. Ambrose JA, Barua RS. The pathophysiology of cigarette smoking and cardiovascular disease: an update. J Am Coll Cardiol. 2004;43:1731–7.
12. Law MR, Wald NJ. Environmental tobacco smoke and ischemic heart disease. Prog Cardiovasc Dis. 2003;46:31–8.
13. Pryor WA, Stone K. Oxidants in cigarette smoke: radicals, hydrogen peroxide, peroxynitrate, and peroxynitrite. Ann N Y Acad Sci. 1993;686:12–28.

14. Glantz SA, Parmley WW. Passive smoking and heart disease: epidemiology, physiology, and biochemistry. Circulation. 1991;83:1–12.
15. Burke A, FitzGerald GA. Oxidative stress and smoking-induced tissue injury. Prog Cardiovasc Dis. 2003;46:79–90.
16. Penn A, Snyder CA. 1,3 butadiene, a vapor phase component of environmental tobacco smoke, accelerates arteriosclerotic plaque development. Circulation. 1996;93:552–7.
17. Quillen JE, Rossen JD, Oskarsson HJ, et al. Acute effect of cigarette smoking on the coronary circulation: constriction of epicardial and resistance vessels. J Am Coll Cardiol. 1993;22:642–7.
18. Kaijser L, Berglund B. Effect of nicotine on coronary blood-flow in man. Clin Physiol. 1995;5:541–52.
19. Celermajer DS, Sorensen KE, Georgakopoulos D, et al. Cigarette smoking is associated with dose-related and potentially reversible impairment of endothelium-dependent dilation in healthy young adults. Circulation. 1993;88:2149–55.
20. Puranik R, Celermajer DS. Smoking and endothelial function. Prog Cardiovasc Dis. 2003;45:443–58.
21. Kojda G, Harrison D. Interactions between NO and reactive oxygen species: pathophysiological importance in atherosclerosis, hypertension, diabetes and heart failure. Cardiovasc Res. 1999;43:562–71.
22. Nedeljkovic ZS, Gokce N, Loscalzo J. Mechanisms of oxidative stress and vascular dysfunction. Postgrad Med J. 2003;79:195–200.
23. Heitzer T, Brockhoff C, Mayer B, et al. Tetrahydrobiopterin improves endothelium-dependent vasodilation in chronic smokers: evidence for a dysfunctional nitric oxide synthase. Circ Res. 2000;86:E36–41.
24. Kayyali US, Budhiraja R, Pennella CM, et al. Upregulation of xanthine oxidase by tobacco smoke condensate in pulmonary endothelial cells. Toxicol Appl Pharmacol. 2003;188:59–68.
25. Heitzer T, Just H, Munzell T. Antioxidant vitamin C improves endothelial dysfunction in chronic smokers. Circulation. 1996;94:6–9.
26. Fennessy FM, Moneley DS, Wang JH, Kelly CJ, Bouchier-Hayes DJ. Taurine and vitamin C modify monocyte and endothelial dysfunction in young smokers. Circulation. 2003;107:410–5.
27. Takajo Y, Ikeda H, Haramaki N, Murohara T, Imaizumi T. Augmented oxidative stress of platelets in chronic smokers: mechanisms of impaired platelet-derived nitric oxide bioactivity and augmented platelet aggregability. J Am Coll Cardiol. 2001;38:1320–7.
28. Chalon S, Moreno H, Benowitz NL, et al. Nicotine impairs endothelium-dependent dilatation in human veins in vivo. Clin Pharmacol Ther. 2000;67:391–7.
29. Sarabi M, Lind L. Short-term effects of smoking and nicotine chewing gum on endothelium-dependent vasodilation in young healthy habitual smokers. J Cardiovasc Pharmacol. 2000;35:451–6.
30. Neunteufl T, Heher S, Kostner K, et al. Contribution of nicotine to acute endothelial dysfunction in long-term smokers. J Am Coll Cardiol. 2002;39:251–6.
31. Krupski WC, Olive GC, Weber CA, et al. Comparative effects of hypertension and nicotine on injury-induced myointimal thickening. Surgery. 1987;102:409–15.
32. Heitzer T, Yla-Herttuala S, Luoma J, et al. Cigarette smoking potentiates endothelial dysfunction of fore-arm resistance vessels in patients with hypercholesterolemia. Role of oxidized LDL. Circulation. 1996;93:1346–53.
33. Ichiki K, Ikeda H, Haramaki N, et al. Long-term smoking impairs platelet-derived nitric oxide re- lease. Circulation. 1996;94:3109–14.
34. Newby DE, McLeod AL, Uren NG, et al. Impaired coronary tissue plasminogen activator release is associated with coronary atherosclerosis and cigarette smoking: direct link between endothelial dysfunction and atherothrombosis. Circulation. 2001;103:1936–41.
35. Simpson AJ, Gray RS, Moore NR, et al. The effects of chronic smoking on the fibrinolytic potential of plasma and platelets. Br J Haematol. 1997;97:208–13.
36. Jensen EJ, Pedersen B, Frederiksen R, et al. prospective study on the effect of smoking and nicotine substitution on leucocyte blood counts and relation between blood leucocytes and lung function. Thorax. 1998;53:784–9.
37. Tracy RP, Psaty BM, Macy E, et al. Lifetime smoking exposure affects the association of C-reactive protein with cardiovascular disease risk factors and subclinical disease in healthy elderly subjects. Arterioscler Thromb Vasc Biol. 1997;17:2167–76.
38. Tuut M, Hense H-W. Smoking, other risk factors and fibrinogen levels: evidence of effect modification. Ann Epidemiol. 2001;11:232–8.
39. Libby P, Ridker PM, Maseri A. Inflammation and atherosclerosis. Circulation. 2002;105:1135–43.

40. Totti III N, McCusker KT, Campbell EJ, et al. Nicotine is chemotactic for neutrophils and enhances neutrophil responsiveness to chemotactic peptides. Science. 1984;223:169–73.
41. Yong T, Zheng MQ, Linthicum DS. Nicotine induces leukocyte rolling and adhesion in the cerebral microcirculation of the mouse. J Neuroimmunol. 1997;80:158–64.
42. Jemal A, Bray F, Center MM, Ferlay J, Ward E, Forman D. Global cancer statistics. CA Cancer J Clin. 2011;61:69–90.
43. Torre LA, Bray F, Siegel RL, et al. Global cancer statistics,2012. CA Cancer J Clin. 2015;65:87–108.
44. Islami F, Torre LA, Jemal A. Global trends of lung cancer mortality and smoking prevalence. Transl Lung Cancer Res. 2015;4(4):327–38.
45. Hecht SS. Tobacco carcinogens, their biomarkers and tobacco-induced cancer. Nat Rev Cancer. 2003;3:733–44.
46. Leon ME, Peruga A, McNeill A, Kralikova E, Guha N, Minozzi S, Espina C, Schuz J. European code against cancer, 4th edition: tobacco and cancer. Cancer Epidemiol. 2015. doi:10.1016/j.canep.2015.06.001 (in press).
47. Wang A, Kubo J, Luo J, Desai M, Hedlin H, Henderson M, et al. Active and passive smoking in relation to lung cancer incidence in the Women's Health Initiative Observational Study prospective cohort. Ann Oncol. 2015;26:221–30.
48. Thomas JL, Guo H, Carmella SG, et al. Metabolites of a tobacco-specific lung carcinogen in children exposed to secondhand or thirdhand tobacco smoke in their homes. Cancer Epidemiol Biomarkers Prev. 2011;20:1213–21.
49. Suwan-ampai P, Navas-Acien A, Strickland PT, et al. Involuntary tobacco smoke exposure and urinary levels of polycyclic aromatic hydrocarbons in the United States, 1999 to 2002. Cancer Epidemiol Biomarkers Prev. 2009;18:884–93.
50. Hackshaw AK, Law MR, Wald NJ. The accumulated evidence on lung cancer and environmental tobacco smoke. BMJ. 1997;315:980–8.
51. Stayner L, Bena J, Sasco AJ, et al. Lung cancer risk and workplace exposure to environmental tobacco smoke. Am J Public Health. 2007;97:545–51.
52. Oberg M, Jaakkola MS, Woodward A, et al. Worldwide burden of disease from exposure to second-hand smoke: a retrospective analysis of data from 192 countries. Lancet. 2011;377:139–46.
53. Yu Y, Liu H, Zheng S, Ding Z, Chen Z, Jin W, Wang L, Wang Z, Fei Y, Zhang S, Ying K, Zhang R. Gender susceptibility for cigarette smoking-attributable lung cancer: a systematic review and meta-analysis. Lung Cancer. 2014;85:351–60.
54. Lee PN, Forey BA, Coombs KJ. Systematic review with meta-analysis of the epidemiological evidence in the 1900s relating smoking to lung cancer. BMC Cancer. 2012;12:385.
55. Toh CK, Gao F, Lim WT, Leong SS, Fong KW, Yap SP, et al. Never-smokers with lung cancer: epidemiologic evidence of a distinct disease entity. J Clin Oncol. 2006;24:2245–51.
56. Okamoto T, Suzuki Y, Fujishita T, Kitahara H, Shimamatsu S, Kohno M, Morodomi Y, Kawano D, Maehara Y. The prognostic impact of the amount of tobacco smoking in non-small cell lung cancer—differences between adenocarcinoma and squamous cell carcinoma. Lung Cancer. 2014;85:125–30.
57. Peto R, Darby S, Deo H, et al. Smoking, smoking cessation, and lung cancer in the UK since 1950: combination of national statistics with two case–control studies. BMJ. 2000;321:323–9.
58. Personal habits and indoor combustions. A review of human carcinogens. International Agency for Research on Cancer. Monogr Eval Carcinog Risks Hum. 2012;1–538.
59. Pirie K, Peto R, Reeves GK, Green J, Beral V. The 21st century hazards of smoking and benefits of stopping: a prospective study of one million women in the UK. Lancet. 2013;381:133–41.
60. Carter BD, Abnet CC, Feskanich D, Freedman ND, Hartge P, Lewis CE, Ockene JK, Prentice RL, Speizer FE, Thun MJ, Jacobs EJ. Smoking and mortality—beyond established causes. N Engl J Med. 2015;372:631–40.
61. Carrozzi L, Falcone F, Carreras G, Pistelli F, Gorini G, Martini A, Viegi G. Life gain in Italian smokers who quit. Int J Environ Res Public Health. 2014;11:2395–406.
62. Ma J, Ward EM, Smith R, et al. Annual number of lung cancer deaths potentially avertable by screening in the United States. Cancer. 2013;119:1381–5.
63. Gallus S, Lugo A, La Vecchia C, et al. Pricing policies and control of tobacco in Europe (PPACTE) project:cross-national comparison of smoking prevalence in 18 European countries. Eur J Cancer Prev. 2014;23:177–85.

64. Gallus S, Lugo A, La Vecchia C, et al. Pricing policies and control of tobacco in Europe (PPACTE) project: smoking prevalence and consumption in 18 European countries. Final report. Dublin: PPACTE Consortium; 2011.
65. World Health Organization. WHO report on the global tobacco epidemic, 2015: raises taxes on tobacco—executive summary. Available online ▶ http://apps.who.int/iris/bitstream/10665/178577/1/WHO_NMH_PND_15.5_eng.pdf?ua=1&ua=1
66. Moolgavkar SH, Holford TR, Levy DT, et al. Impact of reduced tobacco smoking on lung cancer mortality in the United States during 1975–2000. J Natl Cancer Inst. 2012;104:541–8.
67. Cesaroni G, Forastiere F, Agabiti N, et al. Effect of the Italian smoking ban on population rates of acute coronary events. Circulation. 2008;117:1183–8.
68. Pell JP, Haw S, Cobbe S, et al. Smoke-free legislation and hospitalizations for acute coronary syndrome. N Engl J Med. 2008;359:482–91.
69. Mackay DF, Irfan MO, Haw S, et al. Meta-analysis of the effect of comprehensive smoke-free legislation on acute coronary events. Heart. 2010;96:1525–30.

Cancer, Heart Diseases and Common Risk Factors: Diet and Physical Activity

Paolo Tralongo, Chiara Lestuzzi, and Francesco Furlanello

C. Lestuzzi et al. (eds.), *Manual of Cardio-oncology*, DOI 10.1007/978-3-319-40236-9_3

3.1 Background

Lifestyle and diet are recognized as risk factors determinants in the pathogenesis of cancer and cardiovascular disease. There are many epidemiological studies that have documented the correlation between the role of diet and how it's modified in geographical area and migration. Smoke, obesity, diabetes, hypertension, and high blood cholesterol are the most important risk factors for atherosclerosis and coronary artery disease (CAD). A heart-healthy diet contains fruits and vegetables, grains, fish, low-fat dairy, and few sugar-sweetened beverages [1]. It has been known for long time that a healthy diet and regular physical activity, together with avoiding smoking, reduce the recurrence of ischemic heart disease and might improve survival in subjects with CAD or at high risk [2–4]. A diet rich in saturated fatty acids is dangerous also in patients with heart failure [5]. The Mediterranean diet is associated with a significant reduction in overall mortality (9 %), mortality from cardiovascular diseases (CVD) (9 %), and incidence of or mortality from cancer (6 %) [6]. A diet rich in fruits and vegetables reduces the risk of cancer of the digestive tract particularly colorectal cancer. Red meat increases the risk of colorectal cancer. Consumption of sugary drinks too seems to have a strong correlation with the incidence of pancreatic cancer. It is also known that overweight and insufficient physical activity increases the risk of several types of cancer, including breast, colon, lung, prostate, and endometrium [7, 8].

High intake of calories leads to increased body weight and obesity; therefore, it's a factor associated with an increased risk for both cancer and cardiovascular disease. Many studies have documented how reducing caloric intake reduces this risk. The factors that are determinants are hyperinsulinemia, insulin resistance, upregulation of insulin-like growth factor, changes in sex hormones metabolism, chronic inflammation, oxidative stress, increased production of angiogenic growth factors, and immune system impairment. As a result, they will determine alteration of the regulation of cell proliferation with a reduction in apoptosis and increased replicative potential, immunological escape, and favors metastatic process [9, 10].

Some food components have a role such as the direct carcinogenic *nitroso-compounds*-heme iron found in red meat promote colorectal cancer. Heterocyclic amines and polycyclic aromatic hydrocarbons are carcinogens that are formed when red meat is cooked at very high flame for a long time [11].

Each food item and its components has the ability to influence multiple mechanisms of the pathogenesis of cancer. Micronutrients can affect these processes in a single or combined form. In fact, there are multiple and complex links between cancer and diet; hence, it is impossible to ascribe to a single food a causal effect; the combination of various foods and duration of exposure are actually affecting many pathways involved in carcinogenesis and in atherosclerosis [12].

> **Cardiovascular diseases and many cancers share the same risk factors, and the strategies useful to prevent cardiovascular diseases are often useful to prevent various kinds of cancer and vice versa [13] (Figs. 3.1, 3.2, and 3.3).**

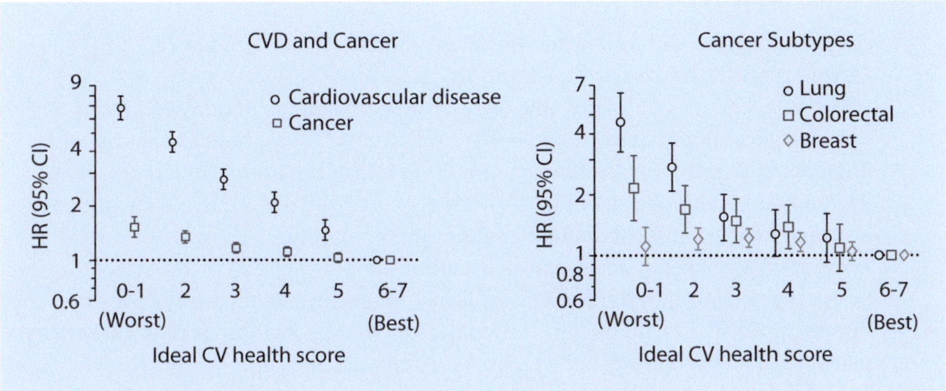

Fig. 3.1 Multivarable-adjusted hazard ratios and 95 % CI for incident cardiovascular disease (CVD) and cancer (*left*) and cancer subtypes (*right*) by ideal cardiovascular health (CVH) score. Reproduced with permission from: Foraker et al. [13]

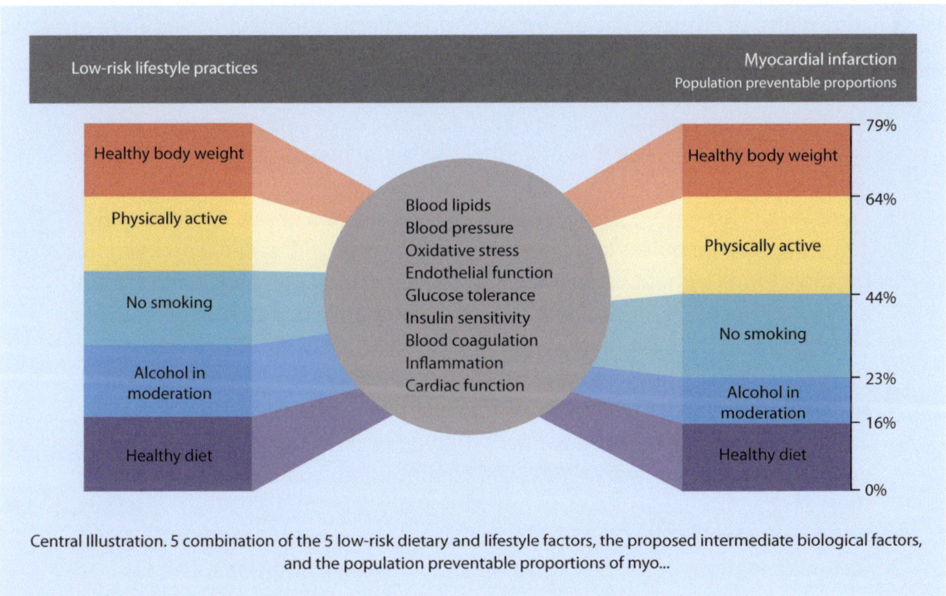

Fig. 3.2 Combined low-risk behaviors and the population preventable proportions of myocardial infarction. Reproduced with permission from: Åkesson A, et al. Low-risk diet and lifestyle habits in the primary prevention of myocardial infarction in men: a population-based prospective cohort study. Journal of the American College of Cardiology 2014; 64: 1299–1306

Practical Suggestions for a Healthy Lifestyle Aimed at Preventing Cancer

1. *Do not smoke*: If smoker, stop smoking.
2. *Body fatness*: be as lean as possible within the normal range of body weight personal recommendations. Ensure that body weight throughout childhood and adolescent growth projects towards the lower end of the normal BMI range at age 21. Maintain body weight within the normal range from age 21. Avoid weight gain and increases in waist circumference throughout adulthood.
3. *Physical activity*: be physically active as part of every day life. Be moderately physically active, equivalent to brisk walking, for at least 30 min every day. As fitness improves, aim for 60 min of moderate or 30 min of vigorous physical activity every day. Limit sedentary habits such as watching television.
4. *Foods and drinks that promote weight gain*: limit consumption of energy-dense foods and avoid sugary drinks. Consume energy-dense foods sparingly. Avoid sugary drinks. Consume fast foods sparingly, if at all.
5. *Plant foods*: eat foods mostly of plant origin. Eat at least five portions/servings (at least 400 g or 14 oz) of a variety of non-starchy vegetables and fruit every day. Eat relatively unprocessed cereals (grains) and/or pulses (legumes) with every meal. Limit refined starchy foods. People who consume starchy roots or tubers as staples should also to ensure sufficient intake of non-starchy vegetables, fruit, and pulses.
6. *Animal foods*: limit intake of red meat and avoid processed meat. People who eat red meat should consume <500 g (18 oz) a week, very little, if any, to be processed.
7. *Alcoholic drinks*: limit alcoholic drinks. If alcoholic drinks are consumed, limit consumption to no more than two drinks a day for men and one drink a day for women.
8. *Preservation, processing, preparation*: limit consumption of salt. Avoid mouldy cereals (grains) or pulses (legumes). Avoid salt-preserved, salted, or salty foods; preserve foods without using salt. Limit consumption of processed foods with added salt to ensure an intake of <6 g (2.4 g sodium) a day. Do not eat mouldy cereals (grains) or pulses (legumes).
9. *Dietary supplements*: aim to meet nutritional needs through diet alone. Dietary supplements are not recommended for cancer prevention.
10. *Breast feeding*: mothers to breastfeed; children to be breastfed. Aim to breastfeed infants exclusively up to 6 months and continue with complementary feeding thereafter.
11. *Cancer survivors*: follow the recommendations for cancer prevention. Personal recommendations. All cancer survivors should receive nutritional care from an appropriately trained professional. If able to do so, and unless otherwise advised, aim to follow the recommendations for diet, healthy weight, and physical activity.

TO BE NOTED: Items 1–9 are valid also for cardiovascular prevention.

Modified with permission from: World Cancer Research Fund/American Institute for Cancer Research, Food, Nutrition, Physical Activity and the prevention of cancer: a global perspective. Washington, DC: world Center Research Fund/American Institute for cancer Research, 2007.

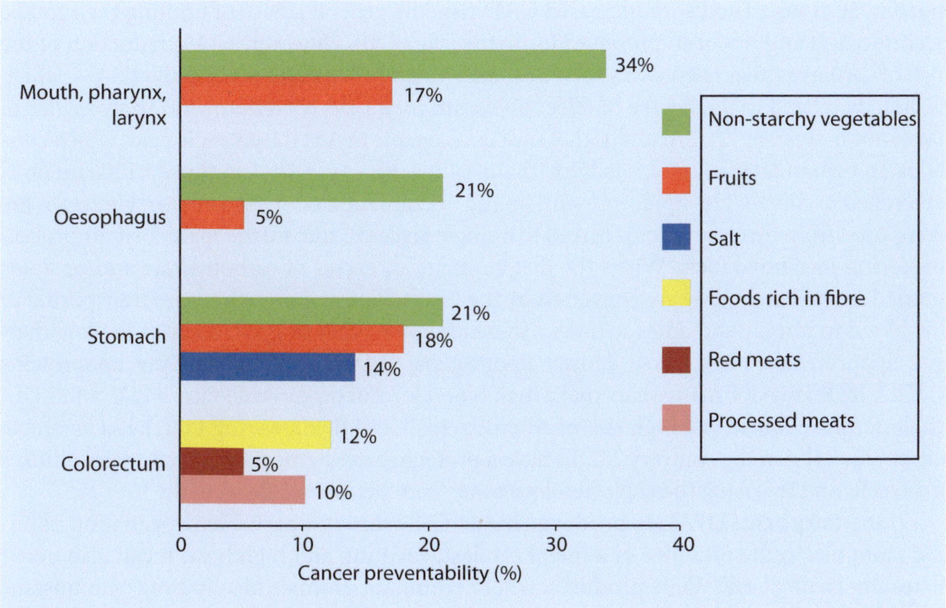

Fig 3.3 Cancer preventability estimates for the United Kingdom for dietary factors judged to be convincingly or probably related to the risk of some cancers. The figure shows the percentage of cancer cases preventable by adequate diet in the United Kingdom. Reproduced with permission from: Norat et al. [14]

3.2 Diet

Sugar

There is a strong association of sugar-sweetened beverage intake with adiposity in children and adults [15]. Diets high in sugar or carbohydrates with high glycemic index promotes diabetes, cardiovascular diseases, and carcinogenesis, by increasing the secretion of insulin and promoting oxidative stress and weight gain [14, 16]. A positive association between sugar-sweetened beverages or high glycemic index food has been linked to CAD and pancreatic, colorectal, and breast cancers [17–19]. Compared with solid foods, calories in liquid form may be less satiating and thereby increase the total amount of daily calories consumed. Sugar-sweetened beverage intake can also displace more healthful beverages, such as milk.

Reduction in sugar-sweetened beverages is an important dietary target for reducing both cardiovascular and cancer risk in individuals.

Fats

Unsaturated fatty acids may be mono-unsaturated (MUFA, as oleic and palmitoleic acids) and poly-unsaturated (PUFA, including omega-3, omega-6 acids). The high content of MUFA in olive oil is considered to be one of the key advantages of the Mediterranean diet. The optimal dietary ratio of omega-6 to omega-3 is 1:1–4:1. Seafood-derived omega-3 PUFAs have strong inverse relations with CHD mortality; the potency of plant-based omega-3 appears weaker. *Saturated fatty acids* (SFA) in the food supply are animal products, such as butter, cows' milk, meat, salmon, and egg yolks, and some plant products, such as chocolate and cocoa butter, coconut, and palm kernel oils. Since a greater SFA consumption has traditionally been associated with increased CAD risk, the general advice of limiting their intake seems logical and has been proposed for many years [20]. However, a 14 % reduction of the risk of cardiovascular events was seen in studies of fat modification (not reduction)—which is directly related to the degree of effect on serum total LDL cholesterol and triglycerides in men, not in women [21]. Actually, the most atherogenic SFA is the palmitic acid, which contains 16 carbon atoms (16C). Medium-chain fatty acids (*MCFAs*), i.e., those <12C are non-atherogenic. *Sterols* are lipids present in the membranes of most cells, *tryglicerides* are composed from three fatty acids linked to a single glycerol, and are the main form or process of storing metabolic fuels. When the diet contains an excess of carbohydrate and/or lipids needed immediately, they are converted by the liver to lipoproteins which are transported in the blood to muscle and adipose tissue. There are three types of lipoproteins: very-low-density lipoproteins (*VLDL*), low-density lipoproteins (*LDL*), and high-density lipoproteins (*HDL*). It's known for many years that a high blood level of trygliceride-rich VLDL and LDL-cholesterol are linked to a high risk of atherosclerosis and that lowering LDL has a favorable effect [22–24]. On the contrary, HDLs have a protective effect, mediating cholesterol effluxes from cells and reversing the cholesterol pathway from peripheral tissue to the liver [25].

Trans-fatty acids (TFA) are produced industrially through partial hydrogenation of liquid plant oils in the presence of a metal catalyst, vacuum, and high heat. It can also occur naturally in meat and dairy products, where ruminant animals bio-hydrogenate unsaturated fatty acids via bacterial enzymes. Consumption of industrial trans-unsaturated fatty acids is associated with a 30 % increase in the risk of CHD events and an 18 % increase in the risk of CHD mortality [26]. However, natural TFA contained in dairy products as *trans*-palmitoleate are associated with higher LDL cholesterol and with lower triglycerides, fasting insulin, blood pressure, and incident diabetes [27]. Trans-fatty acids have also a key role in the pathogenesis of cancer of the breast, colon, stomach, and prostate [28–31].

- Substitution of dietary PUFAs for SFA has been shown to lower CVD risk, but replacing saturated fat with carbohydrate, particularly refined carbohydrate, can exacerbate the atherogenic dyslipidemia associated with insulin resistance and obesity that includes increased triglycerides, small LDL particles, and reduced HDL cholesterol [32].
- The most recent studies state that there is insufficient evidence to determine whether lowering dietary cholesterol reduces LDL cholesterol [33].

Dietary advice should lay emphasis on optimizing the quality of fats (limiting industrial TFA and >12C SFA; increasing the use of MFAs and PUFAs; limiting the omega-6/omega-3 ratio to <5/1; preferring seafood derived omega-3)—rather than limiting total calories intake—and associating physical activity [34].

Integral Foods

Dietary fiber intake is associated with lower levels of inflammation markers, such as C-reactive protein and tumor necrosis factor α receptor 2, which play key roles in chronic inflammatory conditions [35, 36]. Moreover, whole grains and cereal fiber have a high content of antioxidants, vitamins, trace minerals, phenolic acids, lignans, and phytoestrogens, which have been associated with a reduced risk of colorectal cancer [37, 38]. Dietary fiber from vegetables stimulates the fermentation of anaerobia bacteria in the large intestine. This leads to the synthesis of short-chain fatty acids that are able to induce apoptosis and reduce cell proliferation. The fibers reduce the contact time between mucosa and intestinal contents (including carcinogenic substances) and are able to reduce the levels of circulating estrogen and androstenedione and therefore may have a protective role against breast cancer [39]. Dietary fibers have specific and unique impacts on intestinal microbiota composition and metabolism, and gut microbiota have been related with various chronic diseases such as obesity, CVD, diabetes, and cancer [40, 41].

There is consistent epidemiological evidence that whole grain foods substantially lower the risk of CAD, diabetes, and cancer and also play a role in body weight management and digestive health; high consumption of whole grains or cereal fiber was significantly associated with reduced risk of all-cause mortality and death from CVD, cancer, diabetes, respiratory disease, infections, and other causes [42, 43].

Fruits and Vegetables

Regular consumption of fruits and vegetables produce substantial improvements in several risk factors, including blood pressure (BP), lipid levels, insulin resistance, inflammatory biomarker levels, endothelial function, and weight control [44–46]. The polyphenols that are derived from the plant have an important role in the prevention by acting as scavengers of oxidizing agents, anti-inflammatory, antimicrobial, and able to inhibit platelet aggregation [47]. Eating phenol-rich fruits at the end of a meal enhances the antioxidant capacity of the blood. *Legumes*, mostly soy beans, provide an overall package of micronutrients, phytochemicals, and fiber that could plausibly reduce cardiometabolic risk. An advantage of legumes is their content of proteins and that can be used as an alternative to meat [48]. *Nuts*, mostly tree nuts, contain several bioactive constituents that could improve cardiometabolic health, including unsaturated fatty acids, vegetable proteins, fiber, folate, minerals, antioxidants, and phytochemicals. Nut consumption reduces total cholesterol; LDL cholesterol; postprandial hyperglycemia from high-carbohydrate meals; and (variably) oxidative, inflammatory, and endothelial biomarkers [49]. Garlic and other vegetables from the same family act as inhibitor of deacetylase inhibitors increasing the stability of DNA. The resveratrol and curcumin have antioxidant, anti-inflammatory, and anticarcinogenic activities [50, 51].

There is a strong concordant evidence that fruit (both fresh and nuts) and vegetable consumption lowers CVD and cancer risk.

There are significant differences amongst the different types of fruits, vegetables, or their juices, according to the way they are cultivated (open air versus green houses; southern versus northern countries).

To obtain the most beneficial effects, the diet should include a large variety of different fruits and vegetables, preferring season foods.

Meat

Several constituents of red meats could increase cardio-metabolic risks, including saturated fatty acids, cholesterol, heme iron, and also in processed meats—high levels of salt and other preservatives [52]. However, fat composition of meats is about 50 % of MUFAs and PUFAs, beside SFAs. Increased red meat intake is associated with higher fasting glucose, fasting insulin concentrations, and unfavorable plasma concentrations of inflammatory and glucose metabolic biomarkers [53, 54]. Consumption of processed meats but not unprocessed red meats is associated with higher incidence of CVD and diabetes and higher mortality for CVD and cancer [55]. These findings suggest that adverse effects of preservatives (e.g., sodium, nitrites, and phosphates) and/or preparation methods (e.g., high-temperature commercial cooking/frying) could influence health effects of meat consumption [56]. Several studies have shown an association between high intake of processed meat (such as ham, bacon, sausages, and hot dogs), red meat (mainly beef, pork, or lamb) and colorectal, pancreatic cancer [57, 58]. Cooking meat at high temperatures(frying or grilling) generates carcinogenic aromatic amines; marinades with virgin oil, garlic, onions, red wine, and herbs have antioxidant capacity and may inhibit the formation of such amines [59].

The cardiovascular and cancer risk linked to eating meat is mostly due to the quality (fresh or processed) and the type of cooking. A moderate intake of meat seems to be safe.

Dairy Foods

Dairy foods often have a high content of saturated fatty acids, sodium, and calories and thus have been considered as potentially dangerous as regards CVD. Dietary interventions that includes low-fat dairy foods have been suggested and significantly lowered BP, lipid levels, and insulin resistance and improved endothelial function, independent of changes in weight. However, in the most recent studies, there is no evidence that dairy products are associated with risk of CAD or stroke in a generally healthy population [32, 60]. On the contrary, high intakes of dairy products could be associated with a lower risk of CVD, while fermented dairy product may be associated with a reduced risk of stroke [61]. Sheep's and goat's milk are richer in MCFAs compared to cow's milk; the quality of milk fats is also influenced by the animal diet. Milk minerals, especially calcium and potassium, may be responsible for the antihypertensive effect.

Dairy foods are a good source of proteins, calcium, and other nutrients and should not be banned from the diet. However, they should be used as an alternative to meat in the meal.

Alcohol

An excess of alcohol consumption may cause or favor dilated cardiomyopathy; atrial fibrillation; liver cirrhosis; cancers of the mouth, esophagus, pharynx, larynx, and liver, and breast cancer in women [62, 63]. However, moderate quantities (10 to <50 g per day for men and 5 to <25 g per day for women) have a favorable effect, increasing HDL-cholesterol, improving insulin resistance, and reducing the postprandial lipemia [64]. Wine (mostly red wine) contains phenolic compounds, which are cardio-protective. The drinking pattern is also relevant: drinking at meals slows the absorption of alcohol and prevents the production of carcinogenic metabolites.

Regular consumption of one glass of wine (125 ml) at meals is recommended for the prevention of CAD.

Salt

A high consumption of salt (sodium chloride) raises the blood pressure, thereby increasing the risk of stroke and cardiovascular diseases. Dietary salt intake has a synergistic effect with *Helicobacter pylori* infection on gastric carcinogenesis and enhances the carcinogenicity of *nitroso compounds*, increasing the risk of stomach cancer. In North America and in Europe, 75 % of sodium intake is derived from packaged or restaurant foods.

Lowering the sodium intake is beneficial for preventing both cardiovascular diseases and stomach cancer.

Vitamins and dietary supplements, minerals and vitamins Vitamins B6, C, D, E, carotenoids, and selenium have antioxidant activity and antiproliferative and anti-inflammatory properties, acting in a manner protective of DNA [65].

3.2.1 Dietary Supplements

Several dietary supplements have been proposed as effective both for the prevention as well as therapy for cardiovascular diseases and cancer.

- **Some of them actually have a beneficial effect** when used as a complement (not an alternative) to pharmacology:
  - Omega-3 PUFAs are the only supplements suggested to prevent atherosclerosis.
  - Coenzyme Q10 might be useful in reducing the cardiovascular risk in patients with metabolic syndrome and in the elderly, but there are no proven effects on cancer prevention [66, 67].
- **Some supplements have some positive effects theoretically**, but the advantage has not been confirmed by prospective studies. Amongst these are *Folic acid*, *vitamins, and Selenium*. For years, *green tea* has been shown to be a potential cancer-fighting agent. Some researches suggests that in countries where consumption of green tea is increased, cancer incidence are decreased accordingly. *Soy isoflovones* are reported to possess strong antioxidant and anti-angiogenic properties which may prove to be useful in the fight against cancer. *Curcumin* has been reported to offer anti-angiogenesis properties as well as immunity, enhancing benefits in the fight against cancer. It has also been suggested that it may help traditional cancer therapies such that chemotherapy may work better [68].
- **Some supplements may even have harmful side effects** (mostly according to the dose):
  - **Calcium supplements** reduce the risk of colorectal cancer, but increase the risk of myocardial infarction.
  - **Vitamin E** may protect against a number of chronic diseases, such as cardiovascular disease, and an inverse relationship was observed between alpha-tocopherol levels and prostate cancer, but only in current and recent ex-smokers. However, the administration of high doses of vitamin E (alone or with Selenium) results in an increased risk of prostate cancer.
  - High doses of *vitamin C* are usually given intravenously and might have some anticancer effect and potentiate the effect of drugs such as platinum and paclitaxel. However, they may also interfer with other chemotherapeutic drugs such as doxorubicin and bortezomib.
  - High doses of *beta-carotene* can result in pro-oxidant effects, especially in smokers, and increase the risk of lung and prostate cancer.
  - **Amygdalin** (also called Laetrile or vitamin B17) is present in bitter almonds, apple, apricot, peach, plum seeds, fava beans, and other vegetables. It has shown little anticancer activity in animal studies and no anticancer activity in human clinical trials. It contains cyanide and may cause a toxicity mirroring the symptoms of cyanide poisoning, including liver damage, difficulty walking (caused by damaged nerves), fever, coma, and death.
  - Herbs and vitamins with antiplatelet activity that have the potential to prolong bleeding time, includeing garlic (*Allium sativum*), gingko (*Gingko biloba*), cranberry *(Vaccinium macrocarpon)*, vitamin E, ginger *(Zingiber officinale)*, and ginseng (*Panax ginseng*), may be harmful in patients undergoing surgery, and should be avoided 1–2 weeks before [69].
  - Several herbs and foods, as St John's wort (*Hypericum perforatum*), grapefruit juice, gingko, ginseng, and garlic, may interact with drugs interfering with the Cytochrome P450 system [70, 71].

> **Many natural compounds, including vitamins, have beneficial effects in preventing cardiovascular diseases and cancer.**

> **However, the presumption that the greater the intake, the greater the benefit is not true. On the contrary, it can be even harmful.**

> **A diet including a variety of foods (different fruits and vegetables) is likely to provide the necessary amount of vitamins and micronutrients. The intake of dietary supplements (or of "fortified foods") is not recommended.**

3.2.2 Prevention of Cardiotoxicity

We are not able to code, despite many preclinical studies performed on in vitro models and animals, a dietary pattern that can have an absolute value and applicable to all patients who undergo treatment or those who are cured and start a cancer follow-up. Most of the efforts have been directed towards the use of medications of integration and in this context assumes an important role also the nutraceutical in the prevention of cardiotoxicity and other side events of treatments. Although none of them have provided a convincing evidence that agents of nutrition can prevent myocardial damage induced by chemotherapy [72].

- **The prevention of anthracycline cardiotoxicity** has been approached with the use of free radical scavengers such as flavonoids of natural origin, vitamins A, C, and E, endogenous antioxidants, but the available data are limited to preclinical studies.
  - **Flavonoids, polyphenolic benzo-γ-pyrone** present in all plants, possess the property iron-chelating and radical scavenging. Flavonoids derived from spinach or from grape seeds have shown a beneficial role in animal models with heart disease induced by doxorubicin [73, 74].
  - High dose *vitamin supplements* have also been studied in animal models but did not find any application in humans.
  - **Selenium and zinc** in some studies protect against cardiotoxicity in animal models involving the use of rats and rabbits. However, the shortage of this mineral is not itself a factor that can exacerbate cardiac damage induced by the use of anthracyclines.
  - **Endogenous antioxidants**, such as N-acetylcysteine and coenzyme-Q10, obtained conflicting results in studies using animal models and in those conducted with humans. Interesting data—highlighted by studies involving the use of melatonin in rodents—has shown to have an action free-radical scavenger, capable of neutralizing the damaged myocyte induced by doxorubicin. No human data are available at the time.
- **Androgen deprivation therapy**. Dietary supplements (flavonoids, selenium, Vitamine E, omega-3 and omega-6 fatty acids, various herbs) have been suggested to relieve adverse effects related to metabolic syndrome resulting from androgen deprivation therapy (ADT). However, there is no convincing evidence of the effectiveness of most of them. On the contrary, the unregulated self-prescription of active compounds such as soy, Selenium, or Vitamin E may in some cases even prove to be harmful or negatively interfere with cancer treatment [75]. The only suggested supplements in men undergoing ADT are calcium and Vitamin D supplementation to prevent osteoporosis; the isoflavones of soy and flaxseed seem to have little effect on reducing the levels of LDL-cholesterol [76, 77]. Unsaturated fatty acids are effective in reducing some cardiovascular risk factors if given as an alternative to saturated fatty acids rather than a supplement to the diet [78].

3.2.3 Traditional and Alternative Dietary Patterns (▪ Table 3.1)

Several healthy dietary patterns have been identified, sharing several key characteristics [79]:

- **An emphasis on fruits, vegetables, other plant foods such as beans and nuts, and whole grains and fish.**
- **Moderate consumption of dairy products, preferring sheep's, goat's, and fermented products.**
- **Limited red meats or processed meats.**
- **Few refined carbohydrates and other processed foods.**

▪ **Table 3.1** Myths and truth about diet, supplements, and complementary/alternative therapies for cancer

Diet	Hypothesis	The truth
Blood groups	Blood groups (A, B, AB, and O) define a natural predisposition to take advantage/disadvantage of eating different foods	No physiologic rationale, no studies supporting the hypothesis: it's an urban legend All 4 diets (or "ways of eating") are mostly based on healthy food and a huge step up from the standard Western diet of processed junk food
Vegetarian	Avoiding meat and fish may prevent cancer and cardiovascular disease	The advantage of limiting meat intake (mostly processed meat and red meat) is accepted. The superiority of a vegetarian over a mediterranean diet has not been demonstrated
Vegan	Avoiding any animal and animal-derived food may prevent cancer and cardiovascular disease and cure some cancers	There is no advantage compared with vegetarian or Mediterranean diet. Vitamin B12 deficiency may be harmful
Macrobiotic	Avoiding foods containing toxins; cooking and storing foods in pots and utensils made of wood, glass, stainless steel, or ceramics; without electricity or microwave could cure cancer and other serious illenesses	Available scientific evidence does not support claims that a macrobiotic diet can treat or prevent cancer. As vegetarian and Mediterranean diet, it lowers cholesterol level. The intake of calcium, iron, vitamins, and proteins may be insufficient
Gerson and Gonzalez regimens	Organic and vegetarian diets associated to various supplements may cure some cancers	No prospective, peer-reviewed studies confirming the assumption
Alcaline diet	Replacing acid-forming foods with alkaline foods can improve health and fight cancer	It is impossible to change the body pH with foods; food can only change urine pH. Any change in blood pH would be harmful

(continued)

Table 3.1 (continued)

Supplementary, complementary, alternative treatments	Hypothesis	The truth
Folic acid	Reduce oxidative stress	The evidence of a positive effect has not been proven
Beta carotene	Reduce oxidative stress	High doses may have a pro-oxidant effect; increases the risk of lung cancer
Vitamin E	Reduce oxidative stress	High doses may increase the risk of prostate cancer
Mistletoe extracts	May improve cancer survival	They may improve chemotherapy side effects (nausea, vomiting) and reduce fatigue, but there is no clinical evidence of improved survival
Vitamin C	Generating hydrogen peroxide has a cytotoxic effect on various cell lines	High dose of Vitamin C (mostly through the intravenous route) may increase the effect of chemotherapy and radiotherapy in some solid tumors, but may reduce the effect of chemotherapies in leukemia, lymphoma, and multiple myeloma
Cannabis and cannabinoids	Have an antitumor effect inducing apoptosis of tumor cells, inhibiting tumor cell growth and neoangiogenesis. Have antiemetic and analgesic effects, reduce anxiety, stimulate appetite	Their beneficial effect on pain and nausea has been confirmed in clinical studies. Therapeutic use of cannabinoids for prevention of chemotherapy-induced nausea is approved in the USA. Oromucosal administration of cannabis is approved in several countries for cancer pain. There are no clinical data supporting the antineoplastic use
Laetrile (amygdalin)	Has antitumor and radiosensitizing effects	The claimed benefits of laetrile are not supported by controlled clinical trials. There is a risk of serious adverse effects from cyanide poisoning after laetrile or amygdalin, especially after taking it by mouth
Echinacea	Boost the immune system and then fights cancer	No anticancer or immunomodulatory effect. It might reduce some of the side effects of cancer chemotherapy (sore mouth or diarrhea)
St John's worth (*Hypericum*)	It's a non toxic and natural therapy for depression	It is effective in mild to moderate depressive symptoms. It interferes with the absorption and metabolism of many drugs, including anticancer and cardiovascular drugs, anticoagulants, antiepileptic drugs

Further information in
► http://www.cancer.gov/about-cancer/treatment/cam/hp
► http://authoritynutrition.com/search/?q=cancer
► http://authoritynutrition.com/search/?q=cardiovascular+disease
► http://www.cancerresearchuk.org/about-cancer/cancers-in-general/treatment/complementary-alternative/

The *Mediterranean diet* is a good example of a healthy dietary pattern; however, its benefits are mostly evident in the Mediterranean countries, where a large variety of fresh fruits and vegetables are available. In northern countries, the Mediterranean diet should be adapted to the locally available foods.

Vegetarians (lacto-vegetarian, ovo-vegetarians, and lacto-ovo-vegetarian) *diets* have beneficial effects on diabetes, obesity, lipid profile, metabolic syndrome, and cardiovascular diseases [80–82]. However, they did not show any statistically significant advantage, compared to a diet containing meat, as regards the prevention of colon cancer [83]. In a recent study, vegetarians had significantly lower mortality for pancreatic (but not colorectal) and hematologic cancers compared to meat eaters, but similar advantages were observed for fish eaters; the overall all-cause mortality did not differ between vegetarians and nonvegetarians [84].

Vegan diets (excluding eggs and dairy products) cause a vitamin B12 deficiency and require a supplementation. Vitamin B12 deficiency raises plasma homocysteine (increasing thrombotic risk) and the indexes of atherosclerosis [85]. A vegetarian diet should be preferred to a vegan diet.

Several alternative dietary regimens including cocktails of supplements pretending to cure cancer in a "natural" way have been proposed both by physicians and nonphysicians and are often quoted by complementary/alternative medicine (CAM) sites on the web. Given the high prevalence of complementary therapy use (often self-prescribed by the patients), raising a discussion is an excellent opportunity for the physician to demonstrate compassion, understanding, and humanity and to provide high-quality care based on scientific data [86–88].

- **Aloe vera** is a plant from which several compounds are extracted. Some of them have antineoplastic activity on multiple tumor cells involving multi-channel mechanisms, including the disruption of cell cycle, induction of apoptosis, anti-metastasis, antiangiogenic, and strengthening of immune function. However, only in vitro or animal studies have been done so far, and data about its use in clinical oncology are still lacking. Presently, Aloe vera extracts are successfully used as cosmetics and for skin or mucosal protection or healing during radiotherapy and chemotherapy [89].
- **Antineoplastons** are drugs composed of chemical compounds that are naturally present in the urine and blood. They were introduced as a possible cancer treatment in 1976. The hypothesis was that they should provide a natural biochemical substance that is excreted and therefore lacking in people with cancer. No randomized controlled trials showing the effectiveness of antineoplastons have been published in the peer-reviewed scientific literature till date. Their side effects include serious neurologic toxicity.
- **Cannabis.** Chemical components of Cannabis also known as cannabinoids activate specific receptors found throughout the body to produce pharmacologic effects, particularly in the central nervous system and the immune system. Cannabinoids (dronabinol and nabilone) may have benefits in the treatment of some cancer-related side effects, mostly in nausea and pain. There are no published data on the use of *Cannabis* for other cancer-related symptoms. In vitro and animal studies suggests that cannabinoids may cause antitumor effects by various mechanisms, like induction of cell death, inhibition of cell growth, and inhibition of tumor angiogenesis invasion and metastasis. However, no clinical trials of *Cannabis* as a treatment for cancer in humans have been published, except for a single, small study of intratumoral injection of delta-9-THC in patients with recurrent glioblastoma multiforme.

- **Essiac and Flor Essence** are herbal tea mixtures originally developed in Canada by a nurse in 1922 and are marketed worldwide as dietary supplements. Proponents have claimed that Essiac and Flor Essence can help detoxify the body, strengthen the immune system, fight cancer, relieve pain, reduce side effects, improve quality of life and reduce tumor size. No report of a clinical study on Essiac has been published in the peer-reviewed scientific literature. A retrospective review of data voluntarily submitted by physicians for 86 cancer patients who had been treated with Essiac did not show any curative effect.
- **Gerson therapy** is empirically based on observations made by Max Gerson, M.D., in the 1930s–1950s. It is advocated by its supporters as a method of treating cancer patients based on an organic vegetarian diet plus nutritional and biological supplements, pancreatic enzymes, and coffee or other types of enemas. No prospective, controlled study of the use of the Gerson therapy in cancer patients has been reported in a peer-reviewed scientific journal.
- **Gonzalez regimen** combines prescribed diets, nutritional supplements, coffee enemas, and pancreatic enzymes in a cancer management program. The regimen is intended to detoxify the body, correct nervous system imbalances that might lead to impaired general health, and support natural immune processes. There are no data supporting its efficacy: on the contrary, in one and only study published amongst patients who had pancreatic cancer, those who chose gemcitabine-based chemotherapy survived more than three times *as long* (14.0 versus 4.3 months) and had better quality of life than those who chose Gonzalez treatment.
- **Mistletoe** is one of the most widely studied complementary/alternative therapy for cancer. In certain European countries, the preparations made from European mistletoe (*Viscum album*, Loranthaceae) are among the most prescribed drugs offered to cancer patients. The mistletoe extracts and products studied in clinical trials were Iscador, Eurixor, Helixor, Lektinol, Isorel, abnobaVISCUM, and recombinant lectin ML-1. Improvement in chemotherapy-associated fatigue, nausea and vomiting, depression, emotional well-being, and concentration were reported in several randomized trials. There is no clinical evidence of a significant effect on survival, after tests in various kinds of tumors.
- **Sodium bicarbonate** acts by inducing the formation of an alkaline environment adverse to cancer growth. The proton pump inhibitors (PPIs), used in the treatment of gastric ulcer (omeprazole, lansoprazole, and others), have been extensively investigated for their potential role in reducing tumor acidity and overcome the acid-related chemoresistance and because they could have direct tumor cell toxicity by depriving them of a key mechanism for maintaining pHi/pHe gradient [90]. No clinical studies are available.

Dietary supplements are popular and readily available. Patients often use them on their own, without informing their physicians.

Patients are drawn also to natural products lacking anticancer activity, but are marketed with "buzzwords" such as *antioxidant*, *immune booster*, and *detox*. Product claims indicating protection of good cells from damage, restoring suppressed immune function, or removing "toxins" left behind by cancer treatment are not uncommon.

The patients should receive a packet reminding them to discuss any self-prescribed supplements or medications with their physicians and should be asked at each visit

to disclose any herbs and other dietary supplements they are taking on a "home medication list."

- **The caring physician should discuss CAM with the patient, explaining the possible risks of some supplements.**

- **The use of agents that are generally safe and have shown some preliminary evidence of anticancer activity should be tolerated, if it is not in conflict with the prescribed therapies.**

3.3 Physical Activity

Sedentary behavior and limited physical activity are associated with a higher risk of hypertension, diabetes, cardiovascular disease, and some cancers [91]. Physical activity interacts with a plethora of metabolic and health-related functions, independently of energy balance: insulin sensitivity and glucose metabolism, fatty acid metabolism, and endothelial function [92]. There are several mechanism through which physical activity may affect cardiovascular and cancer risk [93, 94].

- Reduced blood pressure, both in men and women [95].
- Reduced adiposity and thus:
  - Reduces inflammatory cytokines, lowering the risk for both atherosclersis and most cancers.
  - Decreased insulin use, insulin resistance, hyperglycemia, and type 2 diabetes (all factors linked to the risk of CAD and of breast, colon, pancreas, and endometrial cancer),
- Reduced HDL cholesterol levels among men and women and triglycerides among men [96].
- In postmenopausal women, it lowers estrogen and progesterone levels, reducing the risk of endometrial and some other types of breast cancers.
- Increases gut motility, leading to a reduced exposure to food carcinogenenic substances, contributing to a reduced risk of colon cancer [97].
- Comorbidities (diabetes, ischemic heart disease, stroke, metabolic syndrome) may increase the overall mortality of patients who have been cured of cancer; these comorbidities may be prevented/controlled by physical activity [98–100].

Various aspects of physical activity should be taken into account:

1. **Physical activity** is any movement that increases energy expenditure above the basal level. It is conventionally classified as: low-intensity if the energy expenditure is between 1.6 and 2.9 metabolic equivalents of task (METs), moderate-intensity 3–5.9 METs), and vigorous-intensity (≥6 METs).
   1. *Physical exercise* is a planned and repetitive physical activity, aimed at improving or maintaining physical fitness. It may be classified as
      i. Aerobic (high volume-low force muscle contractions), leading to increase in heart rate and energy expenditure.
      ii. Anaerobic/resistance (low volume-high force muscle contractions), leading to increase in muscle size and strength.
   2. *Occupational physical activity* is the activity performed during work hours (approximately 6–8 h a day).

   3. *Household activity* includes cleaning, moving objects, walking in home, gardening, child care.
2. **Sedentary behavior** refers to the time spent in activities with a low level of energy expenditure (i.e., ≤1.5 METs), such as sitting, lying down, and watching television and videos.

Physical activity and sedentary behavior are not mutually exclusive.

3.3.1 Physical Activity and Cardiovascular Diseases

- Studies amongst men and women suggest that high level of leisure time PA reduces the risk of CVD in a range of 20–30 %, compared to the risk of those with low level of PA at leisure time, while moderate leisure time PA decreases the risk by about 10–20 %, indicating an obvious dose–response relationship. However, a moderate level of occupational PA is associated with a 10–20 % lower risk of CVD, whereas high PA at work fails to show any stronger protective effect against CVD. These effects are independent of the impact of major cardiovascular risk factors which were considered as confounders [101].
- Volume of physical activity has been inversely associated with both ischemic heart disease and stroke [102].
- In people >65 years of age, there is an inverse association between recreational physical activity and incidence of major vascular events up to about 20 MET-hours per week (equivalent to approximately 1 h of non-vigorous, or half an hour of vigorous, physical activity per day) [103] (Fig. 3.4).
  - At higher levels of physical activity, there is no evidence of further reductions in risk and no evidence of an increase in risk.
- In patients with congestive heart failure, physical training can have beneficial effects on neuro-humoral, inflammatory, metabolic, and central hemodynamic responses, as well as on endothelial, skeletal muscle and cardiovascular functions, leading to:
  - Improvement in functional capacity and quality of life [104].
  - Improved survival [105].
- After an acute myocardial infarction, an exercise intervention based on early progressive exercises, started in the inpatient setting and followed by unsupervised training on discharge, has a positive impact on quality of life and functional capacity [106].

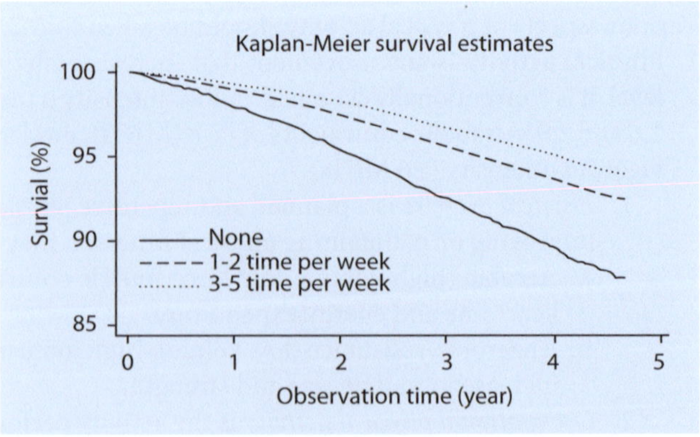

Fig. 3.4 Overall survival of citizens aged ≥65 years according to number of times (0 times/week, 1–2 times/week, and 3–5 times/week) they performed physical activity for ≥30 min. Reproduced with permission from: Wu CY, et al. The association of physical activity with all-cause, cardiovascular, and cancer mortalities among older adults. Prev Med. 2015 Mar;72:23–9

3.3.2 Physical Activity in Cancer Prevention (Fig. 3.5)

Breast Cancer

Convincing epidemiologic evidence indicates that physical activity is inversely associated with breast cancer risk with an average decrease in risk of 25–30 % for women in the highest versus the lowest category of physical activity [107].

- The effect is most evident in postmenopausal women.
- The protective effect is evident in both obese and nonobese women; body mass index (BMI) is directly linked to breast cancer risk, but this risk is independent of physical activity [108].
- The cancer receptors are also relevant: the difference between active and non active women is significant as regards Estrogen receptors (ER) positive and/or HER2 negative cancer [109].
- Dose–response analysis suggests that the risk of breast cancer decreased by 2 % for every 25 metabolic equivalent (MET)-h/week increment in nonoccupational physical activity, 3 % for every 10 MET-h/week (roughly equivalent to 4 h/week of walking in 2 miles/h or 1 h/week of running in 6 miles/h) increment in recreational activity, and 5 % for every 2 h/week increment in moderate plus vigorous recreational activity, respectively [110].

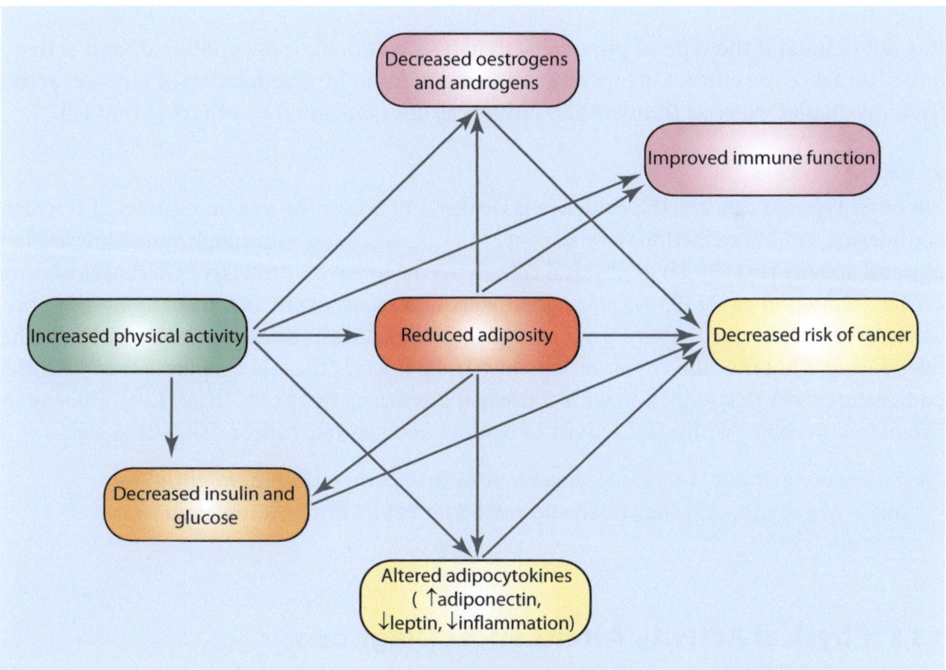

Fig. 3.5 Hypothesized mechanisms linking physical activity to cancer risk or prognosis. Physical activity might work through reducing the amount of adipose tissue, which lowers production of sex hormones, insulin, leptin, and inflammatory markers, thereby decreasing the exposure to these potentially carcinogenic hormones and peptides and reducing cancer risk. Reproduced with permission from: McTiernan [93]

■ Colorectal Cancer

There is convincing evidence linking physical activity and reduced incidence of colon cancer by about 25 %.

- Both occupational and recreational physical activity are protective, and the effect is similar for males and females [111].
- The preventive effect of physical activity does not seem to differ between the colonic subsites (proximal versus distal), but it seem be irrelevant as regards the rectum, perhaps indicating that different mechanisms are operating in the development of colon and rectal cancer [112, 113].
- Whether sedentary behavior and nonaerobic physical activity are associated with the risk of colon cancer is still do be defined.

■ Endometrial Cancer

An increase in leisure-time physical activity by 3 MET-hour/week is associated with 2 % reduced risk of endometrial cancer and by 1 h/week with 5 % reduced risk [114].

■ Gastric Cancer

The risk of gastric cancer is 21 % lower among the most physically active people as compared with the least physically active people.

- The advantage is maintained after adjustment for important confounders, including age, obesity, and other risk factors for gastric cancer (smoking, alcohol, dietary patterns), and socioeconomic status [115].

It is not defined if the type of physical activity (recreational or occupational) and activity levels influence the effect. One meta-analysis suggests an inverse relation of physical activity, in particular exercise frequency, but this was not confirmed by others [116, 117].

■ Other Cancers

For other types of cancers, the evidence is weaker, but according to some studies, it is worth considering. A 12 % reduction in renal cancer risk is associated with a high versus low level of physical activity B [118]. High physical activity seems to have a protective effect against lung cancer (reduction of 22–23 %) among smokers and ex-smokers, but not among the non-smokers [119]. Physical activity is not strongly associated with pancreatic cancer risk, and the relationship is not modified by smoking status or BMI level. There is a suggestion of potential pancreatic cancer risk reduction with consistent physical activity over time [120]. There is an inverse relationship of physical activity to bladder and prostate cancer risk [121, 122].

Sedentary behavior increases the risk of various cancers independently from physical activity—this has been suggested for colon, endometrial, and breast cancers [123].

3.3.3 Physical Activity After Cancer Diagnosis

- In breast cancer patients, physical inactivity was related to reduced health and increased symptoms such as pain, depression, and anxiety [124].
- A meta-analysis of physical activity after breast cancer diagnosis in relation to survival found a 34 % decrease in breast cancer mortality, 41 % decreased risk of all-cause mortality, and 24 % decreased risk of disease recurrence [125].

- Both pre-diagnosis (lifetime and more recent combined) and post-diagnosis physical activities were also associated with reduced risk of breast cancer events (breast cancer progression, new primaries, and recurrence combined) [126].
- However, after breast cancer surgery, many patients are more sedentary and participate in less low intensity activity, both compared to non-cancer control subjects and to their previous habits [127, 128].

3.3.4 Cardiovascular Disease, Cancer, and Physical Activity

- Both antineoplastic treatments (chemotherapy, target therapy, hormone treatment) and lifestyle modifications (physical inactivity, sedentary behavior) after the diagnosis of cancer may negatively impair the cardiovascular function or increase the cardiovascular risk [129–132].
  - The effect may indirectly induce the metabolic syndrome or alter the lipid profile or directly lead to an endothelial dysfunction [133, 134].
  - Patients treated for extragonadal seminomas have an increased risk of cardiovascular disease, while those with testicular seminomas have not [135].
- Physical activity has the rationale for reducing the adverse effects of antineoplastic treatments on the cardiovascular system.
  - Several exercise intervention studies in breast cancer survivors were successful in lowering resting heart rate, systolic and diastolic blood pressure, C-reactive protein, and in improving cardiovascular function [136–139].
  - It has been suggested to ameliorate and/or reverse long-term cardiovascular disease sequelae in germ cell cancer survivors [132].
  - Physical activity improves the quality of life in cancer patients (both during and after treatments) through positive changes in physical functioning, emotional well-being, sleep disturbance, social functioning, anxiety, fatigue, and pain [140, 141].
  - Although the preclinical data supports the importance of exercise to mitigate cardiotoxicity, only one human study has reported specifically the influence of cardiac activity in patients undergoing chemotherapy treatment. A case study by De Palleville has documented that physical exercise a week prior to chemotherapy treatment and continued during treatment can lead to an improvement of heart function parameters in breast cancer patients [142].
  - A prevention program could be divided into two stages: primary and secondary preventions. Primary prevention should include the ability to start physical activity prior to chemotherapy and during treatment. In fact, there are no data supporting the fact that the start of physical activity prior to chemotherapy is likely to speed-up with what is needed to start the treatment and the recovery time after surgery.

References

1. Shay C, Stamler J, Dyer A, et al. Nutrient and food intakes of middle-aged adults at low risk of cardiovascular disease: the international study of macro-/micronutrients and blood pressure (INTERMAP). Eur J Nutr. 2012;51:917–26.
2. Chow CK, Jolly S, Rao-Melacini P, et al. Association of diet, exercise, and smoking modification with risk of early cardiovascular events after acute coronary syndromes. Circulation. 2010;121:750–8.

3. Ford ES, Bergmann MM, Boeing H, et al. Healthy lifestyle behaviors and all-cause mortality among adults in the United States. Prev Med. 2012;55:23–7.
4. Kwagyan J, Retta TM, Ketete M, et al. Obesity and cardiovascular diseases in a high-risk population: evidence-based approach to CHD risk reduction. Ethn Dis. 2015;25:208–13.
5. Colin-Ramirez E, Castillo-Martinez L, Orea-Tejeda A, et al. Dietary fatty acids intake and mortality in patients with heart failure. Nutrition. 2014;30:1366–71.
6. Sofi F, Cesari F, Abbate R, et al. Adherence to Mediterranean diet and health status: meta-analysis. BMJ. 2008;337:a1344. Review.
7. Shephard RJ. Exercise in the prevention and treatment of cancer. An update. Sports Med. 1993;15:258–80. Review.
8. Na HK, Oliynyk S. Effects of physical activity on cancer prevention. Ann N Y Acad Sci. 2011;1229:176–83.
9. Hursting SD, Lavigne JA, Berrigan D, et al. Calorie restriction, aging and cancer prevention: mechanism of action and applicability to humans. Annu Rev Med. 2003;54:131–52.
10. Anderson AS, Key TJ, Norat T, et al. European code against cancer 4th edition: obesity, body fatness and cancer. Cancer Epidemiol. 2015;39 Suppl 1:S34–45.
11. Cross A, Pollock JR, Bingham SA. Haem, not protein or inorganic iron, is responsible for endogenous intestinal N-nitrosation arising from red meat. Cancer Res. 2003;63:2358–60.
12. Diet, nutrition and the prevention of chronic disease. Report of a WHO study group. World Health Organ Tech Rep Ser. 1990;797:1–204.
13. Foraker RE, Abdel-Rasoul M, Kuller LH, et al. Cardiovascular health and incident cardiovascular disease and cancer: the women's health initiative. Am J Prev Med. 2016;50:236–40.
14. Norat T, Scoccianti C, Boutro-Roulat MC, et al. European code against cancer 4th edition: diet and cancer. Cancer Epidemiol. 2015;39 Suppl 1:S56–66.
15. Mozaffarian D, Hao T, Rimm EB, Willett WC, Hu FB. Changes in diet and lifestyle and long-term weight gain in women and men. N Engl J Med. 2011;364:2392–404.
16. Ludwig DS. The glycemic index: physiological mechanisms relating to obesity, diabetes, and cardiovascular disease. JAMA. 2002;287:2414–23. Review.
17. Fung TT, Malik V, Rexrode KM, et al. Sweetened beverage consumption and risk of coronary heart disease in women. Am J Clin Nutr. 2009;89:1037–42.
18. Genkinger JM, Li R, Spiegelman D, et al. Coffee, tea, and sugar-sweetened carbonated soft drink intake and pancreatic cancer risk: a pooled analysis of 14 cohort studies. Cancer Epidemiol Biomarkers Prev. 2012;21:305–18.
19. Choi Y, Giovannucci E, Lee JE. Glycaemic index and glycaemic load in relation to risk of diabetes-related cancers: a meta-analysis. Br J Nutr. 2012;108:1934–47.
20. Mensink RP, Zock PL, Kester AD, Katan MB. Effects of dietary fatty acids and carbohydrates on the ratio of serum total to HDL cholesterol and on serum lipids and apolipoproteins: a meta-analysis of 60 controlled trials. Am J Clin Nutr. 2003;77:1146–55.
21. Hooper L, Summerbell CD, Thompson R, et al. Reduced or modified dietary fat for preventing cardiovascular disease. Cochrane Database Syst Rev. 2012;5:CD002137.
22. Talayero BG, Sacks FM. The role of triglycerides in atherosclerosis. Curr Cardiol Rep. 2011;13:544–52.
23. Chapman MJ, Guérin M, Bruckert E. Atherogenic, dense low-density lipoproteins. Pathophysiology and new therapeutic approaches. Eur Heart J. 1998;19(Suppl A):A24–30. Review.
24. Morris PB, Ballantyne CM, Birtcher KK, et al. Review of clinical practice guidelines for the management of LDL-related risk. J Am Coll Cardiol. 2014;64:196–206.
25. von Eckardstein A, Nofer JR, Assmann G. High density lipoproteins and arteriosclerosis. Role of cholesterol efflux and reverse cholesterol transport. Arterioscler Thromb Vasc Biol. 2001;21:13–27. Review.
26. de Souza RJ, Mente A, Maroleanu A, et al. Intake of saturated and trans unsaturated fatty acids and risk of all cause mortality, cardiovascular disease, and type 2 diabetes: systematic review and meta-analysis of observational studies. BMJ. 2015;351:h3978.
27. Mozaffarian D, de Oliveira Otto MC, Lemaitre RN, et al. Trans-palmitoleic acid, other dairy fat biomarkers, and incident diabetes: the multi-ethnic study of atherosclerosis (MESA). Am J Clin Nutr. 2013;97:854–61.
28. Chajes V, Thiebaut AC, Rotival M, Gaythier E, Maillard V, Bouton Rauault MC, et al. Association between serum trans-monosaturated fatty acids and breast cancer risk in the E3N-EPIC study. Am J Epidemiol. 2008;167:1312–20.
29. Chavarro JE, Stampfer MJ, Campos H, et al. A prospective study of trans fatty acid level in blood and risk of prostate cancer. Cancer Epidemiol Biomarkers Prev. 2008;17:95–101.

30. Chajes V, Jenab M, Romieu I, et al. Plasma phospholipid fatty acid concentrations and risk of gastric adenocarcinomas in the European prospective investigation into cancer and nutrition (EPIC-EURGAST). Am J Clin Nutr. 2011;94(5):1304–13.
31. Vinikoor LC, Schroeder JC, Millikan RC, et al. Consumption of trans fatty acid and its association with colorectal adenomas. Am J Epidemiol. 2008;168:289–97.
32. Siri-Tarino PW, Sun Q, Hu FB, Krauss RM. Meta-analysis of prospective cohort studies evaluating the association of saturated fat with cardiovascular disease. Am J Clin Nutr. 2010;91:535–46.
33. Eckel RH, Jakicic JM, Ard JD, et al. American College of Cardiology/American Heart Association Task Force on Practice Guidelines. 2013 AHA/ACC guideline on lifestyle management to reduce cardiovascular risk: a report of the American College of Cardiology/American Heart Association Task Force on Practice Guidelines. Circulation. 2014;129(25 Suppl 2):S76–99.
34. Mozaffarian D, Ludwig DS. The 2015 US dietary guidelines. Lifting the ban on total dietary fat. JAMA. 2015;313:2421–2.
35. Qi L, van Dam RM, Liu S, et al. Whole-grain, bran, and cereal fiber intakes and markers of systemic inflammation in diabetic women. Diabetes Care. 2006;29:207–11.
36. Wannamethee SG, Whincup PH, Thomas MC, Sattar N. Associations between dietary fiber and inflammation, hepatic function, and risk of type 2 diabetes in older men: potential mechanisms for the benefits of fiber on diabetes risk. Diabetes Care. 2009;32:1823–5.
37. Slavin JL. Mechanisms for the impact of whole grain foods on cancer risk. J Am Coll Nutr. 2000;19:300S–7.
38. Okarter N, Liu RH. Health benefits of whole grain phytochemicals. Crit Rev Food Sci Nutr. 2010;50(3):193–208.
39. Monroe KR, Murphy SP, Henderson BE, et al. Dietary fiber intake and endogenous serum hormone levels in naturally postmenopausal Mexican American women: the multiethnic cohort study. Nutr Cancer. 2007;58:127–35.
40. Yang J, Martínez I, Walter J, et al. In vitro characterization of the impact of selected dietary fibers on fecal microbiota composition and short chain fatty acid production. Anaerobe. 2013;23:74–81.
41. Saura-Calixto F. Dietary fiber as a carrier of dietary antioxidants: an essential physiological function. J Agric Food Chem. 2011;59:43–9.
42. Jonnalagadda SS, Harnack L, Liu RH, et al. Putting the whole grain puzzle together: health benefits associated with whole grains—summary of American Society for nutrition 2010 satellite symposium. J Nutr. 2011;141:1011S–22.
43. Huang T, Xu M, Lee A, et al. Consumption of whole grains and cereal fiber and total and cause-specific mortality: prospective analysis of 367,442 individuals. BMC Med. 2015;13:59.
44. Svendsen M, Blomhoff R, Holme I, Tonstad S. The effect of an increased intake of vegetables and fruit on weight loss, blood pressure and antioxidant defense in subjects with sleep related breathing disorders. Eur J Clin Nutr. 2007;61:1301–11.
45. McCall DO, McGartland CP, McKinley MC, et al. Dietary intake of fruits and vegetables improves microvascular function in hypertensive subjects in a dose-dependent manner. Circulation. 2009;119:2153–60.
46. Dauchet L, Amouyel P, Hercberg S, Dallongeville J. Fruit and vegetable consumption and risk of coronary heart disease: a meta-analysis of cohort studies. J Nutr. 2006;136:2588–93.
47. Yoon JH, Baek SJ. Molecular targets of dietary polyphenols with anti-inflammatory properties. Yonsei Med J. 2005;46:585–96.
48. Paul G, Mendelson GJ. Evidence supports the use of soy protein to promote cardiometabolic health and muscle development. J Am Coll Nutr. 2015;34.sup1:56–9.
49. Kris-Etherton PM, Hu FB, Ros E, Sabate J. The role of tree nuts and peanuts in the prevention of coronary heart disease: multiple potential mechanisms. J Nutr. 2008;138:1746S–51.
50. Dashwood RH, Myzak MC, Ho E. Dietary HDAC inhibitors: time to rethink weak ligands in cancer chemoprevention? Carcinogenesis. 2006;27:344–9.
51. Chung MY, Lim TG, Lee KW. Molecular mechanisms of chemopreventive phytochemicalsa against gastroenterological cancer development. World J Gastroenterol. 2013;19:984–93.
52. Bernstein AM, Sun Q, Hu FB, et al. Major dietary protein sources and risk of coronary heart disease in women. Circulation. 2010;122:876–83.
53. Ley SH, Sun Q, Willett WC, et al. Associations between red meat intake and biomarkers of inflammation and glucose metabolism in women. Am J Clin Nutr. 2014;99:352–60.
54. Fretts AM, Follis JL, Nettleton JA, et al. Consumption of meat is associated with higher fasting glucose and insulin concentrations regardless of glucose and insulin genetic risk scores: a meta-analysis of 50,345 Caucasians. Am J Clin Nutr. 2015;102:1266–78.
55. Rohrmann S, Overvad K, Bueno-de-Mesquita HB, et al. Meat consumption and mortality—results from the European prospective investigation into cancer and nutrition. BMC Med. 2013;11:63.

56. Micha R, Wallace S, Mozaffarian D. Red and processed meat consumption and risk of incident coronary heart disease, stroke, and diabetes: a systematic review and meta-analysis. Circulation. 2010;121: 2271–83.
57. Chan DS, Lau L, Aune D, et al. Red and processed meat and colorectal cancer incidence: meta-analysis of prospective studies. PLoS One. 2011;6:e20456.
58. Rohrmann S, Linseisen J, Nöthlings U, et al. Meat and fish consumption and risk of pancreatic cancer: results from the European prospective investigation into cancer and nutrition. Int J Cancer. 2013;132: 617–24.
59. Gibis M. Effect of oil marinades with garlic, onion, and lemon juice on the formation of heterocyclic aromatic amines in fried beef patties. J Agric Food Chem. 2007;55:10240–7.
60. Dalmeijer GW, Struijk EA, van der Schouw YT, et al. Dairy intake and coronary heart disease or stroke—a population-based cohort study. Int J Cardiol. 2013;167:925–9.
61. Soedamah-Muthu SS, Ding EL, Al-Delaimy WK, et al. Milk and dairy consumption and incidence of cardiovascular diseases and all-cause mortality: dose–response meta-analysis of prospective cohort studies. Am J Clin Nutr. 2011;93:158–71.
62. Laonigro I, Correale M, Di Biase M, Altomare E. Alcohol abuse and heart failure. Eur J Heart Fail. 2009;11:453–62.
63. Thun MJ, Peto R, Lopez AD, et al. Alcohol consumption and mortality among middle-aged and elderly U.S. adults. N Engl J Med. 1997;337:1705–14.
64. Pownall HJ, Rosales C, Gillard BK, Gotto Jr AM. Alcohol: a nutrient with multiple salutary effects. Nutrients. 2015;7:1992–2000.
65. Pathak SK, Sharma RA, Mellon JK. Chemoprevention prostate cancer by diet-derived antioxidant agents and hormonal manipulation (review). Int J Oncol. 2003;22:5–13. [Epub ahead of print]
66. Raygan F, Rezavandi Z, Dadkhah Tehrani S, et al. The effects of coenzyme Q10 administration on glucose homeostasis parameters, lipid profiles, biomarkers of inflammation and oxidative stress in patients with metabolic syndrome. Eur J Nutr. 2015 [Epub ahead of print].
67. Alehagen U, Aaseth J, Johansson P. Reduced cardiovascular mortality 10 years after supplementation with selenium and coenzyme Q10 for four years: follow-up results of a prospective randomized double-blind placebo-controlled trial in elderly citizens. PLoS One. 2015;10:e0141641.
68. ▶ http://www.sarcomacancer.org/index.php?page=adjunctive-treatment. Accessed 22 Dec 2015.
69. Andersen MR, Sweet E, Zhou M, Standish LJ. Complementary and alternative medicine use by breast cancer patients at time of surgery which increases the potential for excessive bleeding. Integr Cancer Ther. 2015;14:119–24.
70. Izzo AA, Ernst E. Interactions between herbal medicines and prescribed drugs: an updated systematic review. Drugs. 2009;69:1777–98.
71. Unger M, Frank A. Simultaneous determination of the inhibitory potency of herbal extracts on the activity of six major cytochrome P450 enzymes using liquid chromatography/mass spectrometry and automated online extraction. Rapid Commun Mass Spectrom. 2004;18(19):2273–81.
72. Rock E, De Michele A. Nutritional approaches to late toxicities of adjuvant chemotherapy in breast cancer survivors. J Nutr. 2003;133:3785S–93.
73. Das DK, Sato M, Ray PS, et al. Cardioprotection of red wine: role of polyphenolic antioxidants. Drugs Exp Clin Res. 1999;25:115–20.
74. Bagchi D, Bagchi M, Stohs S, et al. Molecular mechanism of cardioprotection by a novel grape seed proanthocyanidin extract. Mutat Res. 2003;523–524:87–97.
75. Dueregger A, Heidegger I, Ofer P, et al. The use of dietary supplements to alleviate androgen deprivation therapy side effects during prostate cancer treatment. Nutrients. 2014;6:4491–519.
76. Bloedon LT, Balikai S, Chittams J, et al. Flaxseed and cardiovascular risk factors: results from a double blind, randomized, controlled clinical trial. J Am Coll Nutr. 2008;27:65–74.
77. Pan A, Yu D, Demark-Wahnefried W, Franco OH, Lin X. Meta-analysis of the effects of flaxseed interventions on blood lipids. Am J Clin Nutr. 2009;90:288–97.
78. Vafeiadou K, Weech M, Altowaijri H, et al. Replacement of saturated with unsaturated fats had no impact on vascular function but beneficial effects on lipid biomarkers, E-selectin, and blood pressure: results from the randomized, controlled Dietary Intervention and VAScular function (DIVAS) study. Am J Clin Nutr. 2015;102:40–8.
79. Mozaffarian D, Appel LJ, Van Horn L. Components of a cardioprotective diet: new insights. Circulation. 2011;123:2870–91.

80. Yokoyama Y, Barnard ND, Levin SM, Watanabe M. Vegetarian diets and glycemic control in diabetes: a systematic review and meta-analysis. Cardiovasc Diagn Ther. 2014;4:373–82.
81. Pilis W, Stec K, Zych M, Pilis A. Health benefits and risk associated with adopting a vegetarian diet. Rocz Panstw Zakl Hig. 2014;65:9–14. Review.
82. Crowe FL, Appleby PN, Travis RC, Key TJ. Risk of hospitalization or death from ischemic heart disease among British vegetarians and nonvegetarians: results from the EPIC-Oxford cohort study. Am J Clin Nutr. 2013;97:597–603.
83. Gilsing AM, Schouten LJ, Goldbohm RA, et al. Vegetarianism, low meat consumption and the risk of colorectal cancer in a population based cohort study. Sci Rep. 2015;5:13484.
84. Appleby PN, Crowe FL, Bradbury KE, et al. Mortality in vegetarians and comparable non vegetarians in the United Kingdom. Am J Clin Nutr. 2015;103:218–30.
85. Woo KS, Kwok TC, Celermajer DS. Vegan diet, subnormal vitamin B-12 status and cardiovascular health. Nutrients. 2014;6:3259–73. Review.
86. Saghatchian M, Bihan C, Chenailler C, et al. Exploring frontiers: use of complementary and alternative medicine among patients with early-stage breast cancer. Breast. 2014;23:279–85.
87. ► http://www.cancer.gov/publications/pdq/information-summaries/cam. Accessed 15 Dec 2015.
88. Deng G, Cassileth B. Integrative oncology: an overview. Am Soc Clin Oncol Educ Book. 2014;2014: 233–42.
89. Radha MH, Laxmipriya NP. Evaluation of biological properties and clinical effectiveness of Aloe vera: a systematic review. J Tradit Complement Med. 2014;5:21–6.
90. Fais S, Venturi G, Gatenby B. Microenvironmental acidosis in carcinogenesis and metastases: new strategies in prevention and therapy. Cancer Metastasis Rev. 2014;33:1095–108.
91. Kraus WE, Bittner V, Appel L, American Heart Association Physical Activity Committee of the Council on Lifestyle and Metabolic Health, Council on Clinical Cardiology, Council on Hypertension, and Council on Cardiovascular and Stroke Nursing, et al. The national physical activity plan: a call to action from the American Heart Association: a science advisory from the American Heart Association. Circulation. 2015;131:1932–40.
92. Pahkala K, Heinonen OJ, Lagström H, et al. Vascular endothelial function and leisure-time physical activity in adolescents. Circulation. 2008;118:2353–9.
93. McTiernan A. Mechanisms linking physical activity with cancer. Nat Rev Cancer. 2008;8:205–11.
94. Leitzmann M, Powers H, Anderson AS, et al. European code against cancer 4th edition: physical activity and cancer. Cancer Epidemiol. 2015;39 Suppl 1:S46–55.
95. Pouliou T, Ki M, Law C, et al. Physical activity and sedentary behaviour at different life stages and adult blood pressure in the 1958 British Birth Cohort. J Hypertens. 2012;30:275–83.
96. Ki M, Pouliou T, Li L, et al. Physical (in)activity over 20y in adulthood: associations with adult lipid levels in the 1958 British Birth Cohort. Atherosclerosis. 2011;219:361–7.
97. Quadrilatero J, Hoffman-Goetz L. Physical activity and colon cancer. A systematic review of potential mechanisms. J Sports Med Phys Fitness. 2003;43:121–38. Review.
98. Nechuta S, Lu W, Zheng Y, et al. Comorbidities and breast cancer survival: a report from the Shanghai breast cancer survival study. Breast Cancer Res Treat. 2013;139:227–35.
99. Jung HS, Myung SK, Kim BS, Seo HG. Metabolic syndrome in adult cancer survivors: a meta-analysis. Diabetes Res Clin Pract. 2012;95:275–82.
100. Bao PP, Zheng Y, Nechuta S, et al. Exercise after diagnosis and metabolic syndrome among breast cancer survivors: a report from the Shanghai breast cancer survival study. Cancer Causes Control. 2013;24: 1747–56.
101. Li J, Siegrist J. Physical activity and risk of cardiovascular disease—a meta-analysis of prospective cohort studies. Int J Environ Res Public Health. 2012;9:391–407.
102. Elosua R, Redondo A, Segura A, et al. Dose–response association of physical activity with acute myocardial infarction: do amount and intensity matter? Prev Med. 2013;57:567–72.
103. Lacey B, Golledge J, Yeap BB, Lewington S, Norman PE, Flicker L, Almeida OP, Hankey GJ. Physical activity and vascular disease in a prospective cohort study of older men: the health in men study (HIMS). BMC Geriatr. 2015;15:164.
104. Crimi E, Ignarro LJ, Cacciatore F, Napoli C. Mechanisms by which exercise training benefits patients with heart failure. Nat Rev Cardiol. 2009;6:292–300.
105. Loprinzi PD. The effects of free-living physical activity on mortality after congestive heart failure diagnosis. Int J Cardiol. 2015;203:598–9.

106. Peixoto TC, Begot I, Bolzan DW, et al. Early exercise-based rehabilitation improves health-related quality of life and functional capacity after acute myocardial infarction: a randomized controlled trial. Can J Cardiol. 2015;31:308–13.
107. Friedenreich CM, Cust AE. Physical activity and breast cancer risk: impact of timing, type and dose of activity and population subgroup effects. Br J Sports Med. 2008;42(8):636–47.
108. Bellocco R, Marrone G, Ye W, et al. A prospective cohort study of the combined effects of physical activity and anthropometric measures on the risk of post-menopausal breast cancer. Eur J Epidemiol. 2015;31:395–404.
109. Ma H, Xu X, Ursin G, et al. Reduced risk of breast cancer associated with recreational physical activity varies by HER2 status. Cancer Med. 2015;4:1122–35.
110. Wu Y, Zhang D, Kang S. Physical activity and risk of breast cancer: a meta-analysis of prospective studies. Breast Cancer Res Treat. 2013;137:869–82.
111. Wolin KY, Tuchman H. Physical activity and gastrointestinal cancer prevention. Recent Results Cancer Res. 2011;186:73–100.
112. Boyle T, Keegel T, Bull F, et al. Physical activity and risks of proximal and distal colon cancers: a systematic review and meta-analysis. J Natl Cancer Inst. 2012;104:1548–61.
113. Robsahm TE, Aagnes B, Hjartåker A, et al. Body mass index, physical activity, and colorectal cancer by anatomical subsites: a systematic review and meta-analysis of cohort studies. Eur J Cancer Prev. 2013;22:492–505.
114. Keum N, Ju W, Lee DH, et al. Leisure-time physical activity and endometrial cancer risk: dose–response meta-analysis of epidemiological studies. Int J Cancer. 2014;135:682–94.
115. Singh S, Edakkanambeth Varayil J, et al. Physical activity is associated with reduced risk of gastric cancer: a systematic review and meta-analysis. Cancer Prev Res (Phila). 2014;7:12–22.
116. Behrens G, Jochem C, Keimling M, et al. The association between physical activity and gastroesophageal cancer: systematic review and meta-analysis. Eur J Epidemiol. 2014;29:151–70.
117. Abioye AI, Odesanya MO, Abioye AI, Ibrahim NA. Physical activity and risk of gastric cancer: a meta-analysis of observational studies. Br J Sports Med. 2015;49:224–9.
118. Behrens G, Leitzmann MF. The association between physical activity and renal cancer: systematic review and meta-analysis. Br J Cancer. 2013;108:798–811.
119. Leitzmann MF, Koebnick C, Abnet CC, et al. Prospective study of physical activity and lung cancer by histologic type in current, former, and never smokers. Am J Epidemiol. 2009;169:542–53.
120. Behrens G, Jochem C, Schmid D, et al. Physical activity and risk of pancreatic cancer: a systematic review and meta-analysis. Eur J Epidemiol. 2015;30:279–98.
121. Keimling M, Behrens G, Schmid D, et al. The association between physical activity and bladder cancer: systematic review and meta-analysis. Br J Cancer. 2014;110:1862–70.
122. Hrafnkelsdottir SM, Torfadottir JE, Aspelund T, et al. Physical activity from early adulthood and risk of prostate cancer: a 24 year follow-up study among Icelandic men. Cancer Prev Res (Phila). 2015;8:905–11.
123. Schmid D, Leitzmann MF. Television viewing and time spent sedentary in relation to cancer risk: a meta-analysis. J Natl Cancer Inst. 2014;106(7) pii: dju098.
124. Bränström R, Petersson LM, Saboonchi F, et al. Physical activity following a breast cancer diagnosis: implications for self-rated health and cancer-related symptoms. Eur J Oncol Nurs. 2015;19:680–5.
125. Ibrahim EM, Al.Homaid AA. Physical activity and survival after breast cancer diagnosis: meta-analysis of published studies. Med Oncol (Northwood, London, England). 2011;28:753–65.
126. Lahart IM, Metsios GS, Nevill AM, Carmichael AR. Physical activity, risk of death and recurrence in breast cancer survivors: a systematic review and meta-analysis of epidemiological studies. Acta Oncol. 2015;54:635–54.
127. Sabiston CM, Brunet J, Vallance JK, Meterissian S. Prospective examination of objectively-assessed physical activity and sedentary time after breast cancer treatment: sitting on the crest of the teachable moment. Cancer Epidemiol Biomarkers Prev. 2014;23:1324–30.
128. Phillips SM, Dodd KW, Steeves J. Physical activity and sedentary behavior in breast cancer survivors: new insight into activity patterns and potential intervention targets. Gynecol Oncol. 2015;138:398–404.
129. Gandaglia G, Sun M, Popa I, et al. The impact of androgen-deprivation therapy (ADT) on the risk of cardiovascular (CV) events in patients with non-metastatic prostate cancer: a population-based study. BJU Int. 2014;114(6b):E82–9.

130. Jespersen CG, Nørgaard M, Borre M. Androgen-deprivation therapy in treatment of prostate cancer and risk of myocardial infarction and stroke: a nationwide Danish population-based cohort study. Eur Urol. 2014;65:704–9.
131. Fung C, Fossa SD, Milano MT, et al. Cardiovascular disease mortality after chemotherapy or surgery for testicular nonseminoma: a population-based study. J Clin Oncol. 2015;33:3105–15.
132. Christensen JF, Bandak M, Campbell A, et al. Treatment-related cardiovascular late effects and exercise training countermeasures in testicular germ cell cancer survivorship. Acta Oncol. 2015;54:592–9.
133. Redig AJ, Munshi HG. Metabolic syndrome after hormone-modifying therapy: risks associated with antineoplastic therapy. Oncology (Williston Park). 2010;9:839–44. Review.
134. Patterson RE, Flatt SW, Saquib N, et al. Medical comorbidities predict mortality in women with a history of early stage breast cancer. Breast Cancer Res Treat. 2010;122:859–65.
135. Beard CJ, Travis LB, Chen MH, et al. Outcomes in stage I testicular seminoma: a population-based study of 9193 patients. Cancer. 2013;119(15):2771–7.
136. Fairey AS, Courneya KS, Field CJ, et al. Effect of exercise training on C-reactive protein in postmenopausal breast cancer survivors: a randomized controlled trial. Brain Behav Immun. 2005;19:381–8.
137. Courneya KS, Mackey JR, Bell GJ, et al. Randomized controlled trial of exercise training in postmenopausal breast cancer survivors: cardiopulmonary and quality of life outcomes. J Clin Oncol. 2003;21:1660–8.
138. Sturgeon KM, Ky B, Libonati JR, Schmitz KH. The effects of exercise on cardiovascular outcomes before, during, and after treatment for breast cancer. Breast Cancer Res Treat. 2014;143:219–26.
139. Giallauria F, Maresca L, Vitelli A, et al. Exercise training improves heart rate recovery in women with breast cancer. Springerplus. 2015;4:388.
140. Mishra SI, Scherer RW, Snyder C, et al. Exercise interventions on health-related quality of life for people with cancer during active treatment. Cochrane Database Syst Rev. 2012;15:8.
141. Mishra SI, Scherer RW, Geigle PM, et al. Exercise interventions on health-related quality of life for cancer survivors. Cochrane Database Syst Rev. 2012;8:CD007566.
142. de Paleville DT, Topp RV, Swank AM. Effects of aerobic training prior to and during chemotherapy in a breast cancer patient: a case study. J Strength Cond Res. 2007;21:635–7.

Cardiac Problems as a Consequence of Cancer

Contents

Thromboembolic Disorders as a Consequence of Cancer

Irma Bisceglia and Nicola Maurea

C. Lestuzzi et al. (eds.), *Manual of Cardio-oncology*, DOI 10.1007/978-3-319-40236-9_4

4.1 Introduction

Cancer cells and coagulation system are strictly connected. General prothrombotic mechanisms are related both to the host response to cancer and to the procoagulant activity of cancer cells (◘ Fig. 4.1). Host-related factors include the acute-phase reaction, paraprotein production, inflammation, necrosis, and hemodynamic disorders. Malignant cells can activate blood coagulation in several ways. They can produce: procoagulant factors as tissue factor (TF) and cancer procoagulant factor (CP), which are the most powerful procoagulant observed; microparticles (MP); inflammatory cytokines such as tumor necrosis factor (TNF) and interleukin-1 (IL-1); pro-angiogenic factors as vascular endothelial growth factor (VEGF), which promote both endothelial prothrombotic alterations and angiogenesis. VEGF is an indirect procoagulant that increases microvascular permeability, reprograms gene expression, and promotes the survival of endothelial cells; the resulting increased vascular density plays a key role in the pathophysiology of many cancers. *The same procoagulant factors contribute to tumor progression.* Also platelets, endothelial cells, and neutrophils of host cells are stimulated to express procoagulant activity. *Thus, thromboembolism frequently complicates the course of malignancy and can be the first symptom of cancer* [1, 2].

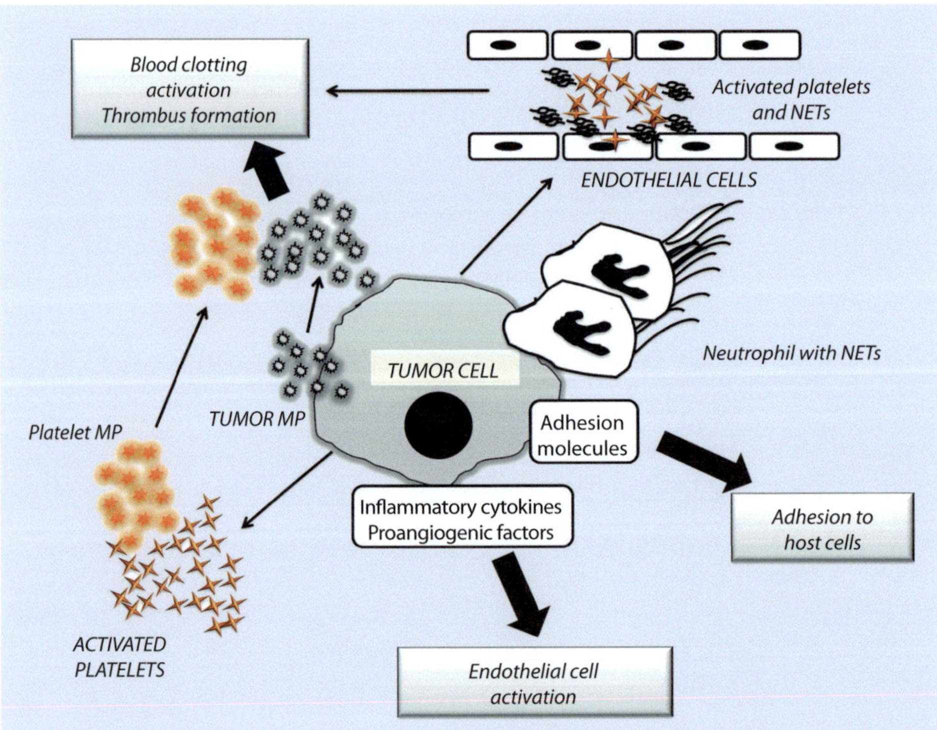

◘ **Fig. 4.1** Cancer-hemostatic system interactions. Tumor cells can activate the hemostatic system in multiple ways. Tumor cells release procoagulant activities, and microparticles (MP), by which the coagulation cascade is activated. Tumor cells also activate the host hemostatic cells (endothelial cells, leukocytes, and platelets), by either release of soluble factors or direct adhesion contact, thus eliciting the expression of a procoagulant phenotype of these cells. In addition, the neutrophils can release neutrophil extracellular trap (NETs), and the adhesion of a large quantity of NETs to the vasculature may initiate thrombosis by providing a scaffold for platelet adhesion, activation, and thrombin generation. Reproduced with permission from [1]

4.2 Clinical Aspects

- The more common events are venous thromboembolism (VTE), including deep venous thrombosis (DVT) and pulmonary embolism (PE). VTE is the second-leading cause of death in patients with malignancy [3].
- The arterial thrombotic events (ATE) in cancer are common after treatment with anti-angiogenic drugs, cisplatin, and hormonal therapies [4, 5].
- The cardiovascular risk factors associated with the hypercoagulability of cancer contribute to the precipitating of thrombotic events. VTE incidence is significantly different ($P < 0.0001$) for the different types of cancer, with the higher rate observed in patients with pancreatic cancer (19.2 %) and the lowest in patients with bladder cancer (8.2 %) [6]. Although DVT is more common in patients with pancreatic cancer (12.6 %), the PE is more common in lung (3.6 %) and gastric cancers (3.3 %).
- VTE is also associated with recurrent VTE as well as bleeding, both at significantly higher rates than seen in non-cancer patients [7].
- Systemic chemotherapy increases the risk of VTE sixfold–sevenfold, and the rise in cancer-associated VTE over recent decades may have been caused in part by the introduction of therapies with direct effects on the vascular endothelium [6].
- Clinically apparent VTE occurs in as many as 10 % of patients with cancer, but autoptic studies have described higher rates of thrombosis in some subgroups: for example the patients who died of pancreatic cancer, [1, 7–9].
- VTE is associated with a threefold increase in hospitalizations and an increased health-care resource utilization and costs. It is vital to adopt appropriate strategies for prevention and treatment of venous thromboembolism in order to reduce its impact in patients with cancer and health care system. [10].

4.3 Screening for Occult Cancer in Patients with Idiopathic VTE

An "idiopathic" VTE may be the first clinical sign of a tumor; up to 10 % of patients with unprovoked VTE receive a cancer diagnosis within the first year subsequent to the event, and more than 60 % of occult cancers are diagnosed shortly after the diagnosis of idiopathic VTE [2, 11]. The utility of using an extensive screening for the purpose of early identification of an occult neoplasm is controversial. In the absence of specific guidelines, clinical practice is very variable and differs depending on the prevailing beliefs of the individual centers. A recently published study compared a limited occult cancer screening (basic blood testing, chest radiography, age screening for breast, cervical, and prostate cancer) to limited occult-cancer screening in combination with computed tomography (CT) of the abdomen and pelvis. There was no significant difference between the two study groups in the mean time to a cancer diagnosis (4.2 months in the limited-screening group and 4.0 months in the limited-screening-plus-CT group, $P = 0.88$) or in cancer-related mortality (1.4 and 0.9 %, $P = 0.75$) at 1-year follow-up [12].

For patients with a first episode of unprovoked VTE, a limited testing for cancer, including a history and physical examination, complete blood count, serum chemistries, liver function tests and urinalysis, routine age-appropriate cancer screening, and chest radiography, is actually suggested [13].

4.4 Primary Thromboprophylaxis and Identification of High-Risk Outpatients

4.4.1 Surgical Prophylaxis

- *After abdominal or pelvic surgery for cancer*, thromboprophylaxis with either unfractionated heparin (UFH) or low molecular weight heparin (LMWH) reduces the risk of deep vein thrombosis by about 15 %.
- *UFH versus LMWH.*
    - In the ENOXACAN study (designed to compare the efficacy and safety of LMWH enoxaparin 40 mg/day versus UFH at low doses, in the prophylaxis in cancer abdominal or pelvic surgery), the incidence of DVT was 18.2 % in patients with UFH and 14.7 % in the group with enoxaparin [14].
    - a meta-analysis that included 16 clinical trials with 12,890 patients with cancer found no major differences between the perioperative thromboprophylaxis with LMWH compared with UFH in their effects on mortality, VTE, and bleeding in patients with cancer.
    - *The advantage of single daily dosing, the most favorable pharmacological profile, and the lower association with heparin-induced thrombocytopenia make the most used LMWH compared with UFH* [15, 16].
- *The benefit of a longer duration of postoperative anticoagulation than typically used for individuals without cancer* was shown in three separate trials that randomized patients undergoing major cancer surgery to 1 week versus 4 weeks of a LMWH.
    - These trials all showed a significant reduction in the incidence of VTE after 4 weeks of anticoagulation compared with 1 week (5 versus 12 %, 7 versus 16 %, and 13 versus 10 %) [17–19].
    - None of the trials showed increased bleeding in the prolonged anticoagulation group. Although it remains to be confirmed that extended thromboprophylaxis improves survival or is cost-effective after surgery for cancer, *extended prophylaxis up to 4 weeks after surgery for cancer is recommended by consensus guidelines.*
- *As regards the laparoscopic surgery, a significant difference in the incidence of postoperative VTE was not observed when compared to traditional open surgery* [20].

4.4.2 High-Risk Cancer Outpatients Identification for Primary Thromboprophylaxis

A recent systematic review estimates the overall risk of VTE to be 13 per 1000 person-years (95% CI, 7-23). The risk of VTE was 68 per 1000 person-years (95% CI, 48 to 96) in patients considered at high risk for metastatic disease or high-risk treatments. The highest risk is in patients with brain cancer (200 per 1000 personyears; 95% CI, 162-247).

Table 4.1 Risk factors for thromboembolism

General Older age Female gender African or Afroamerican ancestry Previous VTE Hypertension Infections Limited mobility	*Treatment related* Hospitalization Surgery Antiangiogenic agents Hormonal therapy Erythropoiesis-stimulating agents Blood transfusions Central venous lines
Cancer related Site (brain, pancreas, kidney, stomach, lung, bladder, gynecologic, hematologic malignancies) Advanced stage Short time after initial diagnosis	*Biomarkers* Platelet count (≥350,000/μL) Leukocyte count (≥11,000/μL) D-dimer TF P selectin TFMP Hyperlipidemia

Modified from Falanga and from ASCO guidelines [1, 22]

An appropriate risk stratification of patients is therefore crucial to highlight which patients should receive prophylaxis [21].

Clinical risk factors, biomarkers, or combinations of the two can be used to estimate VTE risk.

- *Clinical risk factors* include tumor type, location, stage, and time since diagnosis influence VTE risk, along with patient comorbidities and therapeutic interventions (Table 4.1).
  - Factors related to treatment are: surgery, chemotherapy, hormonal therapy, anti-angiogenic agents (thalidomide, lenalidomide, bevacizumab), central venous catheters, erythropoiesis-stimulating agents (ESAs), blood transfusions.
  - VTE risk *after surgery* is 2 times higher in patients with known cancer than in the general population; 1/3 of events occur after discharge, and mortality is more than six times higher in patients with VTE compared to those without VTE (8 versus 1.2 %) [23].
- *Individuals with cancer should be considered high risk for development of postoperative VTE. This increased risk is reflected in the Caprini score for VTE in surgical patients, which assigns two points for the presence of malignancy.*
  - *Chemotherapy* with cisplatin and fluorouracil may induce thrombogenic effects through multiple mechanisms that include the secretion by the tumor cells of pro-angiogenic and immunomodulatory cytokines, increase of TF on endothelial cells, direct toxicity on the endothelium, and reduced synthesis of C protein.
  - *Erythropoiesis-stimulating agents (ESA)* reduce the need for transfusions and improve quality of life but cause an increased incidence of VTE and mortality [23].

Table 4.2 Predictive model for VTE. Points for the risk model are based on the regression coefficients obtained from the final model and divided the population into 3 risk categories based on the score from the risk model: low (score 0), intermediate (score 1-2), and high (score 3; not present)

Patients Characteristic	Score
Site of cancer	
Stomach, pancreas (very high risk)	2
Lung, lymphoma, gynecologic, bladder, testicular	1
Prechemotherapy platelet count 350,000/mm³	1
Hemoglobin level <10 g/dL or use of red cell growth factors	1
Pre chemotherapy leukocyte count >11,000/mm³	1
Body mass index (BMI) ≥35 Kg/m²	1
High-risk score ≥3; intermediate 1–2; low 0	

Modified from Khorana et al. [34]

  - The advent of *novel "targeted" anticancer therapies* has not reduced the risk of VTE. Indeed, drugs targeting angiogenesis such as bevacizumab, sunitinib, sorafenib, and the multi-targeted tyrosine kinase inhibitor ponatinib have been associated with arterial thromboembolism.
  - *Immunomodulatory agents* such as thalidomide and lenalidomide have been associated with very high rates of VTE, and anti-epidermal growth factor antibodies such as cetuximab and panitumumab have also recently been associated with VTE [24–26].
- *A particularly high risk has been reported in patients receiving chemotherapy in combination with antiangiogenic agents. The highest incidence of VTE in myeloma occurs during treatment with thalidomide associated with anthracyclines (12–28 %), thalidomide with dexamethasone at high doses (17–26 %), lenalidomide, and high dose of dexamethasone (18–26 %)* [27–30].
  - *A variety of biomarkers* have also been associated with VTE in malignancy. These include platelet count ≥350,000 before chemotherapy, white blood cell count >11,000 before chemotherapy, hemoglobin value <10 g/dL, elevated tissue factor expression on the surface of cancer cells, high activity of circulating tissue factor, elevated D-dimer, elevated soluble P-selectin, thrombin generation, and levels of TF bearing microparticles (TFMP) [31–33].
  - *A validated model to guide clinical decisions on thromboprophylaxis in patients treated with chemotherapy has been developed by Khorana. The Khorana score is calculated by assigning points for clinical parameters available for patients (i.e., site of primary tumor, hmatologic parameters, and body mass index)* [34] (Table 4.2).
  - This risk score was originally derived from a development cohort of 2701 patients and then validated in an independent cohort of 1365 patients, stratified into three

risk groups to predict the development of VTE. The cumulative incidence of VTE at 2.5 months ranged from 0.3 to 6.7 % in patients with the fewest and most risk factors, respectively.

Subsequently, the score was externally validated prospectively, and modified version of the score was used in an observational cohort study: the *Vienna Cancer and Thrombosis Study (CATS)*. The modified score included:

- Additional high-risk tumor types (brain, myeloma, kidney).
- Two additional laboratory values: soluble P-selectin and D-dimer levels.
- In a retrospective analysis, the cumulative incidence rates of VTE at 6 months were 1 % for the lowest risk group (0 points) and 35 % for the highest risk group (≥5 points) [35].

Recently, the same working group has explored the utility of soluble plasma VEGF-A (sVEGF) as a biomarker for the prediction of VTE in patients with cancer, and elevated sVEGF is proved to be associated with an increased risk of VTE in patients with cancer [36].

In the *PROTECHT score*, the inclusion of chemotherapy with platinum (carboplatin, cisplatin) or gemcitabine over the five variables identified high-risk cancer patients in a post hoc analysis of the PROTECHT study. Patients with higher absolute risk of VTE would derive the most benefit as demonstrated by the analysis of subgroups of two largest randomized trials.. Rates of VTE in high-risk patients enrolled in PROTECHT were 11.1 % in the placebo arm and 4.5 % in the nadroparin arm (NNT = 15 versus 77 for low and intermediate-risk patients) [37].

In the subgroup analysis of SAVE-ONCO, rates of VTE in patients with Khorana risk score ≥3 were 5.4 % in the placebo arm and 1.5 % in the semuloparin arm (NNT = 25 for high-risk patients to 333 for low-risk patients) [38].

Anticoagulant prophylaxis has been shown to reduce the risk of VTE in medical patients, but none of the trials reported the rates of symptomatic venous thromboembolic events or major bleeding episodes according to cancer status; recommendations are therefore made based upon extrapolation of data from randomized trials that included only a small minority of cancer patients [39].

4.4.3 Multiple Myeloma

VTE incidence is about 5 % in myeloma patients treated with conventional chemotherapy. The anti-angiogenic agents for the treatment of multiple myeloma, such as thalidomide and lenalidomide, are known to activate endothelial cells and platelets, and to damage the vascular endothelium, increasing the thrombotic risk. VTE incidence is particularly high when thalidomide or lenalidomide is combined with high-dose dexamethasone (480 mg/month), with doxorubicin or with polichemotherapy. For patients with multiple myeloma, a risk assessment model has been proposed from the Myeloma Working Group. It takes into account individual risk factors, factors linked to the disease and therapy [27].

4

Special Recommendations

- Aspirin is recommended for patients with 0–1 risk factors.
- Enoxaparin 40 mg per day or full-dose warfarin (target INR 2–3) are indicated both for patients with two or more individual risk factors related to myeloma, both for patients treated with thalidomide/lenalidomide associated with high-dose dexamethasone and/or doxorubicin.
- A randomized study compared the effectiveness of low dose aspirin, 1.5 mg/day dose warfarin, and enoxaparin 40 mg in patients with newly diagnosed myeloma treated with thalidomide-based regimens, cortisone and melphalan or bortezomib. Similar efficacy of therapeutic regimens in reducing VTE in elderly patients was observed; however, enoxaparin showed greater efficacy compared to warfarin in reducing major thromboembolic events, acute cardiovascular events, and sudden deaths [40].
- Another study compared low-dose aspirin with enoxaparin 40 mg in patients treated with lenalidomide.
  - The incidence of VTE was 2.27 % in the aspirin group and 1.2 % in the LMWH group, suggesting that aspirin is an effective therapeutic alternative for patients at "standard" risk [41].
- It was also noted that the treatment with bortezomib reduces the 2 % risk of VTE for an antithrombotic effect due to the synthesis of nitric oxide which would result in a reduced platelet activation [42].
- All patients with malignancies undergoing major surgery should be considered for both pharmacological thromboprophylaxis with UFH or with LMWH, unless contraindicated due to active bleeding or high risk of bleeding.
- Once daily LMWH, UFH three times a day or fondaparinux is recommended to prevent postoperative VTE in patients with cancer.
- Pharmacological prophylaxis should be started 12–2 h before surgery and continued for at least 7–10 days. Use of fondaparinux must be made 6 h after surgery.
- The extended prophylaxis for 4 weeks in patients with a high risk of VTE (pelvic and abdominal surgery) and low bleeding risk for patients undergoing abdominal or pelvic surgery for cancer with high-risk features such as reduced mobility, obesity, history of VTE, or other risk factors is recommended.
- The use of LMWH for the prevention of VTE in cancer patients undergoing laparoscopic surgery is recommended as for laparotomy.
- Mechanical methods are used in association with drug therapy in high-risk patients but are not recommended as monotherapy except when pharmacological prophylaxis is contraindicated for active bleeding or high risk of bleeding.

4.5 Appropriate Immediate and Long-Term Treatment for Patients with Acute Thromboembolism and the Role of NOACs

The goal of therapy is to resolve the acute episode and to prevent recurrence, extension, and embolism while minimizing the risk of bleeding. However, treatment of VTE in cancer is complicated due to higher rates of recurrent VTE as well as a higher risk of bleeding with anticoagulation treatment.

4.5.1 Acute Treatment (First 10 Days)

- The therapeutic options for TVE in the acute phase include UFH, LMWH, and Fondaparinux.
  - Few studies have directly compared the anticoagulant therapy for the initial treatment of VTE in cancer patients. In a meta-analysis of 16 randomized controlled trials in cancer patients treated with anticoagulants for VTE, LMWH compared to UHF was associated with a reduction in mortality at 3 months (RR 0.71; 95 % CI 0.52, 0.98) without an increased risk of bleeding [43].
  - LMWH offers other advantages over UFH: cost, ease of dosing and a lower risk of heparin-induced heparin (HIT).

There are no studies in the literature of direct comparison between fondaparinux and LMWH for the initial treatment of VTE.

  - UFH can be used in patients with severe renal impairment (CrCl < 30 mL/min) because the liver is a main site of heparin biotransformation. Other advantages of UFH are the short half-life and the reversibility of effect with protamine sulfate.
  - The initial dose of UFH for VTE treatment is based on weight, with the recommended dose of 80 units/kg bolus followed by 18 units/kg/h infusion.
  - UFH is contraindicated in patients with HIT, and in this situation fondaparinux or a thrombin inhibitor represents a better alternative.
  - Fondaparinux is not the first choice in patients with cancer because of the long half-life, the absence of an effective antidote, and the renal clearance of 100 %.
  - Analysis of Matisse-DVT trial subgroup showed higher rates of recurrent VTE in the fondaparinux group than in the enoxaparin group: 12.7 % compared with 5.4 % with no differences in mortality and bleeding [44].

Currently, the use of LMWH for the initial treatment of VTE patients with cancer is recommended as treatment of choice.

4.5.2 Long-Term (First 3 Months) and Extended Therapy (No Planned Stop Date)

- The minimum duration of anticoagulant therapy for VTE is usually 3 months; this period of treatment is referred to as "long-term therapy." For long-term therapy, the possible options are vitamin K antagonists (VKA), LMWHH, Fondaparinux, and new oral anticoagulants (NOACs) ad dabigatran, rivaroxaban, apixaban.
- A meta-analysis of seven randomized clinical trials involving cancer patients with VTE showed a significant reduction of recurrent VTE in patients treated with LMWH compared with those treated with VKA [45].
- LMWH are preferred to VKA therapy in patients with cancer for several reasons: there is a substantial rate of recurrent VTE in patients with VTE and cancer who are treated with VKA; benefits of LMWH compared to VKA therapy are greater in patients with metastatic disease treated with aggressive chemotherapy [46]; it is often harder to keep patients with cancer who are on VKA in the therapeutic range; LMWH is reliable in patients who have difficulty with oral therapy; and LMWH is easier to withhold or adjust than VKA if invasive interventions are required or thrombocytopenia develops.

- *In the CLOT trial*, the efficacy and safety of immediate dalteparin (200 units/kg daily for 5–7 days) followed by chronic (6 months) therapy with an oral coumarin derivative are compared versus chronic dalteparin therapy (200 units/kg daily for 1 month followed by 150 units/kg for months 2–6) in patients with cancer (most of patients had metastatic disease) after diagnosis of acute proximal DVT, PE, or both. Full dose dalteparin was given for 1 month followed by a reduced dose (75–80 %) for 2–6 months.
- Prolonged treatment with LMWH for 6 months reduced thromboembolic recurrence from 17 to 9 % ($P = 0.0017$), compared to standard therapy without increasing the risk of bleeding [46].
- The CATCH study evaluated the efficacy and safety of *tinzaparin* in patients with active cancer and symptomatic VTE. The patients were randomized to receive tinzaparin 175 IU/kg once a day for 6 months or initial tinzaparin 175 IU/kg once a day for 5–10 days followed by warfarin for 6 months.
- Tinzaparin significantly reduced the risk of recurrent symptomatic DVT, nonfatal and clinically relevant bleeding [47].
- *Fondaparinux* seems to have a similar safety and efficacy profile as LMWH [48].
- Studies focused on the use of *NOAC* in cancer patients are still lacking. Preliminary results of the subgroup analyses and meta-analysis of randomized clinical trials suggest that they have efficacy and safety comparable to anticoagulation with VKA and could represent an alternative for oral anticoagulant therapy.
- A meta-analysis of six RCTs assessed the efficacy and safety of NOACs in patients with cancer-associated VTE. NOACs were shown to be as effective (OR 0.63, 95 % CI 0.37–1.10) and as safe (OR 0.77, 95 % CI 0.41–1.44) as warfarin [49]. The risk reduction for recurrent VTE with the NOACs compared to LMWH has not been assessed but, based on indirect comparisons, LMWH may be more effective that the NOACs in patients with VTE and cancer.
- However, the small number of patients with cancer (5–8 %) enrolled in each study and the use of warfarin or placebo rather than LMWH in the control do not support yet their use for this population [22, 49–61].
- Furthermore, there are interactions with some chemotherapeutic agents [49].
- NOACs have not been compared with VKA in a broad spectrum of patients with VTE and cancer, and indirect comparisons have not shown convincingly different outcomes with different NOACs (◘ Table 4.3).
- A preference for one NOAC over another or for either a NOAC or VKA in patients with cancer cannot presently be expressed.

See ◘ Tables 4.3 and 4.4 for further details on indications and dose of anticoagulant as prophylaxis and therapy, according to different guidelines.

4.5.3 Treatment of Catheter-Related DVT

Permanent central venous catheters (CVC) are usually regularly washed with heparin to maintain their patency. However, symptomatic catheter-related venous thrombosis may occur in 4–8 % of patients. Clinical symptoms include edema, pain, and erythema

Table 4.3 Key points of most recent guidelines

ACCP 2016	ASCO 2015	NCNN 2015	BSH 2015
Thromboprophylaxis			
	Most hospitalized patients with active cancer require thromboprophylaxis throughout hospitalization. Routine thromboprophylaxis may be considered for selected high-risk patients. Patients with multiple myeloma receiving antiangiogenesis agents with chemotherapy and/or dexamethasone should receive prophylaxis with either low-molecular weight heparin (LMWH) or low-dose aspirin to prevent VTE. Extending postoperative prophylaxis up to 4 weeks should be considered in those undergoing major abdominal or pelvic surgery with high-risk features.	Dose adjustments are required for obese patients receiving prophylaxis with dalteparin, enoxaparin, UFH, or fondaparinux. Prophylactic anticoagulation therapy should be considered for all inpatients with cancer without contraindication to such therapy. Following hospital discharge, it is recommended that cancer patients in a high-risk setting for VTE continue to receive VTE prophylaxis, with the duration of anticoagulation determined by the clinical situation. Patients with multiple myeloma who are receiving lenalidomide- or thalidomide-based combination regimens associated with a high thrombotic risk or patients with two or more individual or disease-related risk factors should receive prophylaxis strategy with either LMWH (e.g., enoxaparin 40 mg daily) or dose adjusted warfarin (INR 2–3) Patients with cancer at high risk for VTE (based on Khorana risk assessment score 3 or higher) could be considered for outpatient VTE prophylaxis on an individual basis.	Patients undergoing abdominal and pelvic surgery for cancer should be considered for extended thromboprophylaxis (2B). Thromboprophylaxis should be considered for high-risk outpatients (2B). Patients with active or recent cancer admitted to hospital should receive thromboprophylaxis unless contraindicated (2C). Patients with myeloma receiving thalidomide or lenalidomide should be risk-assessed for VTE and offered thromboprophylaxis unless there is a contraindication (1A). A platelet count of $<50 \times 10^9$/L is a relative contraindication to pharmacological prophylaxis.

(continued)

Table 4.3 (continued)

ACCP 2016	ASCO 2015	NCNN 2015	BSH 2015
Treatment			
LMWH are the preferred long-term treatment for VTE and cancer Extended anticoagulant therapy (no scheduled stop date) over 3 months of therapy (Grade 1B), is recommended in patients who do not have high bleeding risk and suggested in patients who have high bleeding risk (Grade 2B) A reassessment at periodic intervals is recommended in all patients who receive extended an ticoagulant therapy. In patients with VTE and cancer who are not treated with LMWH, a NO AC or VKA could both be considered. Moreover, there isn't any convincing evidence that NOAC is superior to another.	LMWH are recommended for the initial 5–10 days of treatment of established deep vein thrombosis and pulmonary embolism as well as for long-term secondary prophylaxis for at least 6 month Use of novel oral anticoagulants is not currently recommended for patient with malignancy and VTE	LMWHs are preferred for acute management of VTE in cancer patients because they do not require hospitalization or monitoring and are the preferred option for long-term therapy The use of LMWHs as chronic anticoagulation therapy is supported in patients with metastatic disease who are diagnosed with acute VTE Use of novel oral anticoagulants for acute and extended chronic treatment of VTE in patients with cancer remains to be investigated in future prospective trials	Initial treatment should be with LMWH for 6 months, if tolerated (1A). In the presence of active malignancy, anticoagulation should be continued (2B). When the platelet count is <50 × 109/L, platelet support should be given to elevate the count to >50 × 109/L to allow full dose anticoagulation, especially in the immediate period following thrombosis development (2D). Patients with platelet counts between 25 and 50 × 109/L should have frequent assessment to allow decisions on LMWH to be made (2D). If the platelet count remains <25 × 109/L, full anticoagulation should be avoided (1D). Warfarin and other oral anticoagulants are acceptable alternatives if LMWH is impractical and anticoagulation is indicated (1A).

of the affected limb; most of the CVC are inserted in the superior vena cava: thus, there may be swelling of the neck, supraclavicular area, or face. The thrombosis can develop acutely or over a more prolonged period of time. In case of thrombosis, the choice is influenced by the need of maintaining the device for further antineoplastic treatments of the patient [61, 62].

- The removal is recommended if the device is no longer required or when patency cannot be restored by thrombolysis and/or anticoagulation; there are contraindications to anticoagulation (active bleeding, platelet count <50,000/μL, or recent central nervous system bleeding or surgery), if the catheter is infected or dysfunctional.

Table 4.4 Recommended dosing regimens for cancer associated VTE

	Standard dosing	Obese patients (≥40 Kg/m²)
Prophylaxis		
Outpatients		
UFH	5000 UI SC[b] once every 8–12 h	7500 UI every 8 h
Dalteparin Nadroparin Enoxaparin Fondaparinux Tinzaparin	5000 UI SC OD[c] 3800 UI SC OD 4000 UI SC OD 2.5 mg SC OD 4500UI SC OD or 75 units/kg OD	7500 UI SC OD 4000 UI SC OD 5 mg SC every 12 h
Aspirin	81–325 mg (low risk myeloma)	
Inpatients		
Medical patients		
UFH Dalteparin Enoxaparin Fondaparinux	5000 UI SC every 8–12 h 5000 UI SC OD 4000 UI SC OD 2.5 mg SC OD	
Surgical patients		
UFH Dalteparin Enoxaparin Fondaparinux	5000 UI 2–4 h preoperatively and 5000 UIOD postoperatively 2500 UI 2–4 h preoperatively and 5000 UI OD postoperatively 4000 UI 10–12 h preoperatively and 4000 UI OD postoperatively 2.5 mg OD beginning 6–8 h postoperatively	
Warfarin	INR target 2–3	
Treatment		
Initial		
UFH[a] Dalteparin Tinzaparin Enoxaparin Fondaparinux	80 UI/kg IV bolus, then 18 U/kg/h IV; adjust dose based on a PTT 100 UI/kg once every 12 h; 200 U/kg OD 1 mg/kg once every 12 h; 1.5 mg/kg OD 1 mg/kg once every 12 h; 1.5 mg/kg OD <50 kg, 5.0 mg OD; 50–100 kg, 7.5 mg OD;100 kg 10 mg OD	
Long term		
Dalteparin Enoxaparin Tinzaparin	200 UI/kg OD for 1 month, then 150 U/kg OD 1.5 mg/kg OD;1 mg/kg once every 12 h 175 UI/Kg OD	
Warfarin	INR target 2–3	

According to ASCO and NCNN guidelines [22, 58, 59]
[a]Unfractioned Heparin
[b]Subcutaneously
[c]Once a day

   - Before removing the device, a short time (5–7 days) of anticoagulant therapy is recommended to reduce the risk of embolization. Therefore evaluation of the likelihood and consequences of embolization according to the size and location of the thrombus should be carried out.
   - Patients with cancer who have had their CVCs removed and then replaced without anticoagulation often experience recurrent thrombosis.
- Anticoagulant therapy with LMWH is recommended if the catheter must remain in situ for a period of at least 3 months up to 6 months [62].
- Thrombolytic therapy is justified in cases of thrombosis of the superior vena cava with caval syndrome poorly tolerated or complete occlusion of the CVC. Instillation of 2 mg of t-PA or Urokinase 10,000 IU infused in each catheter lumen for 4 h once a week may restore catheter patency.
- In case of symptomatic CVC thrombosis, anticoagulant treatment is recommended for a minimum of 3 months.
- In this setting, LMWHs are suggested. Oral VKA can also be used, in the absence of direct comparisons of these two types of anticoagulants in this setting.
- The CVC can be kept in place if it is functional, well-positioned, and noninfected with good resolution of symptoms under close surveillance.

4.5.4 Vena Cava Filters

- The implantation of inferior vena cava (IVC) filters should be restricted to patients with VTE and/or PE and contraindications to anticoagulation [63].
   - Active bleeding.
   - High risk of bleeding.
   - Undergoing surgery at high risk of bleeding (as major abdominal surgery).
- Their use in patients with recurrent thrombotic events despite anticoagulant therapy does not appear logical because the filters do not treat the condition of thrombosis, and the presence of an intravascular foreign body is likely to promote the formation of a thrombus proximal or distal to the thrombus filter.
   - IVC thrombotic occlusion is the presence of an occluding thrombus in the IVC after filter insertion can be symptomatic or asymptomatic and remains a serious complication of IVC filtration. The reported incidence ranges from 2 to 30 %.
   - Renal failure secondary to renal vein thrombosis has been reported after suprarenal filter placement. Suprarenal filters should be avoided in patients with a single functional kidney, renal insufficiency, or previous renal vein thrombosis.
- The possible complications of inferior vena cava filters are [64]:
   - Penetration of the vein wall by a filter strut or anchor device with transmural incorporation, with secondary lesion to the neighbouring structures.
   - Filter embolization, defined as post-deployment movement of the filter or its components to a distant anatomic site (heart and pulmonary tree).
   - Filter fracture (i.e., breakage or separation); the reported incidence of filter fracture is as high as 2–10 %.
- *Retrievable devices should be used, and possibly be removed, re-starting the anticoagulant therapy, as soon as possible* [63, 64].

Special Recommendations

- Brain tumor in itself is not a contraindication to anticoagulation therapy in VTE. For the treatment of VTE in patients with brain tumor, it is preferable to use LMWH for 6 months in all patients except those with tumors that have a high rate of intracranial hemorrhage (metastases from melanoma, choriocarcinoma, thyroid carcinoma, and renal cell carcinoma).
- There is no evidence to recommend LMWH or UFH over another in elderly patients with active malignancy. Tinzaparin might have a favorable biologic profile using therapeutic dosing in the setting of renal insufficiency.
- In patients with renal insufficiency and Ccr < 30 mL/min, enoxaparin might have a less favorable biologic and the dosage should be reduced a 1 mg/kg sc every 24 h or factor Xa will be monitored UFH, tinzaparin and dalteparin are preferred as agents.
- In cancer patients who are pregnant, standard prophylaxis should be implemented.
- Heparin-induced thrombocytopenia (HIT), due to the formation of antibodies against a complex platelet factor 4 (PF4)/heparin, is a consumptive thrombocytopenia associated with a serious pro-thrombotic state. The treatment of HIT is based on the use of direct thrombin inhibitors, such as lepirudin (0.08 mg/kg/h, to be halved in case of kidney failure), argatroban, and bivalirudin. Fondaparinux may be an alternative, but its use is not consolidated and is considered off-label.

4.6 Management of Recurrent VTE on Anticoagulation Therapy [55, 63–67]

- In patients with thrombosis occurring during treatment with oral anticoagulant, a relapse with INR not in the therapeutic range requires a dose adjustment in order to obtain INR in the range between 2 and 3.
- For recurrent VTE on a non-LMWH anticoagulant, LMWHs are suggested.
- If recurrence occurs in the course of LMWH at subtherapeutic doses (75–80 %), the re-administration of the LMWH at full dose may be effective in more than 90 % of patients and for recurrent VTE on full dose of LMWH; the dose may be increased by about 25 %.
- If the patient is taking medications that increase the risk of thrombosis such as estrogens or chemotherapy, these treatments should be possibly withdrawn.

4.7 Treatment Strategy in Patients with Thrombocytopenia

- In patients with thrombocytopenia, full doses of anticoagulation can be used for VTE treatment if the platelet count is ≥50,000, and there is no evidence of bleeding.
- For patients with a platelet count of 20,000–50,000, a 50 % of full dose must be employed.
- Stop anticoagulants for a count <20,000 always adapting the decision to the individual case.
- If severe cancer or chemotherapy-induced thrombocytopenia is present, platelet transfusions may be used to allow anticoagulation; an experience of few cases reported in the literature suggests that the use of prophylactic doses of LMWH can be tolerated in patients with platelet counts $\leq 20 \times 10^9$/L with associated resolution of thrombotic symptoms [67].

References

1. Falanga A, Marchetti M, Russo L. The mechanisms of cancer-associated thrombosis. Thromb Res. 2015;135 Suppl 1:S8–11.
2. Prandoni P, Falanga A, Piccioli A. Cancer and venous thromboembolism. Lancet Oncol. 2005;6:401–10.
3. Khorana AA, Francis CW, Culakova E, et al. Thromboembolism is a leading cause of death in cancer patients receiving outpatient chemotherapy. J Thromb Haemost. 2007;5(3):632–4.
4. Sanon S, Lenihan DJ, Mouhayar E. Peripheral arterial ischemic events in cancer patients. Vasc Med. 2011;16:119–30.
5. Di Nisio M, Ferrante N, Feragalli B, et al. Arterial thrombosis in ambulatory cancer patients treated with chemotherapy. Thromb Res. 2011;127:382–3.
6. Khorana AA, Dalal M, Lin J, Connolly GC. Incidence and predictors of venous thromboembolism (VTE) among ambulatory high-risk cancer patients undergoing chemotherapy in the United States. Cancer. 2013;119:648–55.
7. Prandoni P, Lensing AW, Piccioli A, et al. Recurrent venous thromboembolism and bleeding complications during anticoagulant treatment in patients with cancer and venous thrombosis. Blood. 2002;100:3484–8.
8. Timp JF, Braekkan SK, Versteeg HH, Cannegieter SC. Epidemiology of cancer-associated venous thrombosis. Blood. 2013;122:1712.
9. Sproul EE. Carcinoma and venous thrombosis: the frequency of association of carcinoma in the body or tail of the pancreas with multiple venous thrombosis. Am J Cancer. 1938;34:566.
10. Khorana AA, Dalal MR, Lin J, Connolly GC. Health care costs associated with venous thromboembolism in selected high risk ambulatory patients with solid tumors undergoing chemotherapy in the United States. Clinicoecon Outcomes Res. 2013;5:101–8.
11. White RH, Chew HK, Zhou H, et al. Incidence of venous thromboembolism in the year before the diagnosis of cancer in 528,693 adults. Arch Intern Med. 2005;165:1782–7.
12. Carrier M, Lazo-Langner A, Shivakumar S, SOME Investigators, et al. Screening for occult cancer in unprovoked venous thromboembolism. N Engl J Med. 2015;373(8):697–70.
13. Khorana AA, Carrier M, Garcia DA, Lee AY. Guidance for the prevention and treatment of cancer-associated venous thromboembolism. J Thromb Thrombolysis. 2016;41(1):81–91. doi:10.1007/s11239-015-1313-4.
14. ENOXACAN Study Group. Efficacy and safety of enoxaparin versus unfractionated heparin for prevention of deep vein thrombosis in elective cancer surgery: a double-blind randomized multicentre trial with venographic assessment. Br J Surg. 1997;84:1099–103.
15. Akl EA, Kahale L, Sperati F, et al. Low molecular weight heparin versus unfractionated heparin for perioperative thromboprophylaxis in patients with cancer. Cochrane Database Syst Rev. 2014;6:CD009447. doi:10.1002/14651858.CD009447.pub2.
16. Akl EA, Kahale LA, Schünemann HJ. Association between perioperative low-molecular-weight heparin vs unfractionated heparin and clinical outcomes in patients with cancer undergoing surgery. JAMA. 2015;313:1364–5.
17. Bergqvist D, Agnelli G, Cohen AT, ENOXACAN II Investigators, et al. Duration of prophylaxis against venous thromboembolism with enoxaparin after surgery for cancer. N Engl J Med. 2002;346:975.
18. Kakkar VV, Balibrea JL, Martínez-González J, Prandoni P, CANBESURE Study Group. Extended prophylaxis with bemiparin for the prevention of venous thromboembolism after abdominal or pelvic surgery for cancer: the CANBESURE randomized study. J Thromb Haemost. 2010;8:1223–9.
19. Rasmussen MS, Jorgensen LN, Wille-Jørgensen P, FAME Investigators, et al. Prolonged prophylaxis with dalteparin to prevent late thromboembolic complications in patients undergoing major abdominal surgery: a multicenter randomized open-label study. J Thromb Haemost. 2006;4:2384–90.
20. Cui G, Wang X, Yao W, Li H. Incidence of postoperative venous thromboembolism after laparoscopic versus open colorectal cancer surgery: a meta-analysis. Surg Laparosc Endosc Percutan Tech. 2013;23:128–34.
21. Horsted F, West J, Grainge MJ. Risk of venous thromboembolism in patients with cancer: a systematic review and meta-analysis. PLoS Med. 2012;9:e1001275.
22. Lyman GH, Bohlke K, Khorana AA, American Society of Clinical Oncology, et al. Venous thromboembolism prophylaxis and treatment in patients with cancer: American society of clinical oncology clinical practice guideline update 2014. J Clin Oncol. 2015;33(6):654–6.
23. Merkow RP, Bilimoria KY, McCarter MD, et al. Post-discharge venous thromboembolism after cancer surgery: extending the case for extended prophylaxis. Ann Surg. 2011;254:131.
24. Choueiri TK, Schutz FA, Je Y, Rosenberg JE, Bellmunt J. Risk of arterial thromboembolic events with sunitinib and sorafenib: a systematic review and meta-analysis of clinical trials. J Clin Oncol. 2010;28:2280–5.

25. Cavo M, Zamagni E, Cellini C, et al. Deep-vein thrombosis in patients with multiple myeloma receiving first-line thalidomide-dexamethasone therapy. Blood. 2002;100:2272–3.
26. Petrelli F, Cabiddu M, Borgonovo K, Barni S. Risk of venous and arterial thromboembolic events associated with anti-EGFR agents: a meta-analysis of randomized clinical trials. Ann Oncol. 2012;23:1672–9.
27. Palumbo A, Rajkumar SV, Dimopoulos MA, International Myeloma Working Group, et al. Prevention of thalidomide- and lenalidomide-associated thrombosis in myeloma. Leukemia. 2008;22:414.
28. Zangari M, Anaissie E, Barlogie B, et al. Increased risk of deep-vein thrombosis in patients with multiple myeloma receiving thalidomide and chemotherapy. Blood. 2001;98:1614.
29. Rajkumar SV, Blood E. Lenalidomide and venous thrombosis in multiple myeloma. N Engl J Med. 2006;354:2079.
30. Rajkumar SV, Jacobus S, Callender N, et al. Phase III trial of lenalidomide plus high-dose dexamethasone versus lenalidomide plus low-dose dexamethasone in newly diagnosed multiple myeloma (E4A03): a trial coordinated by the Eastern Cooperative Oncology Group (abstract). Clin Oncol. 2007;25:968s.
31. Mackman N. Role of tissue factor in hemostasis, thrombosis, and vascular development. Arterioscler Thromb Vasc Biol. 2004;24:1015–22.
32. Khorana AA, Liebman HA, White RH, et al. The risk of venous thromboembolism in patients with cancer. Alexandria, VA: American Society of Clinical Oncology, ASCO Educational Book; 2008. p. 240–8.
33. Carrier M, Le Gal G, Wells PS, et al. Systematic review: the Trousseau syndrome revisited: should we screen extensively for cancer in patients with venous thromboembolism? Ann Intern Med. 2008;149:323–33.
34. Khorana AA, Kuderer NM, Culakova E, et al. Development and validation of a predictive model for chemotherapy-associated thrombosis. Blood. 2008;111:4902–7.
35. Ay C, Dunkler D, Marosi C, et al. Prediction of venous thromboembolism in cancer patients. Blood. 2010;116:5377.
36. Posch F, Thaler J, Zlabinger GJ, et al. Soluble vascular endothelial growth factor (sVEGF) and the risk of venous thromboembolism in patients with cancer: results from the Vienna cancer and thrombosis study (CATS). Clin Cancer Res. 2016;22:200–6.
37. Verso M, Agnelli G, Barni S, et al. A modified Khorana risk assessment score for venous thromboembolism in cancer patients receiving chemotherapy: the Protecht score. Intern Emerg Med. 2012;7:291–2.
38. George D, Agnelli G, Fisher W, et al. Poster presentation: venous thromboembolism (VTE) prevention with semuloparin in cancer patients initiating chemotherapy: benefit risk assessment by VTE risk in SAVE-ONCO. https://ash.confex.com/ash/2011/webprogram/Paper39639.
39. Carrier M, Khorana AA, Moretto P, et al. Lack of evidence to support thromboprophylaxis in hospitalized medical patients with cancer. Am J Med. 2014;127(1):82–6.
40. Palumbo A, Cavo M, Bringhen S, et al. Aspirin, warfarin, or enoxaparin thromboprophylaxis in patients with multiple myeloma treated with thalidomide: a phase III, open-label, randomized tri. J Clin Oncol. 2011;29:986–9381.
41. Larocca A, Cavallo F, Bringhen S, et al. Aspirin or enoxaparin thromboprophylaxis for patients with newly diagnosed multiple myeloma treated with lenalidomide. Blood. 2012;119:933–9.
42. Zangari M, Fink L, Zhan F, Tricot G. Low venous thromboembolic risk with bortezomib in multiple myeloma and potential protective effect with thalidomide/lenalidomide-based therapy: review of data from phase 3 trials and studies of novel combination regimens. Clin Lymphoma Myeloma Leuk. 2011;11:228–36.
43. Akl EA, Kahale L, Neumann I, et al. Anticoagulation for the initial treatment of venous thromboembolism in patients with cancer. Cochrane Database Syst Rev. 2014; 19;(6):CD006649.
44. Van Doormaal FF, Raskob GE, Davidson BL, et al. Treatment of venous thromboembolism in patients with cancer: subgroup analysis of the Matisse clinical trials. Thromb Haemost. 2009;101:762–9.
45. Akl EA, Kahale L, Barba M, et al. Anticoagulation for the long-term treatment of venous thromboembolism in patients with cancer. Cochrane Database Syst Rev. 2014;7:CD006650.
46. Lee AYY, Levine MN, Baker RI, et al. Low-molecular-weight heparin versus a coumarin for the prevention of recurrent venous thromboembolism in patients with cancer. N Engl J Med. 2003;349:146–1539.
47. Lee AY, Kamphuisen PW, Meyer G, CATCH Investigators, et al. Tinzaparin vs warfarin for treatment of acute venous thromboembolism in patients with active cancer: a randomized clinical trial. JAMA. 2015;314(7):677–8.
48. Pesavento R, Amitrano M, Trujillo-Santos J, et al. Fondaparinux in the initial and long-term treatment of venous thromboembolism. Thromb Res. 2015;135:311–7.
49. Bauersachs R, Berkowitz SD, Brenner B, et al. Oral rivaroxaban for symptomatic venous thromboembolism. N Engl J Med. 2010;363:2499–510.

50. Buller HR, Prins MH, Lensin AW, et al. Oral rivaroxaban for the treatment of symptomatic pulmonary embolism. N Engl J Med. 2012;366:1287–97.
51. Buller HR, Decousus H, Grosso MA, et al. Edoxaban versus warfarin for the treatment of symptomatic venous thromboembolism. N Engl J Med. 2013;369:1406–15.
52. Agnelli G, Buller HR, Cohen A, et al. Oral apixaban for the treatment of acute venous thromboembolism. N Engl J Med. 2013;369:799–808.
53. Vedovati MC, Germini F, Agnelli G, Becattini C. Direct oral anticoagulants in patients with VTE and cancer: a systematic review and meta-analysis. Chest. 2015;147:475–83.
54. Franchini M, Bonfanti C, Lippi G. Cancer-associated thrombosis: investigating the role of new oral anticoagulants. Thromb Res. 2015;135:777–81.
55. Lee AY, Peterson EA. Treatment of cancer-associated thrombosis. Blood. 2013;122:2310–7.
56. Carrier M, Cameron C, Delluc A, et al. Efficacy and safety of anticoagulant therapy for the treatment of acute cancer-associated thrombosis: a systematic review and meta-analysis. Thromb Res. 2014;134: 1214–9.
57. Lyman GH, Khorana AA, Kuderer NM, et al. American society of clinical oncology clinical practice. J Clin Oncol. 2013;31:2189–204.
58. Streiff MB, Holmstrom B, Ashrani A, et al. Cancer-associated venous thromboembolic disease, version 1.2015. J Natl Compr Canc Netw. 2015;13:1079–95.
59. Watson HG, Keeling DM, Laffan M, et al. British Committee for Standards in Haematology Guideline on aspects of cancer-related venous thrombosis Guideline on aspects of cancer-related venous thrombosis. Br J Haematol. 2015;170:640–8.
60. Kearon C, Akl EA, Ornelas J, et al. Antithrombotic therapy for VTE disease: CHEST guideline and expert panel report. Chest. 2016;149:315–52.
61. Debourdeau P, Farge D, Beckers M, et al. International clinical practice guidelines for the treatment and prophylaxis of thrombosis associated with central venous catheters in patients with cancer. J Thromb Haemost. 2013;11:71–80.
62. Schiffer CA, Mangu PB, Wade JC, et al. Central venous catheter care for the patient with cancer: American Society of Clinical Oncology clinical practice guideline. J Clin Oncol. 2013;31:1357–70.
63. Abtahian F, Hawkins BM, Ryan DP, et al. Inferior vena cava filter usage, complications, and retrieval rate in cancer patients. Am J Med. 2014;127:1111–7.
64. Casanegra AI, Landrum LM, Tafur AJ. Retrievable inferior vena cava filters in patients with cancer: complications and retrieval success rate. Int J Vasc Med. 2016;2016:6413541.
65. Carrier M, Le Gal G, Cho R, et al. Dose escalation of low molecular weight heparin to manage recurrent venous thromboembolic events despite systemic anticoagulation in cancer patients. J Thromb Haemost. 2009;7:760–5.
66. Heit JA, Mohr DN, Silverstein MD, et al. Predictors of recurrence after deep vein thrombosis and pulmonary embolism: a population-based cohort study. Arch Intern Med. 2000;160:761–8.
67. Herishanu Y, Misgav M, Kirgner I, et al. Enoxaparin can be used safely in patients with severe thrombocytopenia due to intensive chemotherapy regimens. Leuk Lymphoma. 2004;45:1407–11. Review.

Suggested Reading: Society Guidelines

Streiff MB, Holmstrom B, Ashrani A, et al. Cancer-associated venous thromboembolic disease, version 1.2015. J Natl Compr Canc Netw. 2015;13(9):1079–9554.
Lyman GH, Khorana AA, Kuderer NM, et al. American society of clinical oncology clinical practice. J Clin Oncol. 2013;31(17):2189–20455.
Lyman GH, Bohlke K1, Khorana AA, American Society of Clinical Oncology, et al. Venous thromboembolism prophylaxis and treatment in patients with cancer: American society of clinical oncology clinical practice guideline update 2014. J Clin Oncol. 2015;33:654–6.
Watson HG, Keeling DM, Laffan M, et al. British Committee for Standards in Haematology Guideline on aspects of cancer-related venous thrombosis. Guideline on aspects of cancer-related venous thrombosis. Br J Haematol. 2015;170:640–857.
Kearon C, Akl EA, Ornelas J, et al. Antithrombotic therapy for VTE disease: CHEST guideline and expert panel report. Chest. 2016;149:315–5258.
Debourdeau P, Farge D, Beckers M, et al. International clinical practice guidelines for the treatment and prophylaxis of thrombosis associated with central venous catheters in patients with cancer. J Thromb Haemost. 2013;11:71–8059.

Arrhythmias and Electrolyte Imbalances as Consequences of Cancer

Nicola Maurea, Iris Parrini, and Chiara Lestuzzi

C. Lestuzzi et al. (eds.), *Manual of Cardio-oncology*, DOI 10.1007/978-3-319-40236-9_5

Both arrhythmias and electrolyte imbalances are rather frequent consequences of cancer itself and of cancer treatments (and their side effects). Arrhythmias may be also a consequence of electrolyte imbalance.

5.1 Arrhythmias

(See Chap. 11 for more detailed information).

- **Sinus tachycardia** is frequently observed in patients with anemia, pleural or pericardial effusion, mediastinal masses, and lung tumors (both primary and secondary). It is a compensatory mechanism, which does not need any treatment as far as is well tolerated. However, a rest heart rate constantly >110/m', which raises >120–130 at any minimal effort, may be very uncomfortable for the patient.
  - **Treatment:**
    - Try to correct the underlying conditions (anemia, hypoxia…).
    - Low-dose beta-blockers (bisoprolol 1.25 mg/day or more).
    - If beta-blockers are not tolerated because of low blood pressure, ivabradine 5 or 7.5 mg, twice a day, is a good option.
- **Atrial fibrillation (AF)** is more frequent in patients with a cancer history in general, mostly with lung and colorectal cancer, after thoracic surgery, and in neoplastic involvement of the heart [1–4]. A condition possibly linking cancer to AF is chronic inflammation, which increases both cancer and AF risk [5–7]. An association of bisphosphonate use and risk of AF has been reported; bisphosphonate are used in high doses in treatment of bone metastasis and hypercalcemia. In a study of 3981 cancer patients exposed to intravenous bisphosphonate, 128 (3.2 %) developed AF/flutter [8].
- It should be reverted to sinus rhythm, if possible, to avoid the risk of thromboembolism and the need of anticoagulation. Moreover, in a recent prospective single-center study, AF after pulmonary lobectomy for lung cancer affected hospital morbidity and mortality, and long-term outcome in 5-year survivors [9].
  - **Treatment:**
    - In a study on lung cancer patients undergoing lung surgery and who had elevated N-terminal pro-brain natriuretic peptide levels in the perioperative period, both beta-blockers (BBs) and losartan significantly reduced the incidence of postoperative AF [10].
    - Amiodarone is able to lower the incidence of AF from 39.2 to 8.3 % and appeared to be safe with no major complications in patients undergoing lung surgery [11]. It is recommended in patients with low blood pressure.
    - Flecainide, dofetilide, propafenone, and IV ibutilide are useful for cardioversion of AF or atrial flutter, provided contraindications to the selected drug are absent [12].
    - Since many cancer patients are elderly, with possible comorbidities, amiodarone is the drug of choice in case of new onset AF if cardiac function is not known, and in older patients.
- **Ventricular arrhythmias (VA)** are most frequently observed as a consequence of some antineoplastic treatments (see Chap. 11 for more detailed information) or of electrolyte imbalances. Also ventricular tumors may present with VA. In presence of frequent VA, a careful assessment of both possible predisposing factors and risk of sudden death should be carried out [13].

- **Treatment**
  - Check serum electrolytes, including magnesium, and correct any abnormality (see below).
  - Beta-blockers are the first choice in case of frequent and/or symptomatic VA and in patients with ischemic heart disease. Advantages are the rapid effect, the short half-life (should the therapy be changed). The main disadvantage is that BBs are not well tolerated by hypotensive patients.
  - Amiodarone may be a therapeutic choice, unless in presence of QT interval prolongation or thyroid dysfunction. However, the long half-life may be a contraindication in some patients.

5.2 Electrolyte Imbalances

Wide, even rapid, changes in blood electrolytes are rather common in cancer patients, both as a consequence of the disease itself (malnutrition) and of the antineoplastic treatments, both surgical and pharmacological [14]. The sodium and potassium serum level are among the factors predictive of outcome after surgery for gastroesophageal cancer [15, 16].

Electrolyte abnormalities are among the most common causes of cardiac arrhythmias. Of all the electrolyte abnormalities, hyperkalemia and hypercalcemia are the most rapidly fatal.

5.2.1 Hypokalemia

Hypokalemia is a common consequences of vomiting, diarrhea, fluid load, drugs, and some antineoplastic treatments [1]. It may be due to some neuroendocrine tumors [2, 3]. Hypokalemia increases the risk of ventricular arrhythmias [17].

Hypokalemia is defined as a serum potassium level <3.5 mEq/L.

Clinical Manifestations

Hypokalemia may cause weakness, paralysis, muscle cramps, respiratory failure, and constipation.

ECG changes including U waves, T-wave flattening, arrhythmias prevalently ventricular (especially if concomitant digoxin therapy), and asystolia.

Treatment

- Both enteral and parenteral potassium administration are equally effective in restoring serum potassium levels [18].
- Potential adverse effects with enteral administration include unpalatable taste, nausea, and abdominal discomfort.
- Adverse effects with intravenous administration include venous sclerosis, infusion-related pain, and phlebitis when delivered via peripheral vein and the risk of cardiac arrest due to excessive infusion rates when administered via a central intravenous catheter.
- Continuous ECG monitoring is essential during IV infusion, and the dose should be titrated after repeated sampling of serum potassium levels.

- If occurs ventricular arrhythmias or imminent arrest give infusion of 2 mEq/min, followed 10 mEq IV over 5–10 min.
- The mean dose–response per 20 mmol of potassium chloride is 0.25–0.27 mmol/L.

5.2.2 Hyperkalemia

Hyperkalemia may be due to renal insufficiency, tissue breakdown (rhabdomyolysis, tumor lysis, hemolysis), metabolic acidosis, drugs, abnormal erythrocytes, or thrombocytosis. It may cause severe ventricular arrhythmias and cardiac arrest; it is the most common electrolyte disorder associated with cardiopulmonary arrest.

Hyperkalemia is defined as a serum potassium >5.0 mEq/L.

Clinical Manifestations

Severe hyperkalemia may cause weakness, flaccid paralysis, depressed deep tendon reflexes, respiratory failure, and asystolic and cardiac arrest.

ECG changes including peaked T waves (tenting) and-when serum potassium increases-flattened or absent P waves, a prolonged PR interval, widened QRS complex, deepened S waves, merging of S and T waves, idioventricular rhythms, and asystolia.

Treatment [19, 20]

- **Mild hyperkalemia** (serum level <6 mEq/L):
  - Intravenous furosemide: 40–80 mg ev.
  - Potassium exchange resins, i.e., calcium resonium 15–30 g or sodium polystyrene sulfonate (Kayexalate®) 15–30 g in 50–100 mL of 20 % sorbitol, given either orally or by retention enema (onset in 1–3 h, maximal effect at 6 h).
  - Dialysis: hemodialysis is more efficient than peritoneal dialysis at removing potassium (immediate onset, 25–30 mmol potassium h^{-1} removed with hemodialysis).
- **Moderate forms** (serum level 6–7 mEq/L):
  - A solution of glucose 50 mg plus rapid acting insulin 10 units given intravenously over 15–30 min (onset in 15–30 min, maximal effect at 30–60 min; monitoring blood glucose).
  - Intravenous NaCO3 50 mEq ev in 5 min.
  - Use in addition to removal strategies above.
- **In more severe cases** (serum K+ >7 mEq/L):
  - Salbutamol, 5 mg nebulized. Several doses may be required (onset in 15–30 min).
  - Sodium bicarbonate plus glucose/insulin as above (onset in 15–30 min).
  - $CaCl^-$ 10 % (5–10 mL intravenously in 2–5 min) to prevent arrhythmias as membrane stabilizer (to be noticed: this does not lower K+ levels).
- **In case of cardiac arrest,** protect the heart first, then apply shifting and removal strategies using:
  - **Calcium chloride:** 10 mL of 10 % calcium chloride IV by rapid bolus injection to antagonize the toxic effects of hyperkalemia at the myocardial cell membrane.
  - **Sodium bicarbonate:** 50 mmol IV by rapid injection (if severe acidosis or renal failure).

- **Dextrose/insulin:** 10 units short-acting insulin and 50 g glucose IV by rapid injection.
- **Hemodialysis:** consider this for cardiac arrest induced by hyperkalemia, which is resistant to medical treatment.

5.2.3 Hypercalcemia

Hypercalcemia is the most common life-threatening metabolic disorder associated with cancer, occurring in approximately 10–30 % of all patients with neoplastic disease especially with skeletal metastases [21]. It may be humoral due to secretion of the parathormone-like 1,25-dihydroxy vitamin D or PTH-related protein (PTHrP), or secondary to extensive bone lysis (in multiple myeloma, breast cancer bone metastases). PTHrP-secreting tumors may be lymphomas; squamous cancer of the lung, esophagus, head, and neck; gynecologic malignancies, breast cancer, and renal carcinomas. A serum calcium >14 mg/dL may cause acute renal failure and cardiac arrest. It should be promptly treated even in absence of any symptom [22].

Hypercalcemia is defined as serum calcium concentration >10.5 mEq/L.

Clinical Manifestations

Hypercalcemia may cause somnolence, confusion, depression, psychosis, muscle weakness, coma; constipation, anorexia, nausea, abdominal pain, peptic ulcer disease, pancreatitis, polyuria, polydipsia, nephrolithiasis, nephrocalcinosis, and renal failure; hypertension and digitalis sensitivity; and osteoporosis, fracture, and bone pain.

ECG changes including QT interval shortening, atrioventricular block, prolonged PR and QRS intervals, and increased QRS voltage.

Treatment [19, 20]

- **Intravenous isotonic saline** solutions to reverse volume depletion will often lower the serum calcium 1–2 mg/dL as a consequence of expanding the intravascular space. Approximately 3–6 L of intravenous fluid during the initial 24-h period have been recommended.
  - Caution should be exercised in administering large volumes and high rates of intravenous fluid because of the likelihood of producing congestive heart failure and third spacing, particularly in malignancy-associated hypercalcemia, where patients tend to be quite ill and often have concomitant hypoalbuminemia.
- Some authors recommend rehydration with no more than 75–150 mL/h of 0.9 % sodium chloride in this patient population and avoidance of saline-induced diuresis [23].
- Further decreases in the serum calcium can be achieved by infusing intravenous saline to induce a diuresis, though this is not a consistent finding.
- **Furosemide** was used in the past to reduce calcium reabsorption in the loop of Henle and thus augment calciuresis. However it is no longer recommended (unless needed to reverse overly aggressive fluid replacement) as excessive diuresis may lead to volume depletion, hypokalemia, and worsening hypercalcemia.
- **Bisphosphonates** are pyrophosphate analogues that are deposited in bone and lower serum calcium levels via multiple effects on osteoclasts, one of which is inhibition of osteoclastic bone resorption. They are the most used treatment for cancer hypercalcemia, mostly if due to bone lysis.

- Zoledronic acid (3–4 mg intravenously in 100 mL of saline over 15–30 min) is the most powerful biphosphonate and has a rapid and durable effect. In several studies, it performed better than other agents, by reducing the number of skeletal-related events, preventing recurrence of hypercalcemia and exhibiting a longer duration of response. Adverse effects are pyrexia, skeletal pain, nausea, and asthenia [24].
- Pamidronate is also highly effective and show a durable response. It is given at doses of 60–90 mg intravenously in 2–24 h. Its effect is not as prompt as zoledronic acid.
- Salmon calcitonin is useful for treatment of severe hypercalcemia irrespective of etiology, given its early onset of action and relatively mild adverse effects. It begins working within several hours and lowers plasma calcium levels by 1–2 mg/dL only. However, when calcitonin is given along with intravenous fluid therapy, the combination may be sufficient to reverse the immediate risks of severe hypercalcemia. It may be considered in the emergency setting, as an early intervention if biphosphonate are not available. Recommended doses are 4–8 units subcutaneously (or intranasal, less used) every 6–12 h. Side effects include nausea, vomiting, flushing, and injection site reactions, while intranasal form can be associated with rhinitis. Hypersensitivity reactions can occur.

5.2.4 Hypocalcemia

Hypocalcemia may occur in acute pancreatitis, tumor lysis syndrome, rhabdomyolysis, and toxic shock syndrome. Hypocalcemia can exacerbate digitalis cardiotoxicity.

Hypocalcemia is defined as a serum calcium concentration <8 mg/dL.

Clinical Manifestations

Hypocalcemia may cause tetany, seizures, and cardiac arrest.

ECG changes including prolonged QT interval, T-wave inversion, AV heart block, and ventricular fibrillation.

Treatment

- Calcium chloride 10 %: 10–40 mL intravenously
- Magnesium sulfate 50 %: 2–4 g if needed

5.2.5 Hypomagnesemia

Hypomagnesemia is a common consequence of decreased absorption or increased loss of magnesium from the kidneys or intestines such as diarrhea, abnormalities of thyroid hormones, or some drugs (e.g., pentamidine, diuretics, alcohol) and malnourishment.

Hypomagnesemia is defined as a serum magnesium concentration <1.3 mEq/L.

Clinical Manifestations

Hypomagnesemia may cause muscle tremor, nystagmus, tetany, and mental status alterations.

ECG changes including prolonged PR and QT interval, T-wave inversion, widening of QRS, torsades de pointes, and ventricular tachycardias.

Treatment [19, 20]

- 1–2 g of $MgSO_4$ bolus IV in 15 min
- If there are convulsions 2 g of $MgSO_4$ iv in 10 min
- Calcium gluconate when associated hyocalcemia

5.2.6 Hypermagnesemia

Hypermagnesemia is the most common consequences of renal failure but may be iatrogenic with intake of food or continuous use of laxative.

Hypermagnesemia is defined as a serum magnesium concentration >2.2 mEq/L.

Clinical Manifestations

Hypermagnesemia may cause muscular weakness, paralysis, ataxia, drowsiness, confusion, and hypotension. High serum magnesium levels may induce a depressed level of consciousness, hypoventilation, and cardiac arrest.

ECG changes including prolonged PR and QT intervals, bradycardia, block AV, and cardiac arrhythmias.

Treatment

- $CaCl^-$ 10 % (5–10 mL intravenous) to prevent arrhythmias as membrane stabilizer.
- Dialysis is the treatment of choice in severe hypermagnesemia.
- Saline solution 0.9 %.
- Forced diuresis with furosemide 1 mg/kg.

5.2.7 Hyponatremia

Hyponatremia is a common electrolyte disorder representing an excess of water relative to total body solute, may be due to heart failure, liver cirrhosis, renal failure, hypothyroidism, and non-osmotic vasopressin activity determined by malignancies, infections, and drugs as diuretics but also antineoplastic agents as cyclophosphamide, cisplatin, vincristine, and ifosfamide [25–27].

Hyponatremia is defined as a serum sodium concentration <135 mEq/L.

Clinical Manifestations

It is usually asymptomatic, but acute or serious hyponatremia can cause brain edema with severe symptoms as decreased consciousness, seizures, and muscle rigidity. Other symptoms are nausea and vomiting, headache, muscle weakness, cramps, and spasm.

Treatment [25, 26]

Different strategies have been proposed to treat hyponatremia.

- In the setting of severe symptoms, infusion of hypertonic saline intravenous is recommended, having a concentration of 3 % infused at 1 mEq/L/h until restoring neurological symptoms then continue at 0.5 mEq/L/h.

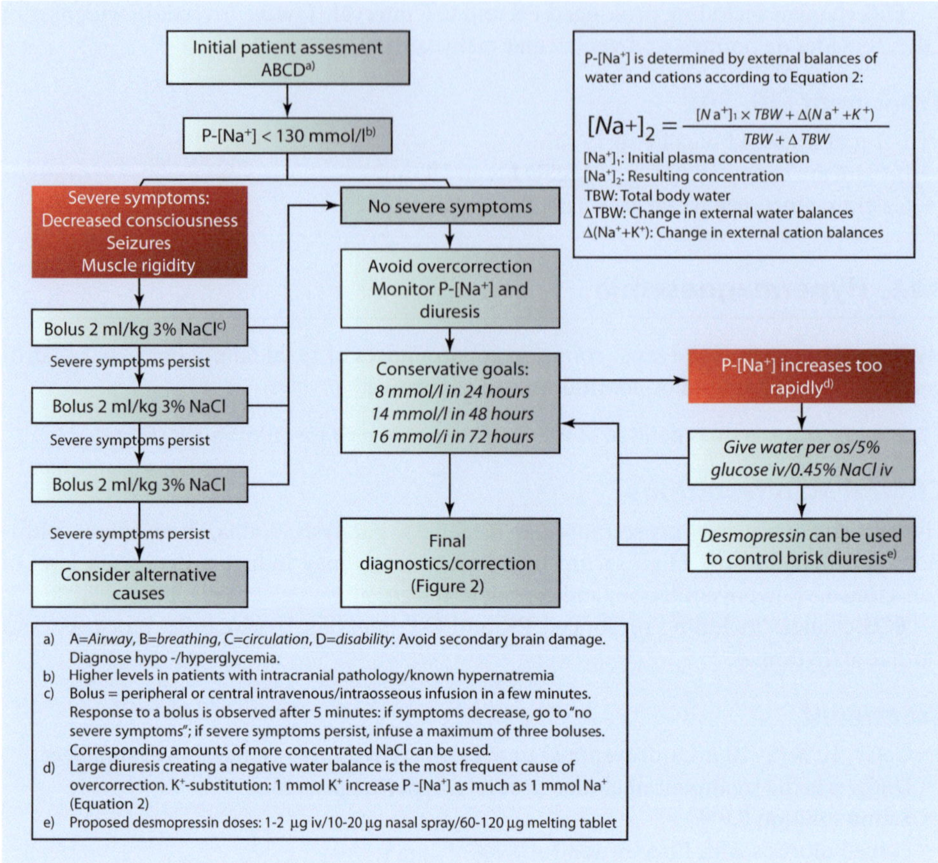

Fig. 5.1 Reproduced from Overgaard-Steensen and Ring [25], published under CC BY 4.0 license ► http://ccforum.biomedcentral.com/articles/10.1186/cc11805

- For euvolemic and hypervolemic asymptomatic hyponatremia fluid restriction are recommended as first treatment.
- Saline solution 0.9 % infusion is recommended calculated with Adrogue–Madias formula (Fig. 5.1).
- Infusion usually varied between 8 and 12 mmol/L during the first 24 h and 18 mmol/L during the first 48 h regardless if hyponatremia was acute or chronic.
- Stricter limit of <8 mmol/L during the first 24 h in cases where the patient was believed to be high risk for developing osmotic demyelination syndrome.

5.2.8 Hypernatremia

Hypernatremia is a rare electrolyte imbalances resulting in three situations [25, 28]:

(a) **Water and solute loss** occurs when hypovolemia is present due to critical illness, sedation, neurological impairment, fever, and gastrointestinal loss of hypotonic fluid.

(b) **Pure water loss** occurs when water balance is negative with reduced water intake as in patients with critical illness and occasionally diabetes insipidus and infants.
(c) **Increased total body solutes** are rare, usually due to infusion of hypertonic potassium-containing solutions, hypertonic saline, and NaHCO3 treatment.

Hypernatremia is defined as a serum concentration above the normal range of 135 to 145 mEq/L.

Clinical Manifestations

Hypernatremia may cause cerebral symptoms as decreased level of consciousness, irritability, hyperreflexia, spasticity, and seizures.

Treatment [28]

(a) **Water and solute loss.**
  - Restoring extracellular volume by infusing intravenous saline (see above).
(b) **Pure water loss.**
  - Restoring of the water loss.
(c) **Increased total body solutes.**
  - Reduce input and increase output with diuretics or rarely dialysis (with caution!). No optimal correction rate has been determined, but it has been suggested that it should not exceed 0.5 mmol/L/h.

5.2.9 Hyperphosphatemia

Hyperphosphatemia may be observed in chronic kidney disease and after cancer treatments; it has been associated to a poorer cancer prognosis [29]. Its more severe form is observed in the tumor lysis syndrome (see below).

Clinical Manifestations

Arrhythmias, lethargy, seizures, nausea, and vomiting.

Treatment

- Diet with no added phosphate in replacement fluids.
- Use of phosphate binders.
- Prevention of oliguria.
- Using diuretics to minimize the risk for calcium phosphate precipitation in renal tubules.
- Dialysis is useful in phosphate removal and continuous venovenous hemofiltration are the therapy of choice.

5.3 Tumor Lysis Syndrome

Tumor lysis syndrome (TLS) is a potentially life-threatening metabolic disorder occurring after massive lysis of tumor cells. It is more frequent after antineoplastic treatments, but it may develop also spontaneously in tumors with rapid tumor cell turnover, such as Burkitt's

Table 5.1 Definitions of laboratory tumor lysis syndrome (LTLS)

Author	Cairo–Bishop	Montesinos	Howard	
			Adults	Children
Uric acid	x ≥ 476 µmol/L or 25 % increase from baseline	>7.5 mg/dL	>8 mg/dL	>ULN
Potassium	x ≥ 6.0 mmol/L or 25 % increase from baseline	>5 mEq/L	>6 mmol/L	
Phosphate	x ≥ 2.1 mmol/L (children), x ≥1.45 mmol/L (adults) or 25 % increase from baseli	>5 mg/dL	>4.5 mg/dL	>6.5 mg/dL
Calcium	x ≤ 1.75 mmol/L or 25 % decrease from baseline	<8 mg/dL	Corrected <7 mg/dL; ionized <1.12	
Creatinine	–	>1.4 mg/dL		

Note: Cairo–Bishop's clinical classification has 5 grades: grade 5 (not reported here) includes death.
Data from Cairo and Bishop [35], Montesinos et al. [37], and Howard et al. [36]
UNL = upper normal limits (for laboratory and/or according to age)

lymphoma and acute leukemias [30–33]. This syndrome may develop in patients with hematologic malignancies or solid tumors, mostly in highly chemosensitive tumors and when the tumor burden is large; also the presence of preexisting renal disease, the use of nephrotoxic drugs, and the presence of disseminated intravascular coagulation are risk factor for TLS [34, 35]. Treatment-induced TLS usually occurs 12–72 h after starting therapy.

- The incidence varies according to the diagnostic method used to define the TLS: laboratory versus clinical presentation; several criteria have been proposed [35–39] (Tables 5.1 and 5.2).
  - Two or more laboratory abnormalities (hyperuricemia, hyperphosphatemia, hyperkalemia, hypocalcemia) are necessary for diagnosis.

It is characterized by the rapid development of:

- **Hyperuricemia,** from rapid release and catabolism of intracellular nucleic acids
- **Hyperkalemia,** caused by the rapid release of potassium from malignant cells and by the renal failure
- **Hyperphosphatemia** from the rapid release of intracellular phosphorous from malignant cells
- **Acute renal failure** as a consequence of calcium phosphate precipitation in the renal tubules

Frequently observed are also:

- **Hypocalcemia**, as a consequence of hyperphosphatemia calcium phosphate precipitation
- **Uremia**, due to uric acid crystal formation in the renal tubules secondary to hyperuricemia, calcium phosphate deposition, tumor infiltration in the kidney, tumor-associated obstructive uropathy, drug associated-nephrotoxicity, and/or acute sepsis.

Table 5.2 Definitions of clinical tumor lysis syndrome (CTLS)

	Cairo–Bishop					Montesinos	Howard
	Grade 0	Grade 1	Grade2	Grade 3	Grade 4		
Renal failure	Creatinine ≤1.5 × UNL	Creatinine >1.5 × UNL	Creatinine >1.5–3 × UNL	Creatinine >3–6 × UNL	Creatinine >6 × UNL	Urine output ≤800 mL/day	Urine output <0.5 mL/kg/h for 6 h
						Dialysis	Increase in serum creatinine of 0.3 mg/dL or >1.5 × ULN
Cardiac arrhythmia	None	No intervention required	Non urgent medical intervention	Symptomatic, incompletely controlled with drugs	With syncope, shock, or life-threatening	Any	If caused by hyperkalemia or hypocalcemia
						ECG signs of hyperkalemia	Hypotension, heart failure
Neuromuscolar irritability	None		One brief seizure; well controlled with anticonvulsivants, focal	Seizure with altered consciousness, poorly medically controlled; generalized	Status epilepticus, intractable epilepsy	Seizures	Seizures
						Tetany	Tetany, paresthesias, carpopedal spasm, Trousseau's sign, laryngospasm, bronchospasm

Note: Cairo–Bishop's clinical classification has 5 grades: grade 5 (not reported here) includes death. Data from Cairo and Bishop [35], Montesinos et al. [37], and Howard et al. [36]
UNL upper normal limits (for laboratory and/or according to age)

5.3.1 Clinical Manifestations

- Renal failure, oliguria
- Seizures, neuromuscular irritability, laryngospasm, bronchospasm
- Cardiac arrhythmias/death
- Heart failure

5.3.2 Treatment [38–40]

- Vigorous hydratation is recommended: target fluid intake of 3 L/day
- Prevent (especially for high risk patients) and treat hyperuricemia choosing amongst these drugs:
  - **Allopurinol** is commonly used in treatment of hyperuricemia. However, it has been associated with several hypersensitivity syndromes. An interaction between allopurinol and azathioprine (often used for immunosuppression in patients with transplants or autoimmune conditions) can lead to severe and life-threatening bone marrow suppression.
  - **Febuxostat** is a novel xanthine oxidase inhibitor that does not appear to have the hypersensitivity profile of allopurinol. In addition, it is metabolized to inactive metabolites in the liver, obviating the need for specific kidney dosing. Its routine use is limited by the higher cost compared to allopurinol.
- **Rasburicase** is an *Aspergillus*-derived recombinant urate oxidase and catalyzes the conversion of uric acid to allantoin, carbon dioxide, and hydrogen peroxide. Recommended dose is 0.15–0.2 mg/kg as a daily intravenous (i.v.) infusion for up to 5 days. It reduces uric acid levels within 4 h, both in pediatric and adult patients, catalyzing the oxidation of uric acid into allantoin, rapidly excreted by the kidneys. It was approved in the EU and in the USA for the management of acute hyperuricemia. *Warning*: it can lead to devastating methemoglobinemia and hemolytic anemia in individuals with glucose-6-phosphate dehydrogenase deficiency [41]. The routine use of Rasburicase in children with cancer is still questionable [42].
- Urine alkalinization, the solubility of uric acid is highly pH dependent. At a typical acidic urine pH of 5.0, the solubility of uric acid is 15 versus 200 mg/dL at a pH of 7.0. *However*, alkalinization of the urine (or serum) can favor the precipitation of calcium phosphate salts in soft tissues and renal tubules, potentially worsening kidney failure. Urinary alkalinization should only be considered in cases of severe hyperuricemia in which recombinant urate oxidase is unavailable.
- Use of diuretics remain controversial.
- Dialysis may be necessary in case of severe renal insufficiency. Continuous modalities are often preferred to intermitted hemodialysis to reduce the risk of "rebound" hyperkalemia or hyperphosphatemia.

References

1. O'Neal WT, Lakoski SG, Qureshi W, et al. Relation between cancer and atrial fibrillation (from the REasons for Geographic And Racial Differences in Stroke Study). Am J Cardiol. 2015;115:1090–4.
2. Erichsen R, Christiansen CF, Mehnert F, et al. Colorectal cancer and risk of atrial fibrillation and flutter: a population-based case–control study. Intern Emerg Med. 2012;7:431–8.

3. Guzzetti S, Costantino G, Sada S, Fundarò C. Colorectal cancer and atrial fibrillation: a case–control study. Am J Med. 2002;112:587–8.
4. Onaitis M, D'Amico T, Zhao Y, et al. Risk factors for atrial fibrillation after lung cancer surgery: analysis of the society of thoracic surgeons general thoracic surgery database. Ann Thorac Surg. 2010;90: 368–74.
5. Ostan R, Lanzarini C, Pini E, et al. Inflammaging and cancer: a challenge for the Mediterranean diet. Nutrients. 2015;7:2589–621.
6. Guo Y, Lip GY, Apostolakis S. Inflammation in atrial fibrillation. J Am Coll Cardiol. 2012;60:2263–70. Review.
7. Guzzetti S, Costantino G, Fundarò C. Systemic inflammation, atrial fibrillation, and cancer. Circulation. 2002;106(9):e40. author reply e40.
8. Erichsen R, Christiansen CF, Frøslev T, et al. Intravenous bisphosphonate therapy and atrial fibrillation/flutter risk in cancer patients: a nationwide cohort study. Br J Cancer. 2011;105:881–3.
9. Imperatori A, Mariscalco G, Riganti G, et al. Atrial fibrillation after pulmonary lobectomy for lung cancer affects long-term survival in a prospective single-center study. J Cardiothorac Surg. 2012;7:4.
10. Cardinale D, Sandri MT, Colombo A, et al. Prevention of atrial fibrillation in high-risk patients undergoing lung cancer surgery: the PRESAGE trial. Ann Surg. 2016;264(2):244–51.
11. Zhang L, Gao S. Systematic review and meta-analysis of atrial fibrillation prophylaxis following lung surgery. J Cardiovasc Pharmacol. 2016;67(4):351–7.
12. January CT, Wann LS, Alpert JS, American College of Cardiology/American Heart Association Task Force on Practice Guidelines, et al. 2014 AHA/ACC/HRS guideline for the management of patients with atrial fibrillation: a report of the American College of Cardiology/American Heart Association Task Force on Practice Guidelines and the Heart Rhythm Society. J Am Coll Cardiol. 2014;64:e1–76.
13. Wellens HJ, Schwartz PJ, Lindemans FW, et al. Risk stratification for sudden cardiac death: current status and challenges for the future. Eur Heart J. 2014;35:1642–51.
14. Melichar B, Králíčková P, Hyšpler R, et al. Hypomagnesaemia in patients with metastatic colorectal carcinoma treated with cetuximab. Hepatogastroenterology. 2012;59:366–71.
15. Dutta S, Horgan PG, McMillan DC. POSSUM and its related models as predictors of postoperative mortality and morbidity in patients undergoing surgery for gastro-oesophageal cancer: a systematic review. World J Surg. 2010;34:2076–82.
16. Filip B, Scarpa M, Cavallin F, et al. Postoperative outcome after oesophagectomy for cancer: nutritional status is the missing ring in the current prognostic scores. Eur J Surg Oncol. 2015;41:787–94.
17. Wahr JA, Parks R, Boisvert D, et al. Preoperative serum potassium levels and perioperative outcomes in cardiac surgery patients. JAMA. 1999;281:2203–10.
18. DeCarolis DD, Kim GM, Rector TS, Ishani A. Comparative dose response using the intravenous versus enteral route of administration for potassium replenishment. Intensive Crit Care Nurs. 2016;36:17–23.
19. Vanden Hoek TL, Morrison LJ, Shuster M, et al. Part 12: cardiac arrest in special situations: 2010 American Heart Association guidelines for cardiopulmonary resuscitation and emergency cardiovascular care. Circulation. 2010;122:S829–61.
20. Soar J, Deakin CD, Nolan JP, European Resuscitation Council, et al. European Resuscitation Council guidelines for resuscitation 2005. Section 7. Cardiac arrest in special circumstances. Resuscitation. 2005;67 Suppl 1:S135–70. Review.
21. Santarpia L, Koch CA, Sarlis NJ. Hypercalcemia in cancer patients: pathobiology and management. Horm Metab Res. 2010;42:153–64.
22. Maier JD, Levine SN. Hypercalcemia in the intensive care unit: a review of pathophysiology, diagnosis, and modern therapy. J Intensive Care Med. 2015;30:235–52.
23. Le Grand SB. Modern management of malignant hypercalcemia. Am J Hosp Palliat Care. 2011;28: 515–7.
24. Sabry NA, Habib EE. Zoledronic acid and clodronate in the treatment of malignant bone metastases with hypercalcaemia; efficacy and safety comparative study. Med Oncol. 2011;28:584–90.
25. Overgaard-Steensen C, Ring T. Clinical review: practical approach to hyponatraemia and hypernatraemia in critically ill patients. Crit Care. 2013;17:206.
26. Nagler EV, Vanmassenhove J, Van der Veer SN, Nistor I, Van Biesen W, Webster AC, Vanholder R. Diagnosis and treatment of hyponatremia: a systematic review of clinical practice guidelines and consensus statements. BMC Med. 2014;12:231.
27. Adrogue HJ, Madias NE. Primary care: hyponatremia. New Engl J Med. 2000;342:1581–9.
28. Adrogue HJ, Madias NE. Primary care: hypernatremia. New Engl J Med. 2000;342:1493–9.
29. Ye Z, Palazzo JP, Lin L, et al. Postoperative hyperphosphatemia significantly associates with adverse survival in colorectal cancer patients. J Gastroenterol Hepatol. 2013;28:1469–75.

30. Mughal T, Ejaz AA, Foringer JR, Coiffier B. An integrated clinical approach for the identification, prevention, and treatment of tumor lysis syndrome. Cancer Treat Rev. 2010;36:164–76.
31. Mika D, Ahmad S, Guruvayoorappan C. Tumour lysis syndrome: implications for cancer therapy. Asian Pac J Cancer Prev. 2012;13:3555–60. Review.
32. Akoz AG, Yildirim N, Engin H, et al. An unusual case of spontaneous acute tumor lysis syndrome associated with acute lymphoblastic leukemia: a case report and review of the literature. Acta Oncol. 2007;46:1190–2. Review.
33. Rasool M, Malik A, Qureshi MS, et al. Development of tumor lysis syndrome (TLS): a potential risk factor in cancer patients receiving anticancer therapy. Bioinformation. 2014;10:703–7.
34. Darmon M, Vincent F, Camous L, Groupe de Recherche en Réanimation Respiratoire et Onco-Hématologique (GRRR-OH), et al. Tumour lysis syndrome and acute kidney injury in high-risk haematology patients in the rasburicase era. A prospective multicentre study from the Groupe de Recherche en Réanimation Respiratoire et Onco-Hématologique. Br J Haematol. 2013;162:489–97.
35. Cairo MS, Bishop M. Tumour lysis syndrome: new therapeutic strategies and classification. Br J Haematol. 2004;127:3–11. Review.
36. Howard SC, Jones DP, Pui CH. The tumor lysis syndrome. N Engl J Med. 2011;364:1844–54. Review.
37. Montesinos P, Lorenzo I, Martín G, et al. Tumor lysis syndrome in patients with acute myeloid leukemia: identification of risk factors and development of a predictive model. Haematologica. 2008;93:67–74.
38. Weeks AC, Kimple ME. Spontaneous tumor lysis syndrome: a case report and critical evaluation of current diagnostic criteria and optimal treatment regimens. J Investig Med High Impact Case Rep. 2015;3:2324709615603199.
39. Wilson FP, Berns JS. Tumor lysis syndrome: new challenges and recent advances. Adv Chronic Kidney Dis. 2014;21:18–26.
40. Malaguarnera G, Giordano M, Malaguarnera M. Rasburicase for the treatment of tumor lysis in hematological malignancies. Expert Rev Hematol. 2012;5:27–38.
41. Browning LA, Kruse JA. Hemolysis and methemoglobinemia secondary to rasburicase administration. Ann Pharmacother. 2005;39(11):1932–5.
42. Cheuk DK, Chiang AK, Chan GC, Ha SY. Urate oxidase for the prevention and treatment of tumour lysis syndrome in children with cancer. Cochrane Database Syst Rev. 2014;8:CD006945.

5

Oncologic Treatments and Cardiotoxicity

Contents

Molecules, Drugs, and First-Line Therapies: A Guide for the Cardiologist

Sandro Barni and Fausto Petrelli

C. Lestuzzi et al. (eds.), *Manual of Cardio-oncology*, DOI 10.1007/978-3-319-40236-9_6

6.1 Introduction: Cardiovascular Toxicity with First-Line Therapy in Solid Tumors, Risk, and Benefit

Neoplastic conditions are diseases of aged subjects, generally already suffering of different medical comorbidities and likely to assume polypharmacy for these conditions. This leads to a potentially increased risk of drug interactions and may increase the likelihood of cardiovascular events when they have to be treated with certain cardiotoxic anticancer drugs.

- Cancer therapy has evolved, becoming more selective and potentially less toxic, sparing normal tissue from acute and chronic damage.
  - However, the "off-target" toxicities (an unexpected toxic effect linked to the presence of the drug target on healthy organs, like the heart, vessels, skin, etc.) may be a problem [1].
- Treatment of main solid tumors encloses more commonly a *combination of cytotoxic drugs* (e.g., chemotherapy) that portend a different but existing risk of cardiovascular side effects, *with molecular targeted agents*, that can be associated with adverse events that are the consequence of critical pathways inhibited by these targeted therapies on vessels and the heart [e.g., vascular endothelial growth factor receptor (VEGFR)] [2].
  - This combination has the potential to delay progression of disease, to increase overall survival (OS), and also to increase the burden of toxicity of cancer patients suffering from various cancers [3].
  - The risk of cardiotoxicity can also be augmented if patients were previously exposed to cardiotoxic drugs during the primary treatment of disease or in the past (in case of relapsing or second cancer). Some classical examples are the treatments with anthracyclines for hematologic malignancies and/or for breast cancer that have a cumulative (cardiotoxic) dosage beyond which the risk of heart failure becomes clinically significant. A pretreatment with these agents can also make a (subclinical) cardiac damage not clinically apparent until a further toxic damage is added in the metastatic phase of cancer.

The scope of oncological treatment, when potentially cardiotoxic drugs have planned to be used, must include a comprehensive clinical history of patient for preexisting medical condition, anticancer treatments, other risk factors and polypharmacy, and a careful cardiologic evaluation.

With these data in mind, any oncologist should estimate the real added benefit of any oncological therapy, as a function of prognosis of metastatic cancer to be treated, balanced with the risk of life-threatening adverse events.

Cancer patients receiving chemotherapy or targeted therapies have an increased risk of developing cardiovascular complications, and the risk is even greater, in particular, if there is a known history of heart disease. Several meta-analyses have demonstrated a small risk of fatal adverse events [approximately 1.5–2.5 %, relative risk (RR) 1.5–2.2] with both anti-angiogenic tyrosine kinase inhibitors (TKIs) and bevacizumab [4–6]. In one analysis, bevacizumab was associated with an increased risk of fatal events when used in combination with taxanes or platinum agents (RR, 3.49) but not in combination with other agents (RR, 0.85) [4]. In two meta-analyses, bleeding was the most common fatal adverse event with both classes of agents; however, other causes of treatment-related death were also cardiac [4,5]. In another meta-analysis examining fatal events with anti-VEGFR TKIs, death due to heart failure were higher on the TKI treatment arms [6].

Among the main serious cardiovascular events that have been reported and will be discussed here, there are:
- Arrhythmias
- Myocardial damage causing a dilated cardiomyopathy
- Angina or myocardial infarction
- Pericardial disease (rare)
- Hypertension
- Arterial or venous thromboembolic events

Drug-associated cardiovascular toxicity in oncology patients treated with upfront treatment for advanced stages of disease is the primary argument of this chapter and will be analyzed according to different types of cancer, taking into consideration in particular the combinations of agents used as first-line therapy.

6.2 First-Line Therapy in Different Cancers: Challenges and Pitfalls with Cardiotoxic Drugs

6.2.1 Breast Cancer

Chemotherapy

Anthracyclines and Taxanes Alone or in Combinations

- Systemic treatment of metastatic breast cancer includes the use of one or more of:
  - Hormonal therapies
  - Cytotoxic agents
  - Target therapies

> **The choice of the strategy is based mostly on the biology of disease, and the extent of lymph node and metastatic burden.**

- Hormonal therapies are used in patients whose cancer expresses estrogen and/or progesterone receptors. The most used drugs are tamoxifen and aromatase inhibitors (as letrozole and fulvestrant.). *Tamoxifen* is given for 5 years in the adjuvant setting.
- Cytotoxic therapies are used in patients whose cancer is not hormone-sensitive and in advanced disease.
  - Anthracyclines (monotherapy or with cyclophosphamide).
  - Doxorubicin, epidoxorubicin, and liposomal doxorubicins (pegylated or non-pegylated).
- Taxanes (paclitaxel, docetaxel)—either as a single agent or in combinations with anthracyclines—is the preferred regimen as first-line therapy for metastatic patients. A taxane-based (anthracycline-free) combination has significantly fewer adverse events of neutropenia, infection/febrile neutropenia, nausea, and vomiting compared to anthracyclivnes/cyclophosphamide [7].
- Combination chemotherapy is preferred with visceral and/or symptomatic disease.
- Combination chemotherapy in metastatic setting is not associated with a significant increase in OS, with response rate and time to progression being moderately increased.
- Cardiac toxicity of anthracyclines has been known for many years and is mostly evident as left ventricular dysfunction possibly leading to congestive heart failure.

  - *Epirubicin* is less cardiotoxic than doxorubicin on a mg per mg basis [8]. In a meta-analysis of 13 studies comparing doxorubicin with epirubicin, use of epirubicin significantly decreased the risks of both clinical and subclinical cardiotoxicity [9].
  - In *liposomal formulations*, doxorubicin is included in liposomes which do not cross healthy capillary vessels and concentrate in tumor. A randomized trial compared *pegylated liposomal doxorubicin* (PLD, 50 mg/m^2 every 4 weeks) with doxorubicin (60 mg/m^2 every 3 weeks) as first-line therapy in patients with metastatic BC; 56 % of them previously received anthracyclines. With a similar PFS and OS for the two arms, risk of cardiotoxicity was significantly higher with doxorubicin than PLD ($P < 0.001$) [10]. Similar results, with low rates of cardiac toxicity, were found with *non-pegylated liposomal doxorubicin* + cyclophosphamide compared to conventional anthracycline + cyclophosphamide combination [11].
    - The limit of liposomal formulations is mostly the high cost.

- Cardiotoxicity of taxanes is rare and asymptomatic. Paclitaxel is mainly associated with bradycardia and heart block.
  - However, they may potentiate the cardiotoxicity of anthracyclines.
  - Heart failure has described in up to 20 % of patients treated with paclitaxel plus doxorubicin in different studies [12,13], although an increased incidence of cardiotoxicity was not seen in all studies, even in patients pretreated with adjuvant anthracyclines [14]. The risk of heart failure is apparent at cumulative doxorubicin doses that are much lower than would be expected with single-agent doxorubicin [15–17]. Even docetaxel is associated with potentially related cardiac events and can potentiate the cardiac toxicity of anthracyclines [18]. In two randomized first-line trials comparing combinations of anthracycline + cyclophosphamide with anthracycline + taxanes, in anthracycline-naïve patients, the rate of grade 3–4 cardiac toxicity is similar and about 3 % in both arms [19,20].

The choice of treatment is according to comorbidities, risk factors, and previous therapies.

- The cardiotoxicity of doxorubicin and epirubicin may become relevant with cumulative doses above 300 and 700 mg/m^2, respectively.

  The added toxicity is evident even for treatments given years apart (i.e., the *cumulative dose of anthracyclines is calculated during the lifespan).*

  To better evaluate the cumulative dose of different anthracyclines, a conversion factor of 0.66 may be used for epidoxorubicin.

- Age, preexisting cardiovascular disease (e.g., cardiomyopathies, coronary artery disease, hypertension, peripheral vascular disease, diabetes), and concurrent or prior chest irradiation increase the risk of cardiotoxicity.
- The concomitant use of trastuzumab also increases the risk of cardiac dysfunction.
- In patients at high risk, an anthracycline-free regimen should be preferred. If anthracyclines are considered necessary, liposomal formulations or epidoxorubicin should be used.

Anti-HER2 Agents

Two drugs are currently approved for treatment of HER2+ breast cancer: the monoclonal antibodies trastuzumab and pertuzumab, which are combined with taxanes in a triplet combination showing a better OS that chemotherapy plus trastuzumab alone.

Both drugs bind to the extracellular domain IV of ErbB2 receptor, belonging to the HER family of tyrosine kinase receptor class. Pertuzumab binds instead the domain II, but both prevent dimerization of HER2 with other receptor members of HER family (homo- or heterodimerization). Pivotal early trials in 2000's association of trastuzumab with chemotherapy lead to a 1–4 % of heart failure and up to 18 % of LVEF drop when used in the adjuvant phase of treatment. Risk factors specific for trastuzumab-associated cardiotoxicity have not been clearly discovered. The analyses of the potential risk factors, including age, weight, hypertension, cumulative dose, and HER2 expression level, have revealed, however, that only age and concurrent doxorubicin therapy were significantly associated with an increased risk of cardiac disease [21]. In particular the risk is higher when the concomitant administration of anthracyclines is planned. After the introduction of trastuzumab therapy in early disease after 2005, almost all patients with HER2+ breast cancer are pretreated with anthracyclines as adjuvant therapy, so few women are anthracycline naive in metastatic setting. In the pivotal phase III trial by Slamon et al., the combination of paclitaxel and trastuzumab leads to a NYHA class III–IV cardiac dysfunction in 2 and 1 % of patients treated with paclitaxel + trastuzumab and paclitaxel alone, respectively [22]. In the pivotal phase III CLEOPATRA trial that randomly assigned 808 patients with HER2+ breast cancer to first-line treatment with trastuzumab and docetaxel plus either pertuzumab or placebo [23], combined therapy arm (triple combination) was not associated with significantly worse cardiac toxicity compared to docetaxel/trastuzumab alone. However, only a few patients had received trastuzumab in adjuvant setting. A decline of ≥10 % age points that resulted in an LVEF of <50 % occurred in 3.8 % of the pertuzumab group versus 6.6 % of the control group. Among them, 72 % of patients in the placebo arm and 87 % of those on the pertuzumab arm recovered to a normal value. The prescribing information package suggests monitoring LVEF about every 3 months. When LVEF fall to value <45 % or 45–50 % but with a ≥10 % absolute decrease below the pretreatment value, both pertuzumab and trastuzumab have to be withhold, and LVEF assessment should be repeated within approximately 3 weeks.

Endocrine Therapy (Tamoxifen, Aromatase Inhibitors, Fulvestrant)

Among hormonal therapies used for treating metastatic breast cancer, the most worrisome side effect is venous thromboembolism due to tamoxifen. It manifests as venous thrombosis or pulmonary embolism. Both aromatase inhibitors and fulvestrant are not known cardiotoxics in studies of advanced disease. Probably the limited time on treatment in metastatic patients limits the risk of vascular events.

6.2.2 Colorectal Cancer and Other Upper Gastrointestinal Malignancies

Fluoropyrimidines

The antimetabolite agents 5-fluorouracil (5-FU) and capecitabine are the cornerstone of all treatments for advanced GI cancers, either alone or in combination with oxaliplatin and irinotecan (plus or minus biological agents). Another similar agent, S-1, is now approved for treatment of advanced gastric cancer in association with cisplatin, but has the potential to be associated with lower risk of cardiotoxicity compared to 5-FU continuous infusion. Cardiotoxicity associated with these drugs is frequently reported in the literature, with rates varying according to the series reported from 1 to 20 %. The most frequent cardiac symptom due to FU is an angina-like syndrome and is associated with ECG changes. Angina is reported up to 45 % of patients with 5-FU-related cardiotoxicity, myocardial infarction, and arrhythmia in 22 % of cases. Symptoms and ECG signs usually appear within 72 h in about 70 % of cases; the mortality rate is the more rare event (up to 8 %) [24,25]. The risk seems to be related to the rate of 5-FU administration, the presence of preexisting coronary artery disease, and the use of concurrent radiation or other potentially cardiotoxic drugs (e.g., anthracyclines). It is to be noted that most cases arising in patients not known for cardiac disease and preexisting cardiac disease are not predictive of cardiotoxicity. The risk is higher with continuous infusion (both long-term and short-term schedules) compared to bolus regimens. In one series, 8 % receiving a high-dose continuous infusion of FU developed cardiotoxicity [26]. In a second study of 106 patients receiving short-term infusional 5-FU with the FOLFOX regimen, nine developed chest pain during treatment [24]. The onset was during courses one, two, six, and eight in three, four, one, and one patient(s), respectively. Rechallenge is not recommended, and substitution with other agents (e.g., raltitrexed) is suggested. A possible alternative to 5-FU in colorectal neoplasms is in fact represented by raltitrexed (Tomudex®); an inhibitor is thymidylate synthesis (TS). *Raltitrexed*, an analogue of folate, was developed as a direct and specific inhibitor of TS. Clinical studies have shown a similar activity to 5-FU in metastatic colorectal cancer although the treatment had been accompanied by gastrointestinal toxicity concerns, particularly in patients with renal failure. *Raltitrexed is currently indicated for the palliative treatment of advanced colorectal cancer where 5-FU and folinic acid are not tolerated or inappropriate.* In particular, raltitrexed seems to be an option for patients with cardiovascular risk factors. A review by Kelly et al. showed that raltitrexed is associated with a significantly reduced incidence of cardiovascular toxicity in patients with a history of cardiac toxicity or cardiac comorbidities [27]. Some case studies had been published in which patients who had experienced cardiac symptoms when treated with 5-FU had been shifted to raltitrexed without further cardiac symptoms. To such similar conclusions come Avallone and collaborators, reviewing the literature of raltitrexed which suggested a resurrection of the drug specifically for those patients who manifest cardiovascular toxicity during therapy with 5-FU or have a positive cardiovascular history [28]. From a pooled analysis of studies with upfront raltitrexed associated with oxaliplatin and irinotecan (TOMOX and TOMIRI), Barni et al. revealed a substantial clinical equivalence with standard FOLFIRI and FOLFOX with an apparent minor hematological and gastrointestinal toxicity [29]. Capecitabine is an oral fluoropyrimidine that is metabolized to 5-FU. The cardiac toxicity of capecitabine is similar to that reported with infusional 5-FU [30]. Also, patients who previously experienced cardiotoxicity with 5-FU have still a risk of toxicity with capecitabine [31,32]. The incidence of cardiotoxicity with capecitabine ranges from 3 to 9 % [33,34]. The most frequent is angina; arrhythmias, myocardial infarction, and death have also been reported [30,35–39]. It is likely that the mechanism of cardiotoxicity is similar to that seen with FU, with coronary vasospasm being the most hypnotized. In particular in a trial in which 153 patients were treated with capecitabine plus oxaliplatin for advanced colorectal cancer, 10 cases of cardiotoxicity were observed (7 %), 80 % of which occurred during the first cycle of treatment [36]. Angina occurred in 70 % of them, and there was one case each of sudden death, heart failure, and ventricular fibrillation. In a retrospective series of 78 patients treated with capecitabine, 7 (9 %) developed symptoms of chest pain or chest discomfort suggestive of cardiotoxicity [37]: none had documented preexisting heart disease. Abnormalities were present in 60 % of patients evaluated by ECG, but no elevations of cardiac enzymes were observed. Recurrent symptoms were observed in one of three patients who were rechallenged with a lower dose. In a literature-based review of 53 patients with reported capecitabine cardiotoxicity, the reaction was fatal in 6 (11 %) [39]. Rechallenge led to symptom recurrence in 10 of the 16 patients, and neither dose reduction nor medical prophylaxis influenced the outcome at rechallenge.

Anti-VEGF Agents

Bevacizumab

Bevacizumab is a monoclonal antibody against VEGF that inhibits binding of the normal VEGF ligand to its receptor. *It is approved, other than for the breast, lung, ovarian, and renal cell carcinoma, for the treatment of advanced colorectal cancer in combination with chemotherapy.* Targeting VEGF is associated with typical class effect adverse events as hypertension, thromboembolism, and more rare left ventricular dysfunction. Some events can be fatal as described by a meta-analysis of bevacizumab trials published by Ranpura et al. [4]. The risk of death (2.5 %) was only increased for combinations of bevacizumab with platinum agents or taxanes (RR = 3.49). The primary vascular adverse event reported with bevacizumab is arterial hypertension. The hypothesis for the etiopathogenesis of hypertension is linked with reduced nitric oxide production with a consequent increase in vascular resistance. In a meta-analysis of 12,949 patients treated with bevacizumab for metastatic tumors, the relative risk (RR) of developing significant rise in blood pressure (G3 or 4) was 5.38 (95 % CI 3.63–7.97) for patients treated with bevacizumab [40]. Among patients receiving bevacizumab, the overall incidence of all raised blood pressure events was 24 %, while the incidence of high-grade hypertension was 8 %. The risk was dose dependent, and the risk of G3-4 was higher for those with renal cell carcinoma (RR 13.77, 95 % CI 2.28–83.15) and breast cancer (RR 18.83, 95 % CI 1.23–292.29) who received bevacizumab at 5 mg/kg/week. In two colorectal cancer studies, the RR was 4.87. Data about the correlation of hypertension development with prognosis are controversial. Data about risk of arterial (but not venous) thromboembolic events (ATEs) are also substantial. In a meta-analyses of more than 13,000 patients, the RR of ATEs in patients receiving bevacizumab for advanced cancers was 1.46 (95 % CI 1.11–1.93) with an incidence of 2.6 % (95 % CI 2–3.5) [41]. The highest rate was seen in patients treated for colorectal cancer (3.2 %, 95 % CI 1.9–5.4). In summary, bevacizumab, at the doses labeled for treatment of advanced colorectal cancer, is associated with a small increased risk of ATEs and with a moderately increased risk of hypertension. Heart failure is rarely observed in patients not treated for breast cancer where taxanes are associated with bevacizumab. All these data have to be taken in mind when elderly or hypertensive patients are planned to be treated.

Anti-EGFR Agents

Cetuximab and Panitumumab

Anti-EGFR agents are presently used for the treatment of RAS-wt metastatic colorectal cancer, but they are not known cardiotoxic agents. They, however, are associated with magnesium wasting, probably by a reduced renal absorption, and hypomagnesemia could trigger arrhythmias [42]. Also, anti-EGFR agents are associated with an increased risk of venous but not arterial thrombosis, but the mechanism is presently unknown [43]. Cases of atrial fibrillation not certainly due to cetuximab have been described.

6.2.3 Lung Cancer

Platinum-Based Chemotherapy

Cisplatin

Cisplatin-based chemotherapy is the current standard of care for first-line treatment of advanced non-small cell lung cancer (NSCLC) in fit, good performance status patients. It is used in combination with other agents, rarely alone. Most frequent combinations used are those with gemcitabine, taxanes, or pemetrexed. Carboplatin is a platinum agent with reduced nephrotoxicity and is combined with the same agents listed above, replacing cisplatin when it is contraindicated for preexisting renal insufficiency, neuropathy, or cardiovascular diseases. Cisplatin, in fact, is a known vasculotoxic agent. Cardiac arrhythmias, myocardial infarction, and other ischemic events have also been described, frequently as a consequence of electrolyte disturbance. Cisplatin has also been associated with Raynaud's phenomenon, hypertension, and ischemic cerebral events, frequently observed in long-term survivors of testicular cancer. Patients receiving cisplatin-based chemotherapy are also at increased risk of venous but not arterial thromboembolic events (RR = 1.67, $P = 0.01$ and 1.36, and $P = 0.19$) [44–48]. In those patients with vascular morbidity, elderly or with reduced renal function substitution of cisplatin with carboplatin can be suggested.

6

Anti-EGFR and Anti-ALK TKIs

Crizotinib, a small molecule anti-ALK inhibitor, is approved for the treatment of ALK-positive advanced NSCLC after one previous treatment. The major event reported in the literature is a sinus bradycardia that is relatively frequent in patients treated with crizotinib with high-grade severity seldom reported [49,50]. In general, patients were asymptomatic, but caution should be used with the concomitant administration of beta blockers in patients treated with crizotinib. In two trials evaluating the efficacy of crizotinib for advanced NSCLC, bradycardia was reported in 12 of 240 patients, and all cases were mild (grade 1 or 2) in severity [49]. In another series of 42 patients receiving treatment with crizotinib for advanced NSCLC, there was a medium decrease of 26 beats per minute (bpm) among all patients; 69 % had at least one episode of sinus bradycardia (heart rate <60 bpm) [50]. Profound sinus bradycardia (heart rate <50 bpm) developed in 31 % of patients. None of the patients who developed bradycardia during treatment was symptomatic or had ECG changes such as QTc interval prolongation.

A QTc interval prolongation was however described with crizotinib, and the drug should be avoided in those patients with congenital long QT syndrome, heart failure, bradyarrhythmias, and electrolyte abnormalities or who are taking other agents known to prolong the QTc interval. Treatment should be temporarily discontinued if severe QTc prolongation develops and definitely discontinued if it reappears or is associated with arrhythmia, heart failure, hypotension, shock, syncope, or torsade de pointes. The suggestion is to perform an ECG at baseline in all patients treated with crizotinib in particular if they have a history of heart failure or cardiac arrhythmias and then regularly check for ECG abnormalities only if the patient develops symptoms (bradycardia) or assumes drugs that are known to cause QTc interval prolongation [51].

6.2.4 Genitourinary Cancers (Renal Cell Carcinoma and Prostate and Bladder Cancer)

Multitarget TKIs Used in Renal Cell Carcinoma

Agents used for the treatment of renal cell carcinoma (RCC) involve the angiogenesis pathway mainly through VEGFR receptor inhibition. Also, further tyrosine kinases associated receptors as PDGF, RET, KIT, and FLT-3 are targeted by a larger spectrum of activity with some drugs. With this in mind, it is expected that arterial hypertension and heart failure, the main cardiovascular effect, even if likely associated with a better outcome (biomarker predictive of efficacy), are the more frequent side effects of agents used for curing advanced RCC and targeting the VEGFR pathway. In the pivotal randomized trial that led to approval of sunitinib for advanced RCC, 21 % of patients experienced a decline in LVEF, but this was symptomatic in only 10 % [52]. All cases were reversible and not associated with an adverse clinical outcome. In a meta-analysis of the published literature that included 6936 patients receiving sunitinib for a variety of oncologic indications and who had regular cardiac function monitoring, the summary incidence of all grades of heart failure was 4.1 % with grade 3 or 4 heart failure of 1.5 % [53]. There were no differences in subgroups of patients receiving sunitinib for RCC versus other cancers. Both hypertension and a history of coronary artery disease are associated with an increased risk of sunitinib cardiotoxicity. Less data on cardiotoxicity are available with sorafenib, but the risk seems to be lower than with sunitinib. In a phase III trial of patients treated for advanced RCC, 2.9 % of patients receiving sorafenib developed cardiac ischemia or infarction compared with 0.4 % of those receiving placebo [54].

In trials of pazopanib, an oral multitarget inhibitor of several cell surface receptors as VEGFR-1, VEGFR-2, VEGFR-3 (PDGFR-alpha and PDGFR-beta), fibroblast growth factor receptor (FGFR-1 and FGFR-3), cKIT, interleukin-2 receptor inducible T-cell kinase, leukocyte-specific protein tyrosine kinase (Lck), and transmembrane glycoprotein receptor tyrosine kinase (c-Fms), approved for the upfront treatment of advanced RCC, cardiac dysfunction (decreased LVEF and clinical heart failure) has been observed. In COMPARZ trial [55], a phase III study that compared head-to-head sunitinib with pazopanib as first-line therapy for advanced RCC, symptoms of cardiac dysfunction were rare in both arms (1 %). Instead absolute decrease of ≥15 % of LEVF or >10 % but below the lower normal limit was not rare, but similar in both arms (9 versus 9 % and 7 versus 5 % with pazopanib and sunitinib, respectively).

Sunitinib and sorafenib are associated with a typical increase of blood pressure, a VEGFR class effect. In a meta-analysis of 13 studies (4999 patients treated with sunitinib for RCC or other malignancies), the overall incidence of all-grade hypertension was 22 %, with severe grades in 7 % [56]. Similar results were reported in a systematic review that analyzed the impact of hypertension in patients treated with sorafenib in nine prospective trials [57]. In a meta-analysis of trials with pazopanib [58], it was associated with higher rates of all-grade hypertension than sorafenib or sunitinib (36 versus 23 and 22 %, respectively). However, both this meta-analysis and the phase III trial led by Motzer and coll. showed similar rates of grade 3–4 events.

Sunitinib more than sorafenib is also associated with QTc prolongation [59].

Systemic Therapy Used for Prostate Cancer

LHRH Agents and Antiandrogen (Chemical Castration)

LHRH analogues alone or with antiandrogen represent the initial treatment of castration-sensitive recurrent or metastatic prostate cancer. Other than the well-known vasomotor and endocrine effects due to reduced testosterone levels, potential cardiac effects are observed. The data are contradictory, with some studies suggesting that androgen deprivation therapy (ADT) increases morbidity and/or mortality in particular in men with a cardiac disease [60–63], while others did not found a statistically significant effect [64,65]. An increased risk may be more pronounced in men who have had several (>2) previous cardiovascular disease events, especially during the first 6 months after initiation of ADT [66]. The potential benefits of ADT when it is being considered as part of the multidisciplinary treatment of prostate cancer have to be balanced with the potential cardiovascular harm, in particular in low-risk disease. No randomized trials have prospectively evaluated the risks of cardiovascular disease associated with ADT, but only retrospective data are available. A meta-analysis of eight phase III trials [67] showed that the incidence of cardiovascular death was not significantly different in those assigned to ADT compared with placebo (11.0 versus 11.2 %, relative risk 0.93, $P = 0.41$). There was no increase in risk of cardiovascular death in those who received ADT for a short (≤6 months) or long (3 years or more) duration. Furthermore, the meta-analysis found that in 11 trials with 4805 patients, both cancer-specific mortality and overall mortality were significantly decreased in those assigned to ADT compared with placebo. Another meta-analysis of eight observational studies that included approximately 415,000 men treated with ADT [68] showed that the RR for any type of cardiovascular disease in men treated with an LHRH was 1.38 (95 % CI 1.29–1.48), with similar events observed for surgical or medical castration. Also men with prostate cancer who are on ADT appear to be at increased risk of thromboembolic events (e.g., deep venous thrombosis, pulmonary embolus, arterial embolism). In a Surveillance, Epidemiology, and End Results (SEER) database analysis that included approximately 155,000 men, 38 % of whom received ADT, there was a significantly increased risk of thromboembolic events compared to those not on ADT (15 versus 7 %, HR = 1.56) [69]. Finally, Swedish authors, in an analysis that included approximately 77,000 men with prostate cancer, showed that the risk of thromboembolic events was increased in all men and that the risk was greatest in those who were treated with endocrine therapy [70]. Androgen deprivation therapy may also prolong the QT/QTc interval. Degarelix, an LHRH antagonist, seems associated to a similar risk of cardiovascular events of leuprolide in a prospective trial [71].

New Antiandrogen (Abiraterone and Enzalutamide)

New antiandrogens as abiraterone acetate and enzalutamide are now being used in the earlier castration-resistant stages, before or after chemotherapy. They reduce testosterone effect on prostate cancer cells by reduction of biosynthesis of adrenal precursors (abiraterone) or reducing its interaction with androgen receptors. The most common adverse events related to abiraterone therapy are fluid retention, hypokalemia, hypertension, and cardiac abnormalities due to 17-a hydroxylase inhibition, an enzyme involved in testosterone synthesis in the testis, adrenal glands, and the tumor itself. In the pivotal phase III trial COU-AA-301 that compared abiraterone and placebo in castration-resistant prostate cancer progressing after docetaxel, adverse effects due to elevated mineralocorticoid levels and cardiac disorders (ischemic heart disease, myocardial infarction, supraventricular arrhythmias, ventricular arrhythmias, cardiac failure, and any signs and symptoms of arrhythmia) were not significantly worse in patients receiving abiraterone than placebo (16 versus 12 %) [72]. In the companion trial in chemotherapy-naïve patients, cardiac disorders of any grade were about 20 % in both arms [73]. In a case series of 51 patients with cardiovascular comorbidities or risk factors, Procopio et al. did not found any evidence of safety alert for patients treated with abiraterone acetate [74]. In enzalutamide phase III trial in pre-docetaxel setting (castrate-resistant prostate cancer), no cardiac concerns were raised [75].

6.2.5 Rare Tumors

Imatinib Used as First-Line Therapy in GIST

Imatinib is a small molecule inhibitor of the Bcr-Abl, Kit, PDGFR, and SRC family of tyrosine kinases, and it *is approved for the treatment of gastrointestinal stromal tumors (GIST)*, which are characterized by mutations in KIT or PDGFR genes. The use of imatinib for GIST but not for chronic myeloid leukemia (another indication of imatinib) is not associated with increased risk of heart failure [76–78]. It seems that Abl inhibition handles cardiac disorders. Usually, cardiac monitoring, baseline and thereafter, is not recommended for all patients on imatinib. NCCN guidelines suggest that patients with cardiac disease or other risk factors for heart failure who are receiving imatinib should be monitored and that any patient with signs or symptoms suggestive of heart failure should be evaluated and treated accordingly [79].

Anti-BRAF Agents (Vemurafenib, Trametinib) Used in BRAF-Mutated Advanced Melanoma

Vemurafenib is an oral BRAF inhibitor approved for treatment of metastatic melanoma with a V600E BRAF mutation. Vemurafenib has been associated with prolongation of the QTc interval. Caution is recommended for use in patients with congenital long QTc syndrome or to those who are assuming drugs known to prolong the QT interval. ECG and electrolytes have to be monitored before treatment and after the start of treatment. For patients commencing vemurafenib therapy for advanced melanoma, ECGs are recommended at day 15, monthly during the first 3 months of treatment, and every 3 months after that or when clinically indicated. If the QTc interval exceeds 500 ms, treatment should be temporarily interrupted, and electrolyte abnormalities evaluated and corrected [80].

Chemotherapy Agents Used Upfront for Metastatic Sarcomas

Single agents that retain activity with more than 20 % of responses in metastatic soft tissue sarcoma are doxorubicin, epirubicin, and ifosfamide. The primary agent used for soft tissue sarcoma is single-agent doxorubicin [81]. The threshold dose for optimal activity appears to be ≥60 mg/m^2 administered every 3 weeks, with lower doses associated with inferior antitumor activity [82]. It was not demonstrated a clinically meaningful dose–response relationship with doxorubicin at doses beyond 75 mg/m^2 per cycle. Doxorubicin is associated with a well-known both acute and chronic cardiotoxicity. Infusional rather than bolus administration reduces the likelihood of cardiotoxicity. Combination chemotherapy, consisting of anthracycline + ifosfamide doublet, increases response rate but not OS, so it indicated only for fit and symptomatic patients when a rapid shrinkage of tumor mass is needed. To overcome cardiotoxicity, a liposomal formulation of doxorubicin (Caelyx ®) or use of epirubicin are indicated in high-risk patients. Although combination chemotherapies are clearly associated with greater toxicity than single-agent doxorubicin, infusional administration of doxorubicin over 3–4 days through a central venous catheter appears to reduce doxorubicin cardiotoxicity.

6.3 Recommendations

Many cytotoxic drugs and not usually for the treatment of solid tumors in first-line setting are associated with cardiovascular adverse events. In particular hypertension, heart failure, and arrhythmias are the most frequently reported. For this reason, selection of patients when starting treatment is of paramount importance. Strict collaboration with a cardiologist is needed, in particular, to reveal subclinical cardiac disease, a cardiac history, and potentially avoidable drugs with cardiac side effect. A regular check of blood pressure including basal and serial ambulatory room visits and home-based blood pressure assessment with immediate recheck or instauration of an adequate therapy is necessary for patients starting drugs with known hypertensive effect. Periodic monitoring of LEVF through an echo- or MUGA-based assessment for those cancer patients commencing agents known to depress ventricular function is also of paramount importance. Finally, avoiding or checking for drugs with known effect of cardiac rate can reduce the risk of the QTc interval prolongation. It has to be recognized that association with other drugs used in medical oncology as supportive therapies (e.g., antibiotics or antiemetics) have the potential to increase QTc interval and those must be avoided or substituted, if possible, if other agents with similar side effect have to be commenced. It is not possible to give a comprehensive indication to how frequently monitoring for cardiac toxicity. For most drugs, this information is included in the drug's package insert, where frequency and type of monitoring are described (e.g., trastuzumab or crizotinib). Another general recommendation is to avoid, if possible, cardiotoxic drugs in patients with preexisting risk factors. Many tumors are incurable in their advanced stage despite modern therapies that can improve outcome and save deaths, so using potentially equal-effective but less toxic drugs is suggested according to personal clinical judgment and after careful discussion with patients. The Hippocratic injunction *primum non nocere* remains a potent message because each medical and pharmacological have a potential risk of harm.

References

1. Kerkela R, Woulfe KC, Durand JB, Vagnozzi R, Kramer D, Chu TF, Beahm C, Chen MH, Force T. Sunitinib-induced cardiotoxicity is mediated by off-target inhibition of AMP-activated protein kinase. Clin Transl Sci. 2009;2(1):15–25.
2. Dy GK, Adjei AA. Understanding, recognizing, and managing toxicities of targeted anticancer therapies. CA Cancer J Clin. 2013;63(4):249–79.
3. Ferlay J, Soerjomataram I, Dikshit R, Eser S, Mathers C, Rebelo M, Parkin DM, Forman D, Bray F. Cancer incidence and mortality worldwide: sources, methods and major patterns in GLOBOCAN 2012. Int J Cancer. 2015;136(5):E359–86.
4. Ranpura V, Hapani S, Wu S. Treatment-related mortality with bevacizumab in cancer patients: a meta-analysis. JAMA. 2011;305(5):487–94.

5. Schutz FA, Je Y, Richards CJ, Choueiri TK. Meta-analysis of randomized controlled trials for the incidence and risk of treatment-related mortality in patients with cancer treated with vascular endothelial growth factor tyrosine kinase inhibitors. J Clin Oncol. 2012;30(8):871–7.
6. Sivendran S, Liu Z, Portas Jr LJ, Yu M, Hahn N, Sonpavde G, Oh WK, Galsky MD. Treatment-related mortality with vascular endothelial growth factor receptor tyrosine kinase inhibitor therapy in patients with advanced solid tumors: a meta-analysis. Cancer Treat Rev. 2012;38(7):919–25.
7. Zheng R, Han S, Duan C, Chen K, You Z, Jia J, Lin S, Liang L, Liu A, Long H, Wang S. Role of taxane and anthracycline combination regimens in the management of advanced breast cancer: a meta-analysis of randomized trials. Medicine (Baltimore). 2015;94(17):e803.
8. Ryberg M, Nielsen D, Skovsgaard T, et al. Epirubicin cardiotoxicity: an analysis of 469 patients with metastatic breast cancer. J Clin Oncol. 1998;16:3502.
9. Smith LA, Cornelius VR, Plummer CJ, et al. Cardiotoxicity of anthracycline agents for the treatment of cancer: systematic review and meta-analysis of randomised controlled trials. BMC Cancer. 2010; 10:337.
10. O'Brien ME, Wigler N, Inbar M, Rosso R, Grischke E, Santoro A, Catane R, Kieback DG, Tomczak P, Ackland SP, Orlandi F, Mellars L, Alland L, Tendler C, CAELYX Breast Cancer Study Group. Reduced cardiotoxicity and comparable efficacy in a phase III trial of pegylated liposomal doxorubicin HCl (CAELYX/Doxil) versus conventional doxorubicin for first-line treatment of metastatic breast cancer. Ann Oncol. 2004; 15(3):440–9.
11. Chan S, Davidson N, Juozaityte E, Erdkamp F, Pluzanska A, Azarnia N, Lee LW. Phase III trial of liposomal doxorubicin and cyclophosphamide compared with epirubicin and cyclophosphamide as first-line therapy for metastatic breast cancer. Ann Oncol. 2004;15(10):1527–34.
12. Gianni L, Munzone E, Capri G, et al. Paclitaxel by 3-hour infusion in combination with bolus doxorubicin in women with untreated metastatic breast cancer: high antitumor efficacy and cardiac effects in a dose-finding and sequence-finding study. J Clin Oncol. 1995;13:2688.
13. Gehl J, Boesgaard M, Paaske T, et al. Combined doxorubicin and paclitaxel in advanced breast cancer: effective and cardiotoxic. Ann Oncol. 1996;7:687.
14. Lluch A, Ojeda B, Colomer R, et al. Doxorubicin and paclitaxel in advanced breast carcinoma: importance of prior adjuvant anthracycline therapy. Cancer. 2000;89:2169.
15. Rahman Z, Champlin R, Rondon G, et al. Phase I/II study of dose-intense doxorubicin/paclitaxel/cyclophosphamide with peripheral blood progenitor cells and cytokine support in patients with metastatic breast cancer. Semin Oncol. 1997;24:S17.
16. Giordano SH, Booser DJ, Murray JL, et al. A detailed evaluation of cardiac toxicity: a phase II study of doxorubicin and one- or three-hour-infusion paclitaxel in patients with metastatic breast cancer. Clin Cancer Res. 2002;8:3360.
17. Biganzoli L, Cufer T, Bruning P, et al. Doxorubicin-paclitaxel: a safe regimen in terms of cardiac toxicity in metastatic breast carcinoma patients. Results from a European Organization for research and treatment of cancer multicenter trial. Cancer. 2003;97:40.
18. Malhotra V, Dorr VJ, Lyss AP, et al. Neoadjuvant and adjuvant chemotherapy with doxorubicin and docetaxel in locally advanced breast cancer. Clin Breast Cancer. 2004;5:377.
19. Nabholtz JM, Falkson C, Campos D, Szanto J, Martin M, Chan S, Pienkowski T, Zaluski J, Pinter T, Krzakowski M, Vorobiof D, Leonard R, Kennedy I, Azli N, Murawsky M, Riva A, Pouillart P, TAX 306 Study Group. Docetaxel and doxorubicin compared with doxorubicin and cyclophosphamide as first-line chemotherapy for metastatic breast cancer: results of a randomized, multicenter, phase III trial. J Clin Oncol. 2003;21(6):968–75. Erratum in: J Clin Oncol. 2003;21(10):2048.
20. Biganzoli L, Cufer T, Bruning P, Coleman R, Duchateau L, Calvert AH, Gamucci T, Twelves C, Fargeot P, Epelbaum R, Lohrisch C, Piccart MJ. Doxorubicin and paclitaxel versus doxorubicin and cyclophosphamide as first-line chemotherapy in metastatic breast cancer: the European Organization for Research and Treatment of Cancer 10961 multicenter phase III trial. J Clin Oncol. 2002;20(14):3114–21.
21. Seidman A, et al. Cardiac dysfunction in the trastuzumab clinical trials experience. J Clin Oncol. 2002;20:1215–21.
22. Slamon DJ, Leyland-Jones B, Shak S, Fuchs H, Paton V, Bajamonde A, Fleming T, Eiermann W, Wolter J, Pegram M, Baselga J, Norton L. Use of chemotherapy plus a monoclonal antibody against HER2 for metastatic breast cancer that overexpresses HER2. N Engl J Med. 2001;344(11):783–92.
23. Swain SM, Ewer MS, Cortés J, et al. Cardiac tolerability of pertuzumab plus trastuzumab plus docetaxel in patients with HER2-positive metastatic breast cancer in CLEOPATRA: a randomized, double-blind, placebo-controlled phase III study. Oncologist. 2013;18:257.

24. Jensen SA, Hasbak P, Mortensen J, Sørensen JB. Fluorouracil induces myocardial ischemia with increases of plasma brain natriuretic peptide and lactic acid but without dysfunction of left ventricle. J Clin Oncol. 2010;28:5280.
25. Saif MW, Shah MM, Shah AR. Fluoropyrimidine-associated cardiotoxicity: revisited. Expert Opin Drug Saf. 2009;8:191.
26. de Forni M, Malet-Martino MC, Jaillais P, et al. Cardiotoxicity of high-dose continuous infusion fluorouracil: a prospective clinical study. J Clin Oncol. 1992;10:1795.
27. Kelly C, Bhuva N, Harrison M, Buckley A, Saunders M. Use of raltitrexed as an alternative to 5-fluorouracil and capecitabine in cancer patients with cardiac history. Eur J Cancer. 2013;49(10):2303–10.
28. Avallone A, Di Gennaro E, Silvestro L, Iaffaioli VR, Budillon A. Targeting thymidylate synthase in colorectal cancer: critical re-evaluation and emerging therapeutic role of raltitrexed. Expert Opin Drug Saf. 2014;13(1):113–29.
29. Barni S, Ghidini A, Coinu A, Borgonovo K, Petrelli F. A systematic review of raltitrexed-based first-line chemotherapy in advanced colorectal cancer. Anticancer Drugs. 2014;25(10):1122–8.
30. Ng M, Cunningham D, Norman AR. The frequency and pattern of cardiotoxicity observed with capecitabine used in conjunction with oxaliplatin in patients treated for advanced colorectal cancer (CRC). Eur J Cancer. 2005;41:1542.
31. Frickhofen N, Beck FJ, Jung B, et al. Capecitabine can induce acute coronary syndrome similar to 5-fluorouracil. Ann Oncol. 2002;13:797.
32. Aksoy S, Karaca B, Dinçer M, Yalçin S. Common etiology of capecitabine and fluorouracil-induced coronary vasospasm in a colon cancer patient. Ann Pharmacother. 2005;39:573.
33. Van Cutsem E, Hoff PM, Blum JL, et al. Incidence of cardiotoxicity with the oral fluoropyrimidine capecitabine is typical of that reported with 5-fluorouracil. Ann Oncol. 2002;13:484.
34. Saif MW, Tomita M, Ledbetter L, Diasio RB. Capecitabine-related cardiotoxicity: recognition and management. J Support Oncol. 2008;6:41.
35. Van Cutsem E, Twelves C, Cassidy J, et al. Oral capecitabine compared with intravenous fluorouracil plus leucovorin in patients with metastatic colorectal cancer: results of a large phase III study. J Clin Oncol. 2001;19:4097.
36. Shields AF, Zalupski MM, Marshall JL, Meropol NJ. Treatment of advanced colorectal carcinoma with oxaliplatin and capecitabine: a phase II trial. Cancer. 2004;100:531.
37. Bajetta E, Di Bartolomeo M, Mariani L, et al. Randomized multicenter phase II trial of two different schedules of irinotecan combined with capecitabine as first-line treatment in metastatic colorectal carcinoma. Cancer. 2004;100:279.
38. Hoff PM, Ansari R, Batist G, et al. Comparison of oral capecitabine versus intravenous fluorouracil plus leucovorin as first-line treatment in 605 patients with metastatic colorectal cancer: results of a randomized phase III study. J Clin Oncol. 2001;19:2282.
39. Manojlovic N, Babic D, Stojanovic S, et al. Capecitabine cardiotoxicity—case reports and literature review. Hepatogastroenterology. 2008;55:1249.
40. An MM, Zou Z, Shen H, Liu P, Chen ML, Cao YB, Jiang YY. Incidence and risk of significantly raised blood pressure in cancer patients treated with bevacizumab: an updated meta-analysis. Eur J Clin Pharmacol. 2010;66(8):813–21.
41. Schutz FA, Je Y, Azzi GR, Nguyen PL, Choueiri TK. Bevacizumab increases the risk of arterial ischemia: a large study in cancer patients with a focus on different subgroup outcomes. Ann Oncol. 2011;22(6):1404–12.
42. Petrelli F, Borgonovo K, Cabiddu M, Ghilardi M, Barni S. Risk of anti-EGFR monoclonal antibody-related hypomagnesemia: systematic review and pooled analysis of randomized studies. Expert Opin Drug Saf. 2012;11 Suppl 1:S9–19.
43. Petrelli F, Cabiddu M, Borgonovo K, Barni S. Risk of venous and arterial thromboembolic events associated with anti-EGFR agents: a meta-analysis of randomized clinical trials. Ann Oncol. 2012;23(7):1672–9.
44. Lee YG, Lee E, Kim I, Lee KW, Kim TM, Lee SH, Kim DW, Heo DS. Cisplatin-based chemotherapy is a strong risk factor for thromboembolic events in small-cell lung cancer. Cancer Res Treat. 2015;47:670–5.
45. Mellema WW, van der Hoek D, Postmus PE, Smit EF. Retrospective evaluation of thromboembolic events in patients with non-small cell lung cancer treated with platinum-based chemotherapy. Lung Cancer. 2014;86(1):73–7.
46. Seng S, Liu Z, Chiu SK, Proverbs-Singh T, Sonpavde G, Choueiri TK, Tsao CK, Yu M, Hahn NM, Oh WK, Galsky MD. Risk of venous thromboembolism in patients with cancer treated with cisplatin: a systematic review and meta-analysis. J Clin Oncol. 2012;30(35):4416–26.

47. Proverbs-Singh T, Chiu SK, Liu Z, Seng S, Sonpavde G, Choueiri TK, Tsao CK, Yu M, Hahn NM, Oh WK, Galsky MD. Arterial thromboembolism in cancer patients treated with cisplatin: a systematic review and meta-analysis. J Natl Cancer Inst. 2012;104(23):1837–40.
48. Moore RA, Adel N, Riedel E, Bhutani M, Feldman DR, Tabbara NE, Soff G, Parameswaran R, Hassoun H. High incidence of thromboembolic events in patients treated with cisplatin-based chemotherapy: a large retrospective analysis. J Clin Oncol. 2011;29(25):3466–73.
49. Ou SH, Azada M, Dy J, Stiber JA. Asymptomatic profound sinus bradycardia (heart rate ≤45) in non-small cell lung cancer patients treated with crizotinib. J Thorac Oncol. 2011;6:2135.
50. Ou SH, Tong WP, Azada M, et al. Heart rate decrease during crizotinib treatment and potential correlation to clinical response. Cancer. 2013;119:1969.
51. ▸ http://ec.europa.eu/health/documents/community-register/2012/20121023124213/anx_124213_it.pdf. Accessed 10 Jun 2015.
52. Motzer RJ, Hutson TE, Tomczak P, et al. Sunitinib versus interferon alfa in metastatic renal-cell carcinoma. N Engl J Med. 2007;356:115.
53. Richards CJ, Je Y, Schutz FA, et al. Incidence and risk of congestive heart failure in patients with renal and nonrenal cell carcinoma treated with sunitinib. J Clin Oncol. 2011;29:3450.
54. Escudier B, Eisen T, Stadler WM, et al. Sorafenib in advanced clear-cell renal-cell carcinoma. N Engl J Med. 2007;356:125.
55. Motzer RJ, Hutson TE, Cella D, et al. Pazopanib versus sunitinib in metastatic renal-cell carcinoma. N Engl J Med. 2013;369(8):722–31.
56. Zhu X, Stergiopoulos K, Wu S. Risk of hypertension and renal dysfunction with an angiogenesis inhibitor sunitinib: systematic review and meta-analysis. Acta Oncol. 2009;48:9.
57. Wu S, Chen JJ, Kudelka A, et al. Incidence and risk of hypertension with sorafenib in patients with cancer: a systematic review and meta-analysis. Lancet Oncol. 2008;9:117.
58. Qi WX, Lin F, Sun YJ, Tang LN, He AN, Yao Y, Shen Z. Incidence and risk of hypertension with pazopanib in patients with cancer: a meta-analysis. Cancer Chemother Pharmacol. 2013;71(2):431–9.
59. Shah RR, Morganroth J, Shah DR. Cardiovascular safety of tyrosine kinase inhibitors: with a special focus on cardiac repolarisation (QT interval). Drug Saf. 2013;36(5):295–316.
60. Nanda A, Chen MH, Braccioforte MH, Moran BJ, D'Amico AV. Hormonal therapy use for prostate cancer and mortality in men with coronary artery disease-induced congestive heart failure or myocardial infarction. JAMA. 2009;302(8):866–73.
61. Tsai HK, D'Amico AV, Sadetsky N, Chen MH, Carroll PR. Androgen deprivation therapy for localized prostate cancer and the risk of cardiovascular mortality. J Natl Cancer Inst. 2007;99(20):1516–24.
62. Saigal CS, Gore JL, Krupski TL, Hanley J, Schonlau M, Litwin MS, Urologic Diseases in America Project. Androgen deprivation therapy increases cardiovascular morbidity in men with prostate cancer. Cancer. 2007;110(7):1493–500.
63. Keating NL, O'Malley AJ, Freedland SJ, Smith MR. Diabetes and cardiovascular disease during androgen deprivation therapy: observational study of veterans with prostate cancer. J Natl Cancer Inst. 2010;102(1):39–46. doi:10.1093/jnci/djp404. Epub 2009 Dec 7. Erratum in: J Natl Cancer Inst. 2012;104(19):1518–23.
64. Keating NL, O'Malley AJ, Smith MR. Diabetes and cardiovascular disease during androgen deprivation therapy for prostate cancer. J Clin Oncol. 2006;24(27):4448–56.
65. Alibhai SM, Duong-Hua M, Sutradhar R, Fleshner NE, Warde P, Cheung AM, Paszat LF. Impact of androgen deprivation therapy on cardiovascular disease and diabetes. J Clin Oncol. 2009;27(21):3452–8.
66. O'Farrell S, Garmo H, Holmberg L, Adolfsson J, Stattin P, Van Hemelrijck M. Risk and timing of cardiovascular disease after androgen-deprivation therapy in men with prostate cancer. J Clin Oncol. 2015;33(11):1243–51.
67. Nguyen PL, Je Y, Schutz FA, Hoffman KE, Hu JC, Parekh A, Beckman JA, Choueiri TK. Association of androgen deprivation therapy with cardiovascular death in patients with prostate cancer: a meta-analysis of randomized trials. JAMA. 2011;306(21):2359–66.
68. Bosco C, Bosnyak Z, Malmberg A, et al. Quantifying observational evidence for risk of fatal and nonfatal cardiovascular disease following androgen deprivation therapy for prostate cancer: a meta-analysis. Eur Urol. 2014;68:386–96.
69. Ehdaie B, Atoria CL, Gupta A, et al. Androgen deprivation and thromboembolic events in men with prostate cancer. Cancer. 2012;118:3397.
70. Van Hemelrijck M, Adolfsson J, Garmo H, et al. Risk of thromboembolic diseases in men with prostate cancer: results from the population-based PCBaSe Sweden. Lancet Oncol. 2010;11:450.

71. Smith MR, Klotz L, Persson BE, Olesen TK, Wilde AA. Cardiovascular safety of degarelix: results from a 12-month, comparative, randomized, open label, parallel group phase III trial in patients with prostate cancer. J Urol. 2010;184(6):2313–9.
72. Fizazi K, Scher HI, Molina A, Logothetis CJ, Chi KN, Jones RJ, Staffurth JN, North S, Vogelzang NJ, Saad F, Mainwaring P, Harland S, Goodman Jr OB, Sternberg CN, Li JH, Kheoh T, Haqq CM, de Bono JS, COU-AA-301 Investigators. Abiraterone acetate for treatment of metastatic castration-resistant prostate cancer: final overall survival analysis of the COU-AA-301 randomised, double-blind, placebo-controlled phase 3 study. Lancet Oncol. 2012;13(10):983–92.
73. Ryan CJ, Smith MR, Fizazi K, Saad F, Mulders PF, Sternberg CN, Miller K, Logothetis CJ, Shore ND, Small EJ, Carles J, Flaig TW, Taplin ME, Higano CS, de Souza P, de Bono JS, Griffin TW, De Porre P, Yu MK, Park YC, Li J, Kheoh T, Naini V, Molina A, Rathkopf DE, COU-AA-302 Investigators. Abiraterone acetate plus prednisone versus placebo plus prednisone in chemotherapy-naive men with metastatic castration-resistant prostate cancer (COU-AA-302): final overall survival analysis of a randomised, double-blind, placebo-controlled phase 3 study. Lancet Oncol. 2015;16(2):152–60.
74. Procopio G, Grassi P, Testa I, Verzoni E, Torri V, Salvioni R, Valdagni R, de Braud F. Safety of abiraterone acetate in castration-resistant prostate cancer patients with concomitant cardiovascular risk factors. Am J Clin Oncol. 2013;38:479–82.
75. Scher HI, Fizazi K, Saad F, Taplin ME, Sternberg CN, Miller K, de Wit R, Mulders P, Chi KN, Shore ND, Armstrong AJ, Flaig TW, Fléchon A, Mainwaring P, Fleming M, Hainsworth JD, Hirmand M, Selby B, Seely L, de Bono JS, AFFIRM Investigators. Increased survival with enzalutamide in prostate cancer after chemotherapy. N Engl J Med. 2012;367(13):1187–97.
76. Verweij J, Casali PG, Kotasek D, et al. Imatinib does not induce cardiac left ventricular failure in gastrointestinal stromal tumours patients: analysis of EORTC-ISG-AGITG study 62005. Eur J Cancer. 2007;43:974.
77. Dematteo RP, Ballman KV, Antonescu CR, et al. Adjuvant imatinib mesylate after resection of localised, primary gastrointestinal stromal tumour: a randomised, double-blind, placebo-controlled trial. Lancet. 2009;373:1097.
78. Trent JC, Patel SS, Zhang J, et al. Rare incidence of congestive heart failure in gastrointestinal stromal tumor and other sarcoma patients receiving imatinib mesylate. Cancer. 2010;116:184.
79. National Comprehensive Cancer Network (NCCN). NCCN clinical practice guidelines in oncology. http://www.nccn.org/professionals/physician_gls/f_guidelines.asp. Accessed 01 May 2015.
80. Kim G, McKee AE, Ning YM, Hazarika M, Theoret M, Johnson JR, Xu QC, Tang S, Sridhara R, Jiang X, He K, Roscoe D, McGuinn WD, Helms WS, Russell AM, Miksinski SP, Zirkelbach JF, Earp J, Liu Q, Ibrahim A, Justice R, Pazdur R. FDA approval summary: vemurafenib for treatment of unresectable or metastatic melanoma with the BRAFV600E mutation. Clin Cancer Res. 2014;20(19):4994–5000.
81. Borden EC, Amato DA, Rosenbaum C, et al. Randomized comparison of three adriamycin regimens for metastatic soft tissue sarcomas. J Clin Oncol. 1987;5:840.
82. Judson I, Radford JA, Harris M, et al. Randomised phase II trial of pegylated liposomal doxorubicin (DOXIL/CAELYX) versus doxorubicin in the treatment of advanced or metastatic soft tissue sarcoma: a study by the EORTC Soft Tissue and Bone Sarcoma Group. Eur J Cancer. 2001;37:870.
83. Van Cutsem E, Findlay M, Osterwalder B, et al. Capecitabine, an oral fluoropyrimidine carbamate with substantial activity in advanced colorectal cancer: results of a randomized phase II study. J Clin Oncol. 2000;18:1337.

The Pharmacologist's Point of View: Mechanisms of Cardiotoxicity

Barbara Bassani, Antonino Bruno, Nicoletta Macrì, Paola Corradino, Douglas M. Noonan, and Adriana Albini

Barbara Bassani and Antonino Bruno contributed equally with all other contributors

C. Lestuzzi et al. (eds.), *Manual of Cardio-oncology*, DOI 10.1007/978-3-319-40236-9_7

7.1 Introduction

Cancer chemotherapy has made remarkable advances in the treatment of both solid and hematologic malignancies, and significant progress has been achieved in the reduction of recurrences. However, many anticancer treatments present a risk of side effects on the cardiovascular system [1]. The phenomenon of cardiovascular toxicity has become more evident with increased survival and longer life expectancy in oncology patients. In this scenario, cardiotoxicity is one of the most important adverse reactions of chemotherapy, leading to an increase in morbidity and mortality [2]. According to the NIH cancer dictionary (▸ www.cancer.gov/dictionary/Cardiotoxicity), "cardiotoxicity" is a general term used to define "toxicity that affects the heart." Nevertheless, a clear and unique definition for "cardiotoxicity," and in particular the identification/clarification of the mechanisms involved, is lacking. Chemotherapy-induced cardiotoxicity refers both to direct effects of the chemotherapy on the entire cardiovascular compartment and also to an indirect effects associated with the thrombogenic status or hemodynamic flow alterations as a consequence of drug administration [3]. Two main categories of cardiotoxicity have been described and conventionally recognized [4]:

1. Type I cardiotoxicity, which is generally induced by anthracycline treatment. It is known to be irreversible, dose related, and caused by free radical formation, oxidant stress, and myofibrillar disarray.
2. Type II cardiotoxicity, observed with some "biological" therapy, mainly studied for trastuzumab, has been described as reversible, not dose related, and not associated with ultrastructural abnormalities.

The major side effects associated with chemotherapy-induced cardiotoxicity include arrhythmias, myocardial ischemia, coronary artery disease, hypertension, and myocardial dysfunction [3]. Heart failure incidence rates associated with the widely prescribed chemotherapy agents range from 0.14 to 48 % for anthracyclines, 7 to 28 % for high-dose cyclophosphamides, 1 % for trastuzumab, and 8 to 12.5 % for tyrosine kinase inhibitors [5]. Cardiotoxicity, which can occur up to 20 years after treatment, is likely to become even more prevalent as the cancer population ages and novel "targeted" treatment regimens, which can cause damage to cardiac myocytes, are more commonly employed [6].

Cardiac dysfunction related chemotherapy associates with cardiomyocyte phenotype alterations, involving cellular and molecular mechanisms. Crucial among these are the induction of cell death (apoptosis/necrosis), formation of autophagic vesicles (AVOS), induction of reactive oxygen species (ROS), senescence, and morphological arrangements [7]. In the era of OMICS, deep sequencing, and personalized medicine, the monitoring of all these cellular and molecular events, occurring during cardiotoxicity, clearly represents a crucial hub either for intervention or preventive approaches. In this scenario, cardio-oncology, the new discipline joining together the oncologist and cardiologist, is a necessary field in cancer therapy and prevention of chemotherapy-associated cardiotoxicity [8]. Here we will discuss the cellular and molecular alterations occurring in the chemotherapy-induced cardiotoxicity, focusing on the main anticancer agent categories clinically employed in cancer treatment and the screening approaches required (◘ Fig. 7.1).

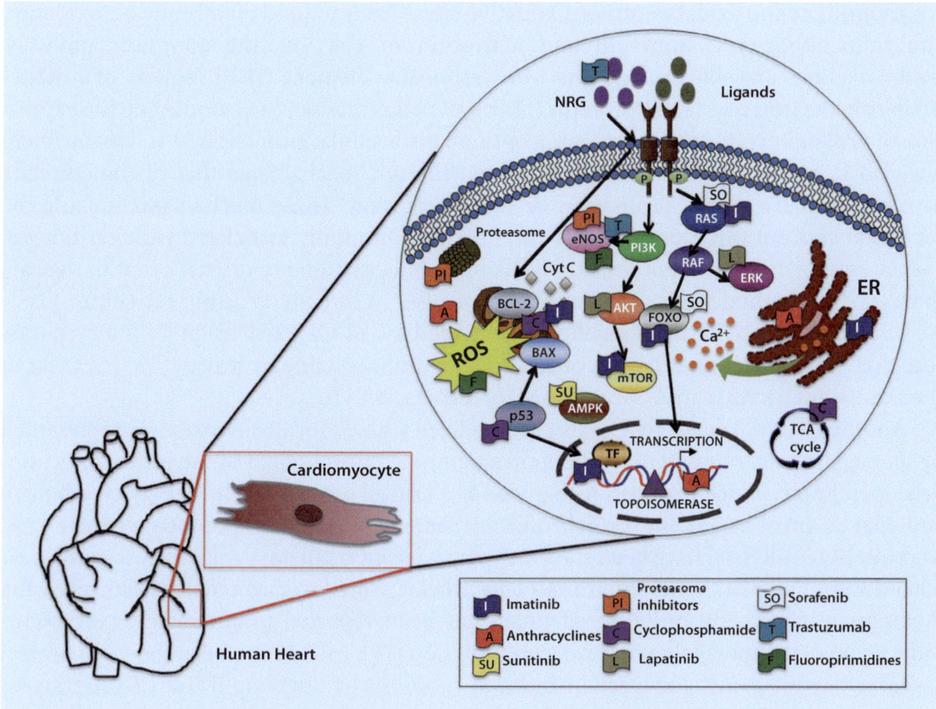

Fig. 7.1 Selected molecular mechanisms associated with chemotherapy-induced cardiotoxicity

7.2 Anticancer Agents Associated with Cardiotoxicity

7.2.1 Anthracyclines

Anthracyclines (doxorubicin, idarubicin, daunorubicin) are antineoplastic agents whose mechanisms of actions include intercalation into the nuclear DNA, affecting the topoisomerase II DNA-repairing activity, thus resulting in cell death [9].

Cardiotoxicity effects associated with the administration of anthracyclines involve left ventricular dysfunction (LVD) and heart failure (HF). It has been reported that anthracycline cumulative doses of 200 mg/m^2 precede left ventricular (LV) systolic dysfunction [10, 11]. Anthracycline single dose, intravenous bolus administration, and combination therapy either with pharmacological or with radiotherapy are relevant risk factors contributing to the induction of cardiotoxicity [12]. Molecular mechanisms associated with anthracycline-induced cardiotoxicity account for impaired protein synthesis, the inhibition of DNA-repair response, formation of ROS, and deregulation of calcium homeostasis [13].

In particular, the enhanced production of ROS due to anthracycline metabolism has been reported as the classical mechanism of cardiotoxicity. Indeed, doxorubicin cycles between the quinone and the semi-quinone radical structure is able to react with oxygen (O_2), generating superoxide (O_2^{-*}) and hydrogen peroxide (OH^-) and directly promoting DNA damage. Moreover, the semi-quinone form of doxorubicin is also able to trigger the release and accumulation of iron, leading to the production of hydroxyl radicals, further contributing to the oxidative stress. Oxidative stress leads to lipid membrane peroxidation and mitochondrial dysfunction and activation of the intrinsic apoptosis pathway. Anthracyclines are able to bind the iron-responsive element (IRE) regions of mRNAs inhibiting the iron regulatory proteins (IRPs)/IREs interaction, thus modifying the expression of proteins crucial for maintaining optimal intracellular iron levels [14]. Doxorubicin has also been reported to induce apoptosis through mechanisms that do not directly involved oxidative stress promotion or ROS formation. These mechanisms include the increased concentration of calcium (Ca^{2+}) that is commonly associated with cardiotoxic events, supporting the hypothesis that calcium dysregulation is a crucial event in the cardiomyopathy pathogenesis. The reduction of SERCA2a (sarcoplasmic reticulum Ca^{2+}-ATPase 2a)-mediated Ca^{2+} reuptake and the increase of Ca^{2+} extrusion by the rynodine receptor (RyR2) were phenomena observed after anthracycline treatment [13, 15] as far as the significant increase in ANF and b-MHC expression [16].

Another relevant factor that is closely correlated with doxorubicin toxicity is represented by the high affinity binding to cardiolipin, an anionic phospholipid of the inner mitochondrial membrane, which has been recognized as a crucial protein for the energy metabolism and that is involved in the cytochrome c release and related apoptosis process [14]. MicroRNAs (miRNAs) have been shown to play relevant regulatory roles in both cardiovascular disease and cancer. Several miRNAs have been related to cardiotoxic effects following doxorubicin treatment. miR208a silencing has been reported to attenuate doxorubicin-induced myocyte apoptosis and cardiac dysfunction [17]. miR-21 has been shown to protect cardiomyocytes against doxorubicin-induced apoptosis by targeting BTG2 (B-cell translocation gene 2) [18]. miR-30 overexpression has been shown to protect cardiac cells from doxorubicin-induced apoptosis, and its maintenance represents a potential cardioprotective strategy to prevent cardiotoxic events associated with anthracyclines [19].

Several antioxidant molecules have been largely used in association with anthracyclines to limit chemotherapy-induced CV damages. The combination of anthracyclines plus the antioxidant dexrazoxane has been reported to reduce cardiotoxic events and the incidence of HF [20]. One rather controversial study showed that it might affect anticancer efficacy [3] although there is a good evidence for its clinical use. Several studies using the antioxidant carvedilol [21], as well as the angiotensin-converting enzyme inhibitor enalapril in combination with anthracyclines, have shown promising prevention activity in treated patients [22, 23].

7.2.2 Fluoropyrimidines

5-Fluorouracil and its prodrugs, capecitabine and tegafur, are cytotoxic agents that belong to the antimetabolite class, widely employed as first-line treatment for various solid tumors (gastrointestinal, gynecological, head and neck, breast carcinomas) [24] and adjuvant treatment of late-stage colon carcinoma and metastatic breast cancer [25]. Fluoropyrimidines act by inhibiting thymidylate synthase (TS), the enzyme-producing thymidine monophosphate (ThMP) that is required for DNA synthesis, leading to the inhibition of DNA replication. Therapy with fluoropyrimidines can have a range of adverse effects: diarrhea, dehydration, abdominal pain, nausea, stomatitis, and hand and foot syndrome. Some patients can also experience different levels of cardiac dysfunctions, including ischemic syndrome, arrhythmias and fibrillation, tachycardia, electrographic alterations, angina, and heart attack, and in a few cases, also sudden cardiac death can occur [26].

The incidence of adverse cardiac events associated with 5-FU is in the range of 1.6–7.6 % [11]. Cardiac toxicities in patients receiving 5-FU varies widely: coronary vasospasms and subsequent calcium antagonist non-responding angina are the most common, followed by myocardial infarction, ischemia, dysrhythmia, cardiomyopathy, takotsubo cardiomyopathy, sinoatrial and atrioventricular nodal dysfunction, QT prolongation with torsades de pointes, ventricular tachycardia, cardiac arrest, and sudden death [3, 4, 25–32]. Clinical manifestations include chest pain, ST-T wave electrocardiogram (ECG) changes, supraventricular/ventricular arrhythmias, and angina [3]. The molecular mechanisms involved in fluoropyrimidine analog-induced cardiovascular toxicity have been widely investigated, and several hypotheses have been proposed, including accumulation of metabolites, global dysfunction, thrombus formation, autoimmune-mediated injury of the myocardium, endothelial damage, and direct cardiomyocyte toxicity [33]. It has also been reported that 5-FU enhances nitric oxide synthase (NOS) activity [34] leading to coronary spasms and endothelium-independent vasoconstriction through protein kinase C induction. Moreover, ROS production has been speculated as a possible molecular mechanism through which 5-FU induces cardiotoxicity. Increased intracellular levels of ROS have been observed after 5-FU and capecitabine treatment [7], leading to cardiomyocyte damage associated with mitochondrial membrane potential impairment, lipid peroxidation, and GSH depletion. These events promote mitochondrial membrane depolarization and cytochrome c release, resulting in caspase-3 activation or necrosis, pending on cellular ATP level. In contrast, 5-FU, but not capecitabine, is able to induce a severe lysosomal membrane damage [35]. Autophagic features, either at the ultrastructural or molecular levels, have been described in 5-FU exposed human cardiomyocytes, and induction of a senescent phenotype has been observed for cardiomyocytes, smooth muscles, and endothelial cells suggesting involvement of the entire CV compartment [7, 36]. Molecularly, the deficiency of dihydropyrimidine dehydrogenase (DPD), a key enzyme involved in 5-FU and capecitabine metabolism, accounts for at least 50 % of 5-FU-induced toxicity [37, 38]. Epidemiological studies described more than 50 genetic polymorphisms that are associated with the impairment of DPD enzymatic activity. Among all, the c.1905+1G>A point mutation is the most commonly observed (52 % of cases), with a prevalence of heterozygosity in the general population ranging between 1 and 2 % [37, 38]. Another common mutation, the IVS14+1G>A, has been associated with a higher risk of 5-FU-induced toxicity [37, 38].

7.2.3 Microtubule-Targeting Agents

Taxanes (paclitaxel and docetaxel) are cytotoxic agents used in the treatment of advanced breast and ovarian cancers and several other solid tumors [11]. These drugs are able to exert their biological activity by impairing microtubule function necessary for cell division. Taxanes have been reported to be associated with early arrhythmia, sinus bradycardia, hypotension, CHF, ischemia and LVD, and HF induction with a 5–15 % incidence with paclitaxel and a 2.3–8 % incidence with docetaxel [10, 39]. The massive histamine release induced by paclitaxel has been proposed as the possible molecular mechanism on the basis of cardiotoxicity. Indeed, in vivo studies demonstrated that stimulation of histamine receptors in cardiac tissues resulted in conduction disorders and arrhythmias [3]. Alternatively, paclitaxel-induced cardiotoxicity could be associated with the induction of cardiac muscle alteration due to subcellular organelle damage [40].

7.2.4 Alkylating Agents

Cyclophosphamide is an alkylating agent employed in the bladder and lung cancer treatment as well as for sarcomas and chronic myelogenous leukemia [41]. This drug has been reported to induce an acute myopericarditis as well as LVD in 7–22% of treated patients [6] and to promote hemorrhagic myocarditis development [42].

Although the precise molecular mechanisms associated with cyclophosphamide-induced cardiotoxicity have not been elucidated, it has been hypothesized that the oxidative stress and related lipid peroxidation caused by its metabolites play a crucial role in the CV toxicity onset. Indeed, ROS production has been observed to induce a direct damage on the endothelial capillary, with an associated extravasation of proteins and erythrocytes. Further, capillary microthrombosis and fibrin deposition in myocardial interstitium have been observed after cyclophosphamide treatment. Ultrastructural analysis by electron microscopy revealed hypercontraction bands, myofibrillar damage, lysis, intramitochondrial electron dense inclusions, and fibrin deposition in the myocyte cytoplasm [43].

An in vivo study suggested that cyclophosphamide treatment is able to increase the mRNA expression levels of several proapoptotic genes, including p53 and Bax and decreases antiapoptotic genes, i.e., Bcl2 in the myocardium. Cyclophosphamide treatment also induces a downregulation of glutathione peroxidase, catalase, and superoxide dismutase antioxidant enzymes in cardiac tissues and decrease ATP levels promoting an alteration of ATP/ADP balance [44]. Moreover, cyclophosphamide administration has been shown to induce a decrease of tricarboxylic acid (TCA) cycle enzymes including succinate dehydrogenase, malate dehydrogenase, and isocitrate dehydrogenase in treated rats and to interfere with lipid metabolizing enzyme activity, inducing an increase of free cholesterol, esterified cholesterol, and triglycerides in the cardiac tissue [45]. Serum low-density lipoprotein (LDL) and very-low-density lipoprotein (VLDL) levels have been reported to significantly increase in response to cyclophosphamide treatment, while a decrease of high-density lipoprotein (HDL) comparing with control animals has been observed following treatment [45, 46].

7.2.5 Proteasome Inhibitors

Proteasome inhibitors, including bortezomib and carfilzomib, are agents approved for the treatment of hematologic malignancies (multiple myeloma and non-Hodgkin lymphoma). Proteasome inhibitors are able to interfere with the degradation of several proteins involved in cell cycle, proliferation, and apoptosis regulation leading to increased smooth muscle cell and endothelial progenitor cell death [47, 48]. The incidence of clinical HF has been stated between 2 and 5% [48] in patients treated with proteasome inhibitors (◘ Table 7.1).

In vitro studies have demonstrated that bortezomib-associated cardiotoxicity produces ultrastructural alterations of cardiomyocyte mitochondria, which lead to decreased ATP synthesis and contractile dysfunction. Proteasome inhibition is also associated with the accumulation of poly-ubiquitinated proteins, which induce ER stress and autophagic processes with increased binding immunoglobulin proteins (BIPs) and microtubule-associated protein light chain 3 (LC3) levels in rat cardiomyocytes treated with bortezomib [49]. Moreover, these drugs have been demonstrated to impair eNOS activity promoting coronary vasospasm induction [48].

Table 7.1 List of some clinical manifestations and selected molecular mechanisms associated with chemotherapy-induced cardiotoxicity

Drug	Some clinical manifestations	Selected molecular mechanisms
Anthracyclines		
Doxorubicin	LVD, HF, and LV	Oxidative stress induction
		Iron accumulation
		Activation of the intrinsic apoptosis
		Calcium dysregulation
		miRNAs
Tyrosine kinase inhibitors		
Trastuzumab	LVD and HF	NRG-1b modulation
		Oxidative and nitrosative stress induction
		Angiotensin II upregulation
		Modulation of Notch and NF-kB pathways
Lapatinib	QT prolongation and LVEF	RAS/RAF and PI3K/AKT inhibition
		ABC inhibition
		Mitochondrial damages and fibrosis induction
Imatinib mesilate	LVEF and HF	Impairment of survival pathways
		ER stress induction
		Induction of proapoptotic signaling
		Mitochondrial dysfunction
VEGFR inhibitors		
Bevacizumab	Hypertension and HF, proteinuria	Decreased eNOS activity
		PAI-1 increased activity
		miRNAs
Tyrosine kinase inhibitors targeting the VEGF pathway		
Sunitinib	Hypertension, QT prolongation, and HF	Inhibition of RSK
		Inactivation of AMPK
		Intrinsic apoptosis induction
		Decrease of PDGFR-b expression and NG2 pericyte markers

(continued)

Table 7.1 (continued)

Drug	Some clinical manifestations	Selected molecular mechanisms
Sorafenib	LVD and HF	RAF1 and BRAF inhibition
		MST2 inhibition
		Activation of JNK, FOXO, BAX, and LATS1 proapoptotic proteins
Other VEGF-targeting TKIs	QTcF interval, QT prolongation	BRAF inhibition
Fluoropyrimidines		
5-FU	Chest pain, ST-T ECG changes, supraventricular/ventricular arrhythmias, and angina	Accumulation of metabolites
		Global dysfunction
		Thrombus formation
		Autoimmune-mediated injury of the myocardium
		Endothelial damage
		Direct cardiomyocytes toxicity
		Increased eNOS activity
		Mitochondrial membrane potential impairment
		Lipid peroxidation
		GSH depletion
		Lysosomal membrane damage
		Autophagic induction
		Senescence induction
Microtubule-targeting agents		
Paclitaxel	Early arrhythmia, sinus bradycardia, hypotension, CHF, ischemia and LVD, and HF	Massive histamine release
		Induction of cardiac muscle alteration
		Subcellular organelle damages

Table 7.1 (continued)

Drug	Some clinical manifestations	Selected molecular mechanisms
Proteasome inhibitors		
Bortezomib	HF	Alterations of cardiomyocyte mitochondria
		Decreased ATP synthesis
		Contractile dysfunctions
		Accumulation of poly-ubiquitinated proteins
		ER stress induction
		Autophagic process induction
		Impairment of eNOS activity
Alkylating agents		
Cyclophosphamide	LVD and hemorrhagic myocarditis	Oxidative stress induction
		Lipid peroxidation
		Direct damage on the endothelial capillary
		Extravasation of proteins and erythrocytes
		Capillary microthrombosis and fibrin deposition
		Hypercontraction bands
		Myofibrillar damages
		Lysis
		Intramitochondrial electron dense inclusions
		Fibrin deposition
		Increased mRNA expression levels of proapoptotic genes
		Downregulation of antioxidant enzymes
		Alteration of ATP/ADP balance
		Alteration of TCA cycle enzymes

7.2.6 Tyrosine Kinase Inhibitors

Trastuzumab

Trastuzumab is a humanized monoclonal antibody, currently employed as first-line treatment for patients with metastatic $HER2^+$ breast cancer. This antibody is able to selectively target the human epidermal growth factor receptor 2 (HER2)/ErbB2 protein, inhibiting the related signaling pathways. The administration of trastuzumab can be associated with the development of LVD and HF with an incidence of 2–28 %, with an increased risk in combination therapy with anthracyclines [6].

Physiologically, the HER2 pathway affected by trastuzumab plays a crucial role in the adaptation and stress response and is essential for cell proliferation during the development and for contractile function in the adult. Thus the ability of the antibody to interfere with this process may explain the induction of CV toxicity [50].

At the molecular level, HER2 has been reported to interfere with the activity of neuregulin-1b (NRG-1b), a protein with antioxidant and antiapoptotic properties, which is further able to enhance eNOS levels in cardiomyocytes through the activation of the PI3K/AKT pathway, preserving cells from apoptosis induced by oxidative stress [14, 51].

Recent studies suggest that trastuzumab treatment induces significant effects on the myocardial gene expression, leading to an increased oxidative and nitro-oxidative stress. These events are correlated with the enhancement of serum troponin I and cardiac myosin light chain-1 (cMLC1) levels, which represents two of the major biomarkers of cardiotoxicity [52, 53]. Enhanced levels of ROS determine an increase of angiotensin II that leads to vasoconstriction and deregulation of NRG in cardiac microvasculature, inducing the activation of nicotinamide adenine dinucleotide phosphate oxidase (NADPH) which further increases the accumulation of ROS [16, 54]. A relevant molecular mechanism of trastuzumab-induced cardiotoxicity is represented by Notch and NF-kB pathways. In the cardiac context, the Notch regulates CV development and homeostasis and plays a role in regulating cardiac hypertrophy, cardiomyopathy, and heart failure [55]. Although the relationship between the Notch and ErbB2 remains still unclear, it has been recently demonstrated that Notch-1 may be considered as a novel target in trastuzumab-resistant breast cancer, suggesting a potential correlation between these two molecular signaling pathways [55].

Lapatinib

The dual tyrosine kinase inhibitor lapatinib, which has been shown to inhibit both ErbB1 and ErbB2 receptors, has been reported to induce QT prolongation and to promote LVEF reduction in 1.6 % of treated patients [11]. In vitro treatment with lapatinib alone induced slight damages on rat cardiomyocytes by inhibiting the signal transduction to RAS/RAF MAPKs, mainly decreasing ERK phosphorylation and PI3K/AKT pathway and affecting ATP-binding cassette (ABC) activity [56]. The inhibition of survival pathways leads to enhanced apoptosis and reduction of cell proliferation. At the ultrastructural level, lapatinib is able to induce mitochondrial damages in the myocardium of treated mice and has been observed to promote cardiac fibrosis [57].

Imatinib

Imatinib mesilate is a TKI approved for the treatment of several solid and hematologic malignancies, in particular chronic myelogenous leukemia (CML) due to its ability to inhibit BCR–ABL-dependent phosphorylation. It has been shown to induce a LVEF reduction in 0.5–1.7 % in treated patients [58]. At the molecular level, the inhibition of

BCR–ABL phosphorylation prevents the activation of related molecular antiapoptotic pathways, including Ras–ERK, phosphatidylinositol 3-kinase (PI3K)–Akt-mTOR, and signal transducer and activator of transcription 5 (STAT5) proteins [13]. These pro-survival signaling pathways physiologically enhance the expression of several antiapoptotic proteins, including *BCL2* and *BCL-X*, and reduce the activity of proapoptotic proteins as BAD and FOXO3A, suggesting a key role for mitochondrial dysfunction in the cardiotoxic response to imatinib [13, 59]. In cardiomyocytes, imatinib has been reported to induce endoplasmic reticulum (ER) stress [60] which enhances the activation of the PKR-like ER kinase (PERK) and IRE1 pathways and the overexpression of protein kinase Cδ (PKCδ). PERK phosphorylation leads to the activation of the eukaryotic translation initiation factor 2α (EIF2α), resulting in Jun N-terminal kinases (JNKs) and 14-3-3-mediated apoptosis [61].

VEGFR Inhibitors

VEGFR inhibitors include antibodies, soluble traps, and small-molecule tyrosine kinase inhibitors (TKIs) that have been reported to affect the cardiovascular system in various ways.

Bevacizumab

Bevacizumab is a monoclonal antibody anti-vascular endothelial growth factor (VEGF) studied for the treatment of colorectal, renal, breast, lung, and ovarian cancers [10] in combination with standard therapy. Hypertension is a common side effect in patients treated with bevacizumab; however, low incidence (1–3%) of clinical HF has been observed after treatment [6]. The mechanisms of anti-VEGF therapy hypertension remain unclear; currently it is thought to be associated with the decreased eNOS activity, which leads to reduced NO levels in the arterioles promoting vasoconstriction and reduced sodium excretion, increasing peripheral vascular resistance and blood pressure. Inhibition of eNOS may enhance plasminogen activator inhibitor-1 (PAI-1) expression, leading to an increased risk of hypertension [3]. Along with hypertension, proteinuria represents a common side effect associated with bevacizumab administration [62]. A significant higher risk of all-grade proteinuria and severe grade bleeding has been observed in patients receiving high-dose of BV compared with patients treated with low-dose BV. When comparing the risk of adverse drug responses between low and high doses of BV, the relative risks of all-grade proteinuria (2.64; 95% CI, 1.29–5.40 versus 9.24; 95% CI, 6.60–12.94) and severe grade bleeding (1.36; 95% CI, 1.05–1.75 versus 2.87; 95% CI, 1.97–4.18) has been found to be significantly increased when switching from 2.5 to 5 mg/kg BV [62, 63].

Several miRNA levels have been found to be modulated as a consequence of bevacizumab treatment associated with CV side effects. miR1254 and miR579 have been reported to be significantly increased in patients with bevacizumab-induced cardiotoxicity compared with healthy bevacizumab-treated controls, suggesting the potential role of miRNAs as relevant biomarkers for cardiotoxicity identification and prevention [64].

Tyrosine Kinase Inhibitors Targeting the VEGF Pathway

Sunitinib, sorafenib, pazopanib, vandetanib, regorafenib, axitinib, and cabozantinib are nonselective tyrosine kinase inhibitors targeting the VEGF pathway as well as other tyrosine kinase pathways, approved for the treatment of renal cell carcinoma, hepatocellular carcinoma, colorectal cancer, medullary thyroid cancer, and gastrointestinal stromal tumors [65, 66]. All agents inhibiting the VEGF pathway show several common side effects, in particular hypertension, venous thrombosis, gastrointestinal perforation, and hemorrhage [65, 67]. Malignant hypertension is the most frequently reported CV toxicity with all VEGF inhibitors, and the mechanisms appear to be the same that for bevacizumab. Sunitinib and sorafenib were the first approved drugs in this category, thus more is known concerning their side effects. Cardiotoxic events, which include hypertension, QT prolongation, and clinical HF, have been observed following sunitinib treatment [10], while sorafenib has been reported to induce LVD and HF [68]. The molecular mechanisms involved in TKI-induced cardiotoxicity remain still unclear; several hypotheses have been proposed.

Sunitinib

Sunitinib cardiotoxic events may be associated with the inhibition of ribosomal S6 kinase (RSK), which promotes the release of the proapoptotic factor BCL2-antagonist of cell death (BAD), resulting in the activation of the intrinsic apoptotic pathway and ATP depletion. In addition, sunitinib mediates the inactivation of AMP-activating kinase (AMPK) [69, 70], by increasing energy consumption due to protein translation and lipid biosynthesis, thus affecting eukaryotic elongation factor-2 (EEF2), mammalian target of rapamycin (mTOR), and/or acetyl-coenzyme A carboxylase (ACC) activity [13]. These effects promote hypertrophy and LV dysfunction. AMPK plays also a crucial role in the hypoxic environment, preserving cardiomyocytes during ischemia [13]; thus, inhibition of AMPK would lead to hypersensitivity to hypoxia-induced cardiomyocyte death. A recent in vivo study has identified pericytes as the key target of sunitinib-induced cardiotoxicity, revealing that the treatment with this drug induced a decrease of PDGFR-β expression and NG2, two pericyte markers [71].

Sorafenib

Sorafenib has been reported to interfere with MAPK signaling, inhibiting RAF1 and BRAF and consequently the extracellular signal-regulated (ERK) kinase cascade, decreasing cardiomyocyte cell survival, mainly under conditions of stress [72]. Moreover, sorafenib has been speculated to inhibit RAF1–mammalian sterile 20 kinase 2 (MST2) protein–protein interaction [73, 74], inducing the activation of Jun N-terminal kinase (JNK), forkhead box O (FOXO), and large tumor suppressor homolog 1 (LATS1), all pro-apoptotic proteins [13]. The parallel inhibition of RAF1–apoptosis signal-regulating kinase 1 (ASK1) interaction might trigger the activation of JNK, JNK-mediated phosphorylation of 14-3-3 proteins, and subsequent release of BCL2-associated X protein (BAX), resulting in cell death [13].

Other VEGF-Targeting TKIs

A randomized, double-blind trial indicated that pazopanib produced a concentration-dependent decrease in the heart rate and caused a small, concentration-independent prolongation of the QTcF interval [75]. QT prolongation has also been associated with BRAF inhibitors [76]. There is a case report for a fatal cardiac event in a patient vandetanib that showed cardiomyocyte hypertrophy and myocyte degeneration [77], although it remains to be determined if this is associated with vandetanib use in a subgroup of patients.

7.3 Cardio-oncological Early Detection and Prevention: The Future

Given the widely recognized CV toxicities associated with chemo-/radiotherapeutic agents, the close interaction/cooperation between cardiologists and oncologists is a necessary and urgent need either for intervention of preventive approaches, aimed at limiting the anticancer-mediated CV damages. In this scenario, the discovery as far as the elucidation of the molecular and cellular mechanisms associated with chemo-/radiotherapy is crucial for the development of alternative/combinatory therapies where the possible side effects, especially in the era of the personalized and precision medicine, still represent a significant limit in cancer therapies. Finally, the development of biomarkers for chemotherapy-induced cardiotoxicities early detection, clearly represent the most relevant need where the oncologist and cardiologist efforts should work together.

Chemotherapy-induced cardiotoxicity is a price of effective therapy, increasing in incidence with long-term survival from cancer therapy. Cardiotoxicity should be precociously detected and prevented, to avoid the risk of curing cancer while irreversibly damaging the heart.

It is also increasingly evident that various compounds, ranging from classical cardioprotective agents such as beta-blockers, dexrazoxane, as well as dietary derivatives, such as resveratrol, could help curve the side effects of therapy on the cardiovascular system, in the field we named "cardio-oncological prevention" [3].

Acknowledgments Antonino Bruno is currently supported by a fellowship from the Fondazione Umberto Veronesi. Barbara Bassani is a participant of the PhD program in Biotechnology, Biosciences and Surgical Technologies, School in Biological and Medical Sciences, University of Insubria. We thank Alessandra Panvini Rosati for the secretariat assistance.

References

1. Brown SA, Sandhu N, Herrmann J. Systems biology approaches to adverse drug effects: the example of cardio-oncology. Nat Rev Clin Oncol. 2015;12:718–31.
2. Bordoni B, et al. Cardiologic evaluation of patients undergoing chemotherapy. Monaldi Arch Chest Dis. 2014;82(2):68–74.
3. Albini A, et al. Cardiotoxicity of anticancer drugs: the need for cardio-oncology and cardio-oncological prevention. J Natl Cancer Inst. 2010;102(1):14–25.
4. Ewer MS, Lippman SM. Type II chemotherapy-related cardiac dysfunction: time to recognize a new entity. J Clin Oncol. 2005;23(13):2900–2.
5. Conway A, et al. The prevention, detection and management of cancer treatment-induced cardiotoxicity: a meta-review. BMC Cancer. 2015;15:366.
6. Wells QS, Lenihan DJ. Reversibility of left ventricular dysfunction resulting from chemotherapy: can this be expected? Prog Cardiovasc Dis. 2010;53(2):140–8.
7. Focaccetti C, et al. Effects of 5-fluorouracil on morphology, cell cycle, proliferation, apoptosis, autophagy and ROS production in endothelial cells and cardiomyocytes. PLoS One. 2015;10(2):e0115686.
8. Albini A, et al. Bringing new players into the field: onco-pharmacovigilance in the era of cardio-oncology. Intern Emerg Med. 2012;7(2):99–101.
9. Lyu YL, et al. Topoisomerase IIbeta mediated DNA double-strand breaks: implications in doxorubicin cardiotoxicity and prevention by dexrazoxane. Cancer Res. 2007;67(18):8839–46.
10. Curigliano G, et al. Cardiac toxicity from systemic cancer therapy: a comprehensive review. Prog Cardiovasc Dis. 2010;53(2):94–104.

11. Monsuez JJ, et al. Cardiac side-effects of cancer chemotherapy. Int J Cardiol. 2010;144(1):3–15.
12. Swain SM, Whaley FS, Ewer MS. Congestive heart failure in patients treated with doxorubicin: a retrospective analysis of three trials. Cancer. 2003;97(11):2869–79.
13. Chen B, et al. Molecular and cellular mechanisms of anthracycline cardiotoxicity. Cardiovasc Toxicol. 2007;7(2):114–21.
14. Rochette L, et al. Anthracyclines/trastuzumab: new aspects of cardiotoxicity and molecular mechanisms. Trends Pharmacol Sci. 2015;36(6):326–48.
15. van Norren K, et al. Direct effects of doxorubicin on skeletal muscle contribute to fatigue. Br J Cancer. 2009;100(2):311–4.
16. Richard C, et al. Oxidative stress and myocardial gene alterations associated with Doxorubicin-induced cardiotoxicity in rats persist for 2 months after treatment cessation. J Pharmacol Exp Ther. 2011;339(3):807–14.
17. Tony H, Yu K, Qiutang Z. MicroRNA-208a silencing attenuates doxorubicin induced myocyte apoptosis and cardiac dysfunction. Oxid Med Cell Longev. 2015;2015:597032.
18. Tong Z, et al. MiR-21 protected cardiomyocytes against doxorubicin-induced apoptosis by targeting BTG2. Int J Mol Sci. 2015;16(7):14511–25.
19. Roca-Alonso L, et al. Myocardial MiR-30 downregulation triggered by doxorubicin drives alterations in beta-adrenergic signaling and enhances apoptosis. Cell Death Dis. 2015;6:e1754.
20. Deng S, et al. Dexrazoxane may prevent doxorubicin-induced DNA damage via depleting both topoisomerase II isoforms. BMC Cancer. 2014;14:842.
21. Elitok A, et al. Effect of carvedilol on silent anthracycline-induced cardiotoxicity assessed by strain imaging: a prospective randomized controlled study with six-month follow-up. Cardiol J. 2014;21(5):509–15.
22. Cernecka H, et al. Enalaprilat increases PPARbeta/delta expression, without influence on PPARalpha and PPARgamma, and modulate cardiac function in sub-acute model of daunorubicin-induced cardiomyopathy. Eur J Pharmacol. 2013;714(1–3):472–7.
23. Colombo A, et al. Cardiac complications of chemotherapy: role of biomarkers. Curr Treat Options Cardiovasc Med. 2014;16(6):313.
24. Grem JL. Mechanisms of action and modulation of fluorouracil. Semin Radiat Oncol. 1997;7(4):249–59.
25. Sorrentino MF, et al. 5-fluorouracil induced cardiotoxicity: review of the literature. Cardiol J. 2012;19(5):453–8.
26. Polk A, et al. Cardiotoxicity in cancer patients treated with 5-fluorouracil or capecitabine: a systematic review of incidence, manifestations and predisposing factors. Cancer Treat Rev. 2013;39(8):974–84.
27. Amstutz U, et al. Hypermethylation of the DPYD promoter region is not a major predictor of severe toxicity in 5-fluorouracil based chemotherapy. J Exp Clin Cancer Res. 2008;27:54.
28. Durak I, et al. Reduced antioxidant defense capacity in myocardial tissue from guinea pigs treated with 5-fluorouracil. J Toxicol Environ Health A. 2000;59(7):585–9.
29. Molteni LP, et al. Capecitabine in breast cancer: the issue of cardiotoxicity during fluoropyrimidine treatment. Breast J. 2010;16 Suppl 1:S45–8.
30. Polk A, et al. A systematic review of the pathophysiology of 5-fluorouracil-induced cardiotoxicity. BMC Pharmacol Toxicol. 2014;15:47.
31. Tsibiribi P, et al. Cardiac lesions induced by 5-fluorouracil in the rabbit. Hum Exp Toxicol. 2006;25(6):305–9.
32. Yeh ET, Bickford CL. Cardiovascular complications of cancer therapy: incidence, pathogenesis, diagnosis, and management. J Am Coll Cardiol. 2009;53(24):2231–47.
33. Calik AN, et al. Initial dose effect of 5-fluorouracil: rapidly improving severe, acute toxic myopericarditis. Am J Emerg Med. 2012;30(1):257 e1–3.
34. Dechant C, et al. Acute reversible heart failure caused by coronary vasoconstriction due to continuous 5-fluorouracil combination chemotherapy. Case Rep Oncol. 2012;5(2):296–301.
35. Eskandari MR, et al. A comparison of cardiomyocyte cytotoxic mechanisms for 5-fluorouracil and its pro-drug capecitabine. Xenobiotica. 2015;45(1):79–87.
36. Filgueiras Mde C, et al. Effects of 5-fluorouracil in nuclear and cellular morphology, proliferation, cell cycle, apoptosis, cytoskeletal and caveolar distribution in primary cultures of smooth muscle cells. PLoS One. 2013;8(4):e63177.
37. Magnani E, et al. Fluoropyrimidine toxicity in patients with dihydropyrimidine dehydrogenase splice site variant: the need for further revision of dose and schedule. Intern Emerg Med. 2013;8(5):417–23.
38. Wei X, et al. Molecular basis of the human dihydropyrimidine dehydrogenase deficiency and 5-fluorouracil toxicity. J Clin Invest. 1996;98(3):610–5.

39. Bonita R, Pradhan R. Cardiovascular toxicities of cancer chemotherapy. Semin Oncol. 2013;40(2): 156–67.
40. Schimmel KJ, et al. Cardiotoxicity of cytotoxic drugs. Cancer Treat Rev. 2004;30(2):181–91.
41. Herrmann J, et al. Evaluation and management of patients with heart disease and cancer: cardio-oncology. Mayo Clin Proc. 2014;89(9):1287–306.
42. Braverman AC, et al. Cyclophosphamide cardiotoxicity in bone marrow transplantation: a prospective evaluation of new dosing regimens. J Clin Oncol. 1991;9(7):1215–23.
43. Dhesi S, et al. Cyclophosphamide-induced cardiomyopathy: a case report, review, and recommendations for management. J Investig Med High Impact Case Rep. 2013;1(1):2324709613480346.
44. Asiri YA. Probucol attenuates cyclophosphamide-induced oxidative apoptosis, p53 and Bax signal expression in rat cardiac tissues. Oxid Med Cell Longev. 2010;3(5):308–16.
45. Mythili Y, et al. Protective effect of DL-alpha-lipoic acid on cyclophosphamide induced hyperlipidemic cardiomyopathy. Eur J Pharmacol. 2006;543(1–3):92–6.
46. Sudharsan PT, et al. Lupeol and its ester exhibit protective role against cyclophosphamide-induced cardiac mitochondrial toxicity. J Cardiovasc Pharmacol. 2006;47(2):205–10.
47. Bockorny M, et al. Severe heart failure after bortezomib treatment in a patient with multiple myeloma: a case report and review of the literature. Acta Haematol. 2012;128(4):244–7.
48. Grandin EW, et al. Patterns of cardiac toxicity associated with irreversible proteasome inhibition in the treatment of multiple myeloma. J Card Fail. 2015;21(2):138–44.
49. Nowis D, et al. Cardiotoxicity of the anticancer therapeutic agent bortezomib. Am J Pathol. 2010; 176(6):2658–68.
50. Criscitiello C, Curigliano G. HER2 signaling pathway and trastuzumab cardiotoxicity. Future Oncol. 2013;9(2):179–81.
51. Odiete O, Hill MF, Sawyer DB. Neuregulin in cardiovascular development and disease. Circ Res. 2012;111(10):1376–85.
52. ElZarrad MK, et al. Trastuzumab alters the expression of genes essential for cardiac function and induces ultrastructural changes of cardiomyocytes in mice. PLoS One. 2013;8(11):e79543.
53. van Boxtel W, et al. New biomarkers for early detection of cardiotoxicity after treatment with docetaxel, doxorubicin and cyclophosphamide. Biomarkers. 2015;20(2):143–8.
54. Richard C, et al. Effects of angiotensin-1 converting enzyme inhibition on oxidative stress and bradykinin receptor expression during doxorubicin-induced cardiomyopathy in rats. J Cardiovasc Pharmacol. 2008;52(3):278–85.
55. Pandya K, et al. Targeting both Notch and ErbB-2 signalling pathways is required for prevention of ErbB-2-positive breast tumour recurrence. Br J Cancer. 2011;105(6):796–806.
56. Aarons RD, et al. Increased human lymphocyte beta-adrenergic receptor density following chronic propranolol treatment. Proc West Pharmacol Soc. 1979;22:175–6.
57. Seemann I, et al. Radiation- and anthracycline-induced cardiac toxicity and the influence of ErbB2 blocking agents. Breast Cancer Res Treat. 2013;141(3):385–95.
58. Kerkela R, et al. Cardiotoxicity of the cancer therapeutic agent imatinib mesylate. Nat Med. 2006;12(8):908–16.
59. Force T, Krause DS, Van Etten RA. Molecular mechanisms of cardiotoxicity of tyrosine kinase inhibition. Nat Rev Cancer. 2007;7(5):332–44.
60. Marchan R, Bolt HM. Imatinib: the controversial discussion on cardiotoxicity induced by endoplasmic reticulum (ER) stress. Arch Toxicol. 2012;86(3):339–40.
61. Lai E, Teodoro T, Volchuk A. Endoplasmic reticulum stress: signaling the unfolded protein response. Physiology (Bethesda). 2007;22:193–201.
62. Ahmadizar F, et al. Efficacy and safety assessment of the addition of bevacizumab to adjuvant therapy agents in cancer patients: a systematic review and meta-analysis of randomized controlled trials. PLoS One. 2015;10(9):e0136324.
63. Lee CS, et al. Routine proteinuria monitoring for bevacizumab in patients with gynecologic malignancies. J Oncol Pharm Pract. 2015. doi: 10.1177/1078155215609987
64. Zhao Z, et al. Dysregulated miR1254 and miR579 for cardiotoxicity in patients treated with bevacizumab in colorectal cancer. Tumour Biol. 2014;35(6):5227–35.
65. Bronte G, et al. Conquests and perspectives of cardio-oncology in the field of tumor angiogenesis-targeting tyrosine kinase inhibitor-based therapy. Expert Opin Drug Saf. 2015;14(2):253–67.
66. Mellor HR, et al. Cardiotoxicity associated with targeting kinase pathways in cancer. Toxicol Sci. 2011;120(1):14–32.

67. Hoy SM. Cabozantinib: a review of its use in patients with medullary thyroid cancer. Drugs. 2014; 74(12):1435–44.
68. Orphanos GS, Ioannidis GN, Ardavanis AG. Cardiotoxicity induced by tyrosine kinase inhibitors. Acta Oncol. 2009;48(7):964–70.
69. Dyck JR, Lopaschuk GD. AMPK alterations in cardiac physiology and pathology: enemy or ally? J Physiol. 2006;574(Pt 1):95–112.
70. Terai K, et al. AMP-activated protein kinase protects cardiomyocytes against hypoxic injury through attenuation of endoplasmic reticulum stress. Mol Cell Biol. 2005;25(21):9554–75.
71. Chintalgattu V, et al. Coronary microvascular pericytes are the cellular target of sunitinib malate-induced cardiotoxicity. Sci Transl Med. 2013;5(187):187ra69.
72. Kyriakis JM, et al. Mitogen regulation of c-Raf-1 protein kinase activity toward mitogen-activated protein kinase-kinase. J Biol Chem. 1993;268(21):16009–19.
73. Chen J, et al. Raf-1 promotes cell survival by antagonizing apoptosis signal-regulating kinase 1 through a MEK-ERK independent mechanism. Proc Natl Acad Sci USA. 2001;98(14):7783–8.
74. O'Neill E, Kolch W. Taming the Hippo: Raf-1 controls apoptosis by suppressing MST2/Hippo. Cell Cycle. 2005;4(3):365–7.
75. Heath EI, et al. A randomized, double-blind, placebo-controlled study to evaluate the effect of repeated oral doses of pazopanib on cardiac conduction in patients with solid tumors. Cancer Chemother Pharmacol. 2013;71(3):565–73.
76. Bronte E, et al. What links BRAF to the heart function? new insights from the cardiotoxicity of BRAF inhibitors in cancer treatment. Oncotarget. 2015;6:35589–601.
77. Scheffel RS, et al. Toxic cardiomyopathy leading to fatal acute cardiac failure related to vandetanib: a case report with histopathological analysis. Eur J Endocrinol. 2013;168(6):K51–4.

Cardiotoxicity: Left Ventricular Dysfunction

Stefano Oliva, Ines Monte, and Daniela Cardinale

C. Lestuzzi et al. (eds.), *Manual of Cardio-oncology*, DOI 10.1007/978-3-319-40236-9_8

8.1 Which Drugs Are Involved

The left ventricular dysfunction (LVD), from asymptomatic reduction of left ventricular ejection fraction (LVEF) up to heart failure (HF), is probably the most studied and feared late effect of anticancer therapy because it is often unpredictable and because it has a poor prognosis. It may result from many anticancer drugs through different mechanisms and often for a different combination of cardiotoxic effects in a polychemotherapy schedule.

8.1.1 Definition and Graduation of LVD

Historically, the LVD from chemotherapy was considered like a synonym of "cardiotoxicity." In literature, there are many definitions and classifications of LVD, but actually, in an expert consensus document, the American Society of Cardiology with the European Association of Cardiovascular Imaging defined LVD as a significant decline of left ventricular performance (from baseline or before anticancer therapy), measured by an LVEF reduction up to 10% points with a final LVEF value <53% [1] independently in the presence or not of heart failure symptoms, with a significant reduction of the global longitudinal strain (GLS) index, measured by 2D echo, up to −19%. This society believes that the value of cardiac troponin I (TnI) is also important to detect the asymptomatic or preclinical LVD, because the high level of TnI reflects the loss of myocardial cells due to drug toxicity.

This last definition seems to be useful because it identifies the LVD not for only one aspect and by a single parameter (LVEF) but by a series of different parameters (biological, LV contractility, kinetics).

Therefore, it is crucial to detect periodically the left ventricular performance or LVEF with echocardiography or, less frequently, with cardiac magnetic resonance (CMR) or MUGA scan (see the next chapter), before, during, and after anticancer therapy administration, maybe for all life. But it is evident that, actually, it's not possible to define LVD only with the LVEF value.

However, the graduation of severity of cardiotoxicity is often based on LVEF. The Common Toxicity Criteria Manual (National Cancer Institute—Cancer Therapy Evaluation Program) version 2.0 (1999) is probably the most simple and balanced classification available (see ◘ Table 8.1). This classification does not consider the GLS or TnI value, but it is quite useful to identify the severity of cardiotoxicity.

◘ **Table 8.1** Grading of LVD

Grade I	Asymptomatic decline in LVEF of >10% from baseline evaluation
Grade II	Asymptomatic decrease in LVEF of <50% or ≥20% compared with baseline value
Grade III	Heart failure responsive to treatment
Grade IV	Severe or refractory heart failure or requiring intensive medical therapy and/or intubation
Grade V	Death related to cardiac toxicity

LVEF left ventricular ejection fraction
Adapted from National Cancer Institute Common Terminology Criteria for Adverse Events 2.0 (1999)

Unfortunately, there is no uniformity of opinion to identify the cardiotoxicity and to define this condition; they do not have permission to do a systematic review or meta-analysis of cardiotoxicity, to learn more about those aspects that are actually still unclear [2].

8.1.2 Anthracycline-Related LVD

The anthracyclines, commonly used to treat many hematologic and solid malignances such as Hodgkin's and non-Hodgkin's lymphomas and breast and gastric cancer, are the most studied and most frequent drugs with established LVD.

In 2005, Lipshultz [3] defined and classified the anthracycline-related LVD in three types depending on the time of appearance:

- **Acute cardiotoxicity:** during chemotherapy administration, usually reversible, and characterized by transient contractile LV depression (low incidence)
- **Early-onset chronic progressive cardiotoxicity:** within 1 year after the end of chemotherapy, dose dependent, not reversible spontaneously, and associated by a poor prognosis
- **Late-onset chronic progressive cardiotoxicity:** more than 1 year after the end of chemotherapy

More recent findings, however, suggest that anthracycline-related cardiotoxicity is most likely a unique and continuous phenomenon that starts with myocardial cell injury and is followed by progressive LVEF decline that, if disregarded and not treated, progressively leads to overt HF [5].

This significant late effect seems to have several mechanisms, but free radical formation and topoisomerase 2B-related DNA damage, are generally accepted as the main mechanisms [6–8].

There are several risk factors that increment the probability of anthracycline-related LVD (summarized in ◘ Table 8.2): firstly, cumulative dose of drugs. In fact, the prevalence of cardiomyopathy increases significantly when patients are given doses of doxorubicin ≥550 mg/m^2 (7 % risk of symptomatic HF; 26 % of symptomatic HF in elderly patients) [4, 9, 10]. Age, cardiac risk factors (e.g., hypertension, diabetes, smoke), concomitant radiotherapy, the type of anthracycline, female gender, and other conditions appear to increase (or decrease) the risk of LVD.

Actually the real incidence of chemotherapy-related cardiotoxicity is unclear, because we have several evidences stating that the incidence of cardiovascular diseases, especially heart failure in elderly patients, increased in cancer survivors, during the follow-up [11, 12].

The liposomal formulations of doxorubicin, usable only in selected conditions, have proven to be less cardiotoxic of the traditional molecule [13].

8.1.3 Non-anthracycline-Related LVD

Anthracyclines are not the only chemotherapy drugs related to LVD. Antimicrotubule and alkylating agents seem to increase the anthracycline-related LVD risk in a concomitant polychemotherapy [14]. The cardiovascular risk in patients treated with other conventional chemotherapy drugs is negligible.

Table 8.2 Risk factors for anthracycline cardiotoxicity

Risk factor	Aspect
Cumulative anthracycline dose	Cumulative doses >500 mg/m^2 associated with significantly elevated long-term risk
Rate of anthracycline administration	Prolonged administration to minimize circulating dose volume may decrease toxicity; results are mixed
Individual anthracycline dose	Higher individual anthracycline doses are associated with increased late cardiotoxicity, even when cumulative doses are limited
Type of anthracycline	Liposomal encapsulated preparations may reduce cardiotoxicity. Conflicting data exist about anthracycline analogues and cardiotoxicity differences
Radiation therapy	Cumulative radiation dose >30 Gy; prior or concomitant anthracycline treatment
Concomitant therapy	Trastuzumab, cyclophosphamide, bleomycin, vincristine, amsacrine, and mitoxantrone may increase susceptibility/toxicity. Others are implicated as well
Preexisting cardiac risk factors	Hypertension; ischemic, myocardial, and valvular heart disease; prior cardiotoxic treatment
Comorbidities	Diabetes, obesity, renal dysfunction, pulmonary disease, endocrinopathies, electrolyte and metabolic abnormalities, sepsis, infection, pregnancy
Age	Both young and advanced age at treatment are associated with elevated risk
Sex	Females are at greater risk than males

Partially modified by Lipshultz, Heart 2008 [4]

8

8.1.4 Targeted Therapy and LVD

Not only chemotherapy can cause LVD but also the new anticancer molecular targeting drugs such as monoclonal antibody-based tyrosine kinase inhibitors (TKI), trastuzumab or bevacizumab, and new TKI small cell sunitinib or sorafenib, from asymptomatic LVEF decrease to a symptomatic heart failure, but different pathophysiological mechanisms are involved.

Trastuzumab

Trastuzumab is a monoclonal antibody directed toward some epidermal growth factor receptors (*HerB2*) overexpressed in about 30 % of breast cancer and increase significantly the efficacy of chemotherapy in HerB2+ patients treated in a metastatic and in adjuvant setting [15, 16]. This efficacy depends on the block of intracellular EGFR signal that induces apoptosis by increasing intracellular calcium level. But the link with the HerB2 receptors present in the surface of cardiomyocytes causes also loss of these cells.

The trastuzumab-related LVD depends on the expression of HerB2 that may be transiently upregulated by a compensatory mechanism following cardiac stress in a myocar-

Table 8.3 Classification of LVD

	TYPE I (myocardial damage)	Type II (myocardial dysfunction)
Characteristic agent	Doxorubicin	Trastuzumab
Clinical course, response to CRCD therapy	May stabilize, but underlying damage appears to be permanent and irreversible; recurrence in months or years may be related to sequential cardiac stress	High likelihood of recovery (to or near baseline cardiac status) in 2–4 months (reversible)
Dose effects	Cumulative, dose related	Not dose related
Mechanism	Free radical formation, oxidative stress/damage	Blocked ErbB2 signaling
Ultrastructure	Vacuoles; myofibrillar disarray and dropout; necrosis (changes resolve over time)	No apparent ultra structural abnormalities
Noninvasive cardiac testing	Decreased ejection fraction by ultrasound or nuclear determination: global decrease in wall motion	Decreased ejection fraction by ultrasound or nuclear determination: global decrease in wall motion
Effect of rechallenge	High probability of recurrent dysfunction that is progressive, may result in intractable heart failure and death	Increasing evidence for the relative safety of rechallenge; additional data needed
Effect of late sequential stress	High likelihood of sequential stress-related cardiac dysfunction	Low likelihood of sequential stress-related cardiac dysfunction

CRCD chemotherapy-related cardiac dysfunction
From Ewer, JCO 2005 [18]

dial cell [17]. For this reasons, it is not prudent to administer trastuzumab concurrently with anthracycline but few weeks after the end of this chemotherapy.

In 2005, Ewer called "type 1" the LVD caused by anthracycline or other chemotherapy, and "type 2" the LVD caused by targeted therapy, after highlighting that a group of HF trastuzumab-related patients with breast cancer would recover LVEF as a result of HF therapy and discontinuation of trastuzumab [18, 19]. Many differences are reported from these two conditions: relationship of cumulative dose, presence of histological abnormalities, and prognosis. Table 8.3 summarizes these differences.

Bevacizumab and TKI Small Cell

Bevacizumab is a monoclonal antibody currently used in gastrointestinal cancer patients. In the literature, HF incidence in bevacizumab-treated patients are reported to be from 1 to 3% [6]. The mechanism of HF associated with bevacizumab may be related to uncontrolled hypertension and inhibition of vascular endothelial growth factor (VEGF)/VEGF receptor signaling that induces compensatory hypertrophy in patients with hypertensive and ischemic disease. The HF that results is a hypertensive failure, so we must carefully control the hypertensive patients. Cardiotoxicity in patients treated with bevacizumab is potentially reversible with discontinuation of drug administration, like the other "type 2" dysfunctions.

Sunitinib and sorafenib are two TKI small cell used in advanced renal cell carcinoma and hepatic tumors. These drugs appear to share the same cardiotoxic mechanism with bevacizumab but act within the cell and not outside. Cardiac dysfunction, manifested as HF or asymptomatic declines in LVEF, has also been noted but widely underestimated in the past; the incidence of HF is estimated to be 4–8 %, while the incidence of asymptomatic LVEF decline is even higher, up to 28 % for LVEF declines ≥10 % [20, 21].

8.2 How to Monitor

Highly effective chemotherapeutic agents may cause cancer therapeutics-related left ventricular dysfunction (LVD). To monitoring of left ventricular function is very important for early detection of LVD and prompt treatment that may prevent LV remodeling and the progression to the HF syndrome.

8

- **Echocardiography (ECHO)** is also a precious tool for the evaluation of left ventricular function, pericardium, valves, and right chambers that all may be damaged by cancer therapy.
- **Cardiac magnetic resonance (CMR)** could be useful for improving echocardiographic information when this is unsatisfactory or when tissue characterization is needed. Contrast-enhanced CMR offers a unique capability to identify subtle myocardial abnormalities, such as diffuse fibrosis, compared with other imaging techniques [22, 23], and anthracycline-related myocardial fibrosis [24, 25]. Although this technique suggests promise for future diagnosis and possibly prediction of risk for cardiomyopathies, its current use is limited to research studies.
- **Radionuclide angiography (MUGA)** has been referred as the "gold standard" to monitor anthracycline-related damage due to its high accuracy and reproducibility of LVEF measurements [26–27], but it has the main disadvantage in radiation exposure. Thus, it is frequently used as an adjunct and a complementary technique to echocardiography.

The ECHO represents the imaging modality of choice for evaluation and monitoring of LVD.

8.2.1 LV Systolic Function

The most commonly used parameter for monitoring LV function with echocardiography is ejection fraction (LVEF). In cancer patients, changes in LVEF indicative of LV damage can be more appropriately identified comparing baseline and follow-up studies.

Accurate calculation of LVEF should be done with the best method available in a given echocardiography lab. Consistency with regard to the method used to determine LVEF should be maintained whenever possible during treatment and surveillance after treatment. Importantly, the digital images obtained to calculate LVEF on follow-up echocardiography should be visually compared with the previous ones to minimize reader variability.

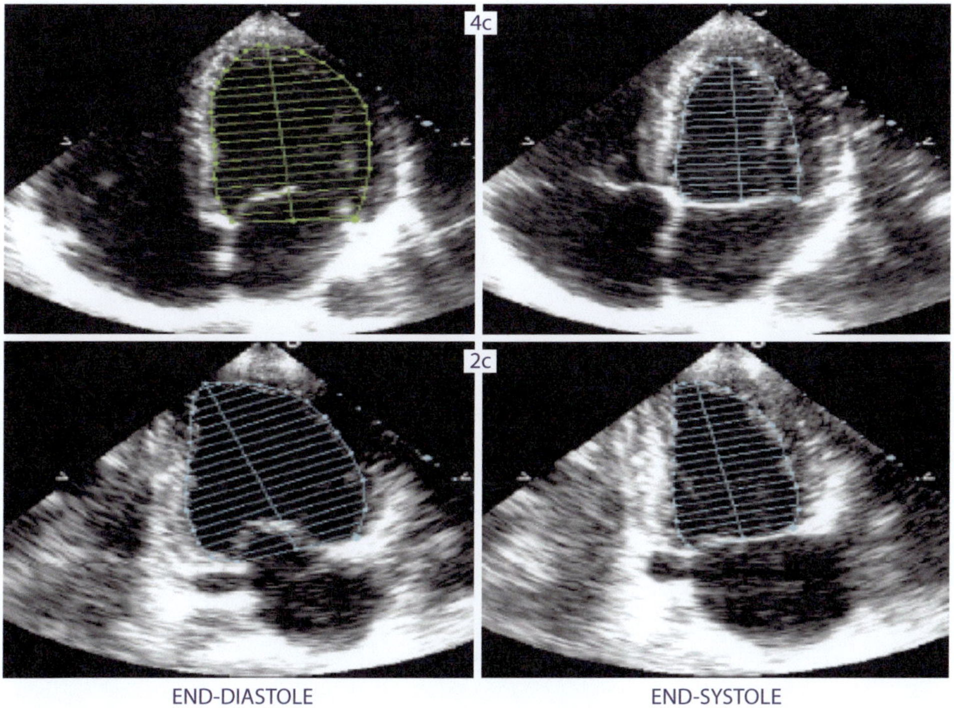

Fig. 8.1 LVEF using biplane Simpson's method

According to joint recommendations from the American Society of Echocardiography (ASE), and the European Association of Echocardiography (EAE) [28], the methods of choice for LV volumes quantitation and LVEF calculation are:

- The modified biplane Simpson's technique (method of disks) by 2DE (Fig. 8.1).
- The use of an automated or semiautomated method for identifying LV endocardium, compared with manual tracing of endocardial contour required by 2D method, provides a more accurate estimation of LV volumes (Fig. 8.2).
- A contrast agent should be used when two contiguous LV segments from an apical view are not seen on non-contrast images.
- 3D evaluation of LVEF is recommended because it is more accurate than 2D modality for LV volume measurement with a precision, which is comparable to that of CMR.
- Advantages: better accuracy in detecting LVEF below the lower limit of normal, better reproducibility, and lower temporal variability than 2DE in patients with cancer treated with chemotherapy.
- Limits: costs, availability, high-quality images, training, and expertise of operators for a clinical application limit the wide application of 3DE in the oncological setting.

A LVEF (assessed by 2D modified Simpson's rule) >52 % for men and >54 % for women is suggestive of normal systolic function [29].

As indicated in previous chapter, consensus of ASE-EACVI [1] proposed for the diagnosis of cardiac toxicity.

- A decrease in the LVEF of >10 % points, to a value <53 %. However, in a recent ESC position Paper [29] the Autors has decided to consider the lower limit of normal of

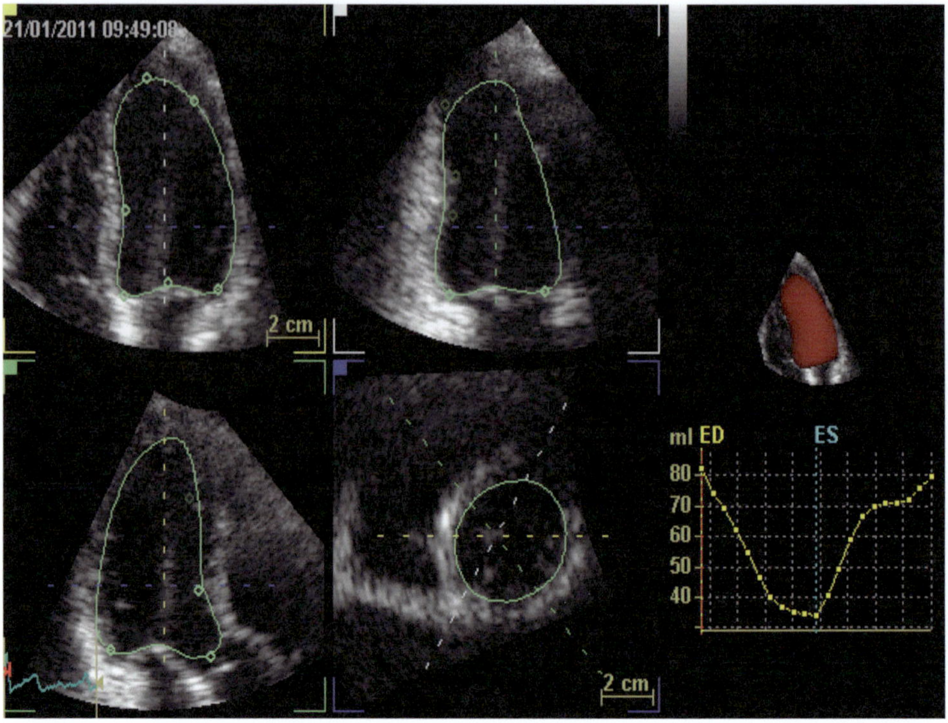

Fig. 8.2 LVEF using automated 3D method

LVEF in echocardiography also 50 %, in line with the definition of cardiotoxicity commonly used in registries and trials in patients with cancer.
- That should be confirmed by repeated cardiac imaging performed 2–3 weeks after the baseline study

The calculation of LVEF should be combined with assessment of the wall motion score index; septal and apical pattern of LV dysfunction have been more frequently found at an early stage of LVD in the presence of a quite normal LVEF; therefore, a careful analysis of regional alterations is strongly worthwhile beyond the LVEF assessment.

8.2.2 LV Diastolic Function

A comprehensive assessment of LV diastolic function should be performed in the oncology setting, although diastolic parameters have not been found to be prognostic of LVD.

According to the joint ASE-EACVI [30], evaluation of LV diastolic function include:
- Diagnosis of LV diastolic dysfunction (Fig. 8.3)
- Estimate of LV filling pressure and grading LV diastolic function (Fig. 8.4)

However, use of the *E*/*e′* ratio remains questionable in the oncological setting, as *E* and *e′* velocities fluctuation in these patients could be the consequence of changes in loading conditions as a result of side effects associated with the chemotherapy (nausea, vomiting, and diarrhea) more than the result of a real change in LV diastolic performance.

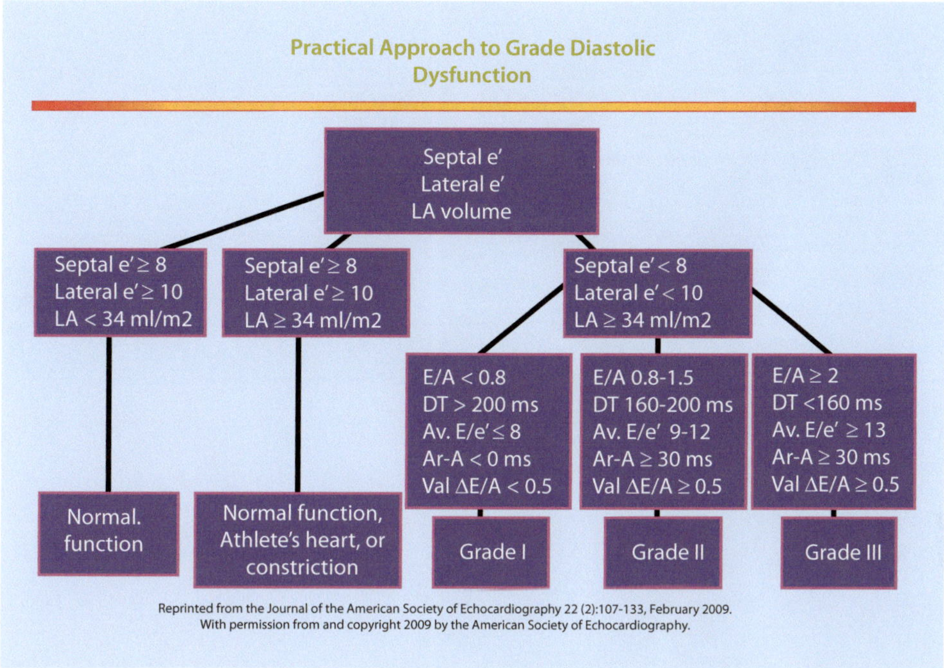

Fig. 8.3 Algorithm for diagnosis of LV diastolic dysfunction if LVEF is normal

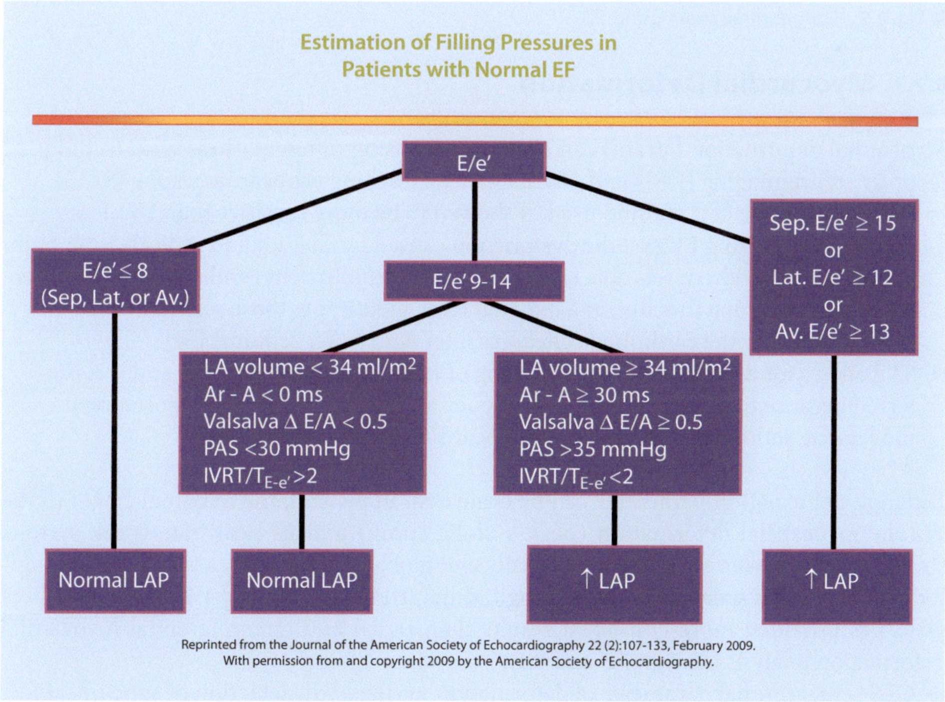

Fig. 8.4 Algorithm for estimation of LV filling pressure and grading diastolic function if LVEF is depressed

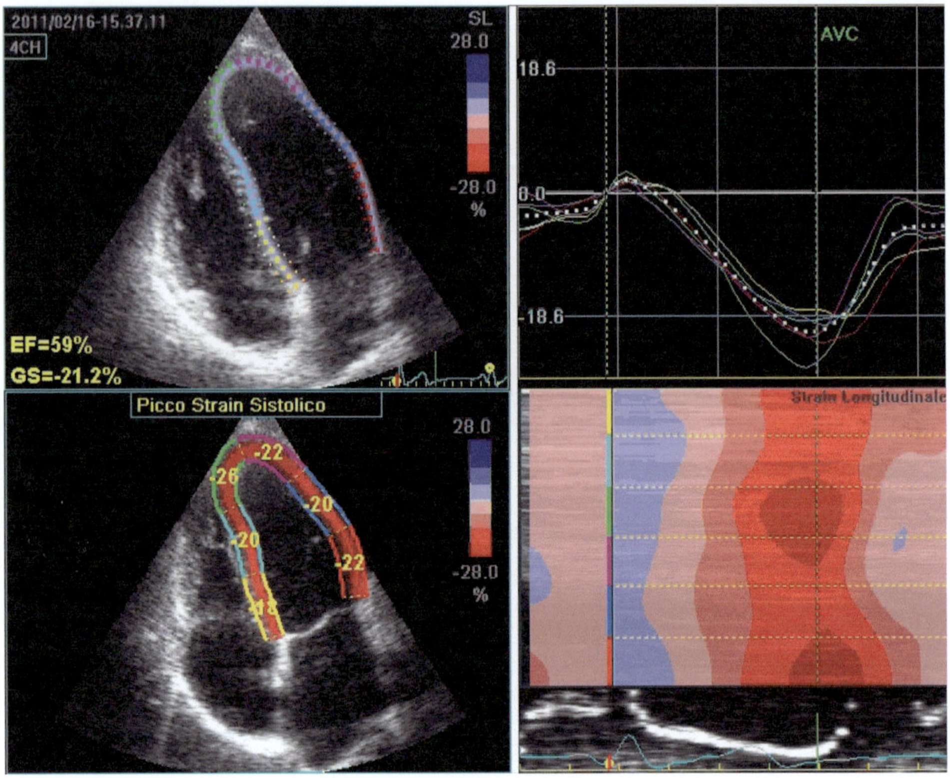

■ **Fig. 8.5** Longitudinal strain using STE

8

8.2.3 Myocardial Deformation

Myocardial deformation (strain) can be measured using different ultrasound techniques: Doppler strain imaging (DSI) and 2D/3D speckle tracking echocardiography (STE).

- DSI has been the first method used. It showed to be more sensitive than LVEF assessment in recognizing LV systolic dysfunction caused by chemo- and radiotherapy, both in adults and children; was able to identify early cardiotoxicity; and could reveal differences in myocardial function at a regional level, identifying those segments that are more affected by the cardiotoxic effect (as interventricular septum) [31].
- STE allows for a frame-by-frame tracking of natural acoustic markers and it is preferred because of a lack of angle dependency and not influenced by translational movement, tethering from adjacent myocardium and signal noise.

Different deformation parameter can be evaluated. In general, the maximal extent of the systolic myocardial deformation (peak systolic strain) and its peak rate (peak systolic strain rate) have been used, both regionally and globally. In general, assessment of longitudinal strain, and specifically global longitudinal strain (GLS) using 4, 2, and 3 chambers view, has provided more consistent results than radial and circumferential myocardial deformation analysis (■ Figs. 8.5 and 8.6).

- GLS is the optimal parameter of deformation for the early detection of subclinical LV dysfunction.

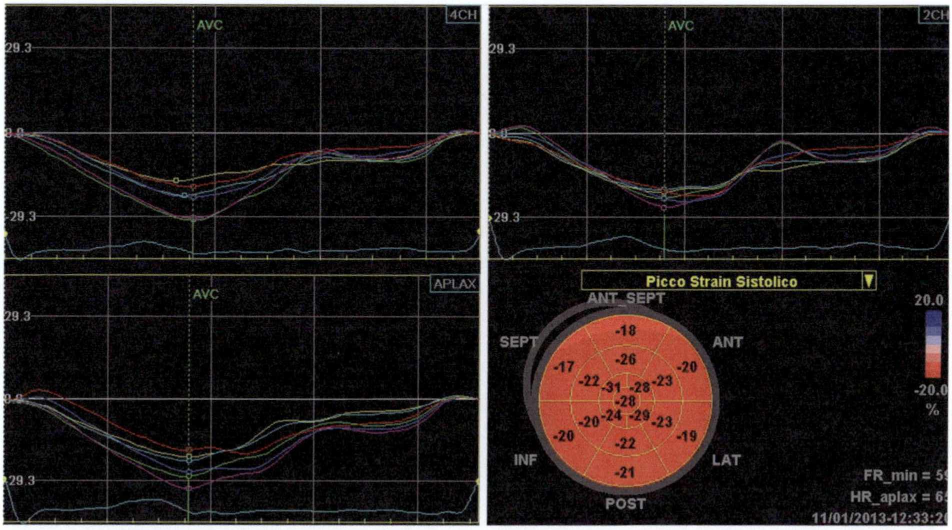

Fig. 8.6 Global longitudinal strain

- The measurements during chemotherapy should be compared with the baseline value. In patients with available baseline strain measurements (Fig. 8.7).
  - a relative percentage reduction of GLS of <8 % from baseline appears not to be meaningful.
  - A relative percentage reduction of GLS of >15 % from baseline are very likely to be abnormal.

When applying STE for the longitudinal follow-up of patients with cancer, the same vendor-specific ultrasound machine and range for sex and age should be used [32] (Table 8.4).

This is important also to detect the reversibility of the myocardial damage.

8.2.4 Use of Biomarkers

Several studies admit the utility of troponins as a robust diagnostic tool for the early identification, assessment, and monitoring of cardiotoxicity [33, 34].

Troponin I (TnI) is a sensitive and specific marker for myocardial injury in adults treated with anthracycline chemotherapy and an elevation of troponin identifies patients at risk for the subsequent development of LVD.

The ASE-EACVI Consensus proposed an integrated approach for baseline assessment and monitoring of LVD [1].

- Baseline assessment (LVEF, GLS, TnI) in patients at high risk for development of LVD.
  - With established risk factors for cardiovascular disease
  - With LV dysfunction
  - >65 years of age
  - Patients scheduled to receive high doses of type I agents (>350 mg/m^2) or combination chemotherapy with both type I and type II agents

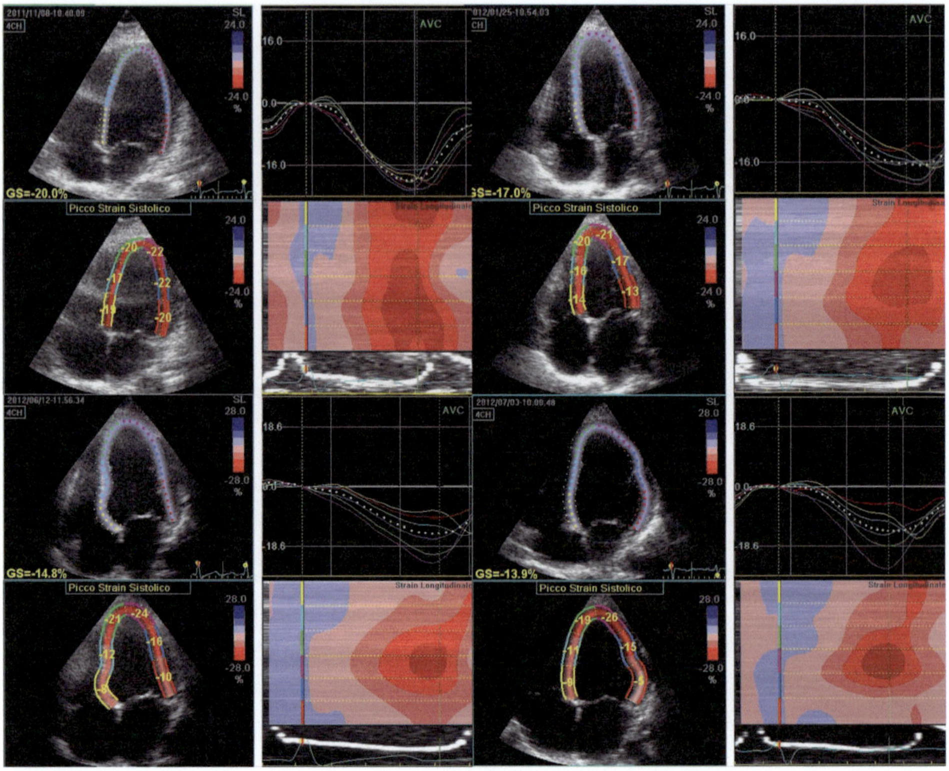

Fig. 8.7 Changes of GLS in a patient with breast cancer treated with anthracyclines (follow-up of 8 months)

Table 8.4 Reference values of global longitudinal strain for vendor, age, and gender

Vendor	Age group (y)					
	0–19	20–29	30–39	40–49	50–59	≥60
Vivid 7 or Vivid E9 (GE Healthcare)						
Male	−21.7 ± 3.1	−20.9 ± 1.9	−20.6 ± 1.9	−20.9 ± 1.8	−21.0 ± 1.9	−19.7 ± 1.4
Female	−22.4 ± 1.6	−22.3 ± 1.6	−22.8 ± 1.8	−22.6 ± 2.1	−23.3 ± 1.9	−20.9 ± 2.1
iE33 (Philips Medical Systems)						
Male	−19.4 ± 2.7	−18.8 ± 2.0	−19.1 ± 2.3	−17.9 ± 2.8	−16.9 ± 2.3	−15.8 ± 1.4
Female	−20.5 ± 2.2	−20.6 ± 2.3	−20.2 ± 2.0	−19.3 ± 0.9	−20.4 ± 1.5	−17.3 ± 2.3
Artida or Aplio (Toshiba Medical Systems)						
Male	−21.6 ± 2.0	−20.2 ± 2.0	−20.4 ± 2.2	−19.8 ± 2.3	−18.7 ± 2.6	−16.3 ± 3.1
Female	−21.2 ± 1.5	−20.2 ± 2.4	−20.4 ± 2.8	−18.7 ± 1.8	−18.3 ± 2.8	−18.6 ± 2.3

Modified from Takigiku, Circ J 2012 [32]

- If the LVEF is <53 %.
- GLS is below the limit of normal.
- Elevated TnI should be considered discussion between the cardiologist and oncologist of the risk/benefit ratio.
  1. **If LVEF, GLS, and TnI are normal**, echocardiographic follow-up is recommended on the basis of the specific type of anticancer agent received.
     a. **For type I agents:** at the completion of therapy and 6 months later for doses of anthracycline <240 mg/m [2] or its equivalent. Once this dose is exceeded, measurements of LVEF, GLS, and troponin are recommended before each additional 50 mg/m [2].
     b. **For type II agents:** every 3 months during therapy for trastuzumab and at 1 month and every 3 months while on therapy with other tyrosine kinase inhibitors.
  2. **The detection of subclinical LVD** is to compare the measurements of GLS obtained during chemotherapy with the one obtained at baseline.
     a. A relative percentage reduction GLS of >15 % is very likely to be abnormal,
     b. A change of <8 % appears not to be of clinical significance.
     c. The abnormal GLS value should be confirmed by a repeat study performed 2–3 weeks after the initial abnormal study.

8.3 How to Treat

Treatment of cardiac dysfunction resulting from anticancer therapy commonly follows the cardiology guideline recommendations for heart failure (HF). This practice, however, is mainly based on extrapolation from other clinical settings rather than on evidence specifically addressing HF in the cancer population.

8.3.1 Left Ventricular Dysfunction Induced by Anthracyclines

Anthracycline-induced cardiac dysfunction (ACD) is believed to be refractory to conventional therapy and to be associated with an especially poor prognosis, with a 2-year mortality rate of up to 60 % [35].

This opinion, however, is based on findings reported in old studies in which standard therapy included only the use of digoxin and diuretics [36–38], and on studies including very small populations (■ Table 8.5), patients with ACD has never been fully investigated because, typically, these patients have been excluded from large randomized trials.

Moreover, data on long-term outcomes of treated and untreated patients with ACD are limited. As a consequence, evidence-based recommendations for the management of cancer patients with asymptomatic and symptomatic ACD are still lacking and no definite guidelines are currently adopted.

The effectiveness of angiotensin-converting enzyme inhibitors (ACEI) and beta-blockers was prospectively assessed only in two studies involving large populations [48]. Evidence coming from these two studies can be outlined as follows:

- Initiation of ACEI and beta-blocker medications promptly after the detection of ACD is a crucial variable for recovery of cardiac function, as a strong inverse relationship

Table 8.5 Clinical studies evaluating heart failure therapy in anthracycline-induced cardiomyopathy

Treatment	Author (year)	Pts (*n*)	Mean age (yrs)	Study	FU (months)	B-LVEF (%)	F-LVEF (%)	Reported event
Dig + Diur	Lefrak (1973) [36]	2	NA	CR	NA	NA	NA	CD
Dig + Diur	Cohen (1982) [37]	1	38	CR	8	23	64	Relief of symptoms
Dig + Diur	Haq (1985) [38]	43	55	R	2–52	NA	NA	Relief of symptoms, HF, CD
Dig + Diur + ACEI	Saini (1987) [39]	3	49	CR	12–16	20	48	Relief of symptoms LVEF↑
Dig + Diur[a] Dig + Diur + ACEI[b]	Jensen (1996) [40]	9	58	PO	26	27	47	CD, HF
Dig + Diur + ACEI[a] BB[b]	Fazio (1998) [41]	1	35	CR	12	14	45	Relief of symptoms
BB BB + ACEI	Noori (2000) [42]	2 6	51	R	32	28	41	LVEF ↑
Dig + Diur[a] Dig + Diur + ACEI[b]	Jensen (2002) [43]	10	54	PO	30	27	41	HF
BB BB + ACEI	Mukai (2004) [44]	3 2	53	CR	27	37	53	LVEF ↑ NYHA ↓
ACEI ACEI + BB	Tallaj (2005) [45]	10 15	47	R	70	25	34	CD, TXS
ACEI + BB	Tabet (2006) [46]	1	52	CR	8	NA	30	HF
ACEI + BB	Cardinale (2010) [47]	201	53	P	12–96	38	46	LVEF ↑ up to ≥50 %
ACEI + BB	Cardinale (2015) [5]	226	50	P	4–228	40	52	LVEF ↑of 5 points + ≥50 %

AC anthracyclines, *ACEI* angiotensin-converting enzyme inhibitors, *B* baseline, *BB* beta-blockers, *CD* cardiac death, *CR* case report, *Dig* digitalis, *Diur* diuretics, *F* final, *HF* heart failure, *impr.* improvement, *LVEF* left ventricular ejection fraction, *NA* not available, *NYHA* New York Heart Association, *O* observational, *P* prospective, *R* retrospective, *TRZ* trastuzumab, *TKI* tyrosine kinase inhibitors, *TXS* cardiac transplantation

[a]First-line therapy

[b]Second-line therapy

exists between the time elapsed from the end of chemotherapy and the beginning of HF therapy for treatment of ACD, and improvement in LVEF—with a fourfold decrease in the chance of complete recovery from cardiac dysfunction for each doubling in time to HF treatment. In particular:
  - The highest chance to recover from ACD is observed in patients treated within 2 months from the end of chemotherapy.
  - No complete recovery in cardiac function is obtained in patients treated after 6 months.
- Cardiac surveillance, exclusively based on symptoms, may miss early detection and effective treatment of ACD.
- ACD recovery is associated with a reduction in cardiac events, when compared with patients who do not recover or who have partially recovered from ACD.
- A greater improvement in cardiac function is observed in patients receiving a combination of ACEI and beta-blockers.

Whether therapy with ACEI and beta-blockers should be either prolonged lifelong or discontinued after complete recovery of LVEF is unknown and needs further investigation.

8.3.2 Left Ventricular Dysfunction Induced by Trastuzumab

Treatment of trastuzumab-induced cardiac dysfunction (TICD) is a controversial issue.

Trastuzumab-related cardiotoxicity seems to have a more favorable outcome than ACD, as cardiac function improves after withdrawal of the drug in most cases [49].

However, the concept that TICD is a reversible condition remains in discussion [50, 51]. Follow-up data from large trials show that:
- In many patients treated with anthracyclines followed by trastuzumab, TICD does not recover.
- Up to two-thirds of patients continue to receive cardiac medication after complete functional recovery.
- Many patients continue to have a LVEF lower than baseline despite optimal HF therapy.

Although favorable data on long-term cardiac outcome of patients with TICD are emerging [52, 53], showing that the risk versus benefit remains in favor of trastuzumab, some uncertainties regarding early diagnosis and management of TICD still remain [49–51].

Guidelines for monitoring patients receiving adjuvant trastuzumab are periodically updated, but they are specifically focused on the continuation/withdrawal/resumption of trastuzumab therapy [51, 54–57].

No evidence-based recommendations for the treatment of patients developing TICD, particularly after the completion of trastuzumab therapy, have been formulated yet. To date, the evidence supporting the use of ACEI and beta-blockers in this setting is limited to case series, and it is not demonstrated in clinical trials (◘ Table 8.6).

In clinical practice, the decision on whether to treat or not treat patients showing asymptomatic decreases in LVEF with trastuzumab is mainly based on the personal clinical experience of both cardiologists and oncologists.

Table 8.6 Clinical studies evaluating heart failure therapy in trastuzumab-induced cardiomyopathy

Treatment	Author (year)	Pts (*n*)	Mean age (yrs)	Study	FU (months)	B-LVEF (%)	F-LVEF (%)	Reported event
ACEI ACEI + BB	Ewer (2005) [18]	38	52	R	10	43	56	LVEF ↑
ACEI ACEI + BB	Cardinale (2010) [47]	251	50	PO	1–79	41	51	LVEF ↑ up to ≥50 %
ACEI ACEI+ BB	Takur (2014) [58]	79	52	R	n.a.	41	53	LVEF ↑

AC anthracyclines, *ACEI* angiotensin-converting enzyme inhibitors, *B* baseline, *BB* beta-blockers, *CD* cardiac death, *CR* case report, *Dig* digitalis, *Diur* diuretics, *F* final, *HF* heart failure, *impr.* improvement, *LVEF* left ventricular ejection fraction, *NA* not available, *NYHA* New York Heart Association, *O* observational, *P* prospective, *R* retrospective, *TRZ* trastuzumab, *TKI* tyrosine kinase inhibitors, *TXS* cardiac transplantation

8

Several algorithms have been proposed for management of TICD but their effectiveness needs to be confirmed in large, prospective trials. To date, the true effectiveness of ACEI and beta-blockers in improving LVEF and favorably impacting cardiac outcome in patients receiving trastuzumab remains unclear [47, 54–57, 59].

TICD recovery rate seems to be higher in patients treated with a combination of ACEI and beta-blockers [47, 59]. On the bases of current evidence, an approach based on the association of these two drugs should be considered in patients developing TICD.

- **Troponin.** The response of TICD to HF treatment may be predicted by assessment of troponin I, a well-recognized marker of myocardial injury in many clinical settings and in cancer patients receiving both old and new antitumor drugs [60].

The rise in troponin I during trastuzumab therapy represents an independent predictor of lack of recovery from TICD—with a threefold decrease in the chance of recovery from cardiac dysfunction, and it is associated with a higher incidence of cardiac events. Therefore, troponin I seems able to discriminate between reversible and irreversible cardiac dysfunction. This information may have relevant clinical implications for the oncologist who has to decide whether to resume trastuzumab or not and allows the cardiologist to distinguish patients with a more favorable cardiac outcome from those in whom a close cardiologic monitoring is mandatory, and prophylactic strategies, for prevention of clinical and subclinical TICD, should be planned [47].

References

1. Plana JC, Galderisi M, Barac A, et al. Expert consensus for multimodality imaging evaluation of adult patients during and after cancer therapy: a report from the American Society of Echocardiography and the European Association of Cardiovascular Imaging. Eur Heart J Cardiovasc Imaging. 2014;15(10):1063–93.
2. Smith LA, Cornelius VR, Plummer CJ, et al. Cardiotoxicity of anthracycline agents for the treatment of cancer: systematic review and meta-analysis of randomized controlled trials. BMC Cancer. 2010;10:337–50.

3. Grenier MA, Lipshultz SE. Epidemiology of anthracycline cardiotoxicity in children and adults. Semin Oncol. 1998;25(10):72–85.
4. Von Hoff DD, Layard MW, Basa P, et al. Risk factors for doxorubicin-induced congestive heart failure. Ann Intern Med. 1979;91(5):710–7.
5. Cardinale D, Colombo A, Bacchiani G, et al. Early detection of anthracycline cardiotoxicity and improvement with heart failure therapy. Circulation. 2015;131(22):1981–8.
6. Yeh ET, Bickford CL. Cardiovascular complications of cancer therapy: incidence, pathogenesis, diagnosis, and management. J Am Coll Cardiol. 2009;53(24):2231–47.
7. Vejpongsa P, Yeh ET. Topoisomerase 2β: a promising molecular target for primary prevention of anthracycline-induced cardiotoxicity. Clin Pharmacol Ther. 2014;95(1):45–52.
8. Zhang S, Liu X, Bawa-Khalfe T, et al. Identification of the molecular basis of doxorubicin-induced cardiotoxicity. Nat Med. 2012;18(11):1639–42.
9. Lipshultz SE, Alvarez JA, Scully RE. Anthracycline associated cardiotoxicity in survivors of childhood cancer. Heart. 2008;94(4):525–33.
10. Swain SM, Whaley FS, Ewer MS. Congestive heart failure in patients treated with doxorubicin: a retrospective analysis of three trials. Cancer. 2003;97(11):2869–79.
11. Bowles EJA, Wellman R, Feigelson HS, et al. Risk of heart failure in breast cancer patients after anthracycline and trastuzumab treatment: a retrospective cohort study. J Natl Cancer Inst. 2012;104(17): 1293–305.
12. Hershman DL, McBride RB, Eisemberger A, et al. Doxorubicin, cardiac risk factors and cardiac toxicity in elderly patients with diffuse B-cell non-Hodgkin's lymphoma. J Clin Oncol. 2008;26(19):3159–65.
13. Batist G, Ramakrishnan G, Rao CS, et al. Reduced cardiotoxicity and preserved antitumor efficacy of liposome-encapsulated doxorubicin and cyclophosphamide compared with conventional doxorubicin and cyclophosphamide in a randomized, multicenter trial of metastatic breast cancer. J Clin Oncol. 2001;19(5):1444–54.
14. Bird BR, Swain SM. Cardiac toxicity in breast cancer survivors: review of potential cardiac problems. Clin Cancer Res. 2008;14(1):14–24.
15. Slamon DJ, Leyland-Jones B, Shak S, et al. Use of chemotherapy plus a monoclonal antibody against HER2 for metastatic breast cancer that overexpresses HER2. N Engl J Med. 2001;344(11):783–92.
16. Dahabreh IJ, Linardou H, Siannis F, et al. Trastuzumab in the adjuvant treatment of early-stage breast cancer: a systematic review and meta-analysis of randomized controlled trials. Oncologist. 2008;13(6): 620–30.
17. de Korte MA, et al. ^{111}Indium trastuzumab visualises myocardial human epidermal growth factor receptor 2 expression shortly after anthracycline treatment but not during heart failure: A clue to uncover the mechanism of trastuzumab-related cardiotoxicity. Eur J Cancer. 2007;43:2046–51.
18. Ewer MS, et al. Changes in left ventricular ejection fraction (LVEF) from baseline to re-treatment with trastuzumab in a selected population. JCO. 2005;23:7820–6.
19. Ewer MS, Lippman SM. Type 2 chemotherapy-related cardiac dysfunction: time to recognize a new entity. J Clin Oncol. 2005;23(13):2900–2.
20. Chu TF, Rupnick MA, Kerkela R, et al. Cardiotoxicity associated with tyrosine kinase inhibitor sunitinib. Lancet. 2007;370:2011–9.
21. Richards CJ, Je Y, Schutz FA, et al. Incidence and risk of congestive heart failure in patients with renal and nonrenal cell carcinoma treated with sunitinib. J Clin Oncol. 2011;29:3450–6.
22. Iles L, Pfluger H, Phrommintikul A, Cherayath J, Aksit P, Gupta SN, et al. Evaluation of diffuse myocardial fibrosis in heart failure with cardiac magnetic resonance contrast-enhanced T1 mapping. J Am Coll Cardiol. 2008;52:1574–80.
23. Ugander M, Oki AJ, Hsu LY, Kellman P, Greiser A, Aletras AH, et al. Extracellular volume imaging by magnetic resonance imaging provides insights into overt and sub-clinical myocardial pathology. Eur Heart J. 2012;33:1268–78.
24. Tham E, Chow K, Spavor M, Pagano JJ, Haykowsky M, Thompson RJ. Degree of diffuse fibrosis measured by MRI correlates with LV remodelling in childhood cancer survivors after anthracycline chemotherapy. J Cardiovasc Magn Reson. 2011;13:P276.
25. Neilan TG, Coelho-Filho OR, Shah RV, Feng JH, Pena-Herrera D, Mandry D, et al. Myocardial extracellular volume by cardiac magnetic resonance imaging in patients treated with anthracycline-based chemotherapy. Am J Cardiol. 2013;111:717–22.
26. Schwartz RG, McKenzie WB, Alexander J, Sager P, D'Souza A, Manatunga A, et al. Congestive heart failure and left ventricular dysfunction complicating doxorubicin therapy. Seven-year experience using serial radionuclide angiocardiography. Am J Med. 1987;82:1109–18.

27. Pinder MC, Duan Z, Goodwin JS, Hortobagyi GN, Giordano SH. Congestive heart failure in older women treated with adjuvant anthracycline chemotherapy for breast cancer. J Clin Oncol. 2007;25:3808–15.
28. Lang RM, Badano LP, Mor-Avi V, et al. Recommendations for cardiac chamber quantification by echocardiography in adults: an update from the American Society of Echocardiography and the European Association of Cardiovascular Imaging. J Am Soc Echocardiogr. 2015;28:1–39.
29. Zamorano JL, Lancellotti P, Munoz DR, et al. 2016 ESC Position Paper on cancer treatments and cardiovascular toxicity developed under auspices f the ESC Committee for Practice Guidelines. Eur Heart J 2016; Aug: 2-34. doi:10.109/eurheartj/ehw.211.
30. Nagueh SF, Smiseth OA, Appleton CP, et al. Recommendations for the evaluation of left ventricular diastolic function by echocardiography: An update from the American Society of Echocardiography and the European Association of Cardiovascular Imaging. J. Am Soc Echocardiogr 2016;29:277–314.
31. Mele D, Rizzo P, Pollina AV, et al. Cancer therapy-induced cardiotoxicity: role of ultrasound deformation imaging as an aid to early diagnosis. Ultrasound Med Biol. 2015;41(3):627–43.
32. Takigiku K, Takeuchi M, Izumi C, Yuda S, Sakata K, Ohte N, et al. Normal range of left ventricular 2-dimensional strain: Japanese ultrasound speckle tracking of the left ventricle (JUSTICE) study. Circ J. 2012;76: 2623–32.
33. Cardinale D, Sandri MT, Colombo A, Colombo N, Boeri M, Lamantia G, et al. Prognostic value of troponin I in cardiac risk stratification of cancer patients undergoing high-dose chemotherapy. Circulation. 2004;109:2749–54.
34. Cardinale D, Sandri MT. Role of biomarkers in chemotherapy-induced cardiotoxicity. Prog Cardiovasc Dis. 2010;53:121–9.
35. Felker GM, Thompson RE, Hare JM, et al. Underlying causes and long-term survival in patients with initially unexplained cardiomyopathy. N Engl J Med. 2000;342(15):1077–84.
36. Lefrak EA, Pitha J, Rosenheim S, Gotilieb JA. A clinicopathologic analysis of adriamycin cardiotoxicity. Cancer. 1973;32:302–14.
37. Cohen M, Kronzon I, Lebowitz A. Reversible doxorubicin-induced congestive heart failure. Arch Intern Med. 1982;142:1570–1.
38. Haq MM, Legha SS, Choksi J, et al. Doxorubicin-induced congestive heart failure in adults. Cancer. 1985;56:1361–5.
39. Saini J, Rich MW, Lyss AP. Reversibility of severe left ventricular dysfunction due to doxorubicin cardiotoxicity. Report of three cases. Ann Intern Med. 1987;106:814–6.
40. Jensen BV, Nielsen SL, Skovsgaard T. Treatment with angiotensin-converting-enzyme inhibitor for epirubicin-induced dilated cardiomyopathy. Lancet. 1996;347:297–9.
41. Fazio S, Calmieri EA, Ferravate B, Bonè F, Biondi B, Saccà L. Doxorubicin-induced cardiomyopathy treated with carvedilol. Clin Cardiol. 1998;21:777–9.
42. Noori A, Lindenfeld J, Wolfel E, Ferguson D, Bristow MR, Lowes BD. Beta-blockade in adriamycin-induced cardiomyopathy. J Card Fail. 2000;6:115–9.
43. Jensen BV, Skovsgaard T, Nielsen SL. Functional monitoring of anthracycline cardiotoxicity: a prospective, blinded, long-term observational study of outcome in 120 patients. Ann Oncol. 2002;13:699–709.
44. Mukai Y, Yoshida T, Nakaike R, et al. Five cases of anthracycline-induced cardiomyopathy effectively treated with carvedilol. Intern Med. 2004;43:1087–8.
45. Tallaj JA, Franco V, Rayburn BK, et al. Response of doxorubicin-induced cardiomyopathy to the current management strategy of heart failure. J Heart Lung Transplant. 2005;24:2196–201.
46. Tabet JY, Meurin P, Ben Driss A, et al. Beta-blockade intolerance in anthracycline-induced cardiomyopathy. Int J Cardiol. 2006;106:132–4.
47. Cardinale D, Colombo A, Torrisi R, et al. Trastuzumab-induced cardiotoxicity: clinical and prognostic implications of troponin I evaluation. J Clin Oncol. 2010;28:3910–6.
48. Cardinale D, Colombo A, Lamantia G, et al. Anthracycline-induced cardiomyopathy. Clinical relevance and response to pharmacologic therapy. J Am Coll Cardiol. 2010;55:213–20.
49. Ewer SM, Ewer MS. Cardiotoxicity profile of trastuzumab. Drug Saf. 2008;31:459–67.
50. Telli ML, Hunt SA, Carlson RW, Guardino AE. Trastuzumab-related cardiotoxicity: calling into question the concept of reversibility. J Clin Oncol. 2007;25:3525–33.
51. Tocchetti CG, Ragone G, Coppola C, Rea D, Piscopo G, Scala S. Detection, monitoring, and management of trastuzumab-induced left ventricular dysfunction: an actual challenge. Eur J Heart Fail. 2012;14: 130–7.
52. Morris PG, Iyengar NM, Patil S, Chen C, Abbruzzi A, Lehman R, Steingart R, Oeffinger KC, Lin N, Moy B, Come SE, Winer EP, Norton L, Hudis CA, Dang CT. Long-term cardiac safety and outcomes of dose-dense

8

doxorubicin and cyclophosphamide followed by paclitaxel and trastuzumab with and without lapatinib in patients with early breast cancer. Cancer. 2013;119:3943–51.

53. de Azambuja E, Procter MJ, van Veldhuisen DJ, Agbor-Tarh D, Metzger-Filho O, Steinseifer J, Untch M, Smith IE, Gianni L, Baselga J, Jackisch C, Cameron DA, Bell R, Leyland-Jones B, Dowsett M, Gelber RD, Piccart-Gebhart MJ, Suter TM. Trastuzumab-associated cardiac events at 8 years of median follow-up in the herceptin adjuvant trial (BIG 1-01). J Clin Oncol. 2014;32:2159–65.
54. Mackey JR, Clemons M, Coté MA, Delgado D, Dent S, Paterson A. Cardiac management during adjuvant trastuzumab therapy: recommendations of the Canadian Trastuzumab Working Group. Curr Oncol. 2008;15:24–35.
55. Sengupta PP, Northfelt DW, Gentile F, Zamorano JL, Khandheria BK. Trastuzumab-induced cardiotoxicity: heart failure at the crossroads. Mayo Clin Proc. 2008;83:197–203.
56. Jones AL, Barlow M, Barrett-Lee PJ, Canney PA, Gilmour IM, Robb SD. Management of cardiac health in trastuzumab-treated patients with breast cancer: updated United Kingdom National Cancer Research Institute recommendations for monitoring. Br J Cancer. 2009;100:684–92.
57. Martin M, Esteva FJ, Alba E, Khandheria B, Pérez-Isla L, Garcìa-Sàenz JA. Minimizing cardiotoxicity while optimizing treatment efficacy with trastuzumab: review and expert recommendations. Oncologist. 2009;14:1–11.
58. Thakur A, Witteles R. Cancer therapy-induced left ventricular dysfunction: interventions and prognosis. J Card Fail. 2014;20:155–8.
59. Ewer MS, Vooletich MT, Durand JB, et al. Reversibility of trastuzumab-related cardiotoxicity. New insight based on clinical course and response to medical treatment. J Clin Oncol. 2005;23:7820–6.
60. Cardinale D, Salvatici M, Sandri MT. Role of biomarkers in cardioncology. Clin Chem Lab Med. 2011;49:1937–48.

Cardiotoxicity: Cardiac Ischemia

Roberto Labianca, Chiara Lestuzzi, Cezar Iliescu, and Laura Ghilardi

C. Lestuzzi et al. (eds.), *Manual of Cardio-oncology*, DOI 10.1007/978-3-319-40236-9_9

9.1 Introduction

- Several antineoplastic treatments have been associated with cardiac ischemia as a side effect. For most of them, however, large studies are lacking and the association is weak.
- Radiation therapy of the mediastinum or of the left chest wall increases by several times the risk of coronary artery disease on the long-term follow-up. This problem will be discussed in the designated chapter.
- The most commonly used drugs that have been involved in cardiac ischemia are the fluoropyrimidines (FP) [5-fluorouracil (5FU) and capecitabine], the vascular endothelial growth factor receptor inhibitors (anti-VEGFR) and the aromatase inhibitors.
  - **In regards to FP and anti-VEGFR, the association with acute ischemia is well recognized.**
  - In regards to aromatase inhibitors, the cause–effect relationship is less clear. Studies are conflicting, and many confounding factors (blood lipid profile, comorbidities) should be taken into account.
  - Other antineoplastic treatments have been associated with acute ischemia during treatment or with an increased risk in medium or long term (◻ Table 9.1).

9.2 Fluoropyrimidines

The fluoropyrimidines (FP) are the antimetabolite 5-fluorouracil (5-FU) and its oral prodrug capecitabine (CAPE).
- 5-FU is used in different schemes (bolus, short- and long-term infusions) with different dosages, as monotherapy or in association with other drugs.
- CAPE is used mostly with the scheme 14 days on therapy, 7 off therapy, alone, or associated to other drugs. As radiosensitizing agent, it may be used daily over 4–5 weeks.

◻ **Table 9.1** Probability of cause–effect relation with antineoplastic therapies and acute myocardial ischemia according to time

	During therapy or within days after	Weeks/months after therapy	Years after therapy
Fluoropyrimidines	Very likely	Very unlikely	Very unlikely
Bevacizumab	Very likely	Possible	Unlikely
TKI (VEGF or BCR-ABL targeted)	Very likely	Unlikely	Unlikely
Platinum	Likely	Likely	Possible
I1-2, IFN	Likely	Unlikely	Very unlikely
Taxanes	Possible	Very unlikely	Very unlikely
Aromatase Inhibitors	Possible	Possible	Possible
Anti-androgen treatments	No data	Likely in patiens with previous cardiovascular risk factors	Likely (mostly linked to metabolic syndrome)
Radiation therapy	Unlikely	Possible	Likely

- The FPs are effective in several carcinomas: colorectal, stomach, esophagus, breast, head/neck and pancreas.
- The principal mechanism of action of FP has been considered to be the inhibition of thymidylate synthase (TYMS), but recent evidence has shown an alternative pharmacodynamic pathway acting through the incorporation of drug metabolites into DNA and RNA.
- Cardiac ischemia due to either 5-FU or capecitabine share the same clinical presentation.

9.2.1 Pathophysiology

The pathophysiology of FP-induced ischemia has not been fully clarified yet. Several mechanisms have been proposed, but a satisfactory hypothesis consistent with all the various clinical aspects is lacking [1].

- The observation of rest angina with ST elevation on ECG suggests a vasospastic (the so-called "variant" or "Prinzmetal" angina) component. Vasospasm of a major coronary artery has been actually described in patients who underwent coronary angiography. However, this is in contrast with the usually low increase in cardiac enzymes and the usually complete recovery of left ventricular kinetics, even after long-lasting episodes. Microvessel spasm has also been suggested as an alternative explanation.
- Impurities in commercial vials leading to accumulation of fluoroacetate as degradation product have been considered as possible cause of 5-FU's cardiotoxicity [2]. However, the frequency of the syndrome has not been reduced in the recent years after this problem has been avoided suggesting that this hypothesis is unlikely; moreover, it does not explain CAPE cardiotoxicity.
- Direct myocardial damage with myocarditis and hemorrhagic infarction has been suggested based on animal studies, but there are no clinical studies supporting this hypothesis.
- 5-FU has a toxic effect on the vascular endothelium and induces a hypercoagulable status. However, this is a common effect, and there is no proof that hypercoagulability is more pronounced in patients with FP-induced angina compared to those who tolerate the therapy without problems [3].
- An intriguing hypothesis is that FP can induce a Kounis syndrome, i.e., an acute coronary syndrome due to hypersensitivity reaction, and mediated by mast cell activation [4, 5]. This mechanism would explain the observation of a subset of patients who have cardiac ischemia at every FP exposure, and also the inconstant response to vasodilator therapy (see below ► Sect. 2.6).

9.2.2 Incidence

The incidence varies from 2 to 3 % in the retrospective studies based on oncological records to 10–18 % in the prospective studies and also varies widely among different scheme of administration [6–9].

- The incidence is higher in the prospective studies as they include the "asymptomatic toxicities" including rest, stress, and/or 24-h (Holter) ECG in the diagnostic work-up [10, 11].
- Cardiac toxicity has been seldom reported for single bolus infusions of 5-FU. It is much more common with *prolonged 5-FU infusions* and with *capecitabine*.

  - Among 5-FU continuous infusions, those lasting >48 h and those with higher daily dosage are at higher risk compared to the shorter and/or lower dosage ones [12].
  - The concomitant use of leucovorin or of cisplatin has been reported as an additional risk [8, 13].
- No individual predisposing factors have been identified so far.
  - Preexisting ischemic heart disease or cardiovascular risk factors have been found by some authors to be more frequent in patients with FP-induced ischemia compared to those without it. However, there might be a bias in evaluating symptoms, mostly atypical chest pain: if a patient with known coronary artery disease complains of chest pain, angina is likely to be considered; the same symptom in a young woman without cardiac history may be easily diagnosed as nonspecific. Moreover, patients with coronary heart disease may have—in case of toxicity—a more severe clinical presentation, and this may lead to an easier recognition.
  - There are studies which did not find any relationship with previous cardiac disease and FP cardiotoxicity. Many cases of even severe cardiotoxicity have been reported in young patients without any cardiovascular risk factor.
- Preexisting heart disease (in particular, coronary artery disease) should be aggressively treated and close follow-up should be performed during cancer treatment, with prompt additional investigation if patient symptomatic.
  - The genetically determined dihydropyridine dehydrogenase (DPD) activity deficit (which can cause severe FP gastrointestinal or hematologic toxicities) seems not to be involved in the cardiac toxicity [14].
  - Patients who developed cardiotoxicity during FP treatment pose a **very high risk of symptoms**/toxicity recurrence at rechallenge, even when shifting from 5-FU to CAPE or vice versa. On the contrary, patients who do not have cardiotoxicity in the first course of therapy seldom have it with further courses.
  - FP-induced ischemia appears mostly patient-related, as a hypersensitivity reaction
  - Cardiac ischemia may be present at rest or be elicited or exacerbated by physical effort [15].

9.2.3 Clinical Presentation

The clinical presentation is variable from case to case, and this may make the recognition of the problem challenging [16, 17].

- Symptoms may appear at rest, under or after effort, and even be completely absent.
- **Typical rest angina** is the best known clinical symptom. The attacks may last from a few minutes to hours. They are usually relapsing and worsening if the infusion/oral assumption is not stopped.
- Atypical symptoms (as jaw pain, sore throat, chest discomfort) are also common in our experience.
- Syncope and sudden death due to ventricular arrhythmias secondary to acute ischemia may be the first symptom, or follow the angina.
  - Effort-induced ischemia may present with typical or atypical angina as well. If it is elicited by physical effort, it usually worsens at higher workloads, but it may also worsen or become evident in the recovery phase (◘ Fig. 9.1).
- The mortality (of myocardial infarction with cardiogenic shock or fatal arrhythmias) is about 8–13 % [17]

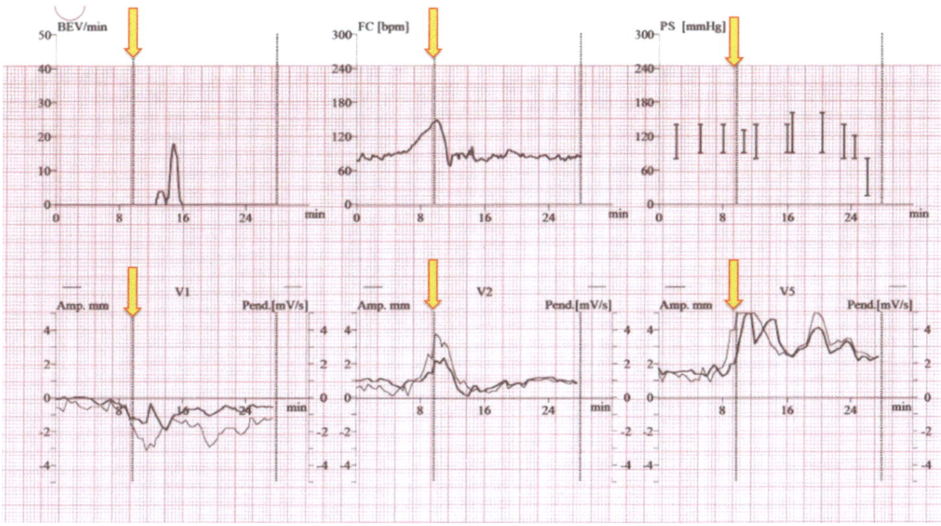

Fig. 9.1 Oligosymptomatic cardiac ischemia during treadmill stress test. The *yellow arrows* sign the end of stress. Ventricular ectopic beats (BEV, *Top left*) are present only in the recovery phase. ST segment elevation (*bottom right*, V5 lead) becomes evident during stress, increases in amplitude during the recovery phase, and lasts more than 30 min, in spite of a rapid reduction on heart rate (FC, *center top*). A mirror ST segment depression may be observed in V1 lead (*bottom left*)

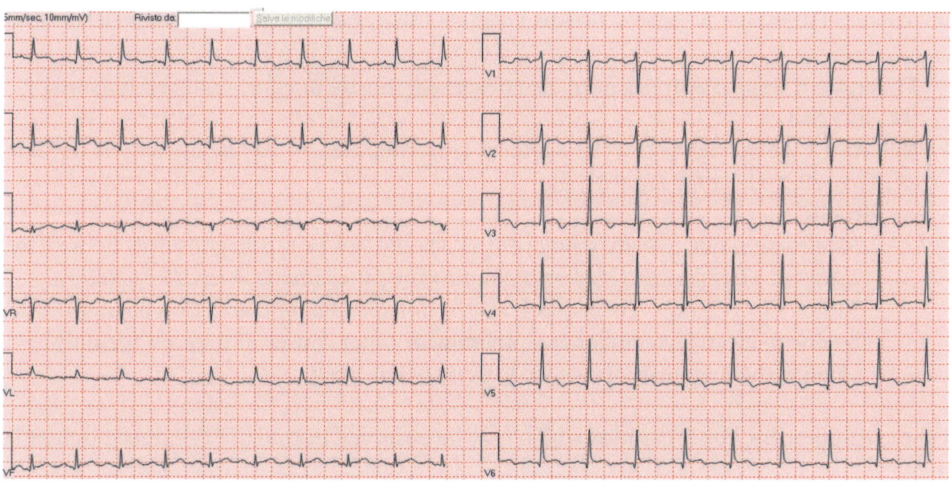

Fig. 9.2 Rest toxicity during fluorouracil infusion: the patient complained of typical chest pain; ECG shows a diffuse ST segment elevation

- The symptoms may last or even appear in the first hours after stopping therapy.
  - **Pitfalls:** Esophageal spasm may mimic anginal pain.

ECG changes may be related to typical or atypical angina symptoms and can even be observed without any symptoms and may last for days after symptoms disappearance.

- **ST segment elevation** is the first and most described ECG change reported for FP cardiac toxicity.
  - It may be diffuse or evident in a limited number of ECG leads (Figs. 9.2 and 9.3a).

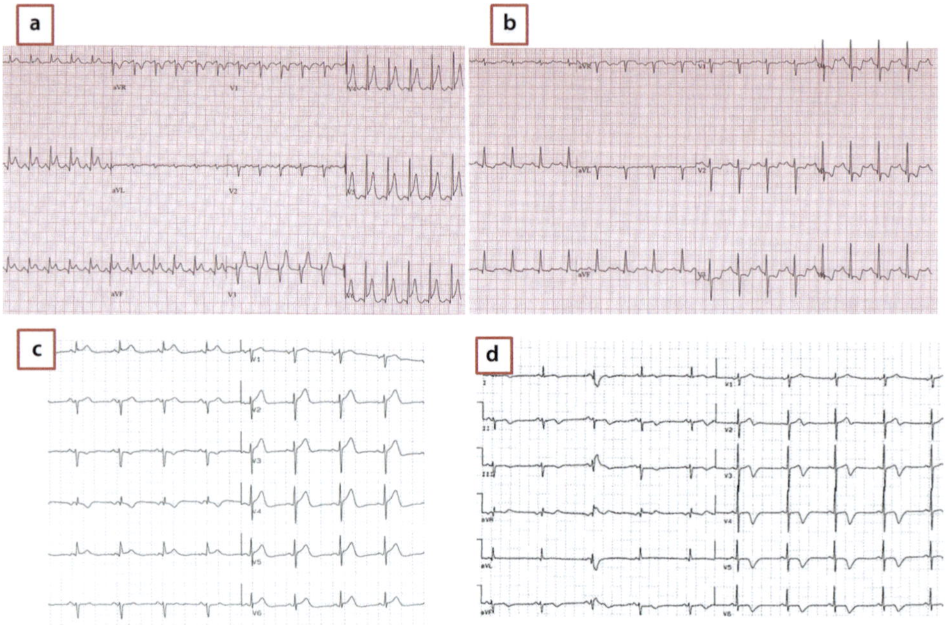

9

Fig. 9.3 Different ECG aspects of fluoropyrimidine cardiac toxicity. **a** ST segment elevation during stress test during 5-FU infusion. **b** ST segment depression during stress test. **c** ST segment elevation at rest during 5-FU infusion. **d** Negative T waves 4 days after stopping 5-FU infusion (same patient as in **c**)

- **ST segment depression** has been also observed, mostly in effort-induced ischemia (Fig. 9.3b).
- **Negative T waves** may follow ST segment abnormalities or may be the only ECG sign of FP cardiotoxicity (Fig. 9.3c, d).
  - **Pitfalls:**
    - ST elevation due to early repolarization should not be misdiagnosed as FP toxicity, *therefore a baseline ECG before chemotherapy, for comparison must be obtained.*
    - Minor ECG changes (negative T waves, nonspecific repolarization changes) may be due to electrolyte imbalance, anemia, or other causes. If they are the only change, the diagnosis of cardiac toxicity is less likely.

Echocardiographic abnormalities which may be observed in case of FP-induced ischemia are:

- Segmental hypoakinesia in the leads corresponding to ECG signs of ischemia
- Apical ballooning like in takotsubo cardiomyopathy [18]
- Diffuse hypokinesia, mimicking myocarditis.
  - All these abnormalities may be transient and disappear before ECG alterations.

9.2.4 Laboratory Analysis Data

- Cardiac necrosis markers (CPK, troponins) may be elevated in cases leading to myocardial infarction but are often within the normal limits or only slightly elevated even in presence of diffuse ST segment elevation and/or chest pain lasting several hours.

- Brain natriuretic factor (BNP) may be elevated in some (but not all) cases of diffuse left ventricular dysfunction [19].
- Blood coagulation tests are usually altered during 5-FU therapy, but this finding is nonspecific.

9.2.5 Challenges in Diagnosis

- FP cardiac toxicity may be underestimated, because of:
  - The variety of clinical presentations (often with only mild or atypical symptoms)
  - The low grade of concordance between symptoms, ECG changes and laboratory analysis data
- Any patient under FP therapy complaining of even mild or atypical symptoms should be thoroughly evaluated for possible ischemia. An ECG performed after some days of therapy may also identify a number of asymptomatic toxicities.
- The diagnostic work up should include (▫ Fig. 9.6):
  - Clinical history with particular attention to angina-like symptoms and their temporal relationship with drug administration.
  - Rest ECG, which should be compared—if possible—with a pre-chemotherapy ECG. In cases with suspect symptoms and normal ECG, a 24-h (Holter) and/or stress ECG should be considered.
  - In cases with typical symptoms and/or ECG alterations the following should be obtained:
    - Echocardiogram.
    - Cardiac enzymes.
    - Blood coagulation tests and D-Dimer.
    - If concern about Kounis syndrome, IgE, histamine, neutral proteases (chymase, tryptase), arachidonic acid products, high sensitivity CRP, and tumor necrosis factor can help in diagnosis.

9.2.6 Therapy

There are no guidelines or large prospective studies on the therapeutic approach. The following suggestions are based on the analysis of the reported case series and literature review, considering the most reliable pathophysiological hypotheses and on our personal experience.

9.2.7 FP Therapy Must Be Stopped Immediately When Cardiotoxicity is Detected

- According to the clinical status (presence of chest pain and/or arrhythmias, heart rate, blood pressure), therapy with nitrates and/or calcium channel blockers (nifedipine, amlodipine, verapamil, or diltiazem) should be started. The effect may be prompt (▫ Fig. 9.4) or even poor (▫ Fig. 9.5). Diltiazem has been proved effective in a small series [20].

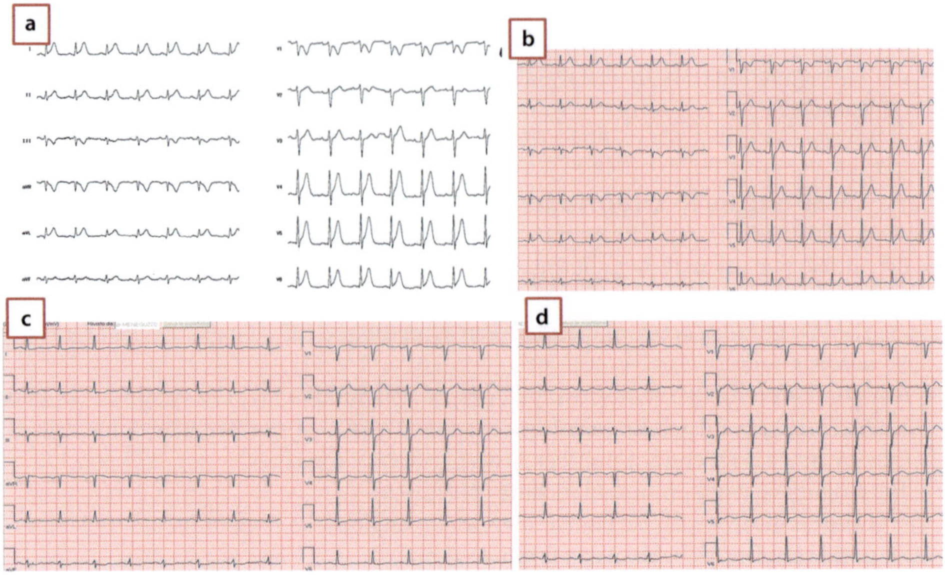

Fig. 9.4 Patient with angina on the 4° day of 5-FU infusion. **a** Diffuse ST segment elevation with tall and peaked T waves and mirror ST segment depression in V1. **b** 20 min later, after nitrates, ECG changes are reduced. **c** After 10 more minutes, pain has disappeared and the ECG changes are reduced. **d** The following day ECG is normal

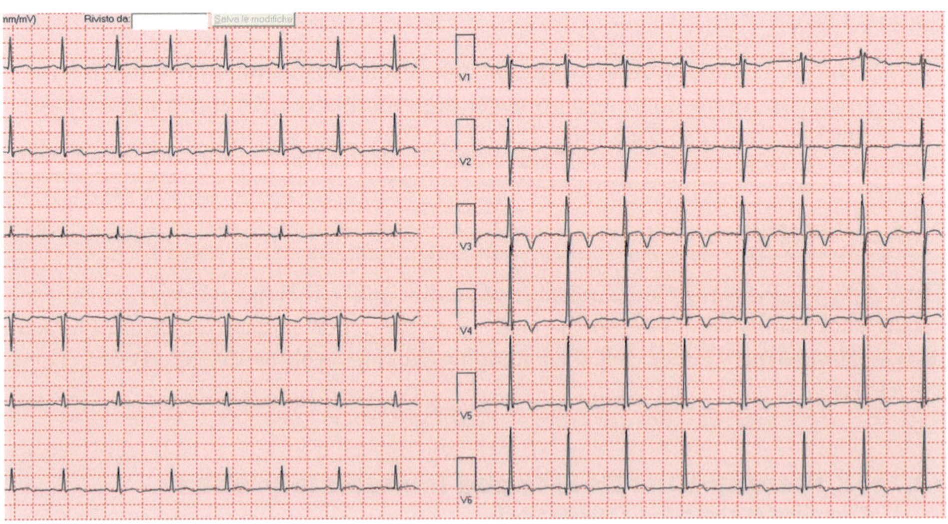

Fig. 9.5 Young female patient with rest toxicity (typical angina and ST segment elevation) during fluorouracil infusion. Mild symptoms and ECG changes (mild ST segment elevation, negative T waves) lasted more than 3 days after stopping the infusion and starting therapy with i.v. nitrates and oral nifedipine

- There are no studies about the use of anticoagulants in this setting. However, if a hypercoagulable status is recognized, the use of low molecular weight heparin seems reasonable and may be considered.
- If a Kounis syndrome is suspected, intravenous hydrocortisone (1–2 mg/Kg/day), anti-histamines (diphenhydramine 1–2 mg/Kg), and ranitidine (1 mg/Kg) may be added to calcium channel blockers and nitrates [4].
- A period of in-hospital observation with cardiac monitoring (cardiac enzymes, ECG) is:
  - Mandatory in all cases presenting with arrhythmias and/or persistent signs/symptoms of ischemia at rest. The monitoring period should be prolonged until complete symptomatic recovery
  - Recommended for at least some hours (preferably 24 h) in all the patients with symptoms at rest or after minimal effort and for those with relevant asymptomatic ECG or echocardiographic changes

9.2.8 Time to Recovery

5-FU disappears rapidly from blood, but active 5FU nucleotide metabolites (also common to capecitabine) responsible for the cytotoxicity of 5FU are retained much more than the 5FU parent drug at the cellular level [21]. Thus, the cardiotoxic effects may last several days after stopping therapy (◘ Fig. 9.5).

9.2.9 Rechallenge

After FP cardiotoxicity, the risk of relapse if the same drug (or even if capecitabine instead of 5FU) is rechallenged is very high, with significant mortality. Thus, *rechallenge should be avoided if possible* (◘ Fig. 9.6).

- Raltitrexed (a thymidylate synthase inhibitor) without the cardiotoxicity spectrum of FP may be considered as an alternative drug [22, 23].
  - Tegafur is another alternative drug which might be considered in particular cases, according to the cancer type and clinical status; in fact, its use is limited, compared to FP [24–27].

In case of strong oncologic indication to FP therapy, the risk/benefit should be assessed together by the caring oncologist and cardiologist (◘ Fig. 9.7). In case of rechallenge, several approaches have been attempted, with variable results [28]:

- Prevention with an association of calcium channel blockers (most used: diltiazem, nifedipine, amlodipine) with/without associated nitrates has been proven useful in some cases [17, 20, 28].
- The most effective strategy is to reduce the dosage and the time of exposure to the drug:
  - 5-FU boluses instead of prolonged infusions or oral capecitabine [14, 15].
  - Reduced total dose. This approach would obviously reduce the therapeutic efficacy of the anticancer treatment: thus the maximum tolerated dose should be

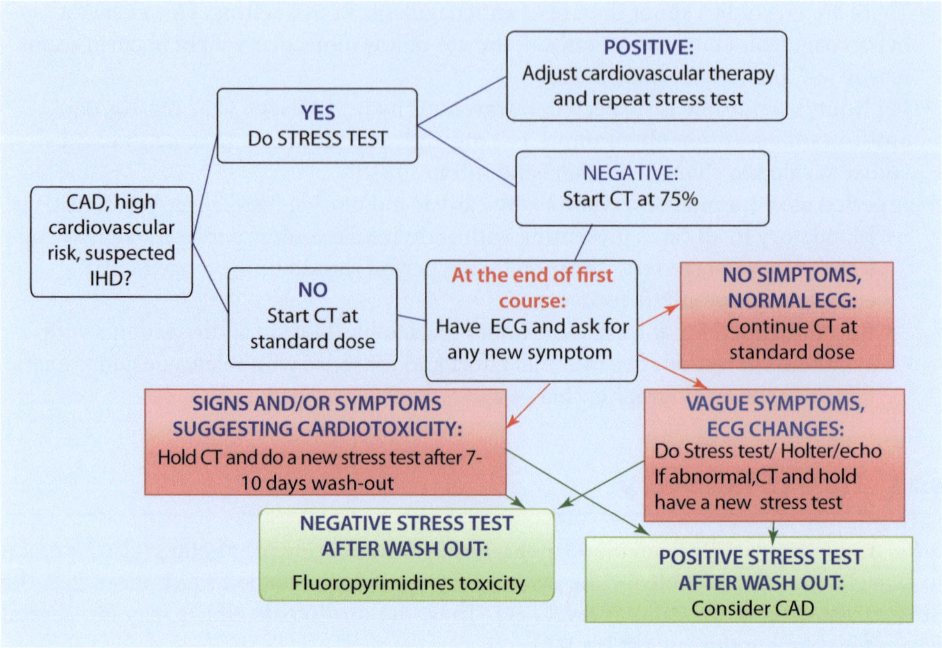

Fig. 9.6 Operative flowchart for selection of patients and screening of cardiotoxicity in fluoropyrimidine-naive patients—*CAD* coronary artery disease, *CT* chemotherapy, *IHD* ischemic heart disease

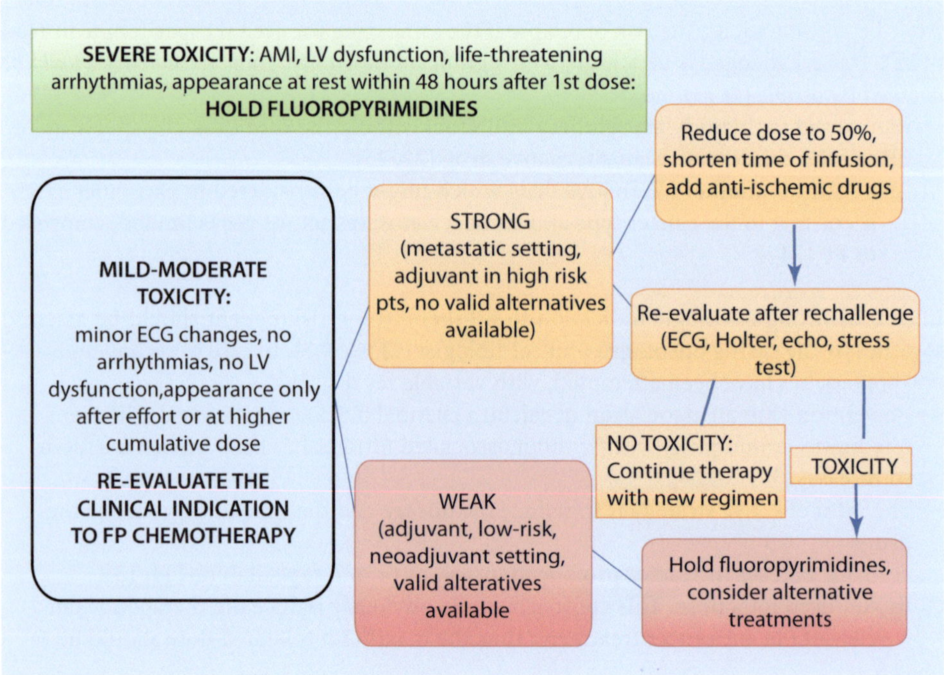

Fig. 9.7 Operative flowchart for rechallenge decision in patients with fluoropyrimidine cardiac toxicity. *AMI* acute myocardial infarction; *LV* left ventricle

identified. A practical approach could be start with a course at 50 % of the original dose, with close monitoring; if the drug is well tolerated, the does can be increased to 70–75 % in the following courses.

- A combination of the two previous approaches (reduced dose with prophylactic treatment and then cautious increase in dose) is the optimal approach in our experience.
- Rechallenge with stress test to assess the efficacy of preventive interventions may be helpful and should be considered in selected cases only [29].

9.3 Anti-VEGFR

Neoangiogenesis, a process involving the proliferation of new blood vessels, plays a crucial role in the growth and metastasis of cancer. This process is mainly driven by the vascular endothelial growth factors (VEGF), whose signaling pathway has been a target of many new antineoplastic agents including bevacizumab, sorafenib, sunitinib, and others. However, these drugs affect also normal vessels leading to a variety of cardiovascular side effects (Fig. 9.8) (see also chapter tot: Hypertension).

- In a meta-analysis published in 2010, the patients treated with bevacizumab (®Avastin) had an increased risk of acute thromboembolic event compared to patients

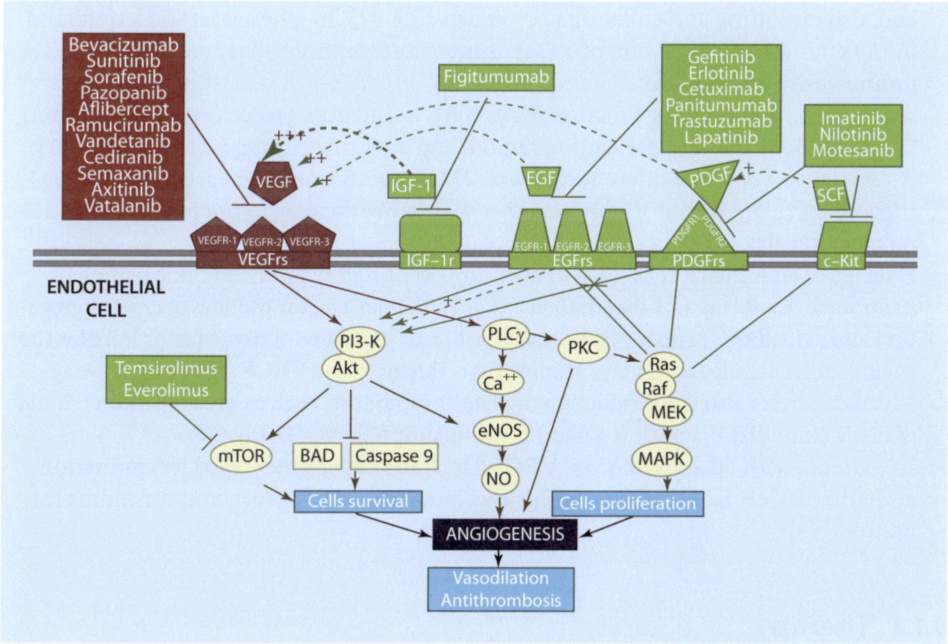

Fig. 9.8 Anti-angiogenic network and inhibitors. In *red*, proper "intended" angiogenic pathways, inhibitors, receptors, and ligand. In *green*, broad unintended or "accidental" angiogenic pathways, inhibitors, receptors and ligands. In *light yellow*, intracellular pathways. In *blue* and *light blue*, final effects on vascular system. *EGF* epidermal growth factor, *EGRFs* EGF receptors, *IGF* insulin-like growth factor-1, *PDGF* platelet-derived growth factor, *PDGFRs* PDGF receptors, *SCF* stem cell factor, *VEGF* vascular endothelial growth factor, *VEGFRs* VEGF receptors (-1, -2, -3). Reproduced with permission from [44]

undergoing conventional chemotherapy, with a 2.2-fold increased risk of acute myocardial ischemia; this risk was observed both in patients with colorectal and renal cancer [30].
- In a more recent study, the risk of ischemic heart disease was significantly increased, with an overall relative risk (RR) 2.49, but varied according to doses (2.1 versus 4.89 RR for doses of 2.5 mg/Kg/week versus 5 mg/Kg/week, respectively) and tumor type: a significant increase was observed in patients with colorectal cancer, not in renal or liver carcinoma [31].
- The anti-VEGF tyrosin kinase inhibitors (TKI) sunitinib and sorafenib have been reported as cause of thromboembolic events and acute coronary syndromes and myocardial infarction [32, 33]. However, in a recent report, the incidence of myocardial ischemia with sorafenib and sunitinib in adjuvant setting was low [34]. TKI have other therapeutic targets beside VEGF, as platelet-derived growth factor receptor (PDGFR), RAF/RAS/MAP kinases.

9.3.1 Pathophysiology

- VEGF family comprises several factors (A, B, C, D, and E, with VEGF-A being the most studied) which can link to several receptors (VEGFR 1, VEGFR 2, and VEGFR 3); they play a crucial role in maintaining endothelial integrity, regulating vasodilation, preventing apoptosis, favoring neoangiogenesis, protecting from oxidative stress, and also exhibiting anti-inflammatory effects [35–37]. In atherosclerotic lesions and in ischemic areas, expression of VEGF is increased; in more advanced lesions, VEGF promotes the growing of collateral vessels [38, 39]. VEGF-B is activated during cardiac ischemia, enhancing functional coronary vascularity, protecting myocytes from the ischemic stress, and preventing remodeling after myocardial infarction [40, 41]. After acute myocardial infarction, blood VEGF significantly increases; this finding suggests a crucial role of VEGF (together with other factors) in the protection and repair of cardiac tissue [42].
- Damage of endothelial cells leads to exposure of the highly prothrombotic basement membrane. Exposure of subendothelial von Willebrand factor induces platelet aggregation and activation (primary hemostasis), whereas exposure of tissue factor initiates the coagulation cascade (secondary hemostasis). Targeting the VEGF signaling pathway adversely affects also the production of platelet inhibitors, such as prostaglandin I-2 and of nitric oxide (NO), which is a natural vasodilator [43, 44] (Fig. 9.7).
- In patients with atherosclerosis, VEGF blockade causes increased inflammation and atherosclerotic instability with subsequent plaque rupture and thrombus formation [45].

9.3.2 Therapy

- Anti-VEGF side effects are both ischemia and bleeding, with hemorrhage being the most common cause of treatment-related mortality with bevacizumab [46, 47]. Thus, the use of antiplatelet and anticoagulant therapy should be done with caution. There are no current guidelines about this topic [48].

- A consensus conference suggested careful selection of patients undergoing anti-VEGF treatments, with particular attention to those with atherosclerotic disease and cardiac ischemia, but no specific therapy for the acute events, besides discontinuing the antineoplastic therapy [49].
- According to the pathophysiology, a reasonable approach might be the use of:
  - Nebivolol, a beta-blocker which increase the release of NO
  - Nitrates, to enhance vasodilatation
  - Low-molecular-weight heparin, according to the bleeding risk
  - Aspirin may also be indicated, since in a retrospective study, its use increased only slightly the bleeding risk in association with bevacizumab [50].
- Antineoplastic therapy with antiangiogenic drugs may cause acute myocardial ischemia or worsen a preexisting ischemic heart disease.
  - A careful clinical history about CAD and cardiovascular risk factors should be obtained before starting therapy.
  - Smoking should be strongly discouraged, and any cardiac therapy for hypertension, dyslipidemia diabetes, and/or cardiac ischemia should be optimized before antineoplastic therapy.
  - VEGFs play a relevant role in restoration of the capillary network after ischemia and revascularization [51, 52]. An inhibition of neoangiogenesis might then be theoretically contraindicated shortly after acute myocardial infarction, an acute coronary syndrome, and/or a revascularization intervention. On the other hand, there are no reported data about the actual clinical risk, and an increase of circulating VEGF after angioplasty might be associated with an increased risk of restenosis [53].
- After an acute coronary syndrome or revascularization, the risk/benefit ratio of starting immediately or postpone for some weeks a required anti-VEGF therapy should be evaluated in the single patient; in either case, a close symptomatic monitoring should be done at least for the first 3 months if possible.

9.4 Other Drugs Which Have Been Involved in Acute Cardiac Ischemia or in Increased Risk of Myocardial Infarction at Medium-Long Term

9.4.1 BCR-ABL-Targeted Tyrosine Kinase Inhibitors

Cardiovascular adverse events occur in patients on *BCR-ABL-targeted tyrosine kinase inhibitors* (nilotinib, ponatinib) [54, 55]. Therefore, in cases of preexisting atherosclerotic changes or ischemic processes presenting with angina pectoris-like symptoms, a coronary angiography should be considered. Ponatinib has a mild inhibitory effect on platelet aggregation. Serious arterial thrombotic events (including cardiovascular, cerebrovascular, and peripheral vascular events) are seen in 8.9 % of the patients who received ponatinib, with an overall incidence of all arterial thrombotic events of 17.1 %. In the “Ponatinib in Newly Diagnosed Chronic Myeloid Leukemia” trial, arterial thrombotic events were observed predominantly in patients with either a documented ischemic condition or the presence of risk factors at baseline [56]. It would be important to close monitor these patients and to investigate whether the use of aspirin or other antiplatelet agents may reduce the risk of events.

9.4.2 All-Trans Retinoic Acid

Catastrophic acute myocardial infarction has been reported in patients with APL treated with *all-trans retinoic acid (ATRA)*, with increased incidence in patients suspected of having ATRA syndrome. Major thrombotic events in APL can happen before, during, or after induction therapy, with more than 80 % of those occurring either before or during induction therapy, at a similar frequency in the two periods [57].

9.4.3 Platinum Compounds

Platinum compounds have been related to an increasing risk of coronary artery disease at long-term follow-up in patients with testicular cancer [58–60].

- Both a direct diffuse endothelial damage (which could be related to the acute toxicity) and an increases of plasma insulin, insulin resistance, total cholesterol and LDL-C, BMI, and a concomitant increase in the volume of the abdominal visceral and subcutaneous fat mass within months after chemotherapeutic treatment (which could lead to coronary artery disease) have been described [61, 62].
- Cisplatin-based treatments for testicular cancer led to a 2.6-fold higher risk of severe atherosclerotic disease at 20-year follow-up compared to surgery alone; the patients who had radiotherapy and chemotherapy had a 4.8-fold higher risk; bleomycin, etoposide, and cisplatin (BEP) was significantly associated to a 5.7-fold higher risk for coronary artery disease and a 3.1-fold increase risk of myocardial infarction, but CVB (cisplatin, vinblastine, bleomycine) was not [63]. Interestingly, another study found an increased incidence of myocardial infarction in patients treated with PVB (platinum, vinblastine, bleomycine) and not in those treated with BEP; in this study the excess risk compared to the general population was particularly evident (twofold increase) in patients with nonseminoma cancer and younger than 45 years [64].
- In a recent large, population-based study of testicular nonseminoma, an excess mortality for noncancer-related causes of 60 % (compared to the general population) after chemotherapy was observed; 24.2 % of these noncancer-related deaths were a result of cardiovascular disease [65]. In this study, significantly elevated cardiovascular mortality was observed only in the first year after cancer diagnosis.
- It is not clearly defined if platinum causes myocardial ischemia directly or inducing metabolic changes which lead to atherosclerosis, and if the effect is due to platinum alone or to the association with other drugs. It should be considered also the possible role of other factors, as subclinical hypogonadism after orchiectomy, radiotherapy and antiemetic treatments with glucocorticoids, leading to a metabolic syndrome [66].

> **There are convincing data that cardiac ischemia is more frequent, both at short- and medium-long term, in patients treated by platin compounds in comparison with general population. This excess risk is mostly remarkable in young men treated for testicular carcinoma.**

> **Patients cured from testicular cancer should be advised to avoid smoking, practice regular physical activity, and check regularly blood glucose and lipids.**

9.4.4 Interleukin-2 (Il-2) and Alpha-Interferon

Acute coronary syndromes during therapy with high-dose *interleukin-2 (Il-2)* and *alpha-interferon (IFN)* cardiac ischemia have been described in the past [67–69].

The mechanisms of *IFN* cardiac toxicity have not been fully explained, and several hypotheses have been proposed: a direct myocite damage, an autoimmune reaction (Kounis syndrome), a toxic effect induced by the increase ein tumor necrosis factor, and cytokines.

Il-2 causes a severe flu-like syndrome, with tachycardia and diffuse edema; the more likely mechanism of ischemia is a capillary leak syndrome leading to interstitial edema.

- The use of these drug in oncology has been changed; their use is now limited, and doses have been reduced. Cardiac ischemia seems to be a very rare side effect nowadays.

9.4.5 Taxanes

Taxanes (paclitaxel and docetaxel) have anticancer effects by promoting polymerization of tubulin, leading to the developments of dysfunctional microtubules and disrupting cell division.

- Paclitaxel causes acute asymptomatic bradycardia in up to 30 % of patients. An early series reported a 5 % incidence of serious arrhythmias and myocardial infarction, including ventricular tachycardia in 5 of 140 patients (3.6 %) [70]. However, a significant risk of cardiac ischemia has not been reported in more recent studies.
- The mechanisms are unknown.
- Docetaxel causes less cardiac toxicity than paclitaxel.
- Taxanes potentiate anthracycline-induced cardiotoxicity, increasing the plasma levels of doxorubicin.

9.4.6 Aromatase Inhibitors

The *aromatase inhibitors (AIs)* are used in adjuvant, neoadjuvant, and metastatic setting.

AIs inhibit the conversion of androgens to estradiol in fat and other tissues, including tumors, and thus reduce estrogen levels in plasma and tissue.

- One large phase III trial (BIG-198) of the AI letrozole versus tamoxifen (TAM) reported a minimal increase in cardiac events in the letrozole arm at a median follow-up of 26 months, which persisted in subgroup analysis at 51 months [71]. Since TAM has a favorable effect on lipid metabolism and reduce the cardiovascular risk, this finding could be due to a lack of beneficial effect from TAM rather than to a true toxicity of AIs [72].
- A meta-analysis of seven trials enrolling 30,023 patients showed that longer duration of AIs use was associated with a statistically significant increase in the odds of developing cardiovascular disease compared with tamoxifen alone or shorter duration of aromatase inhibitor use; however, the magnitude of cardiovascular events was lower for the treatment cohorts where aromatase inhibitors were administered after 2–3 years of treatment with TAM [73]. According to this study, on the other hand, the use of AIs in

postmenopausal women with early-stage breast cancer decreases the odds of venous thrombosis. There were no differences in the odds of cerebrovascular disease, other second cancers, or death without breast cancer recurrence between treatment strategies.
- In a study comparing 2 versus 5 years of TAM therapy, taking TAM for 5 years lowered the risk of CV disease and death as a result of a CV event, particularly among those age 50–59 years [74].
- The meta-analysis of randomized trials of AIs compared with TAM either as initial monotherapy or after 2–3 years of TAM found that AIs produce significantly lower recurrence rates compared with tamoxifen, either as initial monotherapy or after 2–3 years of TAM, without any increase in noncancer-related deaths [75].

There is a general warning in using AIs in patients with heart disease but not a clear contraindication in the overall population.

Switching to AIs after initial TAM therapy might reduce the cardiovascular risk.

The decision on whether to initiate treatment with an AIs or TAM or whether to switch to an AI after 2–3 years of TAM rather than continuing with TAM for 5 years depends on a careful evaluation of the general health issues of each individual and the risk of relapse [76].

9

9.4.7 Androgen Deprivation Therapy

Androgen deprivation therapy (ADT) is the mainstay of treatment for locally advanced and metastatic prostate cancer. Androgen deprivation can be achieved surgically (orchiectomy), medically [gonadotropin-releasing hormone (GnRH) agonists and antagonists, and estrogens], and by inducing androgen resistance (androgen receptor antagonists).
- It has been known for several years that ADT is associated to an increased risk of insulin resistance, diabetes, dyslipidemia, metabolic syndrome, and cardiovascular disease, with the duration of ADT directly associated with the degree of metabolic perturbations [77, 78].
- Venous thromboembolism, peripheral artery disease, and myocardial infarction have been reported as a consequence of ADT and not of orchiectomy [79–82].
- This risk seems to be independent from the presence of traditional cardiovascular risk factors [83].
- A large cohort study found that endocrine medical therapy was associated with increased risk for MI and stroke but did not find a similar association after orchiectomy [84].
- In the most recent study, both orchiectomy and GnRH agonists were associated with an increased risk of CV disease, and men with a previous history of two or more CV events (particularly if the last event occurred within a year) were at a higher risk of CV disease within the first 6 months of therapy [85].

Every patient undergoing orchiectomy or pharmacological treatment for ADT has an increased risk of developing diabetes, insulin resistance, dyslipidemia, and cardiovascular diseases (including CAD) on the medium-long term and should be carefully followed up.

Patients who have already two or more cardiovascular risk factors have an increased risk of myocardial infarction and stroke on the short term.

References

1. Polk A, Vistisen K, Vaage-Nilsen M, Nielsen DL. A systematic review of the pathophysiology of 5-fluorouracil-induced cardiotoxicity. BMC Pharmacol Toxicol. 2014;15:47.
2. Lemaire L, Malet-Martino MC, de Forni M, et al. Cardiotoxicity of commercial 5-fluorouracil vials stems from the alkaline hydrolysis of this drug. Br J Cancer. 1992;66:119–27.
3. Jensen SA, Sørensen JB. 5-fluorouracil-based therapy induces endovascular injury having potential significance to development of clinically overt cardiotoxicity. Cancer Chemother Pharmacol. 2012;69: 57–64.
4. Kounis NG, Tsigkas GG, Almpanis G, Mazarakis A. Kounis syndrome is likely culprit of coronary vasospasm induced by capecitabine. J Oncol Pharm Pract. 2012;18:316–8.
5. Kido K, Adams VR, Morehead RS, Flannery AH. Capecitabine-induced ventricular fibrillation arrest: possible Kounis syndrome. J Oncol Pharm Pract. 2015.
6. Schöber C, Papageorgiou E, Harstrick A, et al. Cardiotoxicity of 5-fluorouracil in combination with folinic acid in patients with gastrointestinal cancer. Cancer. 1993;72:2242–7.
7. de Forni M, Malet-Martino MC, Jaillais P, et al. Cardiotoxicity of high-dose continuous infusion fluorouracil: a prospective clinical study. J Clin Oncol. 1992;10:1795–801.
8. Kosmas C, Kallistratos MS, Kopterides P, et al. Cardiotoxicity of fluoropyrimidines in different schedules of administration: a prospective study. J Cancer Res Clin Oncol. 2008;134:75–82.
9. Lestuzzi C, Vaccher E, Talamini R, et al. Effort myocardial ischemia during chemotherapy with 5-fluorouracil: an underestimated risk. Ann Oncol. 2014;25:1059–64.
10. Rezkalla S, Kloner RA, Ensley J, al-Sarraf M, Revels S, Olivenstein A, Bhasin S, Kerpel-Fronious S, Turi ZG. Continuous ambulatory ECG monitoring during fluorouracil therapy: a prospective study. J Clin Oncol. 1989;7:509–14.
11. Meyer CC, Calis KA, Burke LB, et al. Symptomatic cardiotoxicity associated with 5-fluorouracil. Pharmacotherapy. 1997;17:729–36.
12. Meydan N, Kundak I, Yavuzsen T, et al. Cardiotoxicity of de Gramont's regimen: incidence, clinical characteristics and long-term follow-up. Jpn J Clin Oncol. 2005;35:265–70.
13. Floyd JD, Nguyen DT, Lobins RL, Bashir Q, Doll DC, Perry MC. Cardiotoxicity of cancer therapy. J Clin Oncol. 2005;23:7685–96. Review.
14. Saif MW, Garcon MC, Rodriguez G, Rodriguez T. Bolus 5-fluorouracil as an alternative in patients with cardiotoxicity associated with infusion 5-fluorouracil and capecitabine: a case series. In Vivo. 2013;27:531–4.
15. Lestuzzi C, Viel E, Picano E, Meneguzzo N. Coronary vasospasm as a cause of effort-related myocardial ischemia during low-dose chronic continuous infusion of 5-fluorouracil. Am J Med. 2001;111: 316–8.
16. Robben NC, Pippas AW, Moore JO. The syndrome of 5-fluorouracil cardiotoxicity. An elusive cardiopathy. Cancer. 1993;71:493–509. Review.
17. Saif MW, Shah MM, Shah AR. Fluoropyrimidine-associated cardiotoxicity: revisited. Expert Opin Drug Saf. 2009;8:191–202.
18. Kobayashi N, Hata N, Yokoyama S, et al. A case of takotsubo cardiomyopathy during 5-fluorouracil treatment for rectal adenocarcinoma. J Nippon Med Sch. 2009;76:27–33.
19. Jensen SA, Hasbak P, Mortensen J, Sørensen JB. Fluorouracil induces myocardial ischemia with increases of plasma brain natriuretic peptide and lactic acid but without dysfunction of left ventricle. J Clin Oncol. 2010;28:5280–6.
20. Ambrosy AP, Kunz PL, Fisher PA, Witteles MR. Capecitabine-induced chest pain relieved by diltiazem. Am J Cardiol. 2012;110:1623–6.
21. Miura K, Kinouchi M, Ishida K, et al. 5-fu metabolism in cancer and orally-administrable 5-fu drugs. Cancers (Basel). 2010;2:1717–30.
22. Kelly C, Bhuva N, Harrison M, Buckley A, Saunders M. Use of raltitrexed as an alternative to 5-fluorouracil and capecitabine in cancer patients with cardiac history. Eur J Cancer. 2013;49:2303–10.
23. Ransom D, Wilson K, Fournier M, et al. Final results of Australasian Gastrointestinal Trials Group ARCTIC study: an audit of raltitrexed for patients with cardiac toxicity induced by fluoropyrimidines. Ann Oncol. 2014;25(1):117–21.
24. Deboever G, Hiltrop N, Cool M, Lambrecht G. Alternative treatment options in colorectal cancer patients with 5-fluorouracil- or capecitabine-induced cardiotoxicity. Clin Colorectal Cancer. 2013;12: 8–14.

25. Kroep JR, van Werkhoven E, Polee M, et al. Randomised study of tegafur-uracil plus leucovorin versus capecitabine as first-line therapy in elderly patients with advanced colorectal cancer—TLC study. J Geriatr Oncol. 2015;6:307–15.
26. Ishizuka M, Kubota K, Nemoto T, et al. Administration of adjuvant oral tegafur/uracil chemotherapy post hepatocellular carcinoma resection: a randomized controlled trial. Asian J Surg. 2015.
27. Sadahiro S, Morita S, Sasaki K, et al. Treatment rationale and study design for clinical trial on the efficacy of UFT/LV for stage II colorectal cancer with risk factors for recurrence (JFMC46-1201). Clin Colorectal Cancer. 2015;14:277–80.
28. Sorrentino MF, Kim J, Foderaro AE, Truesdell AG. 5-fluorouracil induced cardiotoxicity: review of the literature. Cardiol J. 2012;19:453–8. Review.
29. Lestuzzi C, Crivellari D, Rigo F, et al. Capecitabine cardiac toxicity presenting as effort angina: a case report. J Cardiovasc Med (Hagerstown). 2010;11:700–3.
30. Ranpura V, Hapani S, Chuang J, Wu S. Risk of cardiac ischemia and arterial thromboembolic events with the angiogenesis inhibitor bevacizumab in cancer patients: a meta-analysis of randomized controlled trials. Acta Oncol. 2010;49:287–97.
31. Chen XL, Lei YH, Liu CF, et al. Angiogenesis inhibitor bevacizumab increases the risk of ischemic heart disease associated with chemotherapy: a meta-analysis. PLoS One. 2013;8:e66721.
32. Schmidinger M, Zielinski CC, Vogl UM, et al. Cardiac toxicity of sunitinib and sorafenib in patients with metastatic renal cell carcinoma. J Clin Oncol. 2008;26:5204–12.
33. Vaklavas C, Lenihan D, Kurzrock R, Tsimberidou AM. Anti-vascular endothelial growth factor therapies and cardiovascular toxicity: what are the important clinical markers to target? Oncologist. 2010;15:130–41. Review.
34. Haas NB, Manola J, Ky B, et al. Effects of adjuvant sorafenib and sunitinib on cardiac function in renal cell carcinoma patients without overt metastases: results from ASSURE, ECOG 2805. Clin Cancer Res. 2015;21:4048–54.
35. Nachman RL, Rafii S. Platelets, petechiae, and preservation of the vascular wall. N Engl J Med. 2008;359:1261–70.
36. Kamba T, McDonald DM. Mechanisms of adverse effects of anti-VEGF therapy for cancer. Br J Cancer. 2007;96:1788–95.
37. Kajdaniuk D, Marek B, Borgiel-Marek H, Kos-Kudła B. Vascular endothelial growth factor (VEGF)—part 1: in physiology and pathophysiology. Endokrynol Pol. 2011;62:444–55. Review.
38. Vuorio T, Jauhiainen S, Ylä-Herttuala S. Pro- and anti-angiogenic therapy and atherosclerosis with special emphasis on vascular endothelial growth factors. Expert Opin Biol Ther. 2012;12:79–92.
39. Toyota E, Warltier DC, Brock T, et al. Vascular endothelial growth factor is required for coronary collateral growth in the rat. Circulation. 2005;112:2108–13.
40. Bry M, Kivelä R, Leppänen VM, Alitalo K. Vascular endothelial growth factor-B in physiology and disease. Physiol Rev. 2014;94:779–94.
41. Kivelä R, Bry M, Robciuc MR, et al. VEGF-B-induced vascular growth leads to metabolic reprogramming and ischemia resistance in the heart. EMBO Mol Med. 2014;6:307–21.
42. Jiménez-Navarro MF, González FJ, Caballero-Borrego J, Investigadores RECAVA (Red Temática de Investigación Cooperativa de Enfermedades Cardiovasculares), et al. Coronary disease extension determines mobilization of endothelial progenitor cells and cytokines after a first myocardial infarction with ST elevation. Rev Esp Cardiol. 2011;64:1123–9.
43. Elice F, Rodeghiero F, Falanga A, Rickles FR. Thrombosis associated with angiogenesis inhibitors. Best Pract Res Clin Haematol. 2009;22:115–28.
44. Conti E, Romiti A, Musumeci MB, et al. Arterial thrombotic events and acute coronary syndromes with cancer drugs: are growth factors the missed link?: what both cardiologist and oncologist should know about novel angiogenesis inhibitors. Int J Cardiol. 2013;167:2421–9.
45. Kuenen BC, Levi M, Meijers JC, et al. Analysis of coagulation cascade and endothelial cell activation during inhibition of vascular endothelial growth factor/vascular endothelial growth factor receptor pathway in cancer patients. Arterioscler Thromb Vasc Biol. 2002;22:1500–5.
46. Hapani S, Sher A, Chu D, Wu S. Increased risk of serious hemorrhage with bevacizumab in cancer patients: a meta-analysis. Oncology. 2010;79:27–38.
47. Hang XF, Xu WS, Wang JX. Risk of high-grade bleeding in patients with cancer treated with bevacizumab: a meta-analysis of randomized controlled trials. Eur J Clin Pharmacol. 2011;67:613–23.
48. Economopoulou P, Kotsakis A, Kapiris I, Kentepozidis N. Cancer therapy and cardiovascular risk: focus on bevacizumab. Cancer Manag Res. 2015;7:133–43. Review.

49. Steingart RM, Bakris GL, Chen HX, et al. Management of cardiac toxicity in patients receiving vascular endothelial growth factor signaling pathway inhibitors. Am Heart J. 2012;163:156–63.
50. Scappaticci FA, Skillings JR, Holden SN, et al. Arterial thromboembolic events in patients with metastatic carcinoma treated with chemotherapy and bevacizumab. J Natl Cancer Inst. 2007;99:1232–9. Erratum in: J Natl Cancer Inst. 2008;100:156. J Natl Cancer Inst. 2008;100:685.
51. Silvestre JS, Smadja DM, Lévy BI. Postischemic revascularization: from cellular and molecular mechanisms to clinical applications. Physiol Rev. 2013;93:1743–802.
52. Ramos C, Napoleão P, Selas M, et al. Prognostic value of VEGF in patients submitted to percutaneous coronary intervention. Dis Markers. 2014;2014:135357.
53. Katsaros KM, Kastl SP, Krychtiuk KA, et al. An increase of VEGF plasma levels is associated with restenosis of drug-eluting stents. EuroIntervention. 2014;10:224–30.
54. Quintas-Cardama A, Kantarjian H, Cortes J. Nilotinib-associated vascular events. Clin Lymphoma Myeloma Leuk. 2012;12:337–40.
55. Brauchli YB, Wais T, Gratwohl A, et al. Fatal myocardial infarction during nilotinib treatment in a 60-year-old male patient. Acta Oncol (Stockholm, Sweden). 2010;49:523–5.
56. Cortes JE, Kim DW, Pinilla-Ibarz J, et al. A phase 2 trial of ponatinib in Philadelphia chromosome-positive leukemias. N Engl J Med. 2013;369:1783–96.
57. Escudier SM, Kantarjian HM, Estey EH. Thrombosis in patients with acute promyelocytic leukemia treated with and without all-trans retinoic acid. Leuk Lymphoma. 1996;20:435–9.
58. Oh JH, Baum DD, Pham S, et al. Long-term complications of platinum-based chemotherapy in testicular cancer survivors. Med Oncol. 2007;24:175–81.
59. Evans C, Williams M, Mazhar D. Long-term cardiovascular risk following platinum-based chemotherapy for germ cell tumors. Future Oncol. 2010;6:1365–8.
60. Fung C, Fossa SD, Williams A, Travis LB. Long-term morbidity of testicular cancer treatment. Urol Clin North Am. 2015;42:393–408.
61. Dieckmann KP, Struss WJ, Budde U. Evidence for acute vascular toxicity of cisplatin-based chemotherapy in patients with germ cell tumour. Anticancer Res. 2011;31:4501–5.
62. Willemse PP, van der Meer RW, Burggraaf J, et al. Abdominal visceral and subcutaneous fat increase, insulin resistance and hyperlipidemia in testicular cancer patients treated with cisplatin-based chemotherapy. Acta Oncol. 2014;53:351–60.
63. Haugnes HS, Wethal T, Aass N, et al. Cardiovascular risk factors and morbidity in long-term survivors of testicular cancer: a 20-year follow-up study. J Clin Oncol. 2010;28:4649–57.
64. van den Belt-Dusebout AW, Nuver J, de Wit R, et al. Long-term risk of cardiovascular disease in 5-year survivors of testicular cancer. J Clin Oncol. 2006;24:467–75.
65. Fung C, Fossa SD, Milano MT, et al. Cardiovascular disease mortality after chemotherapy or surgery for testicular nonseminoma: a population-based study. J Clin Oncol. 2015;33:3105–15.
66. Christensen JF, Bandak M, Campbell A, et al. Treatment-related cardiovascular late effects and exercise training countermeasures in testicular germ cell cancer survivorship. Acta Oncol. 2015;54:592–9.
67. Margolin KA, Rayner AA, Hawkins MJ, et al. Interleukin-2 and lymphokine-activated killer cell therapy of solid tumors: analysis of toxicity and management guidelines. J Clin Oncol. 1989;7(4):486–98.
68. Sonnenblick M, Rosin A. Cardiotoxicity of interferon. A review of 44 cases. Chest. 1991;99:557–61.
69. Kruit WH. Cardiotoxicity as a dose-limiting factor in a schedule of high dose bolus therapy with interleukin-2 and alpha-interferon. An unexpected frequent complication. Cancer. 1994;74:2850–6.
70. Rowinsky EK, McGuire WP, Guarnieri T, et al. Cardiac disturbances during the administration of taxol. J Clin Oncol. 1991;9:1704–12.
71. Coates AS, Keshaviah A, Thurlimann B, et al. Five years of letrozole compared with tamoxifen as initial adjuvant therapy for postmenopausal women with endocrine-responsive early breast cancer: update of study BIG 1-98. J Clin Oncol. 2007;25:486–92.
72. Yang TL, Wu TC, Huang CC, et al. Association of tamoxifen use and reduced cardiovascular events among Asian females with breast cancer. Circ J. 2014;78:135–40.
73. Amir E, Seruga B, Niraula S, et al. Toxicity of adjuvant endocrine therapy in postmenopausal breast cancer patients: a systematic review and meta-analysis. J Natl Cancer Inst. 2011;103:1299–309.
74. Hackshaw A, Roughton M, Forsyth S, et al. Long-term benefits of 5 years of tamoxifen: 10-year follow-up of a large randomized trial in women at least 50 years of age with early breast cancer. J Clin Oncol. 2011;29:1657–63.
75. Dowsett M, Cuzick J, Ingle J, et al. Meta-analysis of breast cancer outcomes in adjuvant trials of aromatase inhibitors versus tamoxifen. J Clin Oncol. 2010;28:509–18.

76. Ribeiro J, Sousa B, Cardoso F. Optimal approach in early breast cancer: adjuvant and neoadjuvant treatment. EJC Suppl. 2013;11:3–22.
77. Basaria S, Muller DC, Carducci MA, et al. Hyperglycemia and insulin resistance in men with prostate carcinoma who receive androgen-deprivation therapy. Cancer. 2006;106:581–8.
78. Shahani S, Braga-Basaria M, Basaria S. Androgen deprivation therapy in prostate cancer and metabolic risk for atherosclerosis. J Clin Endocrinol Metab. 2008;93:2042–9.
79. Keating NL, O'Malley AJ, Smith MR. Diabetes and cardiovascular disease during androgen deprivation therapy for prostate cancer. J Clin Oncol. 2006;24:4448–56.
80. Keating NL, O'Malley AJ, Freedland SJ, Smith MR. Diabetes and cardiovascular disease during androgen deprivation therapy: observational study of veterans with prostate cancer. J Natl Cancer Inst. 2010;102:39–46.
81. Saigal CS, Gore JL, Krupski TL, Urologic Diseases in America Project, et al. Androgen deprivation therapy increases cardiovascular morbidity in men with prostate cancer. Cancer. 2007;110:1493–500.
82. Hu JC, Williams SB, O'Malley AJ, et al. Androgen-deprivation therapy for nonmetastatic prostate cancer is associated with an increased risk of peripheral arterial disease and venous thromboembolism. Eur Urol. 2012;61:1119–28.
83. Keating NL, O'Malley AJ, Freedland SJ, Smith MR. Does comorbidity influence the risk of myocardial infarction or diabetes during androgen-deprivation therapy for prostate cancer? Eur Urol. 2013;64:159–66.
84. Jespersen CG, Nørgaard M, Borre M. Androgen-deprivation therapy in treatment of prostate cancer and risk of myocardial infarction and stroke: a nationwide Danish population-based cohort study. Eur Urol. 2014;65:704–9.
85. O'Farrell S, Garmo H, Holmberg L, et al. Risk and timing of cardiovascular disease after androgen-deprivation therapy in men with prostate cancer. J Clin Oncol. 2015;33:1243–51.

Cardiotoxicity: Hypertension

Maurizio Garozzo, Anna Clementi, and Giorgio Battaglia

C. Lestuzzi et al. (eds.), *Manual of Cardio-oncology*, DOI 10.1007/978-3-319-40236-9_10

10.1 Introduction

Chemotherapy agents have been widely used for a long time in the fight against cancer, improving progression-free survival and reducing mortality of about 20 % in the United States in the last years [1]. Anyway, extensive cancer research has demonstrated that the use of new biologic drugs might be indicated in patients with neoplasia, in particular in the setting of metastatic cancer.

Renal surgery has represented the first line of treatment for renal cancer for years, thus inducing a reduction in the number of nephrons, and consequently the development or the worsening of chronic kidney insufficiency and hypertension. The italian Association of Medical Oncology (AIOM) guidelines have recently reported that the treatment with interferon α and/or interleukin-2 does not improve global survival of patients with renal cancer when compared with surgical intervention. Therefore, renal cancer represents a possible target of biologic chemotherapy drugs, which have been already demonstrated to be effective in case of renal metastatic carcinoma.

Despite a favorable toxicity profile, these new chemotherapeutic agents may present side effects, particularly on cardiovascular and renal systems. In this chapter, we will analyze the cardiovascular and renal adverse events related to the new biologic chemotherapy agents.

10.2 Proteinuria

Agents targeting vascular endothelial growth factor (VEGF) are usually well tolerated, with the most frequently observed adverse events being hypertension, asymptomatic proteinuria, and asthenia [2, 3]. Bevacizumab is a monoclonal antibody against VEGF which has been associated with the development of proteinuria in 23–38 % of patients with colon rectal cancer and in more than 64 % of patients with renal carcinoma [4–6]. In the Avastin for Renal Cell Cancer (AVOREN) study, 95 % of patients treated with bevacizumab (10 mg/kg every 2 weeks) and interferon α (9 MIU 3 times per week) for more than 1 year developed proteinuria, and 6 % of patients presented heavy proteinuria. In the Bevacizumab Expanded Access Trial (BEAT) study, proteinuria was present only in 1 % of patients [7].

A recent meta-analysis of randomized trials on the use of bevacizumab reported a relative risk of 1.4 to develop proteinuria, when low doses of the drug were administered (2.5–7.5 mg/kg). The risk increased to 1.6 when the drug was administered at higher doses (10–15 mg/kg), thus suggesting that the risk for developing proteinuria was dose-dependent [2]. Moreover, it has been demonstrated that the interruption of the therapy with bevacizumab might be associated with a reduction of proteinuria [8].

In the Italian XELBEVOCT study, performed on 45 patients with metastatic endocrine neoplasia treated with octreotide long-acting release, metronomic capecitabine, and bevacizumab, 48 % of patients developed proteinuria and 40 % hypertension [9]. All grades of proteinuria correlated with longer progression-free survival ($p=0.017$), and this correlation was present even after adjustment for bevacizumab therapy duration [9]. Moreover, an inverse relationship between proteinuria and vitamin D levels was observed; in particular 75 % of patients with vitamin D levels <10 ng/ml developed proteinuria. Thus, the authors recommended the administration of vitamin D supplements in patients with hypovitaminosis D [9].

In patients with chronic kidney disease, renal vitamin D activation is progressively lost, and this has been recently associated to an increase in proteinuria and disease progression [10]. The administration of vitamin D analogs in these patients has been demonstrated to have renoprotective effects, similarly to ACE inhibitors and angiotensin receptor blockers [11].

Moreover, the association of bevacizumab with pamidronate seems to increase the risk to develop proteinuria, due to the impairment of podocyte function and the subsequent loss of selective glomerular permeability induced by this drug [8].

Patel et al. have reported a preeclampsia-like syndrome in seven patients treated with the multitargeted kinase inhibitors sunitinib and sorafenib. All the patients developed proteinuria (average 3.8 g/g, range 1.1–10.4 g/g), with peak urine protein excretion occurring at a median of 24 weeks, edema, and hypertension [12]. The reduction of the dose administered or the interruption of the therapy were associated with improved blood pressure control and proteinuria regression in 4 patients with follow-up information [12].

In the kidney, glomerular podocytes express VEGF and glomerular endothelial cells express VEGF receptors. Podocyte-specific deletion of a single VEGF allele causes proteinuria and capillary endotheliosis in rodents, and disrupted glomerular VEGF signaling is strongly implicated in the pathogenesis of human preeclampsia [13, 14]. Therefore, anti-VEGF agents may play a role in the pathogenesis of preeclampsia.

In case of heavy proteinuria or preeclampsia-like syndrome induced by agents targeting VEGF, kidney biopsy is recommended. Izzedine et al. have recently carried out a review on patients treated with anti-VEGF agents undergoing kidney biopsy. They have reported 12 cases of glomerular thrombotic microangiopathy, likely induced by the concomitant administration of pamidronate, one case of cryoglobulinemia glomerulonephritis, one case of proliferative glomerulonephritis, and one case of interstitial nephritis induced by sorafenib [8].

Proteinuria is partially related to the development of hypertension. In a randomized trail performed on 116 patients treated with bevacizumab, the incidence of proteinuria was 16% in case of mild hypertension, reaching 54% in case of moderate-severe hypertension [4]. Moreover, patients treated with bevacizumab and capecitabine with proteinuria developed hypertension more frequently than patients without proteinuria (47.1 versus 16.9%, $p \leq 0.001$) [15].

It is still not known if the risk for developing proteinuria is higher in case of therapy with agents targeting VEGF than with antibodies against VEGF. Anyway, all patients requiring this kind of therapy should be screened for proteinuria and preexisting nephropathy. Therefore, once the treatment is started and before every cycle of therapy, proteinuria and kidney function should be evaluated. In case of proteinuria <1–2 g/24 h, vitamin D supplements or analogs might be administered, in particular in patients with hypovitaminosis D. ACE inhibitors and angiotensin receptor blockers are indicated particularly if hypertension coexists. If proteinuria is higher than 2 g/24 h or acute kidney injury develops, kidney biopsy is strongly recommended and referral to nephrologists is mandatory. It is important, indeed, to investigate the presence of glomerular thrombotic microangiopathy, acute interstitial nephritis, and paraneoplastic glomerulonephritis, which is not related to drug administration but to the type of neoplasm. Pulmonary and gastrointestinal tumors are more frequently associated with paraneoplastic syndromes.

10.3 Hypertension

Hypertension is another side effect of anti-VEGF treatment with an incidence ranging from 9 to 30 % [2, 16–19]. Di Lorenzo et al. carried out a multicenter analysis on cardiac adverse events in 175 patients with metastatic renal cell carcinoma who underwent treatment with sunitinib. Grade 3 hypertension was seen in 17 patients (9.7 %) [16].

Furthermore, the appearance of worsening hypertension (grade 2 or more) was found to be the single independent predictor of a better clinical response to sunitinib in metastatic renal cell carcinoma, as reported by Rixe et al. [18]. In the same study, grade 3 hypertension (requirement of therapy or more intensive therapy than previously) was correlated with a better outcome [18]. Hypertension seems to be a time-dependent and reversible side effect of the anti-VEGF therapy [2, 8, 20, 21]. In a review performed by Zhu et al. on 5000 patients with renal cell carcinoma, gastrointestinal stromal tumor and other malignancies treated with sunitinib, a significantly increased relative risk of high-grade hypertension (RR = 22.72, 95 % CI: 4.48–115.29, $p < 0.001$) was observed [19]. Hypertension was related to left ventricular dysfunction which may represent a side effect of the drug or the result of hypertension [19].

Hypertension is an on-target effect of the VEGF pathway inhibition [21]. In the retrospective analysis of Rini et al., patients with metastatic renal cell carcinoma and sunitinib-induced hypertension (maximum systolic blood pressure ≥140 mmHg or diastolic blood pressure ≥90 mmHg) had better outcomes than those without treatment-induced hypertension (objective response rate: 54.8 versus 8.7 %) [21] (◘ Fig. 10.1).

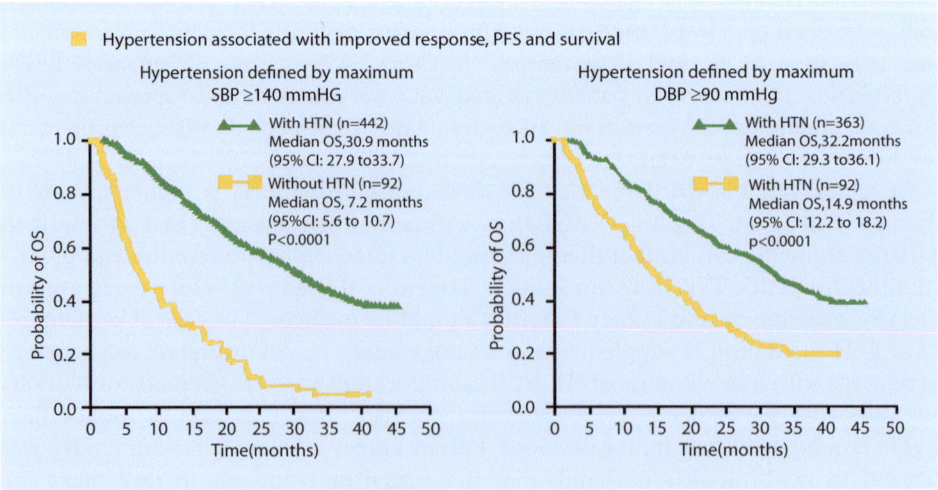

◘ **Fig. 10.1** Hypertension associated with improved response, progression-free survival (PFS) and survival

The inhibition of VEGF plays a pivotal role in the pathogenesis of sunitinib-induced hypertension. It reduces the ability of cell renewal, increases apoptosis in vascular endothelial cells, determines the rarefaction of capillaries and arterioles, and interferes with the cellular production of vasodilators such as nitric oxide and prostacyclin, favoring vasoconstriction, increasing peripheral resistance, and decreasing renal excretion of sodium [22, 23].

All these effects seem to be related to VEGF genotype which has been associated to median overall survival, as well as grade 3 or 4 hypertension, in patients with metastatic breast cancer treated with bevacizumab [24].

Early and intensive antihypertensive therapy with the goal of maintaining the anti-VEGF agents use may improve response rate in these patients. Diuretics, beta-blockers, ACE inhibitors, and angiotensin receptor blockers may be indicated in patients with heart failure, while calcium-channel blockers, nitrates, and beta-blockers may have beneficial effects in patients with ischemic heart disease. Moreover, ACE inhibitors and angiotensin receptor blockers may be useful in patients with nephropathy, with caution in case of renal artery stenosis [17].

10.4 Cardiotoxicity

10.4.1 Anti-vascular Endothelial Growth Factor Agents

Cardiovascular toxicity has been reported among the side effects of anti-VEGF agents. Bevacizumab is a monoclonal antibody acting specifically against VEGF-A, responsible for left ventricular dysfunction in 1 % of treated patients [15]. Conversely, sunitinib and sorafenib are less selective anti-VEGF agents, with an increased risk of cardiotoxicity and an incidence of reduced ejection fraction of 28 % [25].

In a recent trial, Gore et al. enrolled 4371 patients with metastatic renal cell carcinoma treated with sunitinib, reporting heart failure as a side effect of the therapy in <1 % of patients [26]. A higher incidence of cardiac abnormalities was observed among 175 patients with metastatic renal cell carcinoma treated with sunitinib in the study of Di Lorenzo et al. [16]. Twelve patients were classified as grade 3 left ventricular dysfunction and/or congestive heart failure (6.9 %) [16]. Similar data have been reported in two meta-analysis performed on 7000 patients treated with sunitinib and 900 patients treated with sorafenib, demonstrating an incidence of sunitinib-induced heart failure of 4.1 % and of sorafenib-associated cardiac dysfunction of 1 % [16, 27].

In an observational study, Schmidinger et al. found that among 74 eligible patients treated with either sunitinib or sorafenib, 33.8 % experienced a cardiac event, 40.5 % had ECG changes, and 18 % were symptomatic. Seven patients (9.4 %) were seriously compromised and required intermediate care and/or intensive care admission. All patients recovered after cardiovascular management (medication, coronary angiography, pacemaker implantation, heart surgery) and were considered eligible for therapy continuation [28].

Sunitinib and sorafenib belong to the class of small molecule tyrosine kinase inhibitors and are able to block signaling cascades other than the one of VEGF [29]. The higher incidence of cardiotoxicity is indeed explained by the inhibition of off-target kinases, such as ribosomal S6 kinase, with consequent activation of the intrinsic apoptotic pathway, and 5′ AMP-activated protein kinase with worsening of ATP depletion [29]. Therefore, left ventricular dysfunction would occur due to myocyte dysfunction [29].

Moreover, antiangiogenic drugs may interfere with membrane integrity of endothelial cells, thus altering nitric oxide production and inducing hypertension and coagulation disorders [30, 31]. Bevacizumab was found, indeed, to be associated to an increased risk of arterial and venous thromboembolism [30, 32] and hemorrhagic events [33] in patients with renal carcinoma. Sunitinib and sorafenib as well have been reported to induce arterial thromboembolism [16, 34] and hemorrhagic events [35] in patients with renal carcinoma. Furthermore, in a retrospective study on 67 patients with metastatic renal cell carcinoma treated with sorafenib or sunitinib, five patients (7%) died of intracerebral hemorrhage during therapy [31].

Antiangiogenic drugs have been also demonstrated to interfere with potassium channels of myocytes. In particular, the serine/threonine kinase BRAF is responsible for the increased expression of these channels on cellular membrane, with consequent increased intracellular concentration of potassium and action potential. The inhibition of BRAF by chemotherapeutic drugs, such as sorafenib, vemurafenib, regorafenib, and dabrafenib, may induce a QT interval prolongation and an increased risk of cardiac arrhythmias and sudden death [36].

10.4.2 Antihuman Epidermal Growth Factor Receptor 2

Trastuzumab, a recombinant monoclonal antibody against human epidermal growth factor receptor 2 (HER2), has been demonstrated to be effective in case of breast and gastric cancers which overexpress HER2 [37]. Anyway, this drug seems to induce cardiac dysfunction due to reduced myocardial contractility, in particular if it is associated to anthracyclines [37, 38]. Because of the reported cardiotoxicity of both drugs, the association of the two agents is forbidden. Indeed, anthracyclines are responsible for myocytes damage which may be exacerbated by the concomitant administration of trastuzumab [39].

No available data exist about cardiotoxicity of pertuzumab, while lapatinib, an inhibitor of HER2, seems to possess less cardiotoxic effects than trastuzumab [38].

Cardiotoxicity of anti-HER2 agents is related to the inhibition of neuregulin-1 [39, 40]. The neuregulin-1 gene is a member of the epidermal growth factor gene family, abundant in the cardiovascular system. The neuregulin-1 exerts its cardioprotective effects in a paracrine manner and its inhibition by anti-HER2 drugs is responsible for the increased cardiac sensitivity to toxic insults, included anthracyclines [29].

10.4.3 Anti-active Breakpoint Cluster Region Abelson Receptor

Imatinib and dasatinib are new-generation drugs against breakpoint cluster region abelson (BCR-ABL) receptor used in case of chronic myelogenous leukemia and gastrointestinal neoplasia. Even though preliminary data suggested the potential cardiotoxic effects of these drugs, recent studies have not confirmed these results [29].

10.4.4 Prevention and Management of Cardiotoxicity

Before treatment with biologic agents is started, cardiotoxic risk should be evaluated for each patient [29]. Clinical assessment, ECG, and echocardiography performance are recommended in order to identify cardiac disease and arrhythmias. Blood pressure should be monitored and hypertension carefully treated. Thyroid function should be assessed as well, in particular in patients with known cardiac disease or in patients with increased cardiovascular risk factors. In these patients, ejection fraction should be evaluated before the starting of each cycle of therapy for the first four cycles [17]. In patients without cardiovascular risk factors, ejection fraction may be assessed every three cycles [17].

In case of therapy with anti-VEGF agents, coagulation system should be studied to avoid thrombotic events. If patients develop moderate-severe thrombosis or hemorrhagic events, the interruption of treatment is mandatory.

10.5 Renal Dysfunction

Renal function should be always assessed before chemotherapy is started and carefully monitored during all treatment, especially in patients with previous nephrectomy. In these patients, the real incidence of kidney dysfunction might be underestimated, in particular in case of mild reduction of renal function, due to the increased creatinine tubular secretion [19].

Zhu et al. have reported an incidence of renal dysfunction of 65.6 % among patients with renal cell carcinoma treated with sunitinib and of 12.4 % among patients with gastrointestinal neoplasia, when compared with controls (RR 1.359, 95 % CI: 1.197, 1.544; $p < 0.001$). In addition to nephrectomy, renal dysfunction may be also related to hypertension or to the effects of anti-VEGF agents on podocytes and renal tubules [20].

Moreover, nausea, vomiting, and prolonged diarrhea, which are common side effects of chemotherapy, may dehydrate patients, thus triggering acute kidney injury, especially in subjects with chronic kidney disease.

Table 10.1 reports all the side effects of biologic chemotherapy agents.

Table 10.1 Side effects of biological chemotherapy agents

Drug	Target	Action	Indications	Cardiotoxicity	Nephrotoxicity	Indirect neph-rotoxicity	Chronic kidney dis-ease patients	Dialysis patients
Imatinib	c-Kit BCR-ABL receptors	Tyrosine kinase inhibitor	Chronic myeloid leukemia Gastrointestinal stromal tumors	*Common* Edema Hypertension Heart failure Pulmonary hypertension Tachycardia Pulmonary edema *Rare* Arrhythmias Atrial fibrillation Cardiac angina/infarction Pericardial effusion	Hematuria Kidney insufficiency Hypokalemia Hyperkalemia Hypomagnesemia	Diarrhea		
Dasatinib	BCR-ABL receptor	Tyrosine kinase inhibitor	Chronic myeloid leukemia Gastrointestinal stromal tumors	*Common* Edema Heart failure Pericardial effusion Tachycardia *Rare* Ventricular arrhythmias Increased QT interval Pulmonary hypertension Cardiac angina/infarction Ictus cerebri	Kidney insufficiency Proteinuria	Nausea Vomiting Diarrhea Rabdomiolisis Hyperuricemia	No dose adjustment	
Trastu-zumab Lapatinib	EGFR EGFR2 (HER2)	Protein kinase inhibitors	Breast cancer Metastatic gastric cancer	Hypertension Tachycardia Atrial flutter Ejection fraction reduction Heart failure Atrial arrhythmias Cardiomyopathy Pericardial effusion	Membranous nephropathy Kidney insufficiency	Nausea Vomiting Diarrhea	No dose adjustment	

Erlotinib Afatinib	EGFR	Receptors blockers	Pulmonary cancer	Interaction with anticoagulant drugs and statins	Kidney insufficiency	Nausea Vomiting Diarrhea Anorexia	No dose adjustment Not recommended in patients with renal clearance <15 ml/m for Erlotinib and <30 ml/m for Afatinib	
Cetuximab	EGFR	Receptors blockers	Pulmonary cancer	Deep vein thrombosis Cardiac ischemic disease and heart failure if associated with fluoropyrimidine	Hypomagnesemia Hypokalemia Hypocalcemia (in association with cisplatin). Kidney insufficiency	Nausea Vomiting Diarrhea Anorexia	No dose adjustment	
Bevacizumab Aflibercept	VEGF	Antiangiogenesis monoclonal antibodies	Metastatic colorectal carcinoma Metastatic renal carcinoma Breast cancer Pulmonary cancer	Hypertension Arterial and venous thrombosis Heart failure (for bevacizumab)	Proteinuria Nephrotic syndrome kidney insufficiency Thrombotic microangiopathy	Nausea Vomiting Diarrhea	No dose adjustment	
Sunitinib Axitinib Pazopanib	VEGFR2	Tyrosine kinase inhibitor	Metastatic renal carcinoma Gastrointestinal stromal tumors	Hypertension Arterial and venous thrombosis Cardiomyopathy (for sunitinib) Heart failure Increased QT prolongation	Chromaturia (for sunitinib) Proteinuria Nephrotic syndrome acute kidney injury	Nausea Vomiting Diarrhea Rabdomiolisis	No dose adjustment	No dose adjustment
Sorafenib	VEGFR2 VEGFR-3, RET RET/PTC CRAF, BRAF BRAFV600E c-KIT FLT-3 PDGFR-β	Tyrosine kinase inhibitor	Hepatocellular carcinoma Renal carcinoma Differentiated thyroid carcinoma	Hypertension Cardiac angina/infarction Heart failure Interaction with warfarin Increased QT interval prolongation	Proteinuria Nephrotic syndrome Acute kidney injury Hypocalcemia	Nausea Vomiting Diarrhea Rabdomiolisis	No dose adjustment	No data in literature

(continued)

Table 10.1 (continued)

Drug	Target	Action	Indications	Cardiotoxicity	Nephrotoxicity	Indirect nephrotoxicity	Chronic kidney disease patients	Dialysis patients
Cabozantinib	VEGFR2	Tyrosine kinase inhibitor	Medullary thyroid carcinoma not surgically treatable	Hypertension Atrial fibrillation Increased QT interval prolongation Cardiac angina Supraventricular tachycardia Thromboembolism Arterial thrombosis	Proteinuria Hematuria Dysuria Acute kidney injury	Nausea Vomiting Diarrhea Rabdomiolisis	Caution in patients with mild-moderate renal dysfunction	No data for severe chronic renal insufficiency and dialysis patients
Everolimus Temsirolimus	mTOR	Serine threonine-protein kinase inhibitor	Breast cancer Neuroendocrine pancreatic tumors Renal carcinoma	Hypertension *Rare* Heart failure Deep vein thrombosis	Proteinuria Mild renal dysfunction	Diarrhea Nausea High fever	No dose adjustment	No dose adjustment
Trametinib	MEK	MEK inhibitor	Metastatic melanoma positive for BRAF V600	*Hypertension* Increased QT interval prolongation *Reduced ejection fraction* Retinal vein occlusion Deep vein thrombosis Pulmonary embolism	Glomerulonephritis (rare)	Nausea Vomiting Diarrhea High fever Rabdomiolisis Severe dehydration with acute kidney injury	No dose adjustment	No data in literature

c-Kit receptor overexpressed in gastrointestinal stromal tumors, *BCR-ABL R* breakpoint cluster region abelson receptor, *EGFR* epithelial growth factor receptor, *VEGF* vascular endothelial growth factor, *VEGFR* vascular endothelial growth factor receptor, *BRAF* gene encoding for BRAF protein, *PDGFR* platelet derived growth factor receptor, *mTOR* mammalian target of rapamycin, *MEK* protein kinase

References

1. Cancer Treatment & Survivorship Facts & Figures 2014–2015. ► http://www.cancer.org/acs/groups/content/@research/documents/document/acspc-042801.pdf.
2. Zhu X, Wu S, Dahut WL, Parikh CR. Risks of proteinuria and hypertension with bevacizumab, an antibody against vascular endothelial growth factor: systematic review and meta-analysis. Am J Kidney Dis. 2007;49:186–93.
3. Izzedine H, Rixe O, Billemont B, Baumelou A, Deray G. Angiogenesis inhibitor therapies: focus on kidney toxicity and hypertension. Am J Kidney Dis. 2007;50:203–18.
4. Yang JC, Haworth L, Sherry RM, et al. A randomized trial of bevacizumab, an anti-vascular endothelial growth factor antibody, for metastatic renal cancer. N Engl J Med. 2003;349:427–34.
5. Escudier B, Pluzanska A, Koralweski P, AVOREN Trial Investigators, et al. Bevacizumab plus interferon alfa-2a for treatment of metastatic renal cell carcinoma: a randomised, double-blind phase III trial. Lancet. 2007;370:2103–11.
6. Tang P, Cohen SJ, Bjarnason GA, et al. Phase II trial of aflibercept (VEGF Trap) in previously treated patients with metastatic colorectal cancer (MCRC): a PMH phase II consortium trial. J Clin Oncol. 2008;26(Suppl.).
7. Van Cutsem E, Rivera F, Berry S, Kretzschmar A, Michael M, DiBartolomeo M, Mazier MA, Canon JL, Georgoulias V, Peeters M, Bridgewater J, Cunningham D. Safety and efficacy of first-line bevacizumab with FOLFOX, XELOX, FOLFIRI and fluoropyrimidines in metastatic colorectal cancer: the BEAT study. Ann Oncol. 2009;20(11):1842–7. doi:10.1093/annonc/mdp233. Epub 2009 Apr 30.
8. Izzedine H, Massard C, Spano JP, Goldwasser F, Khayat D, Soria JC. VEGF signalling inhibition-induced proteinuria: mechanisms, significance and management. Eur J Cancer. 2010;46(2):439–48.
9. Berruti A, Fazio N, Ferrero A, Brizzi MP, Volante M, Nobili E, Tozzi L, Bodei L, Torta M, D'Avolio A, Priola AM, Birocco N, Amoroso V, Biasco G, Papotti M, Dogliotti L. Bevacizumab plus octreotide and metronomic capecitabine in patients with metastatic well-to-moderately differentiated neuroendocrine tumors: the xelbevoct study. BMC Cancer. 2014;14:184.
10. Goncalves JG, de Braganca AC, Canale D, et al. Vitamin D deficiency aggravates chronic kidney disease progression after ischemic acute kidney injury. PLoS One. 2014;9:e107228.
11. Humalda JK, Goldsmith DJA, Thadhani R, de Borst MH. Vitamin D analogues to target residual proteinuria: potential impact on cardiorenal outcomes. Nephrol Dial Transplant. 2015;30:1988–94.
12. Patel TV, Morgan JA, Demetri GD, et al. A preeclampsia-like syndrome characterized by reversible hypertension and proteinuria induced by the multitargeted kinase inhibitors sunitinib and sorafenib. J Natl Cancer Inst. 2008;100:282–4.
13. Eremina V, Sood M, Haigh J, et al. Glomerular specific alterations of VEGF—a expression lead to distinct congenital and acquired renal diseases. J Clin Invest. 2003;111(5):707–16.
14. Maynard SE, Min JY, Merchan J, et al. Excess placental soluble fms-like tyrosine kinase 1 (sFlt1) may contribute to endothelial dysfunction, hypertension, and proteinuria in preeclampsia. J Clin Invest. 2003;111(5):649–58.
15. Miller KD, Chap LI, Holmes FA, et al. Randomized phase III trial of capecitabine compared with bevacizumab plus capecitabine in patients with previously treated metastatic breast cancer. J Clin Oncol. 2005;23:792–9.
16. Di Lorenzo G, Autorino R, Bruni G, et al. Cardiovascular toxicity following sunitinib therapy in metastatic renal cell carcinoma: a multicenter analysis. Ann Oncol. 2009;20:1535–42.
17. Di Lorenzo G, Porta C, Bellmunt J, Sternberg C, Kirkali Z, Staehler M, Joniau S, Montorsi F, Buonerba C. Toxicities of targeted therapy and their management in kidney cancer. Eur Urol. 2011;59:526–40.
18. Rixe O, Billemont B, Izzedine H. Hypertension as a predictive factor of sunitinib activity. Ann Oncol. 2007;18:1117–25.
19. Zhu X, Stergiopoulos K, Wu S. Risk of hypertension and renal dysfunction with an angiogenesis inhibitor sunitinib: systematic review and meta-analysis. Acta Oncol. 2009;48:9–17.
20. Moreo A, Vallerio P, Ricotta R, Stucchi M, Pozzi M, Musca F, Meani P, Maloberti A, Facchetti R, Di Bella S, Giganti MO, Sartore-Bianchi A, Siena S, Mancia G, Giannattasio C. Effects of cancer therapy targeting vascular endothelial growth factor receptor on central blood pressure and cardiovascular system. Am J Hypertens. 2016 Feb;29(2):158–62.
21. Rini BI, Cohen DP, Lu DR, Chen I, Hariharan S, Gore ME, Figlin RA, Baum MS, Motzer RJ. Hypertension as a biomarker of efficacy in patients with metastatic renal cell carcinoma treated with sunitinib. J Natl Cancer Inst. 2011;103(9):763–73.

22. Porta C, Szczylik C. Tolerability of first-line therapy for metastatic renal cell carcinoma. Cancer Treat Rev. 2009;35(3):297–307.
23. Hicklin DJ, Lee ME. Role of the vascular endothelial growth factor pathway in tumor growth and angiogenesis. J Clin Oncol. 2005;23(5):1011–27.
24. Schneider BP, Wang M, Radovich M, Sledge GW, Badve S, Thor A, Flockhart DA, Hancock B, Davidson N, Gralow J, Dickler M, Perez EA, Cobleigh M, Shenkier T, Edgerton S, Miller KD. Association of vascular endothelial growth factor and vascular endothelial growth factor receptor-2 genetic polymorphisms with outcome in a trial of paclitaxel compared with paclitaxel plus bevacizumab in advanced breast cancer: ECOG 2100. J Clin Oncol. 2008;26(28):4672–8.
25. Chu TF, Rupnick MA, Kerkela R, et al. Cardiotoxicity associated with tyrosine kinase inhibitor sunitinib. Lancet. 2007;370(9604):2011–9.
26. Gore ME, Szczylik C, Porta C, et al. Safety and efficacy of sunitinib for metastatic renal-cell carcinoma: an expanded-access trial. Lancet Oncol. 2009;10:757–63.
27. Richards CJ, Je Y, Schutz FAB, et al. Incidence and risk of congestive heart failure in patients with renal and nonrenal cell carcinoma treated with sunitinib. J Clin Oncol. 2011;29(25):3450–6.
28. Schmidinger M, Zielinski CC, Vogl UM, et al. Cardiac toxicity of sunitinib and sorafenib in patients with metastatic renal cell carcinoma. J Clin Oncol. 2008;26(32):5204–12.
29. Molinaro M, Ameri P, Marone G, Petretta M, Abete P, Di Lisa F, De Placido S, Bonaduce D, Tocchetti CG. Recent advances on pathophysiology, diagnostic and therapeutic insights in cardiac dysfunction induced by antineoplastic drugs. Biomed Res Int. 2015;2015:138148. doi:10.1155/2015/138148. Epub 2015 Oct.
30. Ranpura V, Hapani S, Chuang J, Wu S. Risk of cardiac ischemia and arterial thromboembolic events with the angiogenesis inhibitor bevacizumab in cancer patients: a meta-analysis of randomized controlled trials. Acta Oncol. 2010;49:287–97.
31. Pouessel D, Culine S. High frequency of intracerebral hemorrhage in metastatic renal carcinoma patients with brain metastases treated with tyrosine kinase inhibitors targeting the vascular endothelial growth factor receptor. Eur Urol. 2008;53:376–81.
32. Nalluri SR, Chu D, Keresztes R, Zhu X, Wu S. Risk of venous thromboembolism with the angiogenesis inhibitor bevacizumab in cancer patients: a meta-analysis. JAMA. 2008;300:2277–85.
33. Sher AF, Chu D, Wu S. Risk of bleeding in cancer patients treated with the angiogenesis inhibitor bevacizumab: a meta-analysis. J Clin Oncol. 2009;27:15s.
34. Choueiri TK, Schutz FA, Je Y, Rosenberg JE, Bellmunt J. Risk of arterial thromboembolic events with sunitinib and sorafenib: a systematic review and meta-analysis of clinical trials. J Clin Oncol. 2010;28:2280–5.
35. Je Y, Schutz FA, Choueiri TK. Risk of bleeding with vascular endothelial growth factor receptor tyrosine-kinase inhibitors sunitinib and sorafenib: a systematic review and meta-analysis of clinical trials. Lancet Oncol. 2009;10:967–74.
36. Bronte E, Bronte G, Novo G, Bronte F, Bavetta MG, Lo Re G, Brancatelli G, Bazan V, Natoli C, Novo S, Russo A. What links BRAF to the heart function? New insights from the cardiotoxicity of BRAF inhibitors in cancer treatment. Oncotarget. 2015;6(34):35589–601.
37. Slamon DJ, Leyland-Jones B, Shak S, et al. Use of chemotherapy plus a monoclonal antibody against her2 for metastatic breast cancer that overexpresses HER2. New Engl J Med. 2001;344(11):783–92.
38. Tocchetti CG, Ragone G, Coppola C, et al. Detection, monitoring, and management of trastuzumab-induced left ventricular dysfunction: an actual challenge. Eur J Heart Fail. 2012;14(2):130–7.
39. Ewer MS, Lippman SM. Type II chemotherapy-related cardiac dysfunction: time to recognize a new entity. J Clin Oncol. 2005;23(13):2900–2.
40. Odiete O, Hill MF, Sawyer DB. Neuregulin in cardiovascular development and disease. Circ Res. 2012;111(10):1376–85.

Cardiac Arrhythmias in Cancer Patients

Nicola Maurea, Iris Parrini, and Irma Bisceglia

C. Lestuzzi et al. (eds.), *Manual of Cardio-oncology*, DOI 10.1007/978-3-319-40236-9_11

11.1 Introduction

Patients with cancer may have several kinds of arrhythmias either as an independent comorbidity or as a consequence of the cancer itself or of the antineoplastic therapies.

11.1.1 Incidence of Cardiac Arrhythmias

The real incidence of arrhythmias is difficult to be assessed and can often be underestimated for different reasons:

- Systematic cardiac monitoring is not routinely performed in cancer patients unless symptomatic.
- Some arrhythmias may not be detected during routine monitoring [1, 2]
- Sometimes patients with heart disease or higher risk of cardiotoxicity are excluded in clinical trials
- In many patients, several chemotherapy are administered simultaneously; therefore it is difficult to identify which drug may cause arrhythmia
- Great number of new agents used in the treatment

11.2 Atrial Fibrillation

Atrial fibrillation is a disorganized, rapid, and irregular atrial activation. The ventricular response to the rapid atrial activation is irregular. The rate may vary between 120 and 160 beats/min, but sometimes arrives up to 200 beats/min.Atrial fibrillation is defined as:

- **paroxysmal** if it is self-terminating, usually within 48 h. AF episodes that are cardioverted within 7 days should be considered paroxysmal
- **persistent** if it is present when an AF episode lasts longer than 7 days or requires termination by cardioversion after 7 days or more.
- **permanent** if the presence of the arrhythmia is accepted by the patient (and physician) it lasts for months or years.

The prevalence is 1.5 % to 2 % in the general population, increasing up to 10 % at 80 years of age and to 18 % at 85 years of age [3, 4, 5]

11.2.1 Epidemiology

Most frequent cancer-related AF occurs postoperatively.

- AF is particularly frequent during and after thoracic surgery:
  - Especially in pulmonary resection for lung cancer [6], associated with an increase of postoperative mortality; in patients who underwent elective colectomy for colorectal cancer [7] or esophagectomy for esophageal cancer [8].

The association between cancer and AF is not only limited to the postoperative period but also in some cancers like colorectal of the colon, breast, lung, kidney, and ovary a higher incidence of AF may be observed [9].

11.2.2 Pathophysiology

There are many conditions predisposing to AF in cancer patients:

- A direct manifestation of cancer in case of primary neoplasm such as lung and esophagus involving the heart or metastatic cardiac tumors.
- Electrolyte imbalances, metabolic disorders, an increase in sympathetic tone, paraneoplastic manifestations as in hyperparathyroidism, or autoimmune reactions.
- A consequence of medical therapy such as anthracyclines, taxanes, 5-fluorouracil and capecitabine, cisplatin, ifosfamide, gemcitabine, high-dose corticosteroids, targeted therapies, and bisphosphonates.
- inflammation may lead to AF [10]:
  - Chronic inflammation increases cancer risk and affects all cancer stages, triggering the initial genetic mutation or epigenetic mechanism, promoting cancer initiation, progression, and metastatic diffusion. In fact, a general increase in plasma levels and cell increase of the main inflammatory markers such as C-reactive protein (CRP) and serum amyloid A (A-SAA) are associated with AF [11].

11.2.3 Clinical Considerations

In clinical practice, the approach to atrial fibrillation requires:

- Screening and prophylaxis of AF
- Heart rate control versus restoring sinus rhythm
- Prevention of thromboembolism
- Evaluation of risk of bleeding

- **Consider antiarrhythmic prophylaxis in particular conditions like:**
  - Lung or oesophageal resection
  - In some cancers or chemotherapy
- **Consider pharmacological or electrical cardioversion:**
  - In patients hemodynamically unstable recalling that:
    AF onset <48 h under the cover of UFH administered i.v.
    AF onset >48 h or AF of unknown duration. Anticoagulation or a transesophageal echocardiogram to rule out the presence of atrial thrombi is considered mandatory before elective cardioversion
  - There are evidence in favour of using amiodarone for prophylaxis or rhythm maintenance
- **Consider rate control in patients hemodynamically stable or in metastatic disease**
  - a good ventricular rate is obtained using B-blockers or calcium channel blocker such as verapamil o diltiazem

A balance between thromboembolic and bleeding risks in cancer patients is required. It is known that cancer is itself a pro-thrombotic state increasing the risk of thromboembolic events in patients with AF. Moreover, keep in mind the risk of bleeding of some cancers in oncology patients.

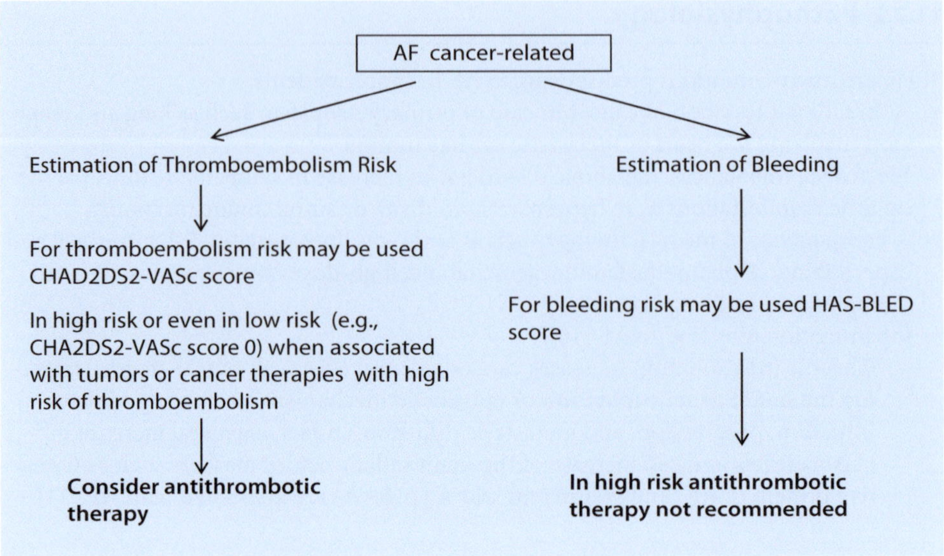

Fig. 11.1 Anticoagulant therapy in patients with cancer-related atrial fibrillation (AF)

Antithrombotic Therapy in Cancer-Related Atrial Fibrillation include evaluation of scores using CHADS2 or CHA2DS2-VASc and HAS-BLED are currently used to guide antithrombotic therapy [3] (Fig. 11.1).

11

In this prediction, scores have not included cancer patients, so may not be adequate: CHA2DS2-VASc rules out previous thromboembolism and HAS-BLED excludes hematological malignancies, coagulation defects, thrombocytopenia, and severe metastatic hepatic disease.

In this context, the antithrombotic therapy should be strictly individualized (see other chapter).

Furthermore, the response to anticoagulant therapy can be complex and may not be predictable for the increased risk of bleeding for concomitant medications or metabolic disorders [12].

11.2.4 Therapy

- Low molecular weight heparin (LMWH) may often be the therapy of choice having a more favorable outcome than vitamin K inhibitors [13].
- To date, there is no evidence for the use of novel anticoagulants in cancer patients [14].
- OAT should be considered, a year after cancer diagnosis [15].
- There are not enough data to use radiofrequency catheter ablation for pulmonary vein isolation in cancer patients, but it may be a good option when it becomes difficult to control the rhythm with therapy considering cancer prognosis.

In 2014 detailed and comprehensive evidence-based guidelines for the prevention and treatment of perioperative/postoperative atrial fibrillation and flutter (POAF) for thoracic surgical procedures have been published [16]. These guidelines may be applied to the general cancer population. However, for patients undergoing

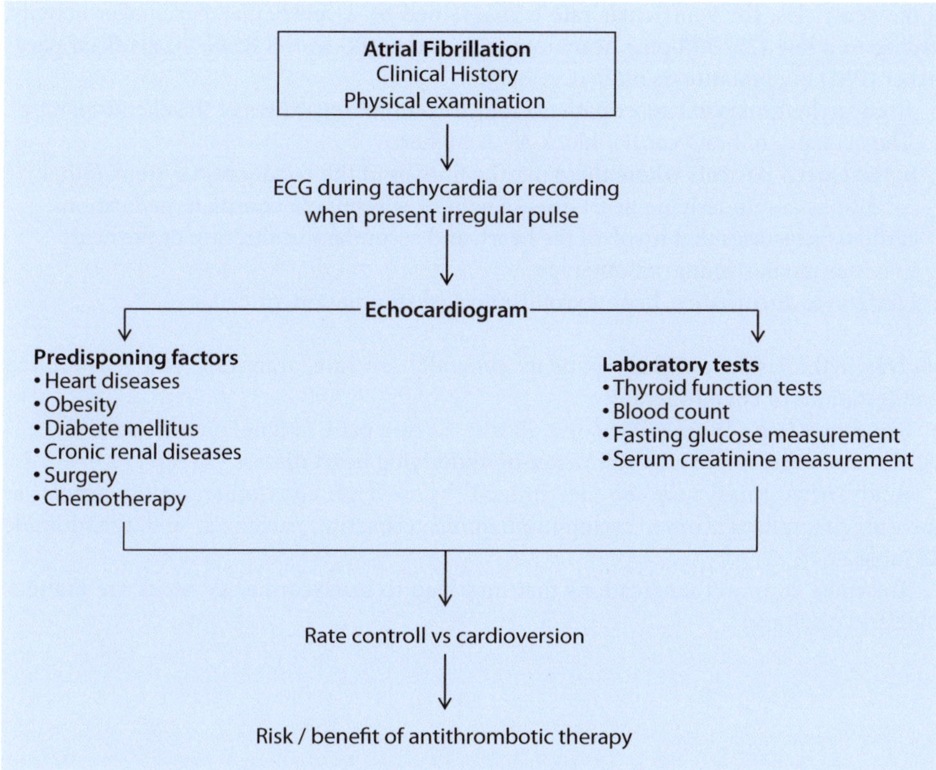

Fig. 11.2 Clinical assessment and theraputic approach for patients with atrial fibrillation

chemotherapy, the possible interaction between cardiologic and oncologic drugs have to be taken into account.

For clinical point of view, see Fig. 11.2.

11.3 Bradyarrhythmias

Bradyarrhythmias are comprised of sinus bradycardia, dysfunction of the sinus node (sinus atrial block to sinus arrest) and atrio-ventricular block.

Sinus bradycardia is a heart rhythm with a ventricular rate of less than 60 beats per minute. Sick sinus syndrome depends on the dysfunctional node sinus where bradycardia is alternating with tachycardia as well as atrial fibrillation.

AV block is a conduction disorder due to failure of impulse conduction over the atrio-ventricular (AV) node/His-Purkinje system. There are three types of AV blocks with increased severity of damage (AV I, II, III degree). In first degree AV block, all the beats are conducted to the ventricles (the ventricular rhythm is the same of the atrial rhythm), but with a delay exceeding 200 msec. In second degree AV block, some atrial impulse are not conducted to the ventricles, and the ventricular rate is slower than the atrial rate. In third degree AV block (also called "Complete AV block"), no atrial impulse is conducted to the ventricles; the ventricular rate is mantained by a ventricular pacemaker activity, leading to a low (25–30/bpm) heart rate with wide QRS in the ECG; an artificial pacemaker (PM) implantation is often necessary.

Bradyarrhythmias in cancer patients may be present regardless of the chemotherapy.

The evidence of bradycardia/ block AV is higher:

- In the elderly patients where there may be fibrosis of the conduction system. Other conditions are underlying heart disease with or without concomitant medications, cardiac metastases that involves the heart, and secondary infiltration of the heart
- Previous mediastinum radiotherapy
- Electrolyte disturbance, hypothyroidism, vagal stimulation, or drugs

Bradyarrhythmias in oncology patients generally are rare, transient, and self-limiting manifestations of chemotherapy.

Symptoms (e.g., dyspnea, syncope, dizziness, chest pain, fatigue) often depend on ventricular rate degree of block or presence of underlying heart disease (Fig. 11.3).

Bradyarrhythmias may be determined by several chemotherapeutic agents as doxorubicin, mitoxantrone, cyclophosphamide, cisplatin, paclitaxel, and thalidomide (Table 11.1).

The most common medications that may lead to bradycardia/AV block are thalidomide and paclitaxel.

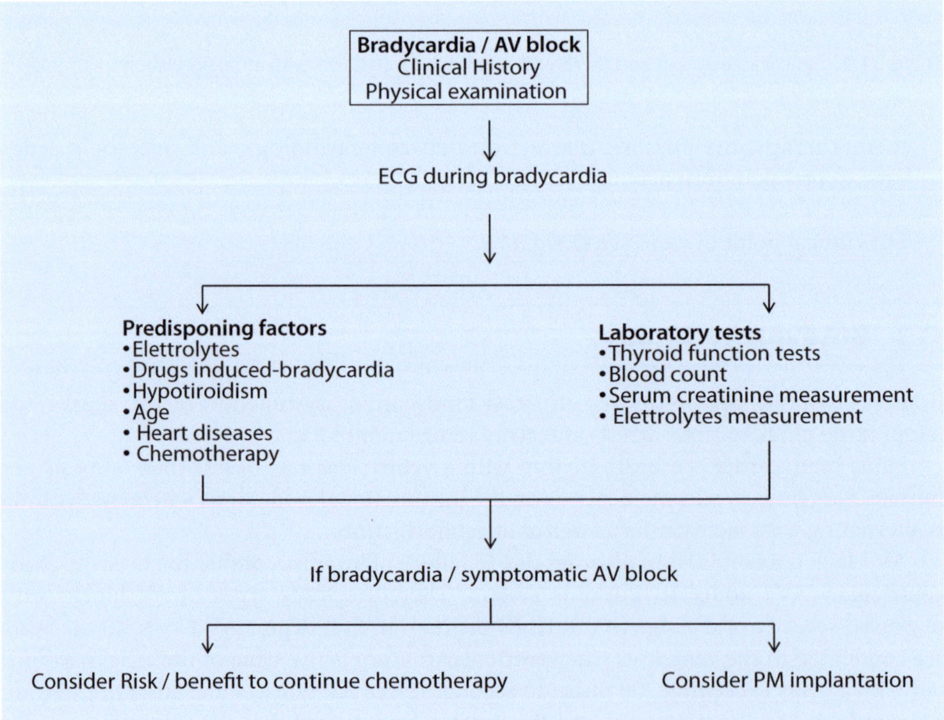

Fig. 11.3 Clinical assessment and therapeutic approach for patients with bradiarrhythmias

Table 11.1 Chemotherapeutic agents induce sinus bradycardia, AV block, intraventricular conduction block

Drug	Sinus bradycardia	AV block	Intraventricular conduction block
Amsacrine	Rare		
Arsenic trioxide	Rare	Rare	Rare
Bortezomib	Rare	Rare	
Capecitabine	Rare	Rare	
Ciplatin	Rare	Rare	Rare
Combretastatin	Rare		
Crizotinib	Rare		
Cyclophosphamide	Rare	Rare	
Cytarabine	Rare		
Daunorubicin	Rare	Rare	
Fludarabine	Rare		
5-Fu	Frequent (*)	Rare	Rare
Mitoxantrone	Rare	Rare	
Paclitaxel	0.1–31 %	25 %	Rare
Polatinib	Rare	Rare	
Rituximab	Rare	Rare	
Taxanes	Rare	Rare	
Thalidomide	27 %	Rare	
Vinca alkaloids	Rare		
Vorinostat	Rare		
Doxorubicin	Rare	Rare	Rare
Epirubicin		Rare	
Ifosfamide		Rare	
IL-2	Rare	Rare	Rare
Interferon-α		Rare	
Trastuzumab			Rare
Imatinib			Rare

11.3.1 Thalidomide

Thalidomide is used for some solid tumors. Sinus bradycardia is observed in about one-third of patients. Third-degree AV block with hypotension and loss of consciousness were reported in a case report [17].

In clinical practice:
- Close monitoring of signs and symptoms of bradycardia (fatigue, syncope, lightheadedness, or dizziness) during the administration of thalidomide
- **Dose reduction or discontinuation in bradycardia with heart rate of 50–60 bpm when symptoms develop**
- **Thalidomide should be interrupted in bradycardia with heart rate of <50 bpm.**
- Bradycardia often recovers after drug discontinuation but sometimes requires a pacemaker implantation [18, 19]
- Particularly in responsive myeloma, requiring a continuous therapy, a pacemaker implantation when third degree AV block occurs should be considered
- Thyroid-stimulating hormone level should be obtained to rule out hypothyroidism

11.3.2 Paclitaxel

Sinus bradycardia and first-degree atrioventricular block, advanced heart block, and conduction abnormalities are rare and often asymptomatic.

In clinical practice:
- Arrhythmias appear within the first 24 h after initiation of infusion and resolve spontaneously over the next 48–72 h [20, 21]
- Cardiac monitoring is generally recommended in the first hours of infusion
- Drug discontinuation should be considered when conduction disturbances occur.
- Pacemaker implantation might be required depending on the severity of symptoms, hemodynamic consequences, and need to continue the therapy [21].
- Pretreatment with antihistamines and corticosteroids prevents the release of histamine and reduces the risk of bradycardia.

11.3.3 Other Drugs

Other drugs that less commonly lead to bradycardia include the following:
- **5-fluorouracil (5-FU) and capecitabine:** Sometimes transient asymptomatic bradycardia has been observed persisting for more than 24 h [21]. Rarely requires pacemaker implantation.
- **Cisplatin:** Bradyarrhythmias are rare, and marked sinus bradycardia may occur during each of the six cycles [22].

In conclusion, the approach to these arrhythmias should be individualized: the decision depends on the drug administered, the need to continue the treatment, and the severity of the arrhythmia and related symptoms.

11.4 Ventricular Arrhythmias Without QT Prolongation

Ventricular tachycardia (VT) is defined as tachyarrhythmia with wide QRS of 3 or more consecutive complexes in duration originating from the ventricles at a rate of ≥ 100 bpm.

Non-sustained VT of 3 or more consecutive complexes in duration, terminating spontaneously in <30 sec.

Sustained VT > 30 sec in duration and /or requiring termination due to haemodynamic compromise in <30 sec.

VT without QT prolongation are rare and may be:

- Manifestations of acute or chronic toxicity, mainly in the presence of predisposing factors (left ventricular dysfunction, ischemia, electrolyte abnormalities, metabolic disorders, or marked bradycardia)
- A direct presentation of a primary neoplasm or cardiac metastasis.

The most common drugs that can induce VT are (Table 11.2):

Table 11.2 Chemotherapeutic agents induce ventricular tachycardia

Drug	Ventricular tachycardia/ fibrillation
Arsenic trioxide	50 %
Capecitabine	2.1 %
Ciplatin	8 %
Cyclophosphamide	Rare
Daunorubicin	Rare
5-FU*	1.1 %
Taxanes	0.26 %
Doxorubicin	6 %
Ifosfamide	Rare
IL-2	05–1.1 %
Interferon-α-ϒ	Rare
Trastuzumab	Rare
Melphalan	Rare
Amsacrine	Rare
Gemcitabine	Rare
Methotrexate	Rare
Dasatinib	Rare
Panobinostat	Rare
Romidepsin	Rare
Alemtuzumab	Rare
Rituximab	Rare

(*) In continuous infusion

- **5-FU and capecitabine**
  - Ventricular arrhythmias and sudden cardiac death often occur during angina or myocardial infarction [23, 24]. Arrhythmias without ischemia are rare.
  - Ischemic-like ECG changes and ventricular arrhythmias appear within 2–5 days and disappear within a few hours to 5 days after drug discontinuation.
- **Interleukin-2** (IL-2). VT during IL-2 administration is rare and described in patients with renal cell carcinoma undergoing treatment with high-dose bolus [25].
- **Ifosfamide** can be associated with malignant arrhythmias when used in high doses [26].
- **Cyclophosphamide** and **cisplatin** seldom cause ventricular arrhythmias [27, 28].
- **Anthracycline** presents serious ventricular arrhythmias which may occur in chronic anthracycline cardiotoxicity even after many years of chemotherapy when patients developed a cardiomyopathy [29].

11.5 Diagnosis of Cardiac Arrhythmias

The first clinical approach is to identify those patients who are more susceptible to developing cardiac arrhythmias optimizing clinical monitoring and therapy (◘ Fig. 11.4).

A careful baseline cardiovascular evaluation should be performed.

- Aggressive treatment of comorbidity before and during therapy is mandatory to reduce the risk of arrhythmias.
- Close monitoring and attention to develop signs or symptoms may improve outcome of those patients.

ECG should be performed before and during the treatment:

- To detect arrhythmias, conduction disturbances, QTc interval prolongation, and signs of myocardial ischemia or LV hypertrophy
- May help in determining the location of the cardiac tumor [30]

ECG Holter monitoring is useful when arrhythmia is suspected in order to prevent it and/or treat.

In conclusion, the approach to these arrhythmias should be individualized; the decision depends on dose and drug administered and the type of cancer. Considering the severity of this arrhythmia the chemotherapy should be discontinued (◘ Fig. 11.4).

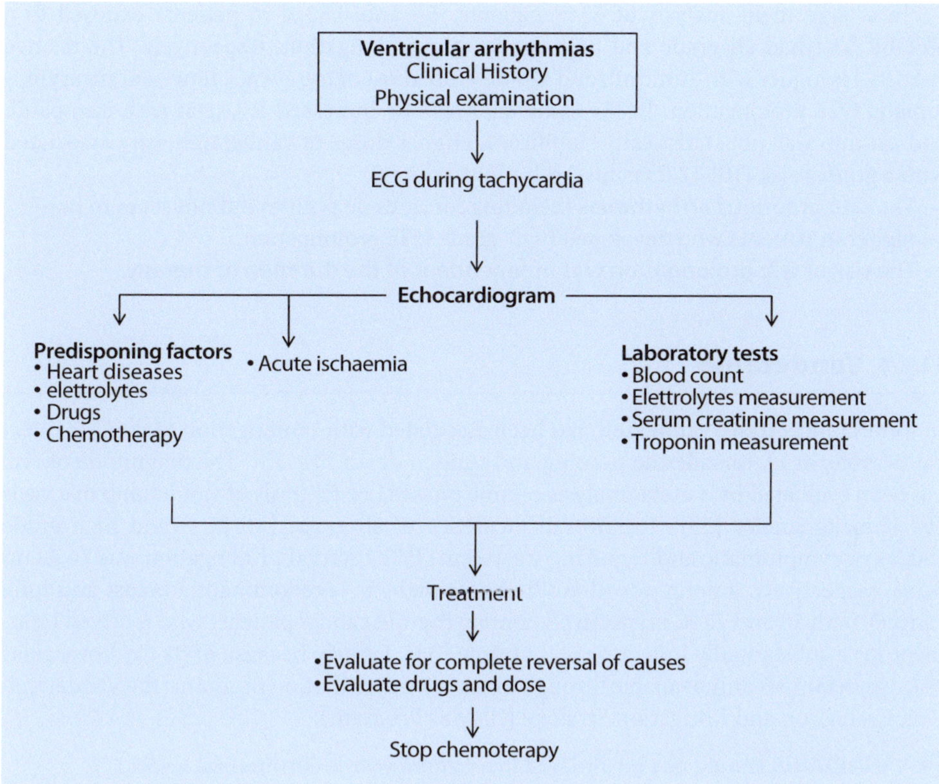

Fig. 11.4 Clinical assessment and theraputic approach for patients with ventricular arrhythmias

11.6 Arrhythmias and Targeted Therapy

Prolongation of the QTc interval and cardiac arrhythmias: Many drugs delay cardiac repolarization—an effect that is reflected on the surface electrocardiogram (ECG) by a prolonged heart rate-corrected QT (QTc) interval. Although a prolonged QTc interval is not immediately harmful, it can be associated with potentially fatal cardiac arrhythmias. The ventricular tachyarrhythmia most typically triggered is of a unique form, known as torsades de pointes, which is most often transient, but when sustained, can give rise to symptoms of impaired cerebral circulation or degenerate into ventricular fibrillation, usually with a fatal outcome.

Of **the vascular endothelial growth factor** (**VEGF**) receptor tyrosine kinase inhibitors (TKIs), **vandetanib** and **sunitinib** have been most convincingly associated with QTc prolongation, although other **VEGF receptor** (**VEGRF**) TKIs including **sorafenib** are less certain [31].

In a large meta-analysis of 6548 patients, 4.4 and 0.83 % of patients exposed to a VEGFR TKI had all-grade and high-grade QTc prolongation, respectively. The relative risk (RR) is higher with Sunitinib and Vandetanib; most of the events, however, are asymptomatic QTc prolongation. In the same analysis, the increased RR seen with pazopanib and axitinib was not statistically significant. Higher doses of vandetanib were associated with a greater risk (RR 12.2 versus 3.6 for lower doses).

- **The rate of serious arrhythmias** including torsades de pointes did not seem to be higher in patients who developed high-grade QTc prolongation.
- **The risk of QTc prolongation was independent of the duration of therapy.**

11.6.1 Vandetanib

In some clinical trials, vandetanib has been associated with prolongation of the QTc interval (waveform 1), torsades de pointes, and sudden death [31–33]. The magnitude of risk has been evaluated by a meta-analysis of nine phase II or III trials of vandetanib in a variety of malignancies [33]. The overall incidence of all-grade (>0.45 s) and high-grade (>0.5 s or symptomatic and requiring treatment) QTc interval prolongation was 16.4 and 3.7 %, respectively, among non-thyroid cancer patients (predominantly breast and lung cancer), with 18 and 12 %, respectively, among thyroid cancer patients who received treatment for a substantially longer period of time [33]. Largely because of its cardiovascular risk, vandetanib is only available through a restricted distribution program (the Vandetanib Risk Evaluation and Mitigation Strategy [REMS] Program).

11

VANDETANIB should not be initiated in a patient with a QTc interval > 450 milliseconds (ms) [34].

Because of the risk of cardiotoxicity, the USA prescribing information includes a black box warning to correct hypocalcemia, hypokalemia, and/or hypomagnesemia prior to drug administration.

In addition, given the long half-life of the drug (19 days), ECGs are recommended to monitor the QT interval.

- At baseline, at two to four weeks, 8 to 12 weeks after starting treatment, and every three months thereafter.
- Monitoring of serum potassium, calcium, and magnesium levels as well as TSH is recommended on the same schedule.
- Concurrent administration of drugs known to prolong the QTc interval should be avoided
- Patients who develop a QTc interval greater than 500 ms during treatment should stop taking the drug until the QTc returns to <450 ms; dosing should be resumed at a reduced dose.

11.6.2 Sunitinib and Sorafenib

Sunitinib also has a dose-dependent effect on the QTc interval [31, 35–37]. In contrast, the effect of sorafenib on changes in the QTc interval appears modest and unlikely to be of clinical significance [31, 38].Specific guidelines for monitoring with ECGs during sunitinib therapy and managing the dose in patients who develop QTc prolongation are lacking.

- In general, we obtain a baseline ECG in patients treated with sunitinib and monitor with ECGs during therapy only if the patient is also receiving therapy with other drugs that have the potential to prolong the QTc interval.

11.6.3 Lenvatinib

In a placebo-controlled trial, approximately 9 % of lenvatinib-treated patients developed QTc interval prolongation versus 2 % in the control group; the incidence of grade 3 or greater QTc prolongation was 2 % versus non in the placebo group.

- The US prescribing information recommends monitoring ECGs in patients with congenital long QT syndrome, heart failure, bradyarrhythmias, or those taking drugs known to prolong the QT interval.

11.6.4 Ponatinib

Approximately, 1 % of patients treated with ponatinib have developed symptomatic bradyarrhythmias and 5 % supraventricular tachyarrhythmias (predominantly atrial fibrillation) [39]. QTc prolongation is not reported.

11.7 Monitoring and Management of Cardiac Arrhythmias Due to Targeted Therapy

Specific guidelines for assessing and monitoring the QTc interval and recommendations for managing the drug based upon the grade of toxicity (◘ Table 11.3) are available for patients receiving vandetanib and lenvatinib. Formal guidelines are not available for any of the other anti-angiogenic TKIs.

Table 11.3 NCI CTCAE v4.0 QT prolongation

Adverseevent	Grade 1	Grade 2	Grade 3	Grade 4
QT intervalprolongation	QTc 450 to 480 milliseconds	QTc 481 to 500 milliseconds	QTc ≥501 milliseconds on at least two separate ECGs	QTc ≥501 milliseconds or >60 milliseconds change from baseline and torsade de pointes or polymorphic ventricular tachycardia or signs/symptoms of serious arrhythmia

Prolongation of the corrected QT interval is found on the electrocardiogram. *NCI CTCAE* National Cancer Institute Common Terminology Criteria for Adverse Events
QTc QT corrected interval, *ECGs* electrocardiograms

11

Recommendations

For any patient receiving therapy with an anti-angiogenic TKI, careful review of concomitant medications is warranted, especially drugs that are associated with increased QTc.

Patients with a history of QT interval prolongation, those who are taking antiarrhythmics, and those with relevant preexisting cardiac disease, bradycardia, or electrolyte disturbances may be more prone to develop a prolonged QTc.

References

1. Senkus E, Jassem J. Cardiovascular effects of systemic cancer treatment. Cancer Treat Rev. 2011;37(4):300–11.
2. Suter TM, Ewer MS. Cancer drugs and the heart: importance and management. Eur Heart J. 2013;34(15):1102–11.
3. Camm AJ, Lip GY, De Caterina R, et al. 2012 focused update of the ESC guidelines for the management of atrial fibrillation: an update of the 2010 ESC guidelines for the management of atrial fibrillation. Eur Heart J. 2012;33:2719–47.
4. Camm AJ, Kirchhof P, Lip GY, et al. Guidelines for the management of atrial fibrillation: the task force for the management of atrial fibrillation of the European Society of Cardiology (ESC). Eur Heart J. 2010;31:2369–42.
5. Driver JA, Djoussé L, Logroscino G, Gaziano JM, Kurth T. Incidence of cardiovascular disease and cancer in advanced age: prospective cohort study. BMJ. 2008;337:a2467.
6. D'Amico T, Zhao Y, O'Brien S, Harpole D. Risk factors for atrial fibrillation after lung cancer surgery: analysis of the Society of Thoracic Surgeons general thoracic surgery database. Ann Thorac Surg. 2010;90:368–74.
7. Siu CW, Tung HM, Chu KW, Jim MH, Lau CP, Tse HF. Prevalence and predictors of new-onset atrial fibrillation after elective surgery for colorectal cancer. Pacing ClinElectrophysiol. 2005;28 Suppl 1:S120–3.19.

8. Bhave PD, Goldman LE, Vittinghoff E, Maselli J, Auerbach A. Incidence, predictors, and outcomes associated with postoperative atrial fibrillation after major non cardiac surgery. Am Heart J. 2012;164:918–24.
9. Guzzetti S, Costantino G, Vernocchi A, Sada S, Fundaro C. First diagnosis of colorectal or breast cancer and prevalence of atrial fibrillation. Intern Emerg Med. 2008;3:227e231.
10. Velagapudi P, Turagam MK, Kocheril AG. Atrial fibrillation in cancer patients: an underrecognized condition. South Med J. 2011;104:667–8.
11. Lainscak M, Dagres N, Filippatos GS, Anker SD, Kremastinos DT. Atrial fibrillation in chronic non-cardiac disease: where do we stand? Int J Cardiol. 2008;128:311–5.
12. Lee AY. Deep vein thrombosis and cancer: survival, recurrence, and anticoagulant choices. Dis Mon. 2005;51:150–7.
13. Klerk CP, Smorenburg SM, Otten HM, et al. The effect of low molecular weight heparin on survival in patients with advanced malignancy. J ClinOncol. 2005;23:2130–5.
14. Connolly SJ, Ezekowitz MD, Yusuf S, et al. For the RE-LY Steering Committee and Investigators. Dabigatran versus warfarin in patients with atrial fibrillation. N Engl J Med. 2009;361:1139–51.
15. Lee Y-J, Park J-k, Uhm J-S, Kim J-Y, Pak H-N, Lee M-H, Sung J-H, Joung B. Bleeding risk and major adverse events in patients with cancer on oral anticoagulation therapy International. J Cardiol. 2016;203:372–8.
16. Frendl G, Sodickson AC, Chung MK, et al.; American Association for Thoracic Surgery. 2014 AATS guidelines for the prevention and management of perioperative atrial fibrillation and flutter for thoracic surgical procedures. J Thorac Cardiovasc Surg. 2014;148(3):e153–93. Epub 2014 Jun 30. Review.
17. Hinterseer M, Becker A, Kaab S, Lang N, Nabauer M, Steinbeck G. Thalidomide-induced symptomatic third-degree atrioventricular block. Clin Res Cardiol. 2006;95:474–6.
18. Fahdi IE, Gaddam V, Saucedo JF, Kishan CV, Vyas K, Deneke MG, et al. Bradycardia during therapy for multiple myeloma with thalidomide. Am J Cardiol. 2004;93(8):1052–5.
19. Barlogie B, Tricot G, Anaissie E, Shaughnessy J, Rasmussen E, van Rhee F, et al. Thalidomide and hematopoietic-cell transplantation for multiple myeloma. N Engl J Med. 2006;354(10):1021–30.
20. Ettinger DS, Armstrong DK, et al. Taxol: a unique antineoplastic agent with significant activity in advanced ovarian epithelial neoplasms. Ann Intern Med. 1989;111(4):273–9.
21. Arbuck SG, Strauss H, Rowinsky E, Christian M, Suffness M, Adams J, et al. A reassessment of cardiac toxicity associated with taxol. J Natl Cancer Inst Mono. 1993;15:117–30.
22. Yavas O, Aytemır K, Celık I. The prevalence of silent arrhythmia in patients receiving cisplatin-based chemotherapy. Turkish J Cancer. 2008;38(1):12–5.
23. Eskilsson J, Albertsson M. Failure of preventing 5-fluorouracil cardiotoxicity by prophylactic treatment with verapamil. Acta Oncol. 1990;29(8):1001–3.
24. Kosmas C, Kallistratos MS, Kopterides P, Syrios J, Skopelitis H, Mylonakis N, et al. Cardiotoxicity of fluoropyrimidines in different schedules of administration: a prospective study. J Cancer Res ClinOncol. 2008;134(1):75–82.
25. Oleksowicz L, Escott P, Leichman GC, Spangenthal E. Sustained ventricular tachycardia and its successful prophylaxis during high-dose bolus interleukin-2 therapy for metastatic renal cell carcinoma. Am J ClinOncol. 2000;23:34–6.
26. Quezado ZM, Wilson WH, Cunnion RE, Parker MM, Reda D, Bryant G, et al. High-dose ifosfamide is associated with severe, reversible cardiac dysfunction. Ann Intern Med. 1993;118(1):31–6.
27. Cazin B, Gorin NC, Laporte JP, Gallet B, Douay L, Lopez M, et al. Cardiac complications after bone marrow transplantation. A report on a series of 63 consecutive transplantations. Cancer. 1986;57(10):2061–9.
28. Kupari M, Volin L, Suokas A, Timonen T, Hekali P, Ruutu T, et al. Cardiac involvement in bone marrow tra nsplantation:electrocardiographic changes, arrhythmias, heart failure and autopsy findings. Bone Marrow Transplant. 1990;5(2):91–8.
29. Steinherz LJ, Steinherz PG, Tan C. Cardiac failure and dysrhythmias 6–19 years after anthracycline therapy: a series of 15 patients. Med Pediatr Oncol. 1995;24(6):352–61.
30. Haqqani HM, Morton JB, Kalman JM. Using the 12-lead ECG to localize the origin of atrial and ventricular tachycardias: part 2--ventricular tachycardia. J Cardiovasc Electrophysiol. 2009;20(7):825–32.
31. Shah RR, Morganroth J, Shah DR. Cardiovascular safety of tyrosine kinase inhibitors: with a special focus on cardiac repolarisation (QT interval). Drug Saf. 2013;36:295.
32. US FDA drug approval summary for vandetanib in medullary thyroid cancer. http://www.accessdata.fda.gov/drugsatfda_docs/label/2011/022405s000lbl.pdf. Accessed 25 Apr, 2011.
33. Zang J, Wu S, Tang L, et al. Incidence and risk of QTc interval prolongation among cancer patients treated with vandetanib: a systematic review and meta-analysis. PLoSOne. 2012;7, e30353.
34. FDA-approved manufacturer's package insert for vandetanib. http://dailymed.nlm.nih.gov/dailymed/lookup.cfm?setid=4dc7f0af-77fb-4eec-46b9-dd1c2dcb4525. Accessed 25 Jan 2013.

35. Schmidinger M, Zielinski CC, Vogl UM, et al. Cardiac toxicity of sunitinib and sorafenib in patients with metastatic renal cell carcinoma. J ClinOncol. 2008;26:5204.
36. Strevel EL, Ing DJ, Siu LL. Molecularly targeted oncology therapeutics and prolongation of the QT interval. J ClinOncol. 2007;25:3362.
37. Bello CL, Mulay M, Huang X, et al. Electrocardiographic characterization of the QTc interval in patients with advanced solid tumors: pharmacokinetic- pharmacodynamic evaluation of sunitinib. Clin Cancer Res. 2009;15:7045.
38. Tolcher AW, Appleman LJ, Shapiro GI, et al. A phase I open-label study evaluating the cardiovascular safety of sorafenib in patients with advanced cancer. Cancer Chemother Pharmacol. 2011;67:751.
39. US Food and Drug Administration (FDA)-approved manufacturer's package insert. http://dailymed.nlm.nih.gov/dailymed/lookup.cfm?setid=807f988e-117b-4497-934d-73aa78baac71. Accessed 03 Jan 2013.

Radiotherapy: Clinical Aspects and Cardiotoxicity

Chiara Lestuzzi, Anju Nohria, Riccardo Asteggiano, and Paola Vallerio

C. Lestuzzi et al. (eds.), *Manual of Cardio-oncology*, DOI 10.1007/978-3-319-40236-9_12

12.1 Pathophysiology

Radiation therapy (RT) causes inflammation, activation of pro-fibrotic cytokines, and endothelial and microvascular damage. Radiation increases oxidative stress through free radical production and results in recruitment of matrix metalloproteinases and pro-inflammatory mediators such as IL-4, IL-13, and TGF-β. After myofibroblasts have been activated, collagen deposition and fibroblast differentiation can continue independent of TGF-β signaling via autocrine induction. These changes may lead to acute toxicity (evident during or shortly after radiotherapy) and start a chronic process leading to delayed dysfunction that is evident several years later. Acute changes largely result from direct radiation damage and the immediate inflammatory response, while long-term changes are due to stem cell loss and late and persistent tissue fibrosis. Thus, chronic radiation-induced damage is irreversible and can affect multiple cardiac structures including the coronary arteries, myocardium, pericardium, cardiac valves, and the conduction system [1] (Table 12.1).

Table 12.1 Reproduced with permission from [74]

	Echo-cardiography	Cardiac CMR	Cardiac CT	Stress echo-cardiography	ERNA/SPECT perfusion
Pericardial disease					
Effusion—screening and positive diagnosis	++++	+	+	–	+/–
Effusion—follow-up	++++	–	–	–	+/–
Constriction—screening and positive diagnosis	++++	++++	++	–	+/–
Myocardial disease					
LV systolic dysfunction	++++ (first-line imaging, contrast echocardiography if poor acoustic window)	++++	+	++++ (contractile reserve assessment)	++++/++++ (used when both function and perfusion are to be analyzed)
LV diastolic dysfunction	++++	+	–	–	++/+
LV dysfunction—follow-up	++++ (first-line imaging, contrast echocardiography if poor acoustic window)	+	–	++ (contractile reserve assessment)	++/++
Myocardial fibrosis	–	++++	+	–	–

Table 12.1 (continued)

Valve disease					
Positive diagnosis and severity assessment	++++	++	–	++	+/–
Follow-up	++++	–	–	++	+/–
Coronary artery disease					
Positive diagnosis	+ (if resting wall-motion abnormalities)	++++ (stress CMRb)	++ (CT angioa)	++++ (exercise or dobutamine)	+/++++
Follow-up	+	+	–	++++ (first-line imaging)	+/++

12.2 Acute Toxicity

12.2.1 Acute Pericarditis

The most common acute toxicity is **acute pericarditis**. It is seen mostly in patients treated with high-dose RT for mediastinal Hodgkin (HL) or non-Hodgkin (NHL) lymphoma, esophageal cancer, lung cancer, and thymoma. It is a consequence of (1) increased production of pericardial fluid due to the increased vascular permeability and (2) impaired drainage due to fibrosis of the lymphatic vessels.

- The incidence of acute pericarditis has decreased over time from 20 % to 2.5 % with modern radiation techniques
- Small, asymptomatic pericardial effusions are the most frequent complication but are usually self-limited and disappear within weeks without requiring any specific therapy [2].

Small pericardial effusions (due probably to impaired lymphatic drainage) are frequently present *before* radiotherapy in patients with lymphoma and large mediastinal masses and should not be considered a complication of RT.

- Acute pericarditis with chest pain, ECG changes, and/or pericardial friction rubs may be observed in some patients during or in the first months after RT over the esophagus or lung cancer. Pericardial effusion is usually mild to moderate or even absent.
- Therapy is the same as for acute viral or idiopathic pericarditis, i.e., nonsteroidal anti-inflammatory drugs. Colchicine may also be considered in refractory cases.

12.2.2 Ventricular Dysfunction

Ventricular dysfunction is a rare event. It is more frequent when an anthracycline or high-dose chemotherapy is administered concurrently, or shortly before RT, since radiation interacts synergistically to induce myocardial damage [3, 4].

- The dysfunction is usually both systolic and diastolic, and a restrictive pattern is usually seen.

12.2.3 Cardiac Ischemia

Cardiac ischemia may also be observed in the first months after RT, especially with radiation fields very close to the heart. In one prospective study, volume-dependent perfusion defects were observed in approximately 40 % of patients within 2 years of RT [5]. Patients with early perfusion defects might have a high incidence of cardiac events at long-term follow-up [6].

12.3 Late Toxicity

Delayed radiation-induced heart disease (RIHD) is a significant problem, especially in long-term survivors of lymphoma and breast cancer. The median time from RT to appearance of clinically significant RIHD is 15 years, with the incidence increasing progressively over time [7–11].

12.3.1 Coronary Artery Disease (CAD)

Coronary Artery Disease (CAD) is the most frequent and relevant form of RIHD. The risk of death due to acute myocardial infarction (AMI) is two- to fourfold higher in patients treated for Hodgkin lymphoma compared with age-matched controls, but can be increased sevenfold or higher in some subgroups [12]. Animal models of radiation-induced atherosclerosis have shown that radiation accelerates the development of atherosclerotic plaques and predisposes to an inflammatory phenotype prone to hemorrhage, as well as increasing the total plaque burden relative to age-matched animals.

- The most relevant risk factors for CAD after chest RT are:
  - Total radiation exposure of the heart: treatments delivered without heart shielding, higher cumulative dose (≥30 Gy), fractional dose ≥ 2 Gy, left vs right chest RT (in breast cancer)
  - Younger age (≤25 years) at the time of RT
  - High blood cholesterol, active cigarette smoking, and other cardiovascular risk factors
- The mechanism involved in plaque formation is thought to mirror spontaneous atherosclerosis; however, plaques in irradiated patients have been found to be more fibrous with decreased lipid content, and the lesions are consistently more proximal, smoother, concentric, tubular, and longer.
- Typically, CAD develops mostly within the radiation field.
  - Ostial stenoses are typical of mediastinal RT. Macroscopically, there is a significantly higher incidence of left main disease, followed by ostial right coronary artery and left anterior descending artery stenoses.
  - After left chest irradiation for breast cancer, the apical segments are more involved; in these patients, there is a damage of the microvasculature, leading to kinetics abnormalities rather than acute myocardial infarction in most cases [13].
- Radiation-induced CAD is often clinically silent and AMI may be the first presenting event (◘ Fig. 12.1). Both silent ischemia and false-negative stress tests have been documented [14]. In our experience, 75 % of patients with inducible ischemia on screening stress tests are asymptomatic.

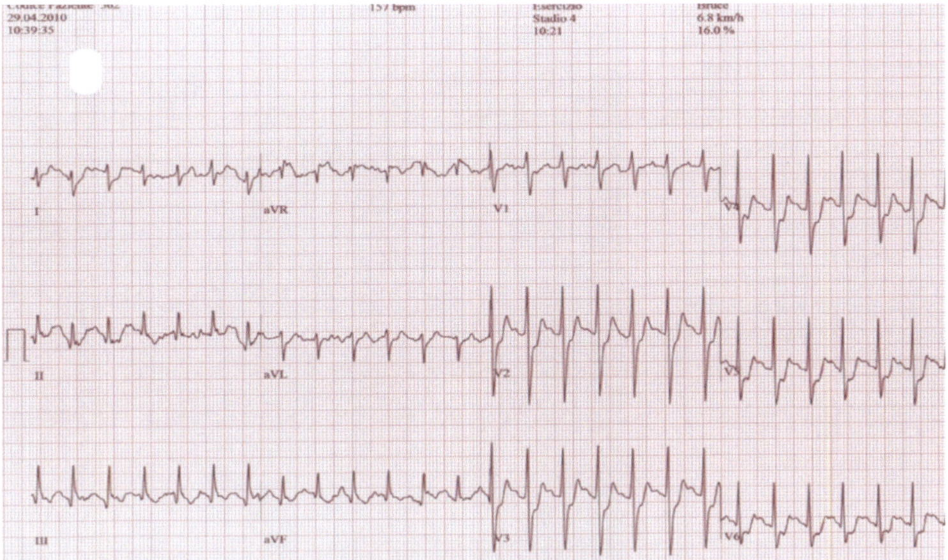

Fig. 12.1 Silent ischemia at stress test in an asymptomatic 48-year-old man, without any cardiovascular risk factor, 22 years after mediastinal radiotherapy. Coronary angiography revealed a stenosis of main left coronary artery, which was successfully treated with percutaneous angioplasty

  - The probable explanation is that radiation damages the cardiac nerves, leading to a functionally denervated heart.
  - Therefore, screening of patients at risk for radiation-induced CAD should be based on functional and/or imaging techniques rather than on symptoms alone.

12.3.2 Left Ventricular (LV) Dysfunction

Left ventricular (LV) dysfunction is a frequent complication of chest RT

- it can occur due to one or more of the following mechanisms:
  - Macroscopic CAD leading to chronic ischemia and myocardial hibernation, stunning, and/or necrosis (Fig. 12.2).
  - Decrease in capillary density resulting in myocyte hypoxia
  - Direct myocyte damage and necrosis, more evident in synergy with anthracycline cardiotoxicity (in the patients treated also with CHOP-like and ABVD chemotherapy), with progressive fibrosis replacing viable myocardial tissue.
  - Increase in type I collagen rather than type III collagen, leading to reduced myocardial distensibility.

The cardiovascular system responds differently to RT-related myocardial damage compared with ischemia-related ventricular dysfunction. Left ventricular dilatation is often limited.

- Strain deformation parameters may be significantly altered before any relevant systolic or diastolic dysfunction (Fig. 12.3).
- Left ventricular diastolic dysfunction is usually predominant, with evolution towards a restrictive cardiomyopathy in most severe cases [15].

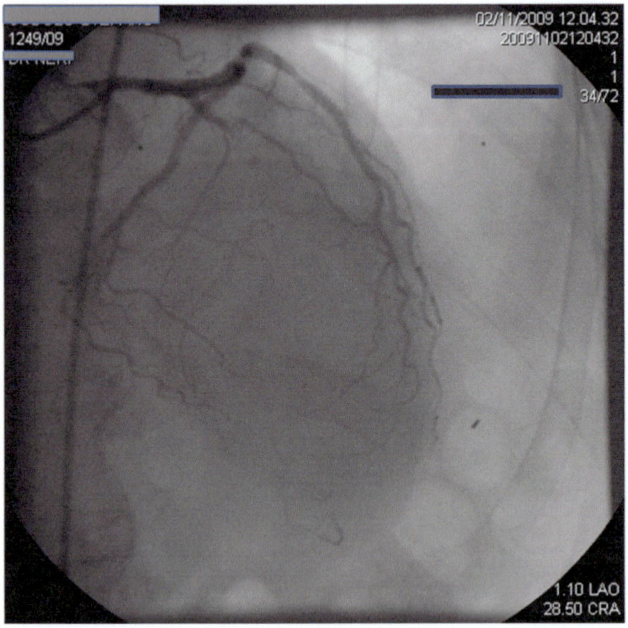

Fig. 12.2 Coronary angiography of a 53-year-old male, former smoker, with high blood pressure and cholesterol. This patient underwent chemoradiotherapy for Non-Hodgkin Lymphoma in 2006. In 2009, a drop of ejection fraction (EF) from 61 % before treatment to 49% was observed. Coronary angiography revealed a 100% stenosis of left anterior descending artery, which was treated by angioplasty. Two years later EF had raised to 59%

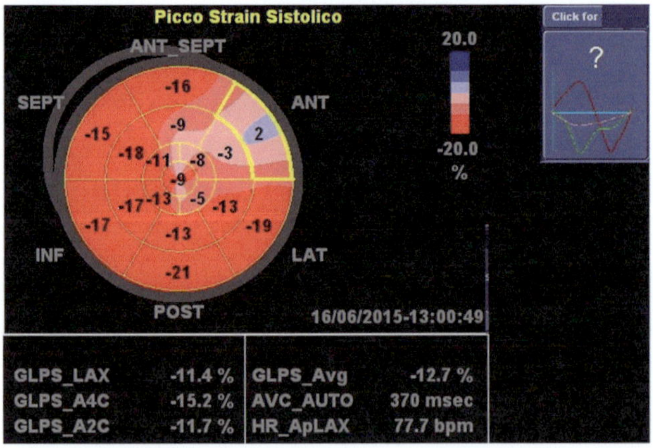

Fig. 12.3 Female patient, age 43, treated by mediastinal radiotherapy for Hodgkin lymphoma at age 17, followed by chemotherapy including doxorubicin at age 18. Ten years later she underwent breast surgery and chemotherapy with epidoxorubicin for radiation-induced breast carcinoma. Ejection fraction is normal (63%) and diastolic function mildly altered (E/A ratio 0.83, E/E' 13), but the global strain is reduced (–13%), with abnormalities most evident at the level of anterior wall

12.3.3 Valvular Heart Disease (VHD)

Valvular heart disease (VHD) ranges from sclerosis to severe, often calcific, valvular stenosis and/or regurgitation. It is more common after mediastinal RT in comparison to chest wall RT for breast cancer. Among breast cancer patients, it is more common after left-sided RT in comparison to right-sided RT [16].

- Screening studies in HL survivors have reported that 32 % of those given mediastinal irradiation developed asymptomatic valvular defects after six years [17].
- In Hodgkin lymphoma patients, the prevalence is 25–40 %, 20 to 30 years after cancer diagnosis (◘ Fig. 12.4).
- The median time between RT and detection of significant valvular heart disease is approximately 20 years, and >50 % of patients require surgery in the following years. Usually the first finding is regurgitation, and stenosis develops years after [18] (◘ Fig. 12.5).
- Aortic valve regurgitation and stenosis is the more frequent finding, followed by mitral valve regurgitation and/or stenosis [19].
- Cardiac doses ≥30 Gy increase the risk of VHD, while at lower doses the increase per Gy is smaller and there may be a threshold dose below which there is no risk.
- The main risk factors include age < 20 years at the time of RT, obesity at HL diagnosis, and hyperlipidemia at the end of follow-up [20, 21] (◘ Fig. 12.1).
- Other potential risk factors include splenectomy at the time of HL diagnosis and hypertension at follow-up (21).
- The use of chemotherapy was not found to be an independent risk factor.

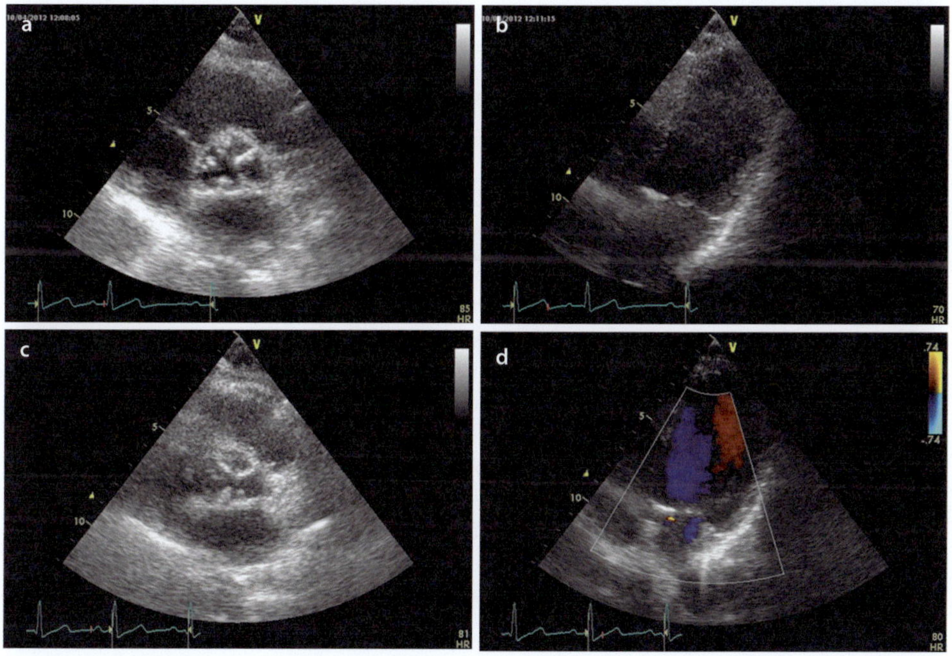

◘ **Fig. 12.4** Same patient of Fig. 12.3: (**a** and **b**): At age 41, the aortic valve leaflets are thickened and mildly calcific, with mild stenosis and regurgitation. Mitral annulus is thickened, with normal leaflets. (**c** and **d**): Three years later, the aortic valve disease is stable, but mitral valve leaflets and mitral annulus are more thickened, with mild regurgitation

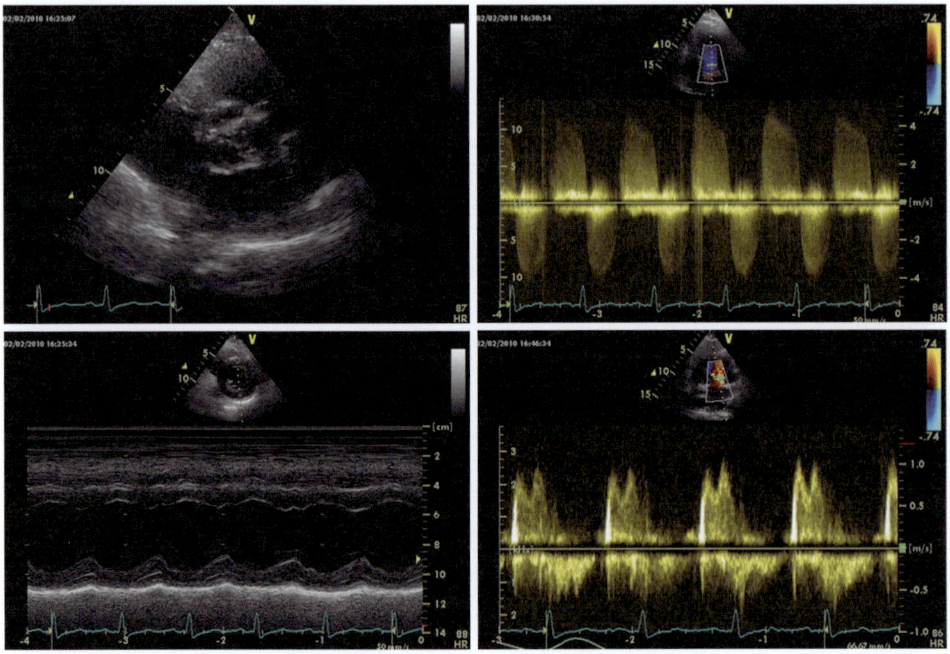

Fig. 12.5 Female patient, 60-year-old, treated with mantle field radiotherapy for Hodgkin lymphoma at age 27. Calcific aortic stenosis (peak gradient 71 mmHg, mean gradient 46 mmHg, area 0.7 cm^2) and moderate regurgitation. Ejection fraction 52 %. NYHA class 2. Pericardium and mitral flow are normal

12.3.4 Chronic Pericarditis

Chronic pericarditis may develop as a consequence of acute pericarditis seen during or shortly after RT and as a delayed complication.

- The pericardium is often thickened and may be calcific.
- The most common clinical presentation is constrictive pericarditis
- Some patients have thickened pericardium with mild to moderate effusion and may become symptomatic when the effusion increases (effusive-constrictive pericarditis).
- Signs and symptoms of pericarditis may be subtle and may change with blood volume.
  - Most patients have a combination of restrictive and constrictive disease and pericardial stripping does not afford similar benefits in RT patients compared to those with constriction due to other causes.

If a constrictive pericarditis is suspected, the intravenous infusion of 300–500 ml of saline is useful to reveal the hemodynamic pattern of constriction.

12.3.5 Arrhythmias

Both brady- and tachyarrhythmias can be seen as a consequence of RT, may be both hyperkinetic and hypokinetic.

- **Inappropriate sinus tachycardia**, both at rest and during effort, is common after thoracic RT and is felt to be a consequence of autonomic dysfunction [22].
- Direct damage and eventually fibrosis of critical structures such as the sinoatrial or atrioventricular nodes may lead to a variety of arrhythmias including all degrees of **atrioventricular block,** including complete heart block, and sick sinus syndrome [23, 24]

Right and left bundle branch blocks may also be observed and are likely due to microvascular damage and ischemia.

12.4 Clinical Presentation

- The clinical presentation differs according to the predominant pathologic change. However, it should be noted that:
  - Pathologies often coexist, thus confounding symptoms. The finding of a severe valvular heart disease in a dyspneic patient may lead to underdiagnosis of an associated pericardial constriction (◘ Fig. 12.6).
  - Patients with RIHD may be asymptomatic for years, even in the presence of significant anatomic changes [25]. This is true mostly for CAD, as stated before.

If a specific RIHD is suspected, a thorough evaluation to rule out any associated pathology affecting other cardiac structures is of outmost importance.

Tip

In patients presenting with symptoms of dyspnea, fatigue, and reduced exercise tolerance, it is important to consider other organs that may be affected by RT or chemotherapy **in the differential diagnosis.**

- **Acute radiation pneumonitis** occurs in the majority of cases between 6 and 12 weeks after the end of thoracic RT. It is characterized by interstitial edema, inflammatory infiltrates, and pneumocyte proliferation. There are often no symptoms or clinical signs appreciated. In some patients, dyspnea and wheezing may occur, sometimes accompanied by a nonproductive cough, and crackles on auscultation. In about half of the cases, chest radiography shows confluent alveolar and interstitial infiltrates in the irradiated field. Rare cases may progress to the development of acute respiratory distress syndrome (ARDS). Rarely, one may observe findings consistent with *bronchiolitis obliterans* with organizing pneumonia (BOOP). The clinical picture is that of a nonspecific pneumonitis, presenting immediately after RT. Imaging depicts sparse and migratory alveolar opacities. Steroid therapy is useful, but relapses have been described after steroid discontinuation [26]. Concomitant chemotherapy with gemcitabine (such as in lung cancer) increases radiosensitivity of the lungs and the incidence of pneumonitis. In breast cancer patients, both paclitaxel and tamoxifen have been reported to increase the rate of pneumonitis.

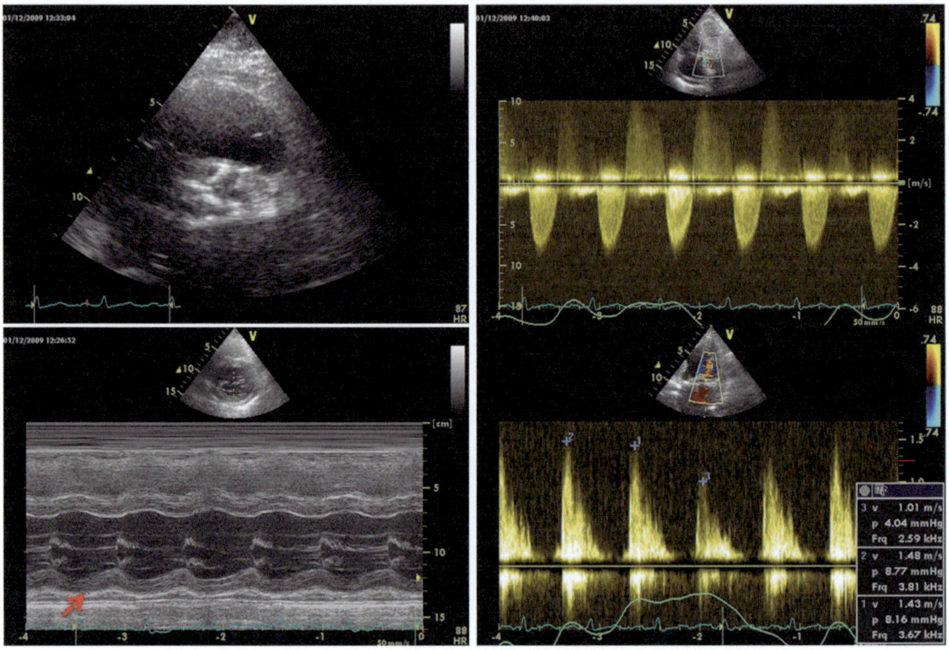

Fig. 12.6 Female patient, 65-year-old, treated with mediastinum radiotherapy for Hodgkin lymphoma at age 35. Calcific aortic stenosis (peak gradient 55 mmHg, mean gradient 30 mmHg, area 0.6 cm^2) and moderate regurgitation. Ejection fraction 51 %. NYHA class 3, with engorged jugular veins, enlarged liver, and ankle edema. The pericardium is thickened (*red arrow*); the diastolic mitral flow is reduced during inspiration (*bottom right*). These findings suggest the presence of constrictive pericarditis

- **Late radiation pneumonitis** occurs approximately 6 months after the end of thoracic RT, even in the absence of acute pneumonia. It is a virtually constant radiological feature which stabilizes two years after the end of treatment. From a pathological point of view, the inflammatory infiltrate is replaced by fibrosis and obliteration of the capillaries, causing chronic ischemia. This fibrosis may lead to chronic restrictive respiratory failure, a rare occurrence.
- **Recall pneumonitis** corresponds to pneumonia in a previously irradiated territory following subsequent chemotherapy (anthracyclines, gemcitabine, etoposide, vinorelbine, taxanes) or after exposure to some targeted therapies [27, 28].
- **Chemotherapy-induced lung disease** may be observed with several agents [29]. Bleomycin, in particular, can cause pulmonary toxicity (from acute pneumonitis to late fibrosis) in 20–40 % of patients [30]. Of note, Bleomycin is part of the ABVD and VEPEB chemotherapy protocols used in lymphomas.
- **Hypothyroidism.** Radiation fields including the neck (such as mantle field used for HL) may cause thyroid dysfunction. The actuarial risk of any thyroid disease is about 67 % at 26 years after therapy for Hodgkin lymphoma that includes irradiation of the thyroid gland. Hypothyroidism, Graves' disease (relative risk, 7.2–20.4), thyroiditis, thyroid nodularity, and thyroid cancer are among the commonly observed thyroid effects of RT [31]. The most frequent effect is hypothyroidism, which may be clinically overt, characterized by low free T4 and high TSH, or subclinical (biochemical or compensated) hypothyroidism with normal free T4 and high TSH. In the majority

of cases, subclinical hypothyroidism evolves to overt hypothyroidism, although up to 20 % of patients experience spontaneous return of TSH to normal levels, or substantial improvement [32].

12.5 Diagnosis of RIHD

Electrocardiography (ECG) and echocardiography are the most widely used tools to screening for RIHD. ECG may be normal or show conduction system and/or repolarization abnormalities. Echocardiography can detect structural cardiac abnormalities (including valvular heart disease and pericardial disease) and measure LV function. Several echocardiographic approaches (M-mode, Doppler, two-/three-dimensional (2D/3D) transthoracic or transesophageal, contrast, or stress echocardiography) can be used according to the clinical indication. **Computed Tomography** (CT) is useful to image the pericardium and coronary arteries and in recognizing cardiac calcifications. **Magnetic Resonance Imaging** (MRI) is the ideal complement to echocardiography: using contrast-enhanced images and dark-blood and bright-blood sequences, it may both give anatomic information and detect signs of inflammation; real-time cine imaging is of great value to assess functional abnormalities. Among the noninvasive tests, standard exercise stress tests, cardiopulmonary stress tests, and pulmonary function tests (for the differential diagnosis between cardiac and lung radiation disease) are also routinely used for screening after RT. **Cardiac catheterization** is useful in assessing CAD and can be used to confirm/distinguish constrictive and restrictive physiologies [33, 34]. See ◘ Table 12.1.

12.5.1 Coronary Artery Disease

- Echocardiography may show segmental abnormalities which suggest the presence of CAD. However, a hypokinetic ventricular region is not necessarily specific for the presence of CAD, but could reflect a myocardial disease process. A stress-induced wall-motion abnormality is a reliable indicator of transient myocardial ischemia and is highly sensitive and specific for angiographically assessed epicardial coronary artery disease. Either dobutamine or exercise echocardiography can be used, but exercise testing is recommended in patients who are able to exercise. In a study enrolling 294 asymptomatic patients with Hodgkin disease treated with mediastinal RT, stress echocardiography had predictive values of 80 and 87 % for detecting ≥70 and 50 % coronary stenoses, respectively. In this study, after a median follow-up of 6.5 years, 23 patients developed symptomatic CAD, including 10 who sustained an acute myocardial infarction. The risk of a cardiac event after screening was related to, among other things, the presence of resting wall-motion abnormalities on echocardiography and ischemia on stress testing [35].
- A cardiac **CT scan** is a noninvasive way to obtain information about the location and extent of calcified plaques in the coronary arteries. In the general population, the presence of coronary calcium is associated with adverse outcomes and can be useful for risk stratification. As with other groups of patients, obstructive CAD is unlikely to be present in the absence of detectable coronary calcium in RT survivors. Thus, **coronary calcium scores using cardiac CT can be used to rule out CAD**. Impaired image

quality and excessive calcification (combined with residual motion artifacts) can lead to overestimation of the severity of obstructive disease. Coronary CT has been used for follow-up in small groups of patients after RT for Hodgkin disease. These studies have demonstrated advanced coronary calcification and obstructive CAD (often requiring revascularization) in relatively young patients, even in the absence of any symptom and with normal stress test [14, 36].

- **MRI** is able to directly image epicardial coronary arteries, microvasculature on myocardial perfusion, ventricular function, and viability. Reversible myocardial ischemia can be assessed through stress-induced myocardial perfusion and/or function. In the last decade, CMR has emerged as the gold standard to evaluate myocardial infarction in both acute and chronic settings [37, 38]. In a recent CMR study of 20-year survivors of Hodgkin disease, perfusion defects were found in 68 % and late myocardial enhancement in 29 % of patients [39].
- **Radionuclide imaging** (SPECT and PET) is an accurate and robust technique to assess myocardial perfusion. The prevalence of myocardial perfusion defects among long-term survivors of chest RT varies widely, depending on the volume of the LV in the radiation field, age and timing of screening, and scintigraphic method used. In a prospective study, the prevalence of stress-induced perfusion abnormalities increased from 5 % to 11 % and 20 % in 2–10 years, 11–20 years, and >20 years after RT, respectively. In this study, myocardial ischemia on SPECT was shown to be associated with a higher risk for subsequent coronary events and prompted myocardial revascularization in a substantial proportion of patients [40].

Tip

There are often discrepancies between imaging techniques and functional studies: no single tool has 100 % sensitivity and specificity in detecting CAD and inducible ischemia after RT [41]. There are limited data comparing the accuracy of different imaging modalities to detect CAD in patients after mediastinal RT. In one head-to-head comparison, SPECT had the highest sensitivity compared with stress echocardiography and exercise stress testing (65 vs. 59 %), albeit at the cost of a higher false-positive rate (89 vs. 11 %). Many of these false-positive findings may actually be caused by microvascular disease, endothelial dysfunction, or vascular spasm [34].

12.5.2 LV Systolic and Diastolic Dysfunction

- LV ejection fraction assessment by **echocardiography** can be regarded as the standard in global systolic function assessment during and after RT. However, subtle changes, particularly due to early treatment effects, may be missed due to measurement variability. Deformation parameters derived by strain imaging can detect subtle changes that may be missed by standard echocardiographic techniques (Fig. 12.3). LV diastolic function is commonly evaluated by conventional Doppler (mitral inflow, pulmonary venous flow) and tissue Doppler techniques (applied to mitral annulus motion). However, it is important to note that diastolic parameters are highly sensitive to any change in loading conditions.

- **MRI** is an adequate alternative technique to assess LV function in patients with poor acoustic windows. Bright-blood cine imaging using the SSFP technique is an accurate and reproducible method to assess ventricular volumes, mass, and systolic function longitudinally. The same set of images can be used to assess regional contractility and contractile patterns [42]. MRI assessment of diastolic function with phase contrast is similar to Doppler echocardiography [43].
- **Radionuclide ventriculography** (RNV), either by the gated-equilibrium or first-pass methods, is an accurate tool to assess and quantify LV systolic and diastolic function at rest and during conditions of stress (for the gated-equilibrium method). The advantage of RNV is the ability to quantify ventricular volumes from total radioactive count density without the need for calculating volumes from 2D slices using assumptions about LV geometry. Diastolic function can be assessed by acquiring data with high temporal resolution and by calculating the peak filling rate and time-to-peak filling rate [44]. The disadvantage is the cost and the radiation burden.

12.5.3 Restrictive Cardiomyopathy

- On ***echocardiography***, classical restrictive cardiomyopathy is characterized by increased stiffness of the myocardium and a small LV with an increased left atrial size. This causes an early rapid rise in LV pressure during LV filling. Systolic function assessed by traditional echocardiographic techniques is usually normal. Doppler measurements of the transmitral flow reveal a typical pattern consisting of a short mitral E deceleration duration and a low A wave velocity resulting in a high E/A ratio [45]. The E′-wave by tissue Doppler imaging is usually decreased. A combined occurrence of constrictive pericarditis and restrictive cardiomyopathy may lead to a more difficult interpretation of the transmitral LV filling pattern.
- **MRI** may add useful information. Restrictive cardiomyopathy occurs as a result of diffuse myocardial fibrosis. $T1$ mapping by MRI may depict diffuse myocardial fibrosis. $T1$ mapping can be used to quantify the concentration of gadolinium-based extracellular contrast agents in the myocardium and in the blood pool. However, the diagnostic power is still limited [46].
- **CTscan and nuclear cardiology** are of little or no value in the diagnosis of restrictive cardiomyopathy.

12.5.4 Valve Disease

- ***Echocardiographic* characteristics** of radiation-induced valve disease include fibrosis and calcification of the aortic root, aortic valve annulus, aortic valve leaflets, aortic-mitral inter-valvular fibrosis, mitral valve annulus, and the base and mid-portions of the mitral valve leaflets (5-8). Typically, these changes spare the mitral valve tips and commissures, which is **the main distinguishing feature between radiation-induced valve disease and rheumatic heart disease.** 3D echocardiography is particularly useful for the assessment of the presence or absence of commissural fusion.

  - **Pitfalls in evaluating valve disease severity:** Planimetry of the mitral valve area at the leaflet tips may underestimate the severity of stenosis since the leaflet tips are spared and there is no commissural fusion. The presence of restrictive cardiomyopathy with significant underlying diastolic dysfunction may lead to shortened pressure half-time and overestimation of the mitral valve area. In addition, increased LV end-diastolic pressure may lead to an elevated mitral E-wave resulting in an elevated velocity–time integral of the mitral inflow CW Doppler signal, which will result in an elevated mean diastolic Doppler gradient tracing. The aortic stenosis gradient may be underestimated in these patients because of significant LV systolic dysfunction. Of note, a low-flow state can also be observed in patients with preserved LV function. When the LV ejection fraction is reduced, dobutamine stress echocardiography can help differentiate pseudo- and fixed severe aortic stenosis. The assessment of the severity of mitral valve regurgitation can be difficult in the presence of significant mitral annular calcification because of acoustic shadowing and difficulties with measuring the diameter of the mitral annulus. Transesophageal echocardiography can be particularly useful in the assessment of mitral valve disease when there is significant mitral valve annular calcification.
- **MRI** provides both anatomic and dynamic evaluation of the diseased valves, including information on the number of leaflets, valve thickness, valve structure, leaflet mobility, and valve orifice. Valvular dysfunction can be quantified by measuring the degree of valvular stenosis (the measurement of transvalvular gradients, assessment of aortic valve area) and/or valvular regurgitation (the measurement of regurgitant volumes and fraction) and by assessing its impact on cardiac chamber size and function [38, 39].

12

12.5.5 Pericardial Disease

- Echocardiography is the first-line imaging modality in patients with suspected or confirmed pericardial disease. **Pericardial effusion** is visualized as an echo-free space, external to the myocardial wall. **Pericardial thickening** appears as increased echogenicity of the pericardium on 2D echocardiography and as multiple parallel reflections posterior to the LV on M-mode recordings. However, the distinction between the normal and thickened pericardium may be difficult. Characteristic echocardiographic findings of **constrictive pericarditis** include:
  - Thickened pericardium.
  - Prominent respirophasic diastolic bounce of the inter-ventricular septum.
  - Restrictive diastolic filling pattern (E/A ratio of >2 and deceleration time of the mitral E-velocity of <140 ms).
  - Significant inspiratory variation of the mitral E-wave velocity (>25 %) (■ Fig. 12.6).
  - Diastolic flattening of the LV posterior wall.
  - Inferior vena cava plethora.
  - Expiratory diastolic flow reversal in the hepatic veins.

- Tissue Doppler interrogation of the medial mitral annulus reveals a normal or increased velocity that can be higher than the lateral annulus velocity.
- The systolic pulmonary pressures are not significantly elevated.

> **Constrictive pericarditis may be differentiated from restrictive cardiomyopathy (also a complication of radiation) by the presence of normal mitral tissue Doppler velocities and a systolic pulmonary artery pressure <50 mmHg.**

- **MRI** allows the detection of indirect signs of constrictive pericarditis, such as unilateral or bilateral atrial enlargement, conical deformity of the ventricles, dilatation of caval/hepatic veins, pleural effusion, and ascites. In pericarditis, the pericardium is typically thickened. Acute, but not chronic, pericarditis is associated with delayed enhancement following contrast administration and this differentiation can have therapeutic implications [47, 48]. **Real-time cine imaging** can be of great value in assessing the impact of respiration on inter-ventricular septal motion, allowing easy detection of pathological (increased) ventricular interdependence [49]. Furthermore, tagged sequencing allows detection of pericardial adhesions. Recently, real-time phase-contrast imaging has been proposed to assess the effects of respiration on cardiac filling [50].
- The pericardial cavity and membranes can be recognized on cardiac **CT** images even without injection of contrast media. Normal pericardium is usually < 3 mm in thickness. Thickening of the pericardium may be difficult to distinguish from small pericardial effusions. **Pericardial calcifications** as well as larger pericardial effusions are also readily identified on non-enhanced CT images. Constrictive pericarditis is not an anatomical diagnosis, although certain CT characteristics such as pericardial calcification, pericardial thickening (>4 mm), narrowing or tubular deformation of the RV, as well as manifestations of venous congestion can be present. Pericardial abnormalities may be regional.

12.6 Prevention Strategies in Subjects Treated By RT

RIHD is the most common nonmalignant cause of death in HL and breast cancer patients treated with RT. Among cured HL patients, it accounts for 25 % of mortality, with myocardial infarction as the most common cause of death. Patients with breast cancer also have an increased cardiovascular mortality if treated with RT, mostly those with left breast cancer [34].

- The first step of prevention is responsibility of the radiation oncologist, who can use radiation techniques (as conformational radiation fields, heart shielding…) at the time of treatment [51]. With modern radiation techniques, probably the problem of RIHD will be reduced in the future.

> **Many of the patients currently aged 40 or more have been treated in the past, before the introduction of new RT techniques, and should be object of an active program of prevention and follow-up. Usually, the HL and breast cancer patients who achieved complete remission are dismissed by the oncological follow-up after 5–10 years. Few patients have the opportunity to be included in a cancer survivor clinic for long-term follow-up of treatment-related disease. The general practitioners and the cardiologists should take care of this problem.**

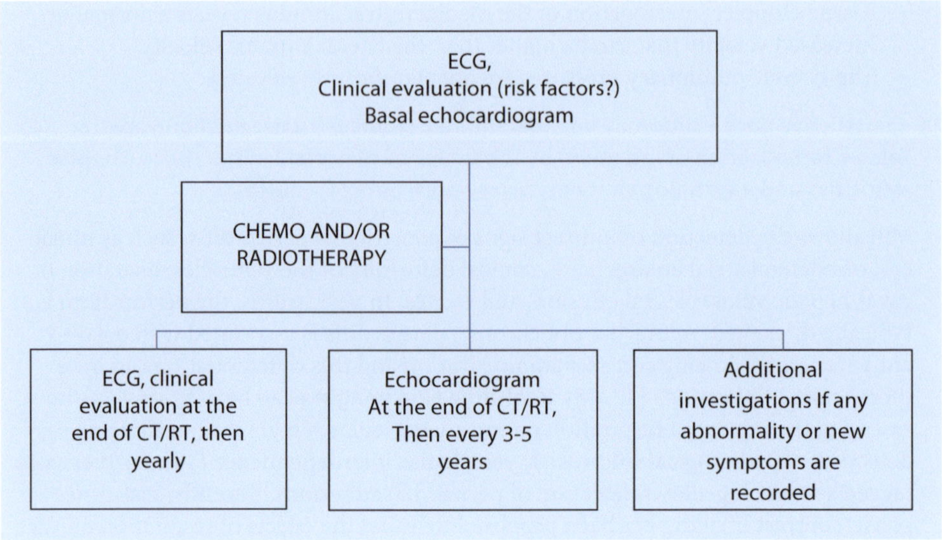

Fig. 12.7 Suggested pretreatment evaluation and short-medium term follow-up for patients without cardiac disease or symptoms undergoing RT

- The group at highest risk is represented by childhood cancer survivors, and this problem has been addressed in Chap. 16 (Cardiotoxicity in children). We will consider here the patients treated in their adulthood. There are no official guidelines about the optimal method and frequency of screening in this group of patients. The following suggestions have been obtained by the synthesis of published recommendations and by the personal experience of the authors.
- **Primary prevention** includes the common strategies for CAD: subjects treated by chest RT should be encouraged to avoid smoking, have a healthy lifestyle (including diet and regular physical activity), and maintain optimal body weight.
- Check regularly patient's blood pressure, blood glucose, and cholesterol, and start appropriate dietary or pharmacological interventions as soon as necessary
  - **Start a cardiac screening** with yearly ECG and clinical visits soon after the end of radiation treatment, and echocardiogram every 3–5 years (Fig. 12.7).
  - The echocardiographic follow-up should be more strict if cardiotoxic chemotherapy was also given.
  - Additional investigations may be planned according to the clinical findings
  - The data about the possible role of biomarkers (natriuretic peptides, troponins), in detecting RT-induced cardiac injury are scarce and conflicting [52].
- **Ten years after RT, noninvasive tests to detect CAD or ischemic heart disease are necessary and should be repeated every 2–3 years thereafter.**
  - In patients with additional risk factors (younger age at RT treatment, other CAD risk factors), the screening should be anticipated (5 years after RT).
- **In the following years, echocardiograms should be performed every 3 years and more often if cardiac valve abnormalities are observed** (Fig. 12.8)
- **The follow-up should last lifelong.**

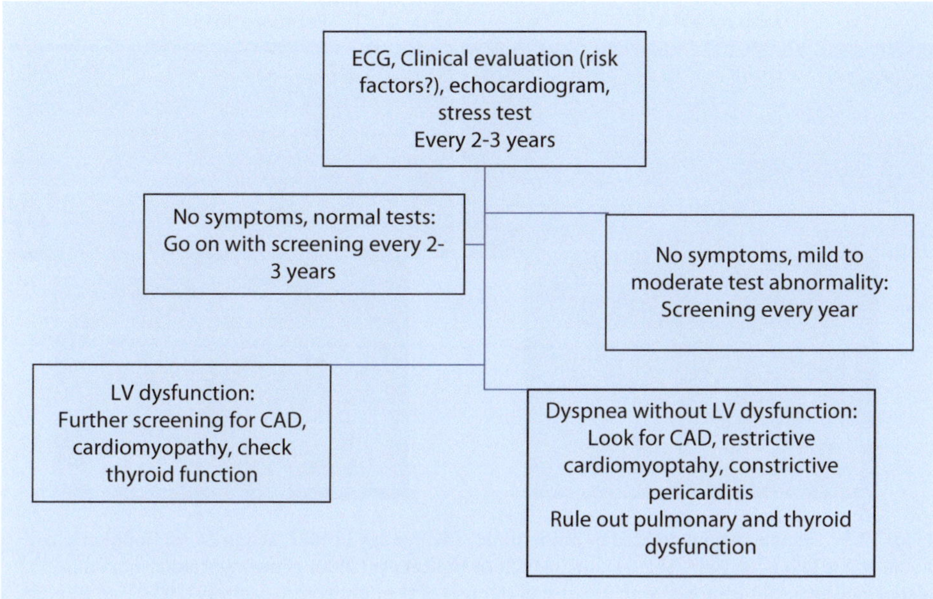

Fig. 12.8 Suggested long-term follow-up for patients without cardiac disease or symptoms. Start after 5 years after RT if the patient has a high cardiovascular risk, after 10 years if he/she haven't

12.7 Therapy

Some particular aspects of RIHD should be considered when planning therapy:

- **Both tachy- and bradyarrhythmias** may affect RT survivors. For advanced atrioventricular block, permanent pacemaker implantation may be necessary. The most common problem, however, is inappropriate sinus tachycardia. Beta blockers are indicated, but often require cautious titration in order to avoid symptomatic hypotension. Ivabradine may be a useful alternative and better tolerated by some patients (Fig. 12.9).
- **Percutaneous angioplasty** (PTCA) for CAD may be technically difficult and followed by early re-stenosis in comparison to non-RT-induced CAD [53].
- **Coronary bypass surgery** may be more difficult or associated with poorer outcomes because the internal mammary arteries may be also be affected by RT, because of poor distal arterial runoff caused by radiation damage [54], or due to the postoperative complications related to RT-induced lung disease and impaired lymphatic drainage.
- **Pericardiectomy** is usually associated with poorer outcomes in RT patients compared to those with non-RT-related causes of pericarditis. This is due to the observation that many RT patients have concomitant myocardial restriction that persists despite pericardiectomy. Pericardial stripping may also be difficult because the visceral pericardium is usually adherent to the epicardium. Pericardiectomy has the highest perioperative and long-term mortality if RT was the underlying cause [55, 56].
- **Cardiac valve repair** is difficult and is associated with suboptimal long-term results compared to **valve replacement**. However, the involvement of multiple valves, pres-

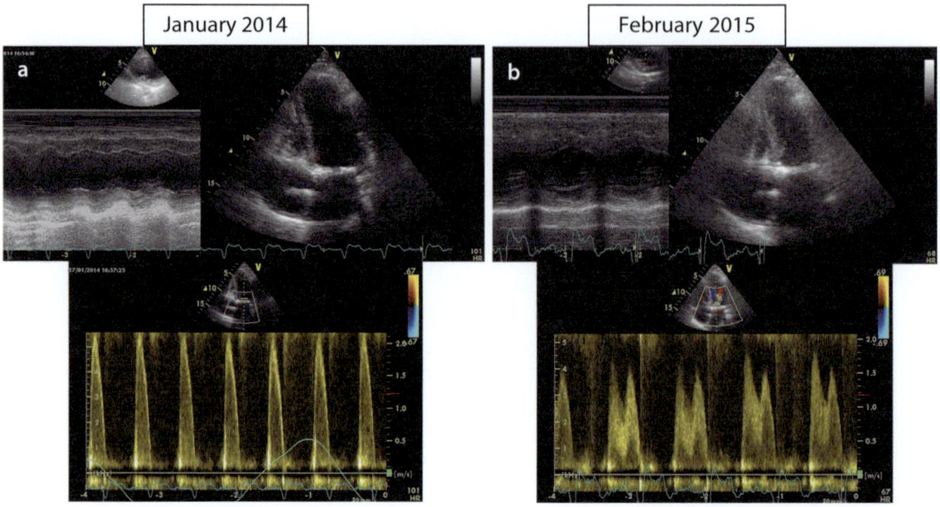

Fig. 12.9 Female patient, treated by mediastinal radiotherapy in 1981, at age 24, for Hodgkin lymphoma. In the following years, she had: thyroidectomy for cancer (2000); acute myocardial infarction (inferior wall and right ventricle) with 95 % ostial stenosis of the right coronary artery (2008) treated with angioplasty; recurring pneumonia; complete atrioventricular block treated by pacemaker (2012); trans-catheter aortic valve replacement for severe stenosis (2013); occlusion of the right coronary artery (2013). (**a**) Systolic four-chamber view, ventricular M-Mode, and diastolic mitral Doppler flow in January 2014: an extensive calcification of the mitral annulus is evident; heart rate 101, ejection fraction 57 %, and restrictive pattern at Doppler. (**b**) One year later, after adding to therapy bisoprolol 2.5 mg and Ivabradine 10 mg the heart rate is reduced to 68, the ejection fraction increased to 62 %, mitral flow has improved, and symptoms have improved from NYHA 3 to NYHA 2

ence of concomitant coronary artery disease, restrictive myocardial disease, aortic abnormalities, and mediastinal fibrosis can increase the length and complexity of the surgery, leading to adverse outcomes. Evolving trans-catheter approaches to valve replacement may be particularly suited to RT patients [19, 57].

- Technical problems during **cardiac operations of any kind** include dense scarring of the mediastinum from radiation-induced mediastinitis and impaired wound healing due to skin changes [58].
- **Due to the multiple cardiac complications seen with RT, patients with RIHD often require repeat cardiac surgery and may even require cardiac transplantation.** However, in two small series published, secondary malignancies, kidney injury, and respiratory failure contribute to significant postoperative morbidity and death [59, 60].

> **According to two large studies, patients with radiation heart disease undergoing cardiothoracic surgery have greater short-term and long-term mortality compared with age- and sex-matched comparison group patients undergoing similar surgeries in the same time frame. Perioperative morbidity and mortality are high mostly because of respiratory dysfunction and multiorgan failure [61, 62].**

  - In radiation heart disease patients undergoing cardiac surgery, the prediction of mortality risk based solely on standard preoperative scores is suboptimal; the extent of exposure is also relevant.

The presence of radiation-induced lung fibrosis is a significant predictor of worse long-term mortality independent of euroSCORE.

It is important to carefully evaluate patients being considered for cardiac surgery using clinical (including detailed pulmonary function testing) and multimodality imaging (echocardiography, multidetector computed tomography, and in select cases, carotid ultrasound) to fully understand the extent of their cardiovascular involvement prior to surgery [63].

12.8 Vascular RT Complications

- The risk from RT has been best characterized in patients with breast cancer or Non-Hodgkin lymphoma. Theoretically, however, any vascular location that is in the radiation field is at increased risk for early atherosclerosis. This is particularly relevant among patients with head and neck cancer because neck RT is a major risk factor for significant carotid disease. In fact, the risk of stroke is increased after mediastinal, cervical, or cranial RT. [64, 65].
- The pathophysiological effects of human cerebrovascular radiation have been shown in vitro or in animal models using non-fractionated, supra-therapeutic radiation [66]. The histological and cellular modifications of the human cerebral vascularization to radiotherapy can be characterized in relation to vessel diameter and time from treatment. Inflammatory response, endothelial damage, intima proliferation, and thrombus formation may occur after irradiation in the cerebral smallest arteries, arterioles, and capillaries, with increased permeability of the blood–brain barrier [67]. Large vessels, carotid arteries, and the circle of Willis are more resistant, but advanced atherosclerosis may occur.
- In the first year after neck irradiation, a certain degree of increase in the thickness of the carotid wall may be shown. In medium and large vessels, vasa-vasorum occlusions with medial necrosis followed by fibrosis, adventitial fibrosis, and accelerated atherosclerosis have been described [68].
  - These alterations lead to increased stiffness and advanced atherosclerosis of carotid arteries also after long time (>10 years after RT) [69].
  - Radiation-induced carotid disease produces carotid lesions that are more extensive than the traditional bifurcation stenosis and often involves atypical areas such as long segments of the carotid artery [70].
  - The global risk of cerebrovascular events is increased and the common atherosclerosis risk factors and preexisting atherosclerotic lesions are exacerbating factors [71]. Thus, a radiation-related increase in vascular disease risk has been confirmed and a dose–response relationship based on individual patient characteristics.
  - Hypertension is a cause and, at the same time, a long-term consequence of the stiffening process that may follow the atherosclerotic disease due to RT.
  - Hypertension can be enhanced by many cancer therapies, including both chemotherapy and targeted agents, should the patient undergo antineoplastic treatments after RT (for a relapsing or a second cancer).
- Similar consequences are reported on the aorta and other peripheral arteries, including subclavian and ilio-femoral arteries, with ischemic limb symptoms [72].

- Frequently, there are no symptoms attributable to carotid disease in patients previously treated with RT. Therefore, clinicians should be proactive about age-appropriate cardiovascular screening for potentially significant yet asymptomatic disease in these patients [73].
  - For patients at risk for carotid artery disease, ultrasound is the safest and most effective screening tool and must be used for follow-up of atherosclerotic damage.
  - During the last years, increasing interest has been placed on methods for assessment of vascular function, such as pulse wave analysis, arterial stiffness, and endothelial dysfunction, able to detect a very early vascular damage, but their role is still debated for the interference with coexisting risk factors.
- It's mandatory to make an estimation of global cardiovascular risk combined with subclinical targeted organ damage, taking into account the increased cardiovascular risk due to the effects of the concomitant oncologic treatment.

Operative Protocol

- In symptomatic patients for stroke/TIA or in the presence of carotid murmurs, it is indicated to perform a study with Doppler ultrasound integrated by MRI angiography or CT angiography.
- These surveys are also indicated for asymptomatic patients who have other manifestations of vascular disease and who have a moderate-to-high cardiovascular risk or for patients exposed to RT by at least 10 years. In the case of proven carotid disease is indicated to carry on an annual survey, otherwise, just a follow-up every 5 years.

References

1. Taunk NK, Haffty BG, Kostis JB, Goyal S. Radiation-induced heart disease: pathologic abnormalities and putative mechanisms. Front Oncol. 2015;5:39.
2. Murthy SC, Rozas MS, Adelstein DJ, et al. Induction chemoradiotherapy increases pleural and pericardial complications after esophagectomy for cancer. J Thorac Oncol. 2009;4:395–403.
3. Murdych T, Weisdorf DJ. Serious cardiac complications during bone marrow transplantation at the University of Minnesota, 1977-1997. Bone Marrow Transplant. 2001;28:283–7.
4. de Ville de Goyet M, Brichard B, et al. Prospective cardiac MRI for the analysis of biventricular function in children undergoing cancer treatments. Pediatr Blood Cancer. 2015;62:867–74.
5. Marks LB, Yu X, Prosnitz RG, et al. The incidence and functional consequences of RT-associated cardiac perfusion defects. Int J Radiat Oncol Biol Phys. 2005;63(1):214–23.
6. Gayed I, Gohar S, Liao Z, et al. The clinical implications of myocardial perfusion abnormalities in patients with esophageal or lung cancer after chemoradiation therapy. Int J Cardiovasc Imaging. 2009;25:487–95.
7. Galper SL, Yu JB, Mauch PM, et al. Clinically significant cardiac disease in patients with Hodgkin lymphoma treated with mediastinal irradiation. Blood. 2011;117:412–8.
8. Darby SC, Ewertz M, McGale P, et al. Risk of ischemic heart disease in women after radiotherapy for breast cancer. N Engl J Med. 2013;368:987–98.
9. Adams MJ, Hardenbergh PH, Constine LS, Lipshultz SE. Radiation-associated cardiovascular disease. Crit Rev Oncol Hematol. 2003;45:55–75. Review.
10. Gaya AM, Ashford RF. Cardiac complications of radiation therapy. Clin Oncol (R Coll Radiol). 2005;17:153–9. Review.
11. van Nimwegen FA, Schaapveld M, Janus CP, et al. Cardiovascular disease after hodgkin lymphoma treatment: 40-year disease risk. JAMA Intern Med. 2015;175:1007–17.

12. Swerdlow AJ, Higgins CD, Smith P, et al. Myocardial infarction mortality risk after treatment for Hodgkin disease: a collaborative British cohort study. J Natl Cancer Inst. 2007;99:206–14.
13. Duma MN, Molls M, Trott KR. From heart to heart for breast cancer patients-cardiovascular toxicities in breast cancer radiotherapy. Strahlenther Onkol. 2014;190:5–7.
14. Daniëls LA, Krol AD, de Graaf MA, et al. Screening for coronary artery disease after mediastinal irradiation in Hodgkin lymphoma survivors: phase II study of indication and acceptance†. Ann Oncol. 2014;25:1198–203.
15. Heidenreich PA, Hancock SL, Vagelos RH, et al. Diastolic dysfunction after mediastinal irradiation. Am Heart J. 2005;150:977–82.
16. McGale P, Darby SC, Hall P, et al. Incidence of heart disease in 35,000 women treated with radiotherapy for breast cancer in Denmark and Sweden. Radiother Oncol. 2011;100:167–75.
17. Cella L, Liuzzi R, Conson M, et al. Dosimetric predictors of asymptomatic heart valvular dysfunction following mediastinal irradiation for Hodgkin's lymphoma. Radiother Oncol. 2011;101:316–32.
18. Wethal T, Lund MB, Edvardsen T, et al. Valvular dysfunction and left ventricular changes in Hodgkin's lymphoma survivors. A longitudinal study. Br J Cancer. 2009;101:575–81.
19. Handa N, McGregor CG, Danielson GK, et al. Valvular heart operation in patients with previous mediastinal radiation therapy. Ann Thorac Surg. 2001;71:1880–4.
20. Schellong G, Riepenhausen M, Bruch C, et al. Late valvular and other cardiac diseases after different doses of mediastinal radiotherapy for Hodgkin disease in children and adolescents: report from the longitudinal GPOH follow-up project of the German-Austrian DAL-HD studies. Pediatr Blood Cancer. 2010;55:1145–52.
21. Cutter DJ, Schaapveld M, Darby SC, et al. Risk of valvular heart disease after treatment for Hodgkin lymphoma. J Natl Cancer Inst. 2015;107(4)
22. Groarke JD, Tanguturi VK, Hainer J, et al. Abnormal exercise response in long-term survivors of hodgkin lymphoma treated with thoracic irradiation: evidence of cardiac autonomic dysfunction and impact on outcomes. J Am Coll Cardiol. 2015;65:573–83.
23. Slama MS, Le Guludec D, Sebag C, et al. Complete atrioventricular block following mediastinal irradiation: a report of six cases. Pacing Clin Electrophysiol. 1991;14:1112–8.
24. Orzan F, Brusca A, Gaita F, et al. Associated cardiac lesions in patients with radiation-induced complete heart block. Int J Cardiol. 1993;39:151–6.
25. Heidenreich PA, Hancock SL, Lee BK, et al. Asymptomatic cardiac disease following mediastinal irradiation. J Am Coll Cardiol. 2003;42:743–9.
26. Chargari C, Riet F, Mazevet M, et al. Complications of thoracic radiotherapy. Presse Med. 2013;42:e342–51.
27. Ding X, Ji W, Li J, Zhang X, Wang L. Radiation recall pneumonitis induced by chemotherapy after thoracic radiotherapy for lung cancer. Radiat Oncol. 2011;6:24.
28. Levy A, Hollebecque A, Bourgier C, et al. Targeted therapy-induced radiation recall. Eur J Cancer. 2013;49:1662–8.
29. Limper AH. Chemotherapy-induced lung disease. Clin Chest Med. 2004;25:53–64.
30. Della Latta V, Cecchettini A, Del Ry S, Morales MA. Bleomycin in the setting of lung fibrosis induction: From biological mechanisms to counteractions. Pharmacol Res. 2015;97:122–30.
31. Hancock SL, Cox RS, McDougall IR. Thyroid Diseases after Treatment of Hodgkin's Disease. N Engl J Med. 1991;325:599–605.
32. Jereczek-Fossa BA, Alterio D, Jassem J, et al. Radiotherapy-induced thyroid disorders. Cancer Treat Rev. 2004;30:369–84. Review.
33. Lancellotti P, Nkomo VT, Badano LP, et al.; European Society of Cardiology Working Groups on Nuclear Cardiology and Cardiac Computed Tomography and Cardiovascular Magnetic Resonance; American Society of Nuclear Cardiology; Society for Cardiovascular Magnetic Resonance; Society of Cardiovascular Computed Tomography. Expert consensus for multi-modality imaging evaluation of cardiovascular complications of radiotherapy in adults: a report from the European Association of Cardiovascular Imaging and the American Society of Echocardiography. Eur Heart J Cardiovasc Imaging. 2013;14:721–40.
34. Jaworski C, Mariani JA, Wheeler G, Kaye DM. Cardiac complications of thoracic irradiation. J Am Coll Cardiol. 2013;61:2319–28.
35. Heidenreich P, Schnittger I, Strauss H, et al. Screening for coronary artery disease after mediastinal irradiation for Hodgkin's disease. J Clin Oncol. 2007;25:43–9.
36. Kupeli S, Hazirolan T, Varan A, et al. Evaluation of coronary artery disease by computed tomography angiography in patients treated for childhood Hodgkin's lymphoma. J Clin Oncol. 2010;28:1025–30.

37. Schwitter J, Arai AE. Assessment of cardiac ischaemia and viability: role of cardiovascular magnetic resonance. Eur Heart J. 2011;32:799–809.
38. Greenwood JP, Maredia N, Younger JF, et al. Cardiovascular magnetic resonance and single-photon emission computed tomography for diagnosis of coronary heart disease (CE-MARC): a prospective trial. Lancet. 2012;379:453–60.
39. Machann W, Beer M, Breunig M, et al. Cardiac magnetic resonance imaging findings in 20-year survivors of mediastinal radiotherapy for Hodgkin's disease. Int J Radiat Oncol Biol Phys. 2011;79:1117–23.
40. Pierga J, Maunoury C, Valette H, et al. Follow-up thallium-201 scintigraphy after mantle field radiotherapy for Hodgkin's disease. Int J Radiat Oncol Biol Phys. 1993;25:871–6.
41. Mulrooney DA, Nunnery SE, Armstrong GT, et al. Coronary artery disease detected by coronary computed tomography angiography in adult survivors of childhood Hodgkin lymphoma. Cancer. 2014;120:3536–44.
42. Grothues F, Smith G, Moon JC, et al. Comparison of interstudy reproducibility of cardiovascular magnetic resonance with two-dimensional echocardiography in normal subjects and in patients with heart failure or left ventricular hypertrophy. Am J Cardiol. 2002;90:29–34.
43. Caudron J, Fares J, Bauer F, Dacher JN. Evaluation of left ventricular diastolic function with cardiac MR imaging. Radiographics. 2011;31:239–59.
44. Brouwer C, Postma A, Vonk J, et al. Systolic and diastolic dysfunction in long-term adult survivors of childhood cancer. Eur J Cancer. 2011;47:2453–62.
45. Nagueh S, Appleton C, Gillebert T, et al. Recommendations for the evaluation of left ventricular diastolic function by echocardiography. Eur J Echocardiogr. 2009;10:165–93.
46. Dickerson JA, Raman SV, Baker PM, Leier CV. Relationship of cardiac magnetic resonance imaging and myocardial biopsy in the evaluation of nonischemic cardiomyopathy. Congest Heart Fail. 2013;19:29–38.
47. Zurick A, Bolen M, Kwon D, et al. Pericardial delayed hyperenhancement with CMR imaging in patients with constrictive pericarditis undergoing surgical pericardiectomy: a case series with histopathological correlation. JACC Cardiovasc Imaging. 2011;4:1180–91.
48. Feng D, Glockner J, Kim K, et al. Cardiac magnetic resonance imaging pericardial late gadolinium enhancement and elevated inflammatory markers can predict the reversibility of constrictive pericarditis after antiinflammatory medical therapy: a pilot study. Circulation. 2011;124:1830–7.
49. Francone M, Dymarkowski S, Kalantzi M, et al. Assessment of ventricular coupling with real-time cine MRI and its value to differentiate constrictive pericarditis from restrictive cardiomyopathy. Eur Radiol. 2006;16:944–51.
50. Thavendiranathan P, Verhaert D, Walls M, et al. Simultaneous right and left heart real-time, free-breathing CMR flow quantification identifies constrictive physiology. JACC Cardiovasc Imaging. 2012;5:15–24.
51. Johansen S, Tjessem KH, Fosså K, et al. Dose Distribution in the Heart and Cardiac Chambers Following 4-field Radiation Therapy of Breast Cancer: a Retrospective Study. Breast Cancer (Auckl). 2013;7:41–9.
52. Tian S, Hirshfield KM, Jabbour SK, et al. Serum biomarkers for the detection of cardiac toxicity after chemotherapy and radiation therapy in breast cancer patients. Front Oncol. 2014;4:277.
53. Schömig K, Ndrepepa G, Mehilli J, et al. Thoracic radiotherapy in patients with lymphoma and restenosis after coronary stent placement. Catheter Cardiovasc Interv. 2007;70:359–65.
54. Brown ML, Schaff HV, Sundt TM. Conduit choice for coronary artery bypass grafting after mediastinal radiation. J Thorac Cardiovasc Surg. 2008;136:1167–71.
55. Ling LH, Oh JK, Schaff HV, et al. Constrictive pericarditis in the modern era: evolving clinical spectrum and impact on outcome after pericardiectomy. Circulation. 1999;100:1380–6.
56. Bertog SC, Thambidorai SK, Parakh K, et al. Constrictive pericarditis: etiology and cause specific survival after pericardiectomy. J Am Coll Cardiol. 2004;43:1445–52.
57. Crestanello JA, McGregor CG, Danielson GK, et al. Mitral and tricuspid valve repair in patients with previous mediastinal radiation therapy. Ann Thorac Surg. 2004;78:826–31.
58. Handa N, McGregor CG, Danielson GK, et al. Coronary artery bypass grafting in patients with previous mediastinal radiation therapy. J Thorac Cardiovasc Surg. 1999;117:1136–42.
59. Uriel N, Vainrib A, Jorde UP, et al. Mediastinal radiation and adverse outcomes after heart transplantation. J Heart Lung Transplant. 2010;29(3):378–81.
60. Saxena P, Joyce LD, Daly RC, et al. Cardiac transplantation for radiation-induced cardiomyopathy: the Mayo Clinic experience. Ann Thorac Surg. 2014;98:2115–21.
61. Chang AS, Smedira NG, Chang CL, et al. Cardiac surgery after mediastinal radiation: extent of exposure influences outcome. J Thorac Cardiovasc Surg. 2007;133:404–13.

62. Wu W, Masri A. Popovic ZBet al. Long-term survival of patients with radiation heart disease undergoing cardiac surgery: a cohort study. Circulation. 2013;127:1476–85.
63. Desai MY, Karunakaravel K, Wu W, et al. Pulmonary fibrosis on multidetector computed tomography and mortality in patients with radiation-associated cardiac disease undergoing cardiac surgery. J Thorac Cardiovasc Surg. 2014;148:475.e3–81.
64. De Bruin ML, Dorresteijn LD, van't Veer MB, et al. Increased risk of stroke and transientischemic attack in 5-year survivors of Hodgkin lymphoma. J Natl Cancer Inst. 2009;101(13):928–37.
65. Plummer C, Henderson RD, O'Sullivan JD, Read SJ. Ischemic stroke and transientischemic attack after head and neck radiotherapy: a review. Stroke. 2011;42:2410–8.
66. Acker JC. Serial in vivo observation of cerebral vasculature after treatment with a large single fraction of radiation. Radiat Res. 1998;149:350.
67. Ye J, Rong X, Xiang Y, et al. A study of radiation-induced cerebral vascular injury in nasopharyngeal carcinoma patients with radiation-induced temporal lobe necrosis. PLoS One. 2012;7(8), e42890.
68. Louis EL, McLoughlin MJ, Wortzman G. Chronic damage to medium and large arteries following irradiation. J Can Assoc Radiol. 1974;25(2):94–104.
69. Hull MC, Morris CG, Pepine CJ, Mendenhall NP. Valvular dysfunction and carotid, subclavian, and coronary artery disease in survivors of Hodgkin lymphoma treated with radiation therapy. JAMA. 2003;290:2831–7.
70. Cheng SW. Carotid stenosis after radiotherapy for nasopharyngeal carcinoma. Arch Otolaryngol Head Neck Surg. 2000;126:517.
71. Steele SR, Martin MJ, Mullenix PS, et al. Focused high-risk population screening for carotid arterial stenosis after radiation therapy for head and neck cancer. Am J Surg. 2004;187:594–8.
72. Jurado JA, Bashir R, Burket MW. Radiation-induced peripheral artery disease. Catheter Cardiovasc Interv. 2008;72:563–8.
73. Zagar TM, Marks LB. Breast cancer radiotherapy and coronary artery stenosis: location, location, location. J Clin Oncol. 2012;30:350.
74. Mousavi N, Nohria A. Radiation-induced cardiovascular disease. Curr Treat Opt Cardiovasc Med. 2013; 15:507–17.

Cardiotoxicity in Children

Francesca Cairello, Sara Pessano, Vera Morsellino, Riccardo Haupt, and Maria Derchi

C. Lestuzzi et al. (eds.), *Manual of Cardio-oncology*, DOI 10.1007/978-3-319-40236-9_13

13.1 General Considerations

- Childhood cancer (age 0–14) is a rare event accounting for <1 % of all newly diagnosed cancers in the general population [1].
- It is estimated that each year about 11,000 new cases of childhood cancer are diagnosed in Europe, and >12,000 children and adolescents in the USA [2, 3].
- During the last decades, advances in cancer treatment strategies led to a substantial improvement in the 5-year survival rate of children (age 0–14) with cancer, moving from less than 60 % in the 1970s to more than 80 % in 2010 [4].
- It has been estimated that a >300,000 childhood cancer survivors are living in the USA [1], and the corresponding number for Europe being between 300,000 and 500,000. Each year >8000 subjects add on to the CCS population in each continent leading to a continuous increase both in terms of total number and in attained age of the CCS population [4–6]. Median age of CCS today is estimated to be of around 30–34 years, with some already beyond the 50 years of age.

Key Point

Currently, it is estimated that about 75–80 % of children newly diagnosed with cancer will be surviving after 10 years from diagnosis, compared to a 65 % probability of 5-year survival of adult patients [1, 7, 8].

- This improvement in outcome came, however, at a price mainly linked to the occurrence of long-term therapy-related morbidities. By the first 30 years after diagnosis, up to 75 % of childhood cancer survivors experience at least one chronic treatment-related condition [4–6, 9].

Key Points

Cardiovascular complications represent the major cause of morbidity and mortality in long-term survivors of childhood cancer, immediately after cancer recurrence and second malignancy [2, 4, 5].

Possible cardiac complications after cancer treatment are progressive cardiomyopathy that may result in Congestive Heart Failure (CHF), valvular, ischemic, conductive system, and pericardial diseases. Among these complications, cardiomyopathy is the most common and life-limiting consequence of post-therapy cardiotoxicity.

Compared with same age and sex general population, childhood cancer survivors have a 15-fold increased risk of developing chronic heart failure (CHF) [1, 8] and a four- to sevenfold higher risk of premature death due to cardiac causes [10, 11].

- Accurate screening and care of cancer survivors are mandatory in order to early diagnose or prevent treatment-related heart damage that might also severely affect their quality of life.
- Counseling about an appropriate lifestyle and cardiologic screening programs are mandatory in order to prevent and/or early identify signs and symptoms of cardiac damage (▪ Table 13.1) [12].

Table 13.1 Relative frequency of malignant childhood tumors

Diagnostic group	Relative (%)
Leukemias	34.1
Acute lymphoid	26.8
Acute myeloid	4.7
Chronic myeloproliferative diseases	0.4
Other	2.2
Lymphomas and reticuloendothelial neoplasms	11.5
Hodgkin lymphoma	4.8
Non-Hodgkin lymphoma	5.3
Burkitt lymphoma	1.3
Miscellaneous/unspecified	0.1
CNS tumors	22.6
Ependymomas and choroid plexus tumors	2.2
Astrocytomas	10.5
Intracranial embryonal tumor	5.0
Other gliomas	1.0
Other/unspecified	3.1
Neuroblastoma and other peripheral nervous cells tumors	7.6
Retinoblastoma	2.1
Renal tumors	5.6
Wilms' tumor (nephroblastoma)	5.5
Other	0.1
Hepatic tumors	1.1
Hepatoblastoma	0.9
Hepatic carcinomas/other	0.2
Malignant bone tumors	4.6
Osteosarcoma	2.3
Ewing' sarcoma	2.1
Other/unspecified	0.2
Soft tissue sarcomas	6.1
Rhabdomyosarcoma	3.4

(continued)

Table 13.1 (continued)

Diagnostic group	Relative (%)
Other soft tissue sarcomas	1.7
Fibrosarcoma/unspecified	1.0
Germ cell tumors	3.1
Malignant gonadal germ cell	1.3
Intracranial germ cell tumors	0.9
Malignant extracranial and extragonadal tumors	0.8
Other malignant epithelial tumors and malignant melanomas	1.5
Thyroid carcinoma	0.8
Other	0.7
Other malignancies	0.1
Total	100

Modified from: Kaatsch P. Epidemiology of childhood cancer. Cancer Treatment Reviews 36: 277–285 (2010)

13.2 Etiology and Pathophysiology

Childhood cancer treatment with anthracycline and/or chest radiotherapy has been correlated with an increased risk of cardiotoxicity.

- Nearly 60 % of all CCS carry a history of prior anthracycline and/or chest radiation exposure [2, 6].

13.2.1 Therapeutic Agents Responsible for Cardiotoxicity

- **Anthracyclines:** (doxorubicin, daunorubicin, epirubicin)
  - The exact mechanism by which anthracyclines can cause heart damage is still not completely understood [1].
  - These drugs play their role by interfering with cell replication through DNA base pair intercalation and disrupting DNA uncoiling through inhibition of topoisomerase 2 activity [7] (Table 13.2) [7, 13].
  - Oxidative stress with generation of free radicals and lipid peroxidation seems to play an important role. Compared to other tissues, cardiac cells are particularly susceptible to oxidative damage due to the relative deficiency of free radical-scavenging enzymes such as catalase and glutathione peroxidase (Table 13.3).
  - The oxidative damage
    - To mitochondrial membranes can cause an impaired energy production reducing the myocytes' ability to contract.
    - To cardiac sarcomeres can lead to myofilament destruction and apoptosis activation, with myocite loss.

Table 13.2 Human Topoisomerase (Top) [7]

In humans, there are two types of Top2 enzymes: Top2α and Top2β
Top2α, found predominantly in proliferating cells, is required for DNA replication and is considered the molecular basis of anthracycline's antitumoral activity.
Top2β, present in all quiescent cells, including cardiomyocytes. Top2 inhibition by anthracycline causes double-stranded breaks in DNA which can lead to cardiomyocyte death.

Table 13.3 Mechanisms involved in anthracycline myocardial susceptibility

Anthracyclines' cardiotoxic effect seems to be related with
Increased generation of reactive oxygen species (ROS), both enzymatically, by a reduction in antioxidant enzymes, Top2β-dependent gene transcription, and through the formation of anthracycline iron complexes, leading to cell membrane damage, increasing permeability, lipid peroxidation, and DNA damage
High affinity for cardiolipin, a phospholipid present in elevated concentration at the level of inner mitochondrial membrane, critical to cell respiration. Cardiolipin's high affinity for anthracyclines allows the drugs to enter cardiomyocytes passively and accumulate in intracellular fluids to concentrations several hundred times higher than that in extracellular fluids.
Changes in mitochondrial metabolism due to iron accumulation and change in mitochondrial gene expression. The cardiac mitochondrial respiratory chain is implicated. There are studies showing mtDNA alteration and respiratory chain defect leading to increased concentrations of reactive oxygen species persisting outside the presence of anthracycline. This may help to explain the potentially prolonged latency of anthracycline-induced cardiotoxicity.
Decrease ATP production by lowering protein expression inducing an alteration of mitochondrial functions.
Induced cell membrane changes that lead to disturbance of intracellular calcium homeostasis with increased intracellular calcium levels. This activates the pathways resulting in apoptosis and cardiac cell death.
Decreased expression of mRNA encoding sarcoplasmic reticulum, inhibition of nucleic acid and sarcomeric proteins synthesis, induced formation of toxic metabolites, and release of vasoactive amines.
Reasons why myocardial cells seem more vulnerable to the anthracycline-induced toxic effect than other tissues:
High metabolic activity
Limited regenerative capability, which increase the susceptibility to long-term adverse effects
Limited antioxidant capacity secondary to lower concentrations of catalase and glutathione peroxidase

Key Point

In CCS, the toxic effect of anthracyclines not only induces apoptotic destruction of myofilaments and loss of myocites, but also influences cardiac repair mechanisms by reducing the pool of cardiac stem cells, compromising the already limited myocardium regenerative capacity [8]. This means that cardiac growth in responses to increasing somatic growth becomes inadequate in these patients, even if the remaining cells try to compensate by becoming hypertrophic to create LV mass. This remodeling process alters the myocardial structure inducing a thinning of the myocardium itself, with resulting increase in wall stress, decreased cardiac contractility, progressive ventricular fibrosis, and progressive ventricular dysfunction [1, 8].

- Polymorphisms in genes involved in different cell metabolic pathways such as in doxorubicin transport and free radical metabolism can play a role in individual susceptibility to anthracycline-induced heart damage [8, 14].
- There is a strong dose-dependent relation between cumulative dose of anthracycline exposure and the risk of developing cardiomyopathy and CHF.
- In addition to cumulative dose, other factors increase the risk of anthracycline-induced cardiotoxicity [8] (Table 13.4).

Key Points

The incidence of anthracycline-related cardiomyopathy and CHF correlates with the cumulative anthracycline dose exposure and is estimated to be:

- <5 % with cumulative anthracyclines dose < 250 mg/m^2;
- Approaching 10 % at doses between 250 and 600 mg/m^2;
- Exceeding 30 % for doses >600 mg/m^2 [6].
  - Currently doses > 250 mg/m^2 are generally considered to be at higher risk.
  - There is no "safe" anthracycline dosage for the development of cardiomyopathy, since also with cumulative doses < 100 mg/m^2 some events have been reported [6].

13

- **Chest irradiation (RT):**
  - Any irradiation in which the heart is in the field of treatment (mediastinal, thoracic, spinal, left or whole upper abdomen, and total body irradiation—TBI) is potentially harmful for the heart leading to possible complications affecting the different cardiac structures: myocardium, valves, coronaries, pericardium, and conduction system [8].
  - The mechanism of this effect is mainly due to microcirculatory injury and inflammation leading to long-term diffuse myocardial fibrosis.
  - There is a dose-dependent effect and a correlation with the area involved in the RT field. Doses ≥15 Gy to the chest clearly increase the risk of developing congestive heart failure. There is little evidence of an increased risk of CHF for doses <15 Gy (Table 13.5).
  - Cumulative incidence of cardiovascular diseases after cardiac radiation in patients receiving ≥ 35 Gy is reported to be around 21 % at a median age of 20 years after cancer diagnosis [2, 15].

Table 13.4 Risk factors that can increase anthracycline-induced cardiotoxicity

Female sex[a]
Young age at the diagnosis[b]
Combination chemotherapy: anthracycline plus other chemotherapeutic agents (i.e., cyclophosphamide, ifosfamide, vincristine, cisplatin, trastuzumab, methotrexate). A combined treatment using anthracycline and cyclophosphamide seems to carry the most relevant risk for acute cardiotoxicity in pediatric population
Concomitant exposure to RT
Trisomy 21
African-American descent

[a]The cause of the "gender effect" is possibly related to the fact that doxorubicin does not concentrate in adipose tissue [4] (which is more represented in female than in male). Then, at same dose levels, female cardiomyocytes are exposed to higher drug concentrations [6, 53].
[b]Children less than 4 years of age at anthracycline exposure showed an increased risk of LV dysfunction [4, 54]. Some studies showed differences in anthracycline pharmacokinetics and clearance in the extreme ages of life as a possible explanation of this "age effect" on the probability of developing therapy-related cardiotoxicity [55].

Table 13.5 Risk factors for RT-induced cardiotoxicity

Radiation dose: any dosage involving the heart exceeding 1,5-3,5 Gy increases the risk for cardiac diseases during long-term follow-up. There is little evidence of an increased risk of CHF for doses < 1,5 Gy [6]
Field of treatment: Mediastinal, thoracic, spinal, left or whole upper abdominal, or TBI are potentially harmful to the heart. Also cranial and cranio-spinal radiotherapy may have an indirect role in cardiovascular damage by affecting the hypothalamic–pituitary axis and thyroid function, thus possibly increasing the risk of MS development.
RT technique
Patient's age, with a higher incidence in younger patients.

Key Point

The association between high-dose anthracyclines and RT further increases the risk of developing heart damage, with a shorter induction period before cardiovascular events develop (CEs).

- **Other Drugs**
  - **Other cancer treatments:** alkylating agents, 5FU, Paclitaxel, Amsacrine, Thyrosine-Kinase inhibitors, and the new therapies with monoclonal antibodies have been reported to be cardiotoxic through different mechanisms, with both direct and indirect consequences on heart cells and structures.

Table 13.6 Preexisting cardiovascular disease or cardiac risk factors and comorbidities

1. Preexisting cardiovascular disease or cardiac risk factors: hypertension, myocardial and valvular diseases, drug hypersensitivity
2. Comorbidities: medical conditions that increase the risk of heart problems such as endocrinopathies, infections, inflammatory conditions, hyperlipidemia, obesity and metabolic diseases, failure to thrive, sedentary lifestyle, pulmonary disease, musculoskeletal disease, renal disease, hepatic disease, prematurity, and genetic disorders (i.e., hereditary hemochromatosis, trisomy 21, ...) as well as smoking may contribute to the increased risk for CVD [56, 57].

Key Point

Independently of these risk factors, not all children and adolescents exposed to toxic treatments, even those who receive the same standardized chemotherapeutic regimens, experience cardiotoxicity. This suggests the possibility of a genetic predisposition [1, 4].

13.2.2 Preexisting Cardiovascular Disease or Cardiac Risk Factors and Comorbidities

- Preexisting cardiovascular disease or cardiac risk factors and comorbidities should be taken into account while deciding to initiate cardiotoxic cancer therapies. This can help identification of high-cardiovascular-risk populations that can benefit from cardioprotective strategies or from reduction/minimization of cardiotoxic therapy use (Table 13.6).

13

13.3 Cardiovascular Manifestations

Cardiovascular complication due to anticancer drug may present soon after drug administration (**acute manifestations**) or months-years after the end of treatment (**chronic manifestations**).

However, CCS population presents, in most cases, a long latency period between cancer treatment and evidence of cardiac disease.

Usually, the first signs of cardiotoxicity are subclinical and can be documented only through appropriate testing (e.g., echocardiogram or ECG). In the second stage, symptoms may become manifest and can also affect the normal daily activities. At a later stage, treatment is indicated to control the disease.

- **Anthracycline-related manifestations**

  Anthracycline-induced cardiotoxicity can be distinguished by the time of presentation as:
  - Acute: symptoms occur during the first week of therapy
  - Early onset: after 1 week and within 1 year after completion of therapy.
  - Late onset: from at least 1 year after completion of therapy, until 10–30 years from the first dose of treatment.

- **Acute cardiotoxicity**
  - Is rare, being reported in about 1.6 % of cases [1, 16].
  - Manifests as

    Intracardiac conduction disturbances, arrhythmias.

    ECG abnormalities can range from minor alterations to fatal arrhythmias: patients can develop atrial tachyarrhythmia, paroxysmal supraventricular tachycardia, and ventricular arrhythmias with or without associated prolongation of QT interval (frequently, there is a combined effect of the anticancer therapies with the concomitant presence of serum ions alterations and administration of other drugs such as antiemetic, antibiotics, antifungal agents).

    Pericarditis

    Acute left ventricular (LV) failure (rare). It is usually only transient, but some fatal cases have also been described.

Key Point

Acute symptoms usually resolve with discontinuation of therapy, though patients may suffer permanent damage.

1. **Early- and late-onset cardiotoxicity**
   - Is the most common and life-limiting consequence in CCS exposed to anthracyclines, with early onset reported in about 1–16 % of cases
   - The incidence increases with the length of follow-up.
   - Is usually a progressive disease, generally irreversible, characterized by initially asymptomatic LV dysfunction that may lead to symptomatic CHF [1], and increased cardiac mortality secondary to pump failure and sudden death.
     - **Asymptomatic stage:** in which the survivor does not complain of any symptom but at an echo examination some early dysfunctions can be detected:
     - *Systolic dysfunction*: characterized by LV dilatation, thinning of the LV wall, and decreased contractility. As contractility diminishes over time, the LV dilates further, with subsequent increase in LV wall stress in order to maintain the cardiac output with a remodeling process similar to the one seen in congenital dilated cardiomyopathy [6, 16].
     - *Diastolic dysfunction*: CCS can develop, during time, a restrictive cardiomyopathy characterized by abnormal diastolic patterns and elevated filling pressures due to rigid ventricular wall, with an almost preserved LV systolic function [6, 8, 17].
     - **Symptomatic stage:** defined by the development of signs and symptoms of CHF; it may appear after a variable period of time.
- **Grading of CHF in children:**

CHF is characterized by the failure of the heart either to supply blood to the systemic and pulmonary circulation (systolic dysfunction) or to receive venous return at an appropriate filling pressure (diastolic dysfunction).

Table 13.7 Symptoms and signs of Heart Failure in children [18, 19]

	Infant/young children	Older children/adolescent
Common symptoms	Tachypnea	Fatigue
	Feeding difficulty	Effort intolerance
	Diaphoresis	Breathlessness, exertional dyspnea, rest dyspnea, orthopnea
	Paleness	Abdominal pain, nausea, and vomiting.
Less common symptoms	Cyanosis	Chest pain
	Palpitation	Palpitation
	Syncope	Dependent edema
	Facial and dependent edema	Ascites
	Ascites	

Symptoms and signs may be different across ages, from infancy through adolescence (Table 13.7) [18].

- Grading of CHF in children derives from a modified NYHA/Ross classification [19]:
  GRADE I: asymptomatic
  GRADE II: mild tachypnea or diaphoresis with feeding in infants; dyspnea on exertion in older children.
  GRADE III: marked tachypnea or diaphoresis with feeding in infants as well as prolonged feeding time with growth failure due to heart failure; in older children marked dyspnea on exertion.
  GRADE IV: tachypnea, retraction, grunting, or diaphoresis at rest.

13

Key Point
Other anthracycline-related cardiovascular complications can also be present [5, 8] (Table 13.8).

Table 13.8 Incidence of symptomatic long-term cardiac events [5, 8]

Congestive heart failure 54 %
Arrhythmias 18 %
Valvular heart diseases 12 %
Ischemia/myocardial infarction 12 %
Pericarditis 4 %

RT-related manifestations:

- Radiation-induced cardiotoxicity usually has a gradual onset, becoming clinically manifest after a decade or more from exposure [2]. As with chemotherapy, the damage appears to be progressive and can become manifest with different clinical scenarios:
- Cardiomyopathy: the most important sequelae of cardiac irradiation is diastolic dysfunction without evidence of systolic dysfunction. Up to 37 % of cases present signs of restrictive cardiomyopathy. Few subjects can develop dilated cardiomyopathy [6, 20]. Often, survivors have no symptoms or only vague fatigue, although in advanced stages they manifest the typical heart failure symptoms.
- Valvular dysfunction: Described in up to 29 % of cases. Is due to the thickening of the valvular endocardium with fibrotic and calcific alterations. It appears to be progressive. The valves of the left side of the heart, the aortic and mitral valves, are most frequently affected with a damage that appears to be progressive. This suggests an important role played by mechanical stress of a high-pressure circulation.

Asymptomatic ventricular dysfunction is usually the first manifestation of cancer treatment-induced cardiotoxicity; it is reported in more than 50 % of cases [1, 7, 8]; thus, appropriate screening should be performed.

During long-term follow-up approximately 5 % of patients develop clinical signs and symptoms of CHF [8, 9].

- Coronary artery disease: Representing up to 10 % of cases. Symptoms range from angina pectoris to myocardial infarction that can lead to sudden death.
- Pericardial disease: This event is less common and may manifest with either constrictive pericarditis or pericardial effusion. The latter is due to the decreased ability of fibrotic venous and lymphatic channels to drain extracellular fluid.
- Arrhythmias: This is a rare event and can manifest as heart block or other arrhythmias caused by both conductive system fibrosis and ischemia.

Cardiac manifestations due to other drugs:

- **Alkylating agents** (e.g., busulfan, cyclophosphamide, ifosfamide, and cisplatin): clinical symptoms in adults range from asymptomatic pericardial effusion to cardiac failure and myopericarditis [2].

  The risk of cardiac toxicity for this class of drugs appears to be related more to the amount of a single administered dose than to the total cumulative dose.

  - **Cyclophosphamide:** symptoms usually appear 1–2 weeks after the initial dose; the cardiac effects may persist for several days and, in some patients, resolve without problems. In children population, the combination treatment with anthracyclines seems to increase the risk of acute cardiotoxicity. High dose (>60 mg/kg/day) may cause acute heart failure. Bolus doses >180 mg/kg have been reported to cause pericardial effusion. The estimated incidence of cyclophosphamide myocarditis, for doses >150 mg/kg in children, is 5 %.

  - **Ifosfamide:** can induce acute dose-related cardiac complication such as arrhythmias and heart failure. It can also alter renal function and this may contribute to worsen the cardiac function.
  - **Cisplatin:** toxicity occurs during the infusion or several months after therapy. Episodes of myocardial ischemia have been described in young boys. Cisplatin can also induce electrolyte disturbances, hypomagnesemia, platelet aggregation, and vascular endothelial damage.
- **Vincristine**, a drug commonly used to treat several malignancies, can be involved in rhythm alterations through autonomic nervous system dysfunction.
- **Antimicrotubule agents (Etoposide, Paclitaxel):** can cause conduction system abnormalities, reversible sinus bradycardia through action on Purkinje system, arrhythmias, hypotension, hypertension, and angina [21].
- **Amsacrine:** not frequently used in children. Two acute forms of cardiotoxicity have been described: ECG changes (prolonged QT interval and nonspecific ST and T-wave alterations) and arrhythmias (atrial and ventricular) [22]. Both occur within minutes to hours after treatment.
- **Antimetabolites (5-Fluorouracil):** 5-FU is not commonly used to treat pediatric tumors. From adult experience, this drug may cause ischemic syndrome secondary to coronary spasm in addition to prolonging QTc interval. Preexisting coronary artery disease and chest radiation are risk factors for 5-FU toxicity [2].
- **Tyrosine kinase inhibitors** (Bevacizumab, Imatinib, dasatinib..): their use in pediatric oncology is still limited [2]. From adult experience, they have been associated with QT interval prolongation, promoting arterial thrombotic activity leading to possible myocardial ischemia subsequent to coronary spasm or thrombosis [23]. Increases in systemic blood pressure have been observed. The pathogenic mechanism is not completely understood, but it is likely related to VEGF receptor inhibition. LV dysfunction has been detected in adults treated with Imatinib.
- **Biological Agents (rituximab):** can cause left ventricular dysfunction, arrhythmias.
- **Miscellaneous chemotherapeutic agents: (asparaginase, all-trans-retinoic acid, arsenic trioxide):** electrocardiographic changes, QT prolongation, torsade de pointes, other arrhythmias, and hypotension.

Other clinical scenarios

It should also be remembered that CCS are at risk of developing premature atherosclerosis, secondary to the early onset of modifiable cardiovascular risk factors that identify the Metabolic Syndrome (MS) (dyslipidemia, systemic hypertension, obesity, insulin resistance, and other endocrine dysfunction).

Cranial RT, total body irradiation, hypothalamic surgery, endocrinologic deficiencies (GH, hypogonadism), wrong dietary habits acquired during treatment, high doses of steroid therapy, and difficulties in the practice of regular physical activity (amputation, bone surgery, neurologic or cardiopulmonary sequelae) are the main factors affecting this risk.

Key Point
In this high-risk population, premature atherosclerosis further increases the global cardiac risk of developing symptomatic disease.

In the presence of metabolic problems it is extremely important to start primary intervention programs as soon as possible. If an healthy lifestyle isn't enough to normalize the metabolic status, it is necessary to address the patients to a specialist in dysmetabolic diseases [24].

Focus on Systemic Hypertension during and after cancer treatment
Systemic hypertension is a common complication among CCS.

Cancer treatment can lead to damage on vascular system, endothelial dysfunction, and autonomic system dysfunction resulting in blood pressure abnormalities.

Systemic Hypertension:
- It may develop during cancer therapy, usually transiently or years later, not only as direct consequence of treatment but also for reasons unrelated with cancer treatment such as lifestyle behavior and genetic predisposition. The literature reports a 16% incidence of patients requiring antihypertensive therapy during the acute phase of treatment. This percentage drops down to 1% at the end of maintenance therapy.
- It increases the risk of global CVD and is one of the five defining criteria of MS. For this reason, blood pressure should be monitored regularly.

Key Point
The Children's Oncology Group recommends annual measurements of blood pressure for survivors treated with anthracycline, cisplatin, methotrexate, chest and cranial RT, and nephrectomy. The recommendation extends also to patients with at least one criterion for MS.

13.4 Cardiologic Clinical Setup of a Childhood Cancer Patient or Survivor

- **Patient's history**
  - Personal health history.
  - Cancer treatment summary: information on the received cumulative dose of chemo- and/or radiotherapy with main focus on anthracyclines' exposure and chest radiotherapy
  - Information on lifestyle habits
  - Family history

- **Physical examination:**
  - State of peripheral perfusion (skin color and temperature, capillary refill time), assessment of peripheral pulse (volume and rate), blood pressure, weight gain.
  - Chest evaluation: pattern work and rate of breathing, pulmonary crepitation.
  - Heart evaluation to detect abnormal rhythms, abnormal sounds, significant murmur, pericardial friction rub.
  - Abdominal evaluation: liver and spleen assessment
  - Other signs of fluid retention.
- **Instrumental investigations:** Preference and priority should be based on medical history, and/or clinical presentation
  - **Chest radiography**

    Is indicated only in children with suspected heart failure [18].
  - **ECG**

    Is nonspecific; can be used to detect arrhythmias and conduction system abnormalities and to measure the QT interval that has been suggested as a noninvasive predictor of patients at high risk for cardiotoxicity [8].
  - **Echocardiography:**

    Is the recommended modality for surveillance, early identification of asymptomatic cardiac dysfunction, and monitoring of symptomatic patients [6, 17, 25].
    Is a noninvasive, cost-effective, and widely available imaging tool.
    2-dimensional echocardiography, M-mode, and Doppler are the most common techniques used to assess heart structure (cavity size, wall thickness, valvular apparatus) and ventricular systolic and diastolic functions (in particular, Fractional Shortening—FS—and Ejection Fraction—EF—are the most frequent echocardiographic measurements used for assessing left ventricle systolic function) (Table 13.9). Additional echocardiographic measurements for evaluation of systolic function can also be used (Table 13.10).

13

Key Points [8]

FS and EF reference values in pediatric population

	EF (%)	FS (%)
Normal	55–60	>29
Borderline	50–54	25–28
Abnormal	<50	<25

After cancer treatment, it is considered as clinically relevant a decrease of EF, compared to previous examinations, by:
- 15 % for values within normal range
- 10 % if the value is below the lower limits of normal

▫ **Table 13.9** Most frequent and relevant echocardiographic measurements for assessing left ventricle systolic function

Echocardiography assessment of left ventricular systolic function [6, 17, 25, 58, 59]:
Ejection Fraction (EF): measures left ventricle end-diastole volume (LV EDV) and end-systole volume (LV ESV).
EF (%) = (LVEDV − LVESV/LVEDV) × 100
Echo technique: 2-D measurements for volume calculations using biplane method of disks (modified Simpson's rule)
Normal Value (n.v.): 55–60 %
Limitations:
Foreshortening of apex will result in overestimation of EF
If asymmetry of ventricular geometry or wall motion abnormality in a single plane—reduced accuracy
Endocardial definition
Dependent on: HR, preload, and afterload
Time-consuming
Ejection Fraction (EF): measures left ventricle end-diastole volume (LV EDV) and end-systole volume (LV ESV).
EF (%) = (LVEDV − LVESV/ LVEDV) × 100
Echo technique: 2-D measurements for volume calculations using biplane method of disks (modified Simpson's rule)
Normal Value (n.v.): 55–60 %
Limitations:
Foreshortening of apex will result in overestimation of EF
If asymmetry of ventricular geometry or wall motion abnormality in a single plane—reduced accuracy
Endocardial definition
Dependent on: HR, preload, and afterload
Time-consuming

- Relevant echocardiographic measurements used for assessing left ventricle diastolic function are mitral valve inflow patterns (E/A report), deceleration time (DT), and isovolumetric relaxation time (IVRT) (▫ Table 13.11). These measurements are useful for the identification of diastolic dysfunction patterns (▫ Table 13.12) [26].
- More sophisticated echocardiography modalities may offer improved sensitivity and specificity. These include:
  - Tissue Doppler imaging measures:
    - Pulsed tissue Doppler may be easily performed during a standard Doppler echocardiographic examination; it has been successfully applied in several clini-

Table 13.10 Additional echocardiography measurement used for the evaluation of left ventricle systolic function

1. 16 segments visual analysis for identifying regional wall motion abnormality (Grading each segment as 1—normal 2—hypokinetic, 3—akinetic, 4—dyskinetic)
2. Volumetric method: based on hydraulic principle that flow rate (Q) is directly proportional to cross-sectional area (CSA) of tube and mean velocity of moving fluid is constant:
Stroke volume (SV) = VTI × CSA
Cardiac output = SV × HR/1000
Cardiac Index = CO/BSA (CI n.v: 3.5 l/min/m^2)
3. Left ventricle Dp/Dt
Normal > 1200 mmHg/s
Borderline 1000–1200 mmHg/s
Abnormal < 800 mmHg/s
4. TEI index: isovolumetric contraction time + isovolumetric relaxation time/ejection time (v.n 0.39 ± 0.05)
5. Tissue Doppler imaging (pulse/color) [60]: pulsed wave TDI measures instantaneous peak velocity from the myocardium (S wave at basal lateral/septal wall of the left ventricle); this parameter shows a good correlation with LVEF
6. Other variables: Left ventricle wall stress, left ventricular mass, velocity of shortening corrected for heart rate, left ventricle thickness-to-dimension ratio.

Table 13.11 Relevant echocardiographic measurements used during clinical practice for assessing left ventricle diastolic function

Echo Assessment of Left Ventricular Diastolic Function [5, 22, 31, 33, 34],
1. 2D observation: LV wall thickness, cavity, size; LA size, pericardium
2. Doppler of Mitral inflow:
Peak E (cm/s): 73 ± 9 in children (peak early filling of the left ventricle) Peak A (cm/s): 38 ± 8 in children (peak late filling of the left ventricle)
E/A ratio (ratio of to) n.v: 2.0 ± 5
3. Deceleration time DT n.v: 100 ± 22 (ms) in children
4. Isovolumetric relaxation time (IVRT) n.v: 55 ± 10 (ms) in children
5. Pulmonary vein flow pattern:
Peak S (cm/s): 44 ± 10 (age > 1 year)
Peak D (cm/s): 61 ± 10 (age > 1 year)
S/D velocity ratio: 0.7 ± 0.3 (age > 1 year)
6. Tissue Doppler imaging TDI [60]:
E/e′ lateral n.v. < 10–12
E/e′ septal n.v. < 15
7. Myocardial deformation parameters: evaluation with Strain and strain rate.

Table 13.12 Patterns of diastolic dysfunction

1. Normal
2. Altered Relaxation (grade I)
Reduced mitral E wave velocity, reduced E/A ratio <1
Prolonged DT, Prolonged IVRT
Pulmonary veins Doppler S/D ratio >1 S > D.
Mitral valve A duration > pulmonary vein AR duration
TDI: E (mitral inflow peak early filling)/e′ (mitral early septal annular velocity) < 10
3. Pseudonormal (grade II)
Mitral inflow is apparently normal (Valsalva maneuver to unmask) E/A ratio 1.1–1.5
DT similar to normal
Pulmonary veins Doppler S/D ratio < 1 (reduced S peak wave velocity S < D),
Mitral valve A duration < Pulmonary vein AR duration
TDI E/e′ > 10
4. Restrictive (grade III)
Prominent E wave and markedly reduced A wave (E/A ratio >1.5)
Reduced DT, reduced IVRT
Pulmonary veins S component is markedly reduced or even absent, Ar wave is prominent
Mitral valve A duration < pulmonary vein AR duration
TDI E/e′ > 10

Modified from "Echocardiography in pediatric and congenital heart disease from fetus to adult": Lai, Mertens, Cohen, Geva [26]

cal settings and appears reliable in providing quantitative information on myocardial diastolic relaxation and systolic performance (E′ wave, A′ wave, and S wave velocity)
  - Tissue Doppler of LV lateral mitral annulus, in combination with PW Doppler of mitral inflow, provides accurate information about the degree of LV filling pressure.
- Myocardial velocity and deformation imaging (strain and strain rate—SR—imaging), torsion analysis, and three-dimensional measures of cardiac size have potential value for early quantification of global and regional systolic and diastolic myocardial dysfunction [27] (Table 13.13).

Table 13.13 Newer echocardiographic techniques for evaluating ventricular function have been introduced during the past decade [61]

Strain and strain rate imaging—using color-coded tissue Doppler imaging—has emerged as a quantitative technique to estimate myocardial function and contractility.
Myocardial strain is a dimensionless measure of regional and global ventricular deformation.
Myocardial strain rate, a time derivative of strain, correlates with LV peak elastance, which is a load-independent global measure of ventricular function.
The speckle-tracking echocardiography-estimated strain and strain rate can detect early cardiac dysfunction, both systolic and diastolic, in asymptomatic patients with normal conventional measures of cardiac function. It should be taken into account, however, that these new techniques depend on the imaging system and on image quality.
3-D—regional and global LV systolic function: good correlation with MRI.

Key Point

The predictive value of standard echocardiography measurements in detecting early cardiac dysfunction is limited by the intrinsic variability in echocardiographic measurements themselves.

Changes in those parameters are considered "late changes," indicating that a significant myocardial damage is already occurred.

There is growing evidence in the literature supporting the complementary role of cardiac biomarkers and echocardiographic imaging studies in early detection of asymptomatic cardiac dysfunctions.

13

- **Cardiac Magnetic Resonance Imaging (CMR):**
  - Is a noninvasive, safe, sensitive, and reproducible technique
  - It has diagnostic potential for detection of early ventricular involvement, giving information regarding both heart structure and function.
  - It has advantages over echocardiography since it allows assessment of ventricular mass and function in a more reproducible and standardized way, and is especially useful when ultrasound evaluation is not technically feasible or optimal.
  - When contrast enhancement is used, it provides information not available by echocardiography on perfusion abnormalities and sub-endocardial damage through identification of delayed enhancement.
  - It might be useful to determine the prognosis and the timing of treatment in children with slowly progressive ventricular dysfunction [6].
  - It may be useful in borderline patients with EF (calculated by echocardiography) between 50 and 59 %.
  - Cost, time, and need of sedation in younger patient are the major limitations for wide employment of CMR [6, 28].

- **Radionucleotide angiography:**
  - Can be used to study myocardial perfusion, when CMR is not technically possible.
- **Holter ECG:**
  - Can be useful for monitoring patient with chronic heart failure and/or patients with previous arrhythmic events, providing additional information.
- **Cardiopulmonary exercise test:**
  - Test used for cardiac functional evaluation; can be useful for detecting asymptomatic cardiac dysfunction.
  - CCS may have adequate cardiac function at rest but may decompensate if metabolic demand increases.
  - In patients with congestive heart failure, maximum oxygen consumption (VO_2 max) closely corresponds with prognosis.
  - Since in CCS it may be difficult to distinguish early/mild heart disease from lack of fitness, the response to an aerobic work may help to differentiate between these two clinical situations.
  - It has been suggested that if CCS show normal response to cardiopulmonary exercise testing, they can take part in dynamic sporting activities. Survivors who exhibit a reduced VO_2 max should be reevaluated after an aerobic training program and should undergo tailored dynamic physical activity if the VO_2 max does not normalize [6, 29, 30]
- **Focus: Physical activity in Pediatric Oncology patients:** [31–34]

Regular participation in physical activity is one of the strategies recommended by the American Heart Association for promoting cardiovascular health in childhood. Physical activity is a key factor in the development of healthy children.

Diagnosis of cancer in children and adolescent interrupts their daily life, changing drastically the capacity of normal physical activity.

The growing CCS population may develop, during and after therapy, physical and psychosocial side effects including:

- Diminished muscular strength, peripheral neuropathy, decreased functional capacity, and increased fatigue;
- Elevated levels of fear and anxiety, poor social functioning, and decreased health-related quality of life.

Exercise capacity is reduced in a large percentage of survivors due to several factors other than cardiac toxicity, such as respiratory or musculoskeletal dysfunction, psychological attitude and lack of physical fitness, endocrine deficiencies, chronic fatigue, or peripheral neuropathies. Most of these, however, not only do not contraindicate but can even be positively affected by a regular physical activity, even if of moderate intensity. Physical activity has emerged as a promising adjuvant therapy to mitigate the negative effects of cancer and its treatment. The importance of physical activity in childhood cancer patients and survivors is very high, as they are at a greater risk (compared to healthy children) to develop a sedentary lifestyle that can aggravate and accelerate the development of physical inactivity-related diseases such as hypertension, diabetes, obesity cardiovascular disease, coronary artery disease, and osteoporosis and cancer recurrence. These are all factors for which this population presents already at higher risk.

A full program for physical activity during maintenance treatment and during follow-up after the end of treatment is recommended [35]. Recently, some authors have documented the integration of physical exercise into primary care of cancer-affected children already during acute phase of treatment with evidence of positive outcome [31]. Evidence suggests that promoting a mild/moderate physical activity is safe, beneficial, and feasible in pediatric cancer experience.

Key Point
With regard to limitations in the intensity of exercise in childhood cancer survivors, according to AHA and ESC, the intensities of exercise (high-, moderate-, low-intensity) are determined by the severity of existing cardiac dysfunction. Cardiologic consultation is recommended for survivors with asymptomatic cardiomyopathy to define limits and precautions for exercise [33, 34]. For high-risk survivors, cardiology consultation might be reasonable for those who plan to be engaged in high-intensity exercise [6].

- **Lab tests**
  - Routine laboratory testing is not recommended for screening
  - In case of symptoms, a complete blood count and RCP, acid–base status, electrolytes (Na^{++}, K^{+}, Cl^{-}, Ca^{2}), glucose, renal and hepatic function, as well as thyroid hormone levels should be evaluated, together with cardiac-specific serum biomarkers.
    Troponin I, T: reflecting acute heart damage
    BNP, NT-pro-BNP reflecting acute and chronic heart damage

- **Focus on specific cardiac serum biomarkers**
  - **Cardiac troponin T (cTnT), cardiac troponin I (cTnI), B-type natriuretic peptide (BNP), and N-terminal pro-BNP (NT-pro-BNP):**
  - BNP, NT-pro-BNP, and cardiac troponins T and I are currently widely recognized as essential part of adult cardiologic evaluation. In adult patients treated with anthracyclines, several studies have reported a correlation between the levels of cardiac biomarkers and abnormalities seen by echocardiography [36]. Evident data, however, are not available in children.
  - **Troponin:** Cardiac troponins I and T are cardiac proteins that control calcium-mediated interaction of actin and myosin. Troponins are specific and sensitive marker for the diagnosis of myocardial injury.
  - **BNP and NT-pro-BNP** [36–39]. In children with congestive heart failure, BNP and NT-pro-BNP levels correlate with functional capacity [39]. Both peptides can differentiate cardiac from pulmonary causes in infants with respiratory distress. It is known that the N-terminal form of BNP is the most discerning neurohumoral marker of early cardiac dysfunction [40, 41]. Children with CHF show high plasma N-BNP concentrations that correlate with the severity of clinical symptoms [29, 41]. Their use and evaluation in pediatric age is complex since their normal levels are age, assay, and gender dependent [19, 36, 38]. They are elevated in

the first few days after birth [37, 41, 42]; thereafter, their levels decrease and remain relatively constant throughout childhood until 10 years, with no differences between boys and girls. During pubertal age, a sex-related difference is found, with higher plasma concentrations in girls [38]. Infants and children with heart disease that causes significant pressure or volume overload of the right or the left ventricles show elevated BNP and NT-pro-BNP levels.

13.5 Preventive Strategies

The need for effective prevention and treatment strategies to limit or avoid cardiotoxicity without reducing oncological efficacy has been widely studied. Several strategies have been tested [8], but only few have been evaluated in the specific contest of pediatric randomized controlled trials.

▪ Primary Cardioprotective strategies under investigation include

- **Limiting the dose of anthracyclines:**
  - Ideally, the primary prevention to avoid cardiac consequences should be not to expose patients to potentially cardiotoxic treatments, but these drugs are so far considered as pivotal for the treatment of several childhood cancers.
  - The cumulative dose of anthracycline used in cancer protocols has been progressively reduced in order to minimize the cardiotoxic effect (while maintaining the same therapeutic efficacy), even if it has been shown that there is no "safe" dose of anthracyclines.
- **Continuous versus bolus anthracycline infusion:**
  - Studies on adult populations showed a reduction in anthracycline-related cardiotoxicity with continuous versus bolus infusion [43, 44]. However, these results were not replicated in children. A study of continuous infusion compared with bolus infusion in children with ALL did not show a better long-term cardioprotection nor improvement in survival [45, 46].
- **Structurally Modified Anthracyclines:** Anthracyclines analogues (i.e., epirubicin, idarubicin, mitoxantrone, etc.)
  - Liposomal anthracyclines: In the last years, new pharmaceutical formulations of anthracyclines (either via a liposomal or pegylated vector) have been developed in order to allow slow release of the drug after injection. These drugs seem to have a better and safer oncological profile than conventional anthracyclines because of their longer circulation times, longer half-lives, slower clearance from plasma, and their impossibility to penetrate cardiac cell tight junctions. However, the cost of these drugs is still high, and for this reason, they are usually used in relapsing patients who had already received anthracyclines as part of their front-line treatment [47]. Their use in children is thus limited and there are no conclusive results.
  - Anthracycline analogues (e.g., epirubicin, idarubicin): in adults, they seem to demonstrate a better and safer oncological profile compared to conventional anthracyclines even if there are not conclusive results regarding the risk of cardiovascular effects, since the doxorubicin equivalent conversion score used in some guidelines is based on hematological toxic effects and not on cardiotoxic effects [6, 48]. In children, there are no conclusive results; more research is needed.

Key Point

It is important to note that based on hematologic toxicity data, the anthracycline dose equivalence ratio with doxorubicin and daunorubicin has been typically assumed to be 1:1, while it is 1:5 for idarubicin and 1:0.67 for epirubicin. However, a recent report based on joint analyses of Dutch and American series has demonstrated that, with regard to the cardiotoxic effect, daunorubicin appears to be substantially less cardiotoxic than doxorubicin (cardiotoxic effect ratio 1:0.5) [62]. Thus, this conversion should be taken into account when calculating the anthracyclines' cumulative dose received by each patient.

- **Use of Cardioprotective Agents**
  - **Dexrazoxane**
    - Is an iron-chelating agent that reduces the formation of iron–anthracycline complexes and is the most widely studied cardioprotective strategy in adult populations.
    - Controversies about the use of dexrazoxane in children have emerged due to fear of reducing treatment efficacy and increasing the number of second cancers, thus compromising overall survival rates [49]. This leads The European Medicines Agency to not recommend the use of dexrazoxane in children.
    - However, some studies suggest with low-to-moderate confidence that there are cardiac beneficial effects in children treated with dexrazoxane, without compromising long-term survival [50, 51].
  - **Nutritive Agents (i.e., Coenzyme Q, Vitamins C, E, A) and antioxidant drugs (i.e., L–Carnitine, glutathione):**

    There is no conclusive evidence supporting their use [52].
  - **ACE inhibitors, Beta-Blockers, ARBs:**

    The use of these drugs as primary prevention during cancer treatment shows a possible beneficial hemodynamic effect. However, their usefulness in reducing the incidence of asymptomatic changes in echocardiographic parameters and the development of symptomatic dysfunction remains uncertain.

Secondary cardioprotective strategies

- **Early identification**
  - Cardiac screening protocols for high-risk patients based on full and sequential cardiology assessment of early signs of myocardial damage in order to initiate adequate treatment and improve prognosis.
- **Pharmacologic treatment**
  - Currently, there are no recommendations for starting cardiac treatment in asymptomatic patients with decreased left ventricular ejection fraction documented by echocardiography.
  - For what concerns the treatment of patients who develop signs and symptoms of heart failure, there is evidence that in the adult population the use of ACE inhibitors and beta-blockers improves cardiac function and decreases mobility and mortality. The benefit from the use of these drugs in pediatrics is controversial, but seems promising. There are no conclusive data at the moment because the studies conducted so far are based on small groups and with short follow-up periods [2, 7, 8, 18].

Key Point
In summary, the evidence for the use of ACE inhibitors and beta-blockers in clinical practice for pediatric population with heart failure has been extrapolated from adult experience and seems to improve cardiac outcome, at least in the short term.

Treatment with ACE inhibitors (captopril, enalapril) is indicated.

Treatment with beta-blockers (carvedilol, metoprolol, or bisoprolol) might be initiated in the treatment of moderate to severe systolic dysfunction.

13.6 Practical Surveillance Program

- **Pretreatment cardiology screening:**
  - Systematic baseline clinical and instrumental cardiologic evaluation (clinical history with attention to cardiovascular risk factors or comorbidities, clinic cardiovascular evaluation, blood pressure, ECG, echocardiography)
- **During treatment, cardiology evaluation** should be repeated:
  - If there is a history suggesting a cardiologic high risk before the treatment.
  - If the patient received a high cumulative anthracycline dose and/or high radiation dose.
  - If patient develops cardiac clinical symptoms and signs and/or if there is a suspected infectious complication or any other cardiac complication.

Key Point
If any grade of myocardial dysfunction is found, the evaluation must be repeated after each therapy cycle. In these patients, it might be reasonable to consider evaluation of specific cardiac biomarkers.

Treatment interruption should be considered if there is severe myocardial dysfunction.

- **Posttreatment cardiology screening:**

Recently, guidelines, and recommendations for cardiac long-term follow-up of children exposed to cardiotoxic treatments have been developed by the International Guidelines Harmonization group, with the contribution of the most important European and North American cooperative groups [6].

According to these guidelines, the risk of developing cardiomyopathy varies based on the cumulative doses received of anthracyclines and/or chest irradiation:

- CCS should be stratified as at low, moderate, or high risk of developing cardiomyopathy based on the received cumulative dose of anthracyclines and chest radiation:

Cardiomyopathy risk	Anthracycline dose	Chest irradiation dose	Anthracycline + chest radiation
High	≥250 mg/m^2	≥35 Gy	≤100 mg/m^2 + ≥15 Gy
Moderate	100–250 mg/m^2	≥15–<35 Gy	
Low	≤100 mg/m^2		

- A screening program is strongly recommended for high-risk patients, while for those at intermediate or low risk the recommendation is less strong
- If a screening program is planned, the recommendations are as follows:

Question	Strength of recommendation
What surveillance modality should be used?	
Echocardiography is recommended as the primary cardiomyopathy surveillance modality	Strong
In particular situations in which ultrasound evaluation is not technically feasible or optimal for cardiac surveillance, CMR or radionuclide studies should be used. If available, a CMR might be preferred in these cases since: It does not use any radiation It presents an increasing diagnostic potential for detection of early ventricular involvement, giving information regarding both heart structure and function. It has advantages since it allows assessment of ventricular mass and function in a more reproducible and standardized way and is especially useful when ultrasound evaluation is not technically feasible or optimal. When contrast enhancement is used, it provides information not available by echocardiography on perfusion abnormalities and subendocardial damage through identification of delayed enhancement Limitations are: Cost, time, and need of sedation in younger patient. The equipment and the expertise needed for its use in this field are not available in all centers.	Moderate
Cardiac blood biomarkers are not recommended as the only modality of surveillance of cardiac dysfunction in asymptomatic CCS	Not recommended
Cardiac blood biomarkers may be useful for further investigation in case that at imaging investigations some sign of cardiomyopathy has emerged	Moderate
It might be reasonable to consider the use of serum cardiac biomarkers for monitoring Symptomatic patients with preserved systolic function Patient with borderline cardiac function during primary surveillance	Moderate
When should cardiac surveillance begin and how long should it continue?	

Question	Strength of recommendation
For CCS included in the high-risk group cardiology surveillance should be: Performed within 2 years from the end of chemotherapy treatment; Repeated at 5 years after diagnosis; Continued every 5 years thereafter	Strong
For CCS included in the moderate- and low-risk group cardiology surveillance should be: Performed within 2 years from the end of chemotherapy treatment; Repeated at 5 years after diagnosis; Continued every 5 years thereafter.	Moderate
A more frequent surveillance is reasonable for high-risk group and may be reasonable in moderate- and low-risk survivors.	Moderate
Lifelong cardiomyopathy surveillance is reasonable in high-risk group and may be reasonable for moderate- and low-risk groups	Moderate/Low
What should be done when abnormalities are identified?	
The recommendations reported above are for primary surveillance. If an asymptomatic cardiomyopathy is detected, the subsequent investigative steps and the follow-up frequency should be defined by the cardiologist	Strong
What to do in case of pregnancy in female survivors treated with anthracycline or chest radiation?	
It is reasonable to perform a cardiology evaluation before pregnancy or during the first trimester of pregnancy to make sure that heart function is normal.	Moderate
If no alterations in heart function are detected during the first evaluation, there are no specific recommendations about the need and/or frequency of further cardiac surveillance during the whole pregnancy.	No recommendation
Survivors and their healthcare provider should pay attention to symptoms such as shortness of breath, fatigue, and ankle swelling. These are commonly reported during pregnancy, but can also be the expression of progressive cardiac dysfunction.	Strong
Recommendations on physical activity	
Exercise is usually beneficial for everybody and as long as the tests don't show any alterations in heart function, regular physical activity is recommended.	Strong
In case of desire to practice high-intensity exercise, a cardiologist consultation is recommended	Moderate
If cardiac tests show alterations in heart function, a cardiologist consultation is recommended to give advice on the limits and precautions of a personal exercise regimen.	Strong

Screening for modifiable cardiovascular risk factors and MS is also strongly suggested in order to set the stage and establish if lifestyle modifications are sufficient or a pharmacology therapy is necessary.

If a cardiac dysfunction is detected at an early stage, a therapeutic approach may significantly increase quality of life and life expectancy. This is even more important in children than in adults, considering the long latency between cardiotoxic exposure and clinically evident disease and the long life expectancy.

The future of childhood malignancies therapy should be based on new biological and molecularly targeted agents, together with a risk-adapted approach basing the intensity of therapy on clinical, biological, and genetic factors and on treatment response, in order to minimize the cardiotoxic complications and contemporarily maintain and enhance the anticancer effect.

References

1. Barry E, Alvarez JA, Scully RE, Miller TL, Lipshultz SE. Anthracycline-induced cardiotoxicity: course, pathophysiology, prevention and management. Expert Opin Pharmacother. 2007;8:1039–58.
2. Lipshultz SE, et al. Long-term cardiovascular toxicity in children, adolescents, and young adults who receive cancer therapy: pathophysiology, course, monitoring, management, prevention, and research directions: a scientific statement from the American Heart Association. Circulation. 2013;128: 1927–95.
3. Mariotto AB, et al. Long-term survivors of childhood cancers in the United States. Cancer Epidemiol Biomark Prev. 2009;18:1033–40.
4. Lipshultz SE, et al. Cardiotoxicity and cardioprotection in childhood cancer. Acta Haematol. 2014;132:391–9.
5. van der Pal HJ, et al. High risk of symptomatic cardiac events in childhood cancer survivors. J Clin Oncol. 2012;30:1429–37.
6. Armenian SH, et al. Recommendations for cardiomyopathy surveillance for survivors of childhood cancer: a report from the International Late Effects of Childhood Cancer Guideline Harmonization Group. Lancet Oncol. 2015;16:e123–36.
7. Vejpongsa P, Yeh ETH. Prevention of anthracycline-induced cardiotoxicity: challenges and opportunities. J Am Coll Cardiol. 2014;64:938–45.
8. Dillenburg RF, Nathan P, Mertens L. Educational paper: decreasing the burden of cardiovascular disease in childhood cancer survivors: an update for the pediatrician. Eur J Pediatr. 2013;172:1149–60.
9. Oeffinger KC, et al. Chronic health conditions in adult survivors of childhood cancer. N Engl J Med. 2006;355:1572–82.
10. Geenen MM, et al. Medical assessment of adverse health outcomes in long-term survivors of childhood cancer. JAMA. 2007;297:2705–15.
11. Armstrong GT, et al. Late mortality among 5-year survivors of childhood cancer: a summary from the Childhood Cancer Survivor Study. J Clin Oncol. 2009;27:2328–38.
12. Kaatsch P. Epidemiology of childhood cancer. Cancer Treat Rev. 2010;36:277–85.
13. Vejpongsa P, Yeh ETH. Topoisomerase 2β: a promising molecular target for primary prevention of anthracycline-induced cardiotoxicity. Clin Pharmacol Ther. 2014;95:45–52.
14. Visscher H, et al. Validation of variants in SLC28A3 and UGT1A6 as genetic markers predictive of anthracycline-induced cardiotoxicity in children. Pediatr Blood Cancer. 2013;60:1375–81.
15. Schellong G, et al. Late valvular and other cardiac diseases after different doses of mediastinal radiotherapy for Hodgkin disease in children and adolescents: report from the longitudinal GPOH follow-up project of the German-Austrian DAL-HD studies. Pediatr Blood Cancer. 2010;55:1145–52.
16. Krischer JP, et al. Clinical cardiotoxicity following anthracycline treatment for childhood cancer: the Pediatric Oncology Group experience. J Clin Oncol. 1997;15:1544–52.
17. Santin JC, Deheinzelin D, Junior SPC, Lopes LF, de Camargo B. Late echocardiography assessment of systolic and diastolic function of the left ventricle in pediatric cancer survivors after anthracycline therapy. J Pediatr Hematol Oncol. 2007;29:761–5.
18. Kantor PF, et al. Presentation, diagnosis, and medical management of heart failure in children: Canadian Cardiovascular Society guidelines. Can J Cardiol. 2013;29:1535–52.
19. Ross RD, Bollinger RO, Pinsky WW. Grading the severity of congestive heart failure in infants. Pediatr Cardiol. 1992;13:72–5.

20. Armstrong GT, et al. Modifiable risk factors and major cardiac events among adult survivors of childhood cancer. J Clin Oncol. 2013;31:3673–80.
21. Chatterjee K, Zhang J, Tao R, Honbo N, Karliner JS. Vincristine attenuates doxorubicin cardiotoxicity. Biochem Biophys Res Commun. 2008;373:555–60.
22. Simbre VC, Duffy SA, Dadlani GH, Miller TL, Lipshultz SE. Cardiotoxicity of cancer chemotherapy: implications for children. Paediatr Drugs. 2005;7:187–202.
23. Lipshultz SE, et al. Managing chemotherapy-related cardiotoxicity in survivors of childhood cancers. Paediatr Drugs. 2014;16:373–89.
24. Bizzarri C, Bottaro G, Pinto RM, Cappa M. Metabolic syndrome and diabetes mellitus in childhood cancer survivors. Pediatr Endocrinol Rev. 2014;11:365–73.
25. Cheitlin MD, et al. ACC/AHA/ASE 2003 Guideline update for the clinical application of echocardiography: summary article. A report of the American College of Cardiology/American Heart Association Task Force on Practice Guidelines (ACC/AHA/ASE Committee to Update the 1997 Guidelines for the Clinical Application of Echocardiography). J Am Soc Echocardiogr. 2003;16:1091–110.
26. Lai WW, Mertens LL, Geva T, Cohen MS. Echocardiography in pediatric and congenital heart disease: from fetus to adult. Chichester: Wiley; 2012.
27. Ganame J, et al. Myocardial dysfunction late after low-dose anthracycline treatment in asymptomatic pediatric patients. J Am Soc Echocardiogr. 2007;20:1351–8.
28. de Ville de Goyet M, et al. Prospective cardiac MRI for the analysis of biventricular function in children undergoing cancer treatments. Pediatr Blood Cancer. 2015;62:867–74.
29. De Caro E, et al. Exercise capacity in apparently healthy survivors of cancer. Arch Dis Child. 2006;91:47–51.
30. De Caro E, et al. Subclinical cardiac dysfunction and exercise performance in childhood cancer survivors. Pediatr Blood Cancer. 2011;56:122–6.
31. Baumann FT, Bloch W, Beulertz J. Clinical exercise interventions in pediatric oncology: a systematic review. Pediatr Res. 2013;74:366–74.
32. San Juan AF, Wolin K, Lucía A. Physical activity and pediatric cancer survivorship. Recent Results Cancer Res. 2011;186:319–47.
33. Maron BJ, et al. Recommendations for physical activity and recreational sports participation for young patients with genetic cardiovascular diseases. Circulation. 2004;109:2807–16.
34. Pelliccia A, et al. Recommendations for participation in competitive sport and leisure-time physical activity in individuals with cardiomyopathies, myocarditis and pericarditis. Eur J Cardiovasc Prev Rehabil. 2006;13:876–85.
35. Viña CC, Wurz AJ, Culos-Reed SN. Promoting physical activity in pediatric oncology. Where do we go from here? Front Oncol. 2013;3:173.
36. Mavinkurve-Groothuis AMC, Kapusta L, Nir A, Groot-Loonen J. The role of biomarkers in the early detection of anthracycline-induced cardiotoxicity in children: a review of the literature. Pediatr Hematol Oncol. 2008;25:655–64.
37. Koch A, Singer H. Normal values of B type natriuretic peptide in infants, children, and adolescents. Heart. 2003;89:875–8.
38. Nir A, et al. NT-pro-B-type natriuretic peptide in infants and children: reference values based on combined data from four studies. Pediatr Cardiol. 2009;30:3–8.
39. Nir A, Nasser N. Clinical value of NT-ProBNP and BNP in pediatric cardiology. J Card Fail. 2005;11:S76–80.
40. Mir TS, et al. Plasma concentrations of N-terminal pro-brain natriuretic peptide in control children from the neonatal to adolescent period and in children with congestive heart failure. Pediatrics. 2002;110:e76.
41. Soker M, Kervancioglu M. Plasma concentrations of NT-pro-BNP and cardiac troponin-I in relation to doxorubicin-induced cardiomyopathy and cardiac function in childhood malignancy. Saudi Med J. 2005;26:1197–202.
42. Lipshultz SE, et al. Changes in cardiac biomarkers during doxorubicin treatment of pediatric patients with high-risk acute lymphoblastic leukemia: associations with long-term echocardiographic outcomes. J Clin Oncol. 2012;30:1042–9.
43. Levitt GA, Dorup I, Sorensen K, Sullivan I. Does anthracycline administration by infusion in children affect late cardiotoxicity? Br J Haematol. 2004;124:463–8.
44. Wouters KA, Kremer LCM, Miller TL, Herman EH, Lipshultz SE. Protecting against anthracycline-induced myocardial damage: a review of the most promising strategies. Br J Haematol. 2005;131:561–78.

45. Lipshultz SE, et al. Doxorubicin administration by continuous infusion is not cardioprotective: the Dana-Farber 91-01 Acute Lymphoblastic Leukemia protocol. J Clin Oncol. 2002;20:1677–82.
46. Lipshultz SE, et al. Continuous versus bolus infusion of doxorubicin in children with all: long-term cardiac outcomes. Pediatrics. 2012;130:1003–11.
47. Gabizon AA, Lyass O, Berry GJ, Wildgust M. Cardiac safety of pegylated liposomal doxorubicin (Doxil/Caelyx) demonstrated by endomyocardial biopsy in patients with advanced malignancies. Cancer Invest. 2004;22:663–9.
48. van Dalen EC, Michiels EM, Caron HN, Kremer LC. Different anthracycline derivates for reducing cardiotoxicity in cancer patients. Cochrane Database Syst Rev. 2010. CD005006. doi:10.1002/14651858.CD005006.pub4
49. Kremer LCM, van Dalen EC. Dexrazoxane in children with cancer: from evidence to practice. J Clin Oncol. 2015;33:2594–6. doi:10.1200/JCO.2015.61.7928.
50. Chow EJ, et al. Late mortality after dexrazoxane treatment: a report from the Children's Oncology Group. J Clin Oncol. 2015. doi:10.1200/JCO.2014.59.4473.
51. Lipshultz SE, et al. Assessment of dexrazoxane as a cardioprotectant in doxorubicin-treated children with high-risk acute lymphoblastic leukaemia: long-term follow-up of a prospective, randomised, multicentre trial. Lancet Oncol. 2010;11:950–61.
52. van Dalen EC, Caron HN, Dickinson HO, Kremer LC. Cardioprotective interventions for cancer patients receiving anthracyclines. Cochrane Database Syst Rev. 2011. CD003917. doi:10.1002/14651858.CD003917.pub4
53. Lipshultz SE, et al. Female sex and drug dose as risk factors for late cardiotoxic effects of doxorubicin therapy for childhood cancer. N Engl J Med. 1995;332:1738–43.
54. Grenier MA, Lipshultz SE. Epidemiology of anthracycline cardiotoxicity in children and adults. Semin Oncol. 1998;25:72–85.
55. Li J, Gwilt PR. The effect of age on the early disposition of doxorubicin. Cancer Chemother Pharmacol. 2003;51:395–402.
56. Bhatia S. Long-term health impacts of hematopoietic stem cell transplantation inform recommendations for follow-up. Expert Rev Hematol. 2011;4:437–52.
57. Armenian SH, et al. Long-term health-related outcomes in survivors of childhood cancer treated with HSCT versus conventional therapy: a report from the Bone Marrow Transplant Survivor Study (BMTSS) and Childhood Cancer Survivor Study (CCSS). Blood. 2011;118:1413–20.
58. Lopez L, et al. Recommendations for quantification methods during the performance of a pediatric echocardiogram: a report from the Pediatric Measurements Writing Group of the American Society of Echocardiography Pediatric and Congenital Heart Disease Council. J Am Soc Echocardiogr. 2010;23:465–95.
59. Steinherz LJ, et al. Guidelines for cardiac monitoring of children during and after anthracycline therapy: report of the Cardiology Committee of the Children's Cancer Study Group. Pediatrics. 1992;89:942–9.
60. Eidem BW, et al. Impact of cardiac growth on Doppler tissue imaging velocities: a study in healthy children. J Am Soc Echocardiogr. 2004;17:212–21.
61. Stoodley PW, et al. Two-dimensional myocardial strain imaging detects changes in left ventricular systolic function immediately after anthracycline chemotherapy. Eur J Echocardiogr. 2011;12:945–52.
62. Feijen EA, et al. Equivalence ratio for Daunorubicin to Doxorubicin in relation to late heart failure in survivors of childhood cancer. J CLin Oncol 2015;33:3774–3780.

Cardiotoxicity in the Elderly

Lucia Fratino and Massimiliano Berretta

C. Lestuzzi et al. (eds.), *Manual of Cardio-oncology*, DOI 10.1007/978-3-319-40236-9_14

14.1 Introduction

The age distribution of population greatly affects its burden of disease and disability, including cancer incidence and mortality. Cancer is now the leading cause of death. Actually, cancer cases reported over the world have doubled in the past 25 years and could even triple by 2030. In fact, the elderly population is rapidly increasing, in Europe 15 % of the population is elderly, and 55 % of cancers are in this group of age [1, 2]. Therefore, age is an important risk factor for cancer. And, as we know, the cancer is forty times higher after 65 years, than when you are aged between 20 and 44 years. Older adults with cancer have different needs than younger adults with the disease. So treatment for older adults needs to consider many issues because they have unique needs by reason of their complex medical histories, numerous drugs taking, their social situations, possible problems with cognitive dysfunction related to age, and general diminution of organ function that occurs naturally in the older population. In contradiction with the fact that the risk of cancer increases with age, there is little interest in their clinical problem. In fact, clinical trial guidelines for treatment of cancer were mainly based on assessment for young age and rarely in elders. That disparity is demonstrated by a low percentage of research in this area. But now there's a big shift in the way oncologists approach treatment for elderly, and oncology management began to raise the consciousness that age was not a contraindication per se and starting in the mid-1980s the need of data and information [3, 4]. Ageing is associated with the decline in organ function that occurs over time and even in the eventual presence of injury, illness or poor lifestyle choices (e.g. unhealthy diet, lack of exercise, substance abuse). Initially, the changes in organ function do not affect baseline function; the first manifestations are a reduced capacity of each organ to maintain homeostasis under stress (e.g. illness, like cancer and, injury, like chemotherapy). The cardiovascular, renal and central nervous systems are usually the most vulnerable (the weakest links) [5].

14.2 Characteristics of Elderly People

The ageing process is characterised, for both acute and chronic diseases, by a progressive decline in physical and cognitive functioning whose underlying causes are only partially understood. As a consequence, one of the most characteristic aspects of ageing is the great variability from person to person: some persons maintain their physical and cognitive abilities throughout a long life (successful ageing), while others lose these abilities rather early in adult life. In a very small subgroup of individuals, the functional status even appears to improve over time The basis for this heterogeneity is largely unknown and probably is affected by the interaction of genetic, environmental, functional, social and psychological factors that make up the individual ageing process [5].

Key Points: Characteristics of Elderly People

- Having multi-morbidity or co-morbidity
- Having unusual presentations of illness
- Experiencing organ physiologic change
- Being functional or psychological a risk of dependency
- Having frailty syndrome

14.3 Evaluating Older Patients for Screening Purpose: The Comprehensive Geriatric Assessment (CGA)

Among the elderly patients, to identify the best candidate to receive potential cardiotoxicity chemotherapy assumes a crucial role [6].

As age from a clinical perspective is highly heterogeneous and poorly reflected by chronological age, the clinical evaluation of the older person is influenced by several factors and is a **key step** in the clinical decision process . A geriatric consultation provides a variety of relevant information and enables the healthcare team to manage the complexity of health care in the elderly; this process is named **Comprehensive Geriatric Assessment (CGA).**

CGA is defined as a multidimensional, often interdisciplinary, diagnostic process aimed at determining the medical, psychological and functional capabilities of elderly persons in order to develop an overall plan for treatment and long-term follow-up. It differs from the standard medical evaluation because (1) it focuses on frail elderly people with their complex problems, (2) it puts emphasis on the functional status and on their quality of life and (3) it benefits from the use of an interdisciplinary team. In the geriatric setting, several studies have supported the effectiveness of CGA in improving functional status, reducing hospitalisation, decreasing medical costs and prolonging survival. The meta-analysis by Stuck and colleagues showed a positive effect of the CGA, and the authors recommended its use within interdisciplinary units [7, 8].

Aim of CGA is the study of the complexity of many aspects of old age and the application of knowledge related to the biological, biomedical, behavioural and social aspects of ageing to diagnosis, treatment and care of older persons.

The onco-geriatric approach is specifically targeted towards patients with multiple, interacting problems brought on by disease or ageing and resulting in a progressive reduction of reserve of multiple organ systems, disability (i.e. functional impairment and dependency), co-morbidity, frailty and geriatric syndromes. Such patients are not simply old, but are "geriatric" patients because of interacting psychosocial and physical problems. In addition, diseases in the elderly may appear with atypical signs and symptoms, a silent presentation may occur, and they are extremely susceptible to iatrogenic disease. Chronicle diseases are common and their contribution makes the picture more complex [9–11].

As a consequence, the health status of old persons cannot be evaluated by merely describing the single disease and/or by measuring the response or survival after treatment. Conversely, it is necessary to conduct a more comprehensive investigation of the "functional status" of the aged person. The assessment of the functional status is defined as the measurement of a patient's ability to complete functional tasks, which range from simple self-care in activities of daily living (ADL) [12] to more complex instrumental activities of daily living (IADL) [13], and fulfil social roles. ADL includes feeding, grooming, transferring and toileting. IADL includes shopping, managing finances, housekeeping, laundry, meal preparation, ability to use transportation and telephone and ability to take medications. Independence, or the degree of dependence in the ADL and IADL scales, determines whether an older person can eventually live alone without a caregiver. As for social roles, these include the ability to use transportation, the ability of requiring help in cases of urgent need and the ability of living in an interpersonal context. Each impairment in the physical, social or psychological dimension which gives rise to functional limitations is defined as disability.

In the early 1990s, Monfardini and colleagues designed and validated a comprehensive geriatric assessment instrument tailored on oncological setting [14]. Such instrument included an evaluation of functional status (ADL, IADL), co-morbidity condition (Cumulative Ilness Rating Scale CIRS) [15], cognitive function (Mini-mental state evaluation) [16], depressive symptoms [17], polypharmacy and nutrition.

Such "geriatric" approach may help in the management of older individuals with cancer in at least three areas: detection of frailty, treatment of unsuspected conditions and to design personalised treatment plan [11, 18].

Key Points

In the case of the older cancer patient, the CGA presents the following advantages:

- Estimate of life expectancy
- Estimate of functional reserve and tolerance of chemotherapy
- Recognition of reversible co-morbidity conditions that may interfere with cancer treatment.
- Recognition of special social economic needs that may interfere with cancer treatment.
- Management of nutrition and medications.

The SIOG included CGA in the guidelines for the management of elderly cancer patients: the main recommendation was that these scales are applied to all elderly cancer patients regardless of age to estimate functional status in order to determine a treatment course, assess eligibility for clinical trials and predict treatment toxicity [19] (◘ Table 14.1).

The further evolution on application of such approach was to use the Geriatric Multidimensional Assessment as a milestone in screening process and in decision-making. Oncologists should be able to intervene and to target interventions by choosing between aggressive or palliative treatments and to prevent toxicity. To assess global health and age-related problem recognition could lead to a stratification of elderly cancer patients for entering optimal treatment strategies and/or clinical trials. Usually according to CGA elderly cancer patients evaluated to treatment course are classified in three risk groups: fit, unfit and frail patients (◘ Fig. 14.1).

Table 14.1 SIOG recommendations for the management of anthracyclines' cardiovascular risk. Reproduced with permission from [19]

Recommendations	Proposal
Rigorous screening to exclude patients at unacceptably high cardiac risk (level 1a)	Comprehensive patient history: Current signs or history of CHF Cardiovascular co-morbidity (i.e. hypertension, diabetes or coronary artery disease) Prior exposure to anthracyclines for this or previoumalignancy (level 1a)
Not exceeding the recommended upper cumulative dose (level 1a)	Reduction in maximum cumulative dose (level 5)
Use of less cardiotoxic therapy (level 1a)	Use of continuous infusion (level 1a) Epirubicin (level 1a) Dexrazoxane (level 1b, Elderly: level 5) Liposomal anthracycline formulations (level 1b, elderly: level 5) Sequential administration of conventional anthracyclines and trastuzumab in HER2-positive breast cancer (level 1b, elderly:level 5)
Regular monitoring of cardiac function, signs and symptoms (level 1a)	Measure of LVEF by ultrasound (preferred, level 5) or MUGA scan, every two to three cycles of anthracyclines (level 1a) Special attention needed if drop in LVEF exceeds 10 %, even if remaining within normal range (level 5) Long-term follow-up (level 1a)
Cardiovascular risk reduction interventions (level 1a)	Early management of dysfunction (level 1a) Lifestyle modifications (i.e. smoking cessation, regular exercise, weight loss where appropriate) (level 1a) Beta blockers and ACE inhibitors (level 1a) Reduced lipid levels (level 1a)

CHF congestive heart failure, *MUGA* multiple uptake gated acquisition, *ACE* angiotensin-converting enzyme

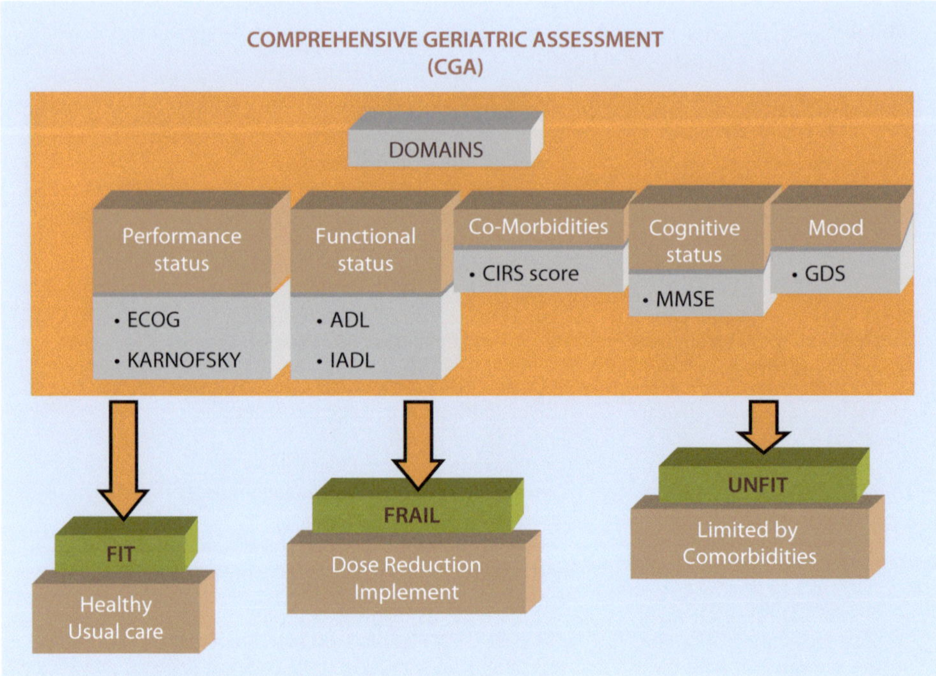

Fig. 14.1 Aspects of comprehensive geriatric assessment

14.4 The Frail Cancer Patient: Definition and Identification

A key step in the patient evaluation in the onco-geriatric setting is the definition and identification of frailty that represents a major issue in clinical geriatrics. Although the term frailty has been increasingly used since the 1980s in the medical literature, its actual meaning is still not well defined.

14

Different authors emphasise different aspects of frailty [5], and frailty includes the following notions:

- Being at a substantial risk of dependency and other adverse health outcomes
- Experiencing the loss of "physiological reserves"
- Having complex medical and psycho-social problems

In the oncological setting, Balducci firstly defined frailty condition as to be over 80 years old, to have some ADL disability or to be affected by more of three co-morbidities or by a geriatric syndrome [4]. Frailty is a reversible condition characterised by a high degree of susceptibility to external changes that require adaptation and compensation. On these bases, when cancer is the "external change" the main objective of frail detection is to adopt compensatory strategies acting at different levels. For instance, the cellular biology level (e.g. growth factors, erythropoietin), the physiologic level (e.g. supportive therapies) and the metabolic pathways (nutritional support) interplay between functional status and social behaviours. With regard to social behaviours, a particular role is played by caregivers whose presence assures adherence to therapeutic plans.

For all these reasons, the effects of ageing must be taken into account during diagnosis and treatment of the elderly [20].

Clinicians should:

- Assess older people according to multidimensional approach by means of validated geriatric assessment tool.

Clinicians should not:

- Mistake pure ageing for disease (e.g. slow information retrieval is not dementia)
- Mistake disease for ageing (e.g. ascribe debilitating arthritis, tremor or dementia to old age)
- Ignore the increased risk of adverse drug effects on weak-link systems stressed by illness
- Forget that the elderly often have multiple underlying disorders (e.g. hypertension, diabetes, atherosclerosis) that accelerate the potential for harm

In addition, clinicians should be alert for diseases that are much more common among the elderly (e.g. diastolic heart failure, Alzheimer disease, incontinence, normal pressure hydrocephalus).This approach enables clinicians to better understand and manage the complexity of the diseases that often coexist in older patients (Fig. 14.2).

Geriatric Multidimensional Assessment Tool

DOMAINS	ASSESSMENT SCALE	
Functional status	PS, ADL, IADL	I Level Total Clinician'Time: 30'-40'
Comorbidity	CIRS,	
Cognitive status	MMS	
Depression	GDS	
Nutrition	MNA	II Level
Polypharmacy	Multifarmacoterapia	
Socio -economics issues	Living conditions, Caregiver, Income, access to trasportation	
Geriatric syndromes	Demenza, Delirium, Depression,	

Fig. 14.2 First and second level assessment of geriatic patients

The unmodifiable effects of ageing may be less dramatic than thought, and healthier, more vigorous ageing may be possible for many people. Today, people >65 are in better health than their ancestors and remain healthier longer. Because health has improved, decline tends to be most dramatic in the oldest old.

14.5 Selected Physiologic Age-Related Changes

Evaluation of the elderly usually differs from a standard medical evaluation. For elderly patients, especially those who are very old or frail, history taking and physical examination may have to be done at different times, and physical examination may require two sessions because patients become fatigued.

The elderly also have different, often more complicated healthcare problems, such as multiple disorders, which may require use of many drugs (sometimes called polypharmacy) and thus greater likelihood of a high-risk drug being prescribed.

14.5.1 Multi-morbidity and Co-morbidity

Diseases interact with pure ageing effects to cause geriatric-specific complications, particularly in the weak-link systems—even when those organs are not the primary ones affected by a disease. Typical examples are delirium complicating pneumonia or UTIs and the falls, dizziness, syncope and weight loss that often accompany many minor illnesses in the elderly [21].

14.5.2 Unusual Presentations of Illness in the Elderly

In the elderly, many common conditions can exist without their characteristic features. Instead, the elderly may have ≥1 non-specific geriatric syndromes (e.g. delirium, dizziness, syncope, falling, weight loss, incontinence). These syndromes result from multiple disorders and impairments; nonetheless, patients may improve when only some of the precipitating factors are corrected. An even better strategy is to identify risk factors for these syndromes and correct as many as possible, thus reducing the likelihood of the syndrome's developing at all.

Although virtually any illness or drug intoxication can cause geriatric syndromes, the following disorders are especially likely to trigger one or more of them, sometimes instead of causing the typical symptoms and signs:

- **Heart failure** may cause confusion, agitation, anorexia, weakness, insomnia, fatigue, weight loss or lethargy; patients may not report dyspnoea. Orthopnoea may cause nocturnal agitation in patients who also have dementia. Peripheral oedema is less specific as a sign of heart failure in elderly than in younger patients. In bed-bound patients, oedema may occur in the sacral area rather than in the lower extremities.
- **Hyperparathyroidism** may cause non-specific symptoms: fatigue, cognitive dysfunction, emotional instability, anorexia, constipation and hypertension. Characteristic symptoms are often absent.

- **Hyperthyroidism** may not cause the characteristic signs (e.g. eye signs, enlarged thyroid gland). Instead, symptoms and signs may be subtle and may include tachycardia, weight loss, fatigue, weakness, palpitations, tremor, atrial fibrillation and heart failure. Patients may appear apathetic rather than hyperkinetic.
- **Hypothyroidism** may manifest subtly in elderly patients. The most common symptoms are non-specific (e.g. fatigue, weakness, falling). Anorexia, weight loss and arthralgias may occur. Cold intolerance, weight gain, depression, paraesthesias, hair loss and muscle cramps are less common than among younger patients; cognitive dysfunction is more common. The most specific sign—delayed tendon reflex relaxation—may not be detectable in elderly patients because of decreased amplitude or absent reflexes [21–24].

14.6 Drug Therapy in the Elderly

Prevalence of prescription drug use among older adults increases substantially with age. Among people ≥65, 90 % use at least 1 drug per week, > 40 % use at least five different drugs per week and 12 % use ≥10 different drugs per week. Women take more drugs, particularly psychoactive and arthritis drugs. Drug use is greatest among the frail elderly, hospitalised patients and nursing home residents; typically, a nursing home resident is given 7–8 different drugs on a regular basis [25].

Providing safe, effective drug therapy for the elderly is challenging for many reasons:

- They use more drugs than any other age group, increasing risk of adverse effects and drug interactions, and making adherence more difficult.
- They are more likely to have chronic disorders that may be worsened by the drug or affect drug response.
- Their physiologic reserves are generally reduced and can be further reduced by acute and chronic disorders.
- Ageing can alter pharmacodynamics) and pharmacokinetics.
- They may be less able to obtain or afford drugs.

There are two main approaches to optimising drug therapy in the elderly:

- Using appropriate drugs as indicated to maximise cost-effectiveness
- Avoiding adverse drug effects

Because the risk of adverse drug effects is higher, overprescribing (polypharmacy) has been targeted as a major problem for the elderly. However, underprescribing appropriate drugs must also be avoided.

14.7 Drug-Related Problems in the Elderly

Drug-related problems are common in the elderly and include drug ineffectiveness, adverse drug effects, overdosage, underdosage and drug interactions.

14.7.1 Before Starting a New Drug

To reduce the risk of adverse drug effects in the elderly, clinicians should do the following before starting a new drug:
- Consider nondrug treatment
- Discuss goals of care with the patient
- Document the indication for each new drug (to avoid using unnecessary drugs)
- Consider age-related changes in pharmacokinetics or pharmacodynamics and their effect on dosing requirements
- Choose the safest possible alternative (e.g. for non-inflammatory arthritis, acetaminophen instead of an NSAID)
- Check for potential drug–disease and drug–drug interactions
- Start with a low dose
- Use the fewest drugs necessary
- Note coexisting disorders and their likelihood of contributing to adverse drug effects
- Explain the uses and adverse effects of each drug
- Provide clear instructions to patients about how to take their drugs (including generic and brand names, spelling of each drug name, indication for each drug and explanation of formulations that contain more than one drug) and for how long the drug will likely be necessary
- Anticipate confusion due to sound-alike drug names and pointing out any names that could be confused (e.g. Glucophage® and Glucovance®)

14.7.2 After Starting a Drug

The following should be done after starting a drug:
- Assume a new symptom may be drug related until proved otherwise (to prevent a prescribing cascade).
- Monitor patients for signs of adverse drug effects, including measuring drug levels and doing other laboratory tests as necessary.
- Document the response to therapy and increase doses as necessary to achieve the desired effect.
- Regularly re-evaluate the need to continue drug therapy and stop drugs that are no longer necessary.

14.7.3 Ongoing

The following should be ongoing:
- **Medication reconciliation** is a process that helps ensure transfer of information about drug regimens at any transition point in the healthcare system. The process includes identifying and listing all drugs patients are taking (name, dose, frequency, route) and comparing the resulting list with the physician's orders at a transition point. Medication reconciliation should occur at each move (admission, transfer and discharge).

- **Computerised physician ordering programs** can alert clinicians to potential problems (e.g. allergy, need for reduced dosage in patients with impaired renal function, drug–drug interactions). These programs can also cue clinicians to monitor certain patients closely for adverse drug effects.

14.7.4 Cardiac Effect of Anticancer Therapy in the Elderly

The elderly are historically underrepresented in clinical trials, with patients older than age 65 years representing only 38 % of enrolled patients. For this reason, less is known about long-term risks in this population of cancer survivors.

Cancer treatments, including chemotherapy, targeted therapy and hormonal therapy, have multiple short- and long-term toxicities, but one of the most concerning is cardiac toxicity. Anticancer therapies can also have indirect effects, such as alterations in blood pressure, or can cause metabolic abnormalities that subsequently increase risk for cardiac events [6, 18, 26–28].

14.7.5 Anthracycline

Anthracyclines are part of most chemotherapeutic regimens for the treatment of many malignancies encountered in the elderly. Toxicity that is observed more frequently is a form of cardiomyopathy that manifests itself during the therapy with doxorubicin in the greatest part of the cases, 86, and it has been reported that the incidence of congestive heart failure following treatment with anthracyclines increases progressively with age after 70 years; these results are confirmed by a multivariate analysis [29].

This may explain why many elderly patients are either excluded from anthracycline treatment or receive less-aggressive chemotherapy.

However, anthracyclines remain the cornerstone of first-line therapy for non-Hodgkin's lymphoma (NHL) and metastatic cancers, and the decision to treat involves balancing likely benefit against possible risks [30, 31].

Anthracycline administration techniques and modality may also affect cardiac risk in the elderly:

Duration and Frequency of Administration

- A Cochrane review of five randomised controlled trials predominantly involving adult patients concluded that continuous infusion of 6 h or longer significantly reduced the risk of clinical heart failure (and probably also subclinical cardiac damage) when compared with infusions of 1 h or less [relative risk (RR) 0.27; 95 % confidence interval (CI) 0.09–0.81] [32].
- In the early retrospective study of Von Hoff et al. [33], weekly administration was associated with less CHF than a 3-week schedule.

Type of Anthracycline

- **Epirubicin** is less cardiotoxic than **doxorubicin** and the Cochrane Review of the evidence from controlled trials has recently confirmed a lower rate of CHF with no difference in response rate and survival observed in patients treated with epirubicin compared with doxorubicin [34].

Table 14.2 Preventable causes of drug-related problems

Category	Definition
Drug interactions	Use of a drug results in a drug–drug, drug–food, drug–supplement or drug–disease interaction, leading to adverse effects or decreased efficacy
Inadequate monitoring	A medical problem is being treated with the correct drug, but the patient is not adequately monitored for complications, effectiveness or both
Inappropriate drug selection	A medical problem that requires drug therapy is being treated with a less-than-optimal drug
Inappropriate treatment	A patient is taking a drug for no medically valid reason
Lack of patient adherence	The correct drug for a medical problem is prescribed, but the patient is not taking it
Overdosage	A medical problem is being treated with too much of the correct drug
Poor communication	Drugs are inappropriately continued or stopped when care is transitioned between providers and/or facilities
Underprescribing	A medical problem is being treated with too little of the correct drug
Untreated medical problem	A medical problem requires drug therapy, but no drug is being used to treat that problem

- **Pegylated liposomal doxorubicin** has shown similar efficacy and improved cardiac safety compared with that of conventional doxorubicin (HR = 3.16, 95 % CI 1.58– 6.31, $P < 0.001$) [35, 36] (Table 14.2).

14

References

1. Baili P, Di Salvo F, Marcos-Gragera R, et al. (2015). EUROCARE-5 Working Group, Age and case mix-standardised survival for all cancer patients in Europe 1999–2007: results of EUROCARE-5, a population-based study. Eur J Cancer. 2015;51:2120–9.
2. Levi F, et al. Changed trends of cancer mortality in the elderly. Ann Oncol. 2001;12:1467–77.
3. Fratino L, Ferrario L, Redmond K, et al. Global Health care: the role of geriatrician, general practitioner and oncology nurse. Crit Rev Oncol Hematol. 1998;27:101–9.
4. Balducci L, Yates J. General guidelines for the management of older patients with cancer. Oncology (Huntingt). 2000;14:221–7.
5. Ferrucci L, et al. The frailty syndrome: a critical issue in geriatric oncology. Crit Rev Oncol Hematol. 2003;46:127–37.
6. Hurria A, Togawa K, Mohile SG, et al. Predicting chemotherapy toxicity in older adults with cancer: a prospective multicentre study. J Clin Oncol. 2011;29(25):3457–65.
7. Solomon DH, Judd HL, Sier HC, Rubenstein LZ, Morley JE. New issues in geriatric care. Ann Intern Med. 1988;108(5):718–32.
8. Stuck AE, Wieland GD, Adams J, Rubenstein LZ. Comprehensive geriatric assessment: a metaanalysis of controlled trials. Lancet. 1993;342(8878):1032–6.

9. Extermann M. Studies of comprehensive geriatric assessment in patients with cancer. Cancer Control. 2003;10:463–8.
10. Repetto L, et al. Comprehensive geriatric assessment adds information to Eastern Cooperative Oncology Group performance status in elderly cancer patients: an Italian Group for Geriatric Oncology Study. J Clin Oncol. 2002;20:404–502.
11. Repetto L, Venturino A, Fratino L, et al. Geriatric oncology: a clinical approach to the older patient with cancer. Eur J Cancer. 2003;39:870–80.
12. Katz S, et al. Studies of illness in the age. The index of ADL: a standardised measure of biological and psychological function. JAMA. 1963;185:914–9.
13. Lawton MP, Brody EM. Assessment of older people: self-maintaining and instrumental activities of daily living. Gerontologist. 1969;9:179–86.
14. Monfardini S, et al. Validation of a multidimensional evaluation scale for use in elderly cancer patients. Cancer. 1996;77:395–401.
15. Miller MD, et al. Rating chronic medical illness burden in gero-psychiatric practice and research: application of the Cumulative Illness Rating Scale. Psychiatry Res. 1992;41:237–48.
16. Folstein MF, et al. "Mini Mental State": a practical method for grading the cognitive state of patients for the clinician. J Psichiatr Res. 1975;12:189–98.
17. Hickie C, Snowdon J. Depression scales for the elderly: GDS. Clin Gerontol. 1987;6:51–3.
18. Extermann M, Aapro M, Bernabei R, et al. Use of the comprehensive geriatric assessment in older cancer patients: recommendations from the task force on CGA of the International Society of Geriatric Oncology (SIOG). Crit Rev Oncol Hematol. 2005;55(3):241–55.
19. Aapro M, Bernard-Marty C. Brain EG, et al:Anthracycline cardiotoxicity in the elderly cancer patient: A SIOG expert position paper. Ann Oncol. 2011;22:257–67.
20. Extermannb M, Boler I, Reich RR, et al. Predicting the risk of chemotherapy toxicity in older patients: the chemotherapy risk assessment scale for high-age patients (CRASH) score. Cancer. 2012;118(13):3377–86.
21. Ritchie CS, Kvale E, Fisch MJ. Multimorbidity: an issue of growing importance for oncologists. J Oncol Pract Am Soc Clin Oncol. 2011;7:371–4.
22. Jørgensen TL, Hallas J, Friis S, Herrstedt J. Comorbidity in elderly cancer patients in relation to overall and cancer-specific mortality. Br J Cancer. 2012;106(7):1353–60.
23. Koroukian SM, Murray P, Madigan E. Comorbidity, disability, and geriatric syndromes in elderly cancer patients receiving home health care. J Clin Oncol Off J Am Soc Clin Oncol. 2006;24:2304–10.
24. Guiding principles for the care of older adults with multimorbidity: an approach for clinicians: American Geriatrics Society Expert Panel on the Care of Older Adults with Multimorbidity. *J Am Geriatr Soc*. 2012;60(10):E1–E25
25. Steinman MA, Seth Landefeld C, Rosenthal GE, Berthenthal D, Sen S, Kaboli PJ. Polypharmacy and prescribing quality in older people. J Am Geriatr Soc. 2006;54(10):1516–23.
26. Sogaard M, Thomsen RW, Bossen KS, Sorensen HT, Norgaard M. The impact of comorbidity on cancer survival: a review. Clin Epidemiol. 2013;5:3–29.
27. Luciani AB, Battisti N, Romanato G, Caldiera S, Bergamo F, Roma A, Zagonel V, Foa P. The assessment of chemotherapy risk in elderly cancer patients: validation of the CRASH score in an Italian cohort. J Clin Oncol. 2015; 33 (suppl; abstr e20521).
28. Maggiore RJ, Dale W, Gross CP, Feng T, Tew WP, Mohile SG, et al. Polypharmacy and potentially inappropriate medication use in older adults with cancer undergoing chemotherapy: effect on chemotherapy-related toxicity and hospitalization during treatment. J Am Geriatr Soc. 2014;62:1505–1512 ([Epub 2014/07/22]).
29. Zauderer M, Patil S, Hurria A. Feasibility and toxicity of dose-dense adjuvant chemotherapy in older women with breast cancer. Breast Cancer Res Treat. 2009;117:205–10.
30. Giordano SH, Pinder M, Duan Z, et al. Congestive heart failure (CHF) in older women treated with anthracycline (A) chemotherapy (C). J Clin Oncol. 2006; 24 (abstr 521)
31. Balducci L, Beghe C. Pharmacology of chemotherapy in the older cancer patient. Cancer Control. 1999;6:466–70.
32. Van Dalen EC, van der Pal HJ, Caron HN, Kremer LC. Different dosage schedules for reducing cardiotoxicity in cancer patients receiving anthracycline chemotherapy. Cochrane Database Syst Rev. 2006;4, CD005008.
33. Van Dalen EC, Michiels EMC, Caron HN, Kremer LCM. Different anthracycline derivates for reducing cardiotoxicity in cancer patients. Cochrane Database Syst Rev. 2006;4, CD005006. doi:10.1002/14651858.CD00506.pub2.
34. Fumoleau P, Roché H, Kerbrat P, et al. Long-term cardiac toxicity after adjuvant epirubicin-based chemotherapy in early breast cancer: French Adjuvant Study Group results. Ann Oncol. 2006;17:85–92.

35. Giotta F, Lorusso V, Maiello E, et al. Liposomal-encapsulated doxorubicin plus cyclophosphamide as first line therapy in metastatic breast cancer: a phase II multicentric study. Ann Oncol. 2007;18: vi66–69.
36. O'Brien MER, Wigler N, Inbar M, et al. Reduced cardiotoxicity and comparable efficacy in a phase III trial of pegylated liposomal doxorubicin HCl (CAELYX/Doxil) versus conventional doxorubicin for first-line treatment of metastatic breast cancer. Ann Oncol. 2004;15:440–9.

Treatments in Patients with Cancer and Cardiac Diseases

Iris Parrini, Chiara Lestuzzi, Cezar Iliescu, and Brigida Stanzione

C. Lestuzzi et al. (eds.), *Manual of Cardio-oncology*, DOI 10.1007/978-3-319-40236-9_15

15.1 Introduction

The incidence and the prevalence of both cardiovascular and the neoplastic diseases are increasing, as are the therapeutic possibilities and survival. Thus, identifying the best cardiovascular care in a patient ready to start an antineoplastic treatment is becoming a rather common problem.

The coexistence of two different diseases may rise several problems:

- The presence of the tumor might worsen the cardiac status
- The antineoplastic treatments might directly or indirectly worsen the preexisting cardiac problems or may limit the cardiac therapeutic options.
- There are pharmacological interactions between cardiac and antineoplastic drugs
- The prognosis of either cardiac or neoplastic disease might influence the therapeutic choices

These points will be analyzed in summary here (for more details go to the relative chapters).

15.1.1 Risk of Worsening of Cardiac Status Due to the Tumor

- Several tumors induce a hypercoagulable status and might increase the risk of thromboembolism [1, 2]. In patients with atrial fibrillation (AF), history of deep vein thrombosis, and/or pulmonary embolism, mechanical prosthetic cardiac valves anticoagulant therapy should be optimized and followed strictly unless actively bleeding.
- A change in the anticoagulant strategy may be required in particular cases: oral anticoagulants (OA) may be less effective in patients with bowel disease, or—on the other hand—be less tolerated in case of bleeding. Low molecular weight heparins (LMWH) are the first choice in treatment and prophylaxis of venous thromboembolism in cancer, since they are more effective and safe compared to OA. To date, there are insufficient evidence to recommend NOACs in cancer patients [3–5]. (See also Chap. 6: "Thromboembolic disorders")

> **In patients with chronic AF or mechanical prosthetic valves, LMWH at dosage of 100 UI/kg twice a day should be considered as the optimal alternative to OA until the cancer has been cured.**

15

- New onset or recurrence of AF is rather common in lung cancer patients, mostly after thoracic surgery, and affects negatively the clinical outcome.
  - ECG and possible Holter monitoring are useful to early detection of arrhythmias. In patients at high risk (clinical history of recurring AF, enlarged left atrium, depressed left ventricular function), antiarrhythmic prophylaxis may be necessary. Unless contraindicated in patients with thyroid dysfunction or by drug–drug interactions, betablockers and amiodarone are the preferred agents.
- Severe anemia (as observed in some **hematologic** malignancies or in solid tumors with severe bleeding) may decompensate a patient with ischemic heart disease or a patient with dilated cardiomyopathy. Secondary tachycardia may also cause angina or precipitate heart failure in patients with both systolic and diastolic dysfunction.
  - Try to correct anemia as far as possible.

  - Persistent sinus tachycardia should be treated if not well tolerated: low dose beta-blockers (bisoprolol, starting with 1.25 mg once a day and carefully titrating the dose according to blood pressure) or ivabradine (5 to 7.5 mg twice a day) in case of hypotension are useful.

15.1.2 Antineoplastic Treatments Interfering with the Cardiovascular Function

- Several antineoplastic treatments are associated with an increased risk of thromboembolism, which may be life-threatening [6].
  - Patients with other thrombosis risk factors should receive appropriate prophylaxis [7].
- Some antineoplastic drugs (as platinum, for instance) require the infusion of large amount of fluid to prevent nephrotoxicity. **In patients with dilated cardiomyopathy, or with diastolic dysfunction, the volume overload may precipitate acute decompensation and pulmonary edema.**

> **In patients with left ventricular dysfunction, a careful balance of fluid loads is necessary.**

- Some antineoplastic treatments may cause an electrolyte imbalance (even indirectly, because of emesis, or of bone or tumor lysis) or may prolong the QT interval. In patients with a clinical history of arrhythmias or with ischemic heart disease, this might be harmful.
  - Baseline routine examinations in any neoplastic patient should include an ECG; cardiologic evaluation should be asked if it is abnormal.
  - In patients at risk, the possibly precipitating factors (anemia, electrolyte changes…) should be prevented or promptly corrected.
- Following abdominal surgery or antineoplastic treatments inducing prolonged emesis, some patients may be unable to take regularly their prescribed cardiologic drugs.
  - Oncologists and surgeons should ask a cardiologist's consult before therapy in any case there is such a risk. Some treatments (lipid lowering drugs, acetylsalicylic acid, anticoagulants in patients with recurring atrial fibrillation but in sinus rhythm, drugs with very long blood half-life as amiodarone, for instance) may be temporarily discontinued; other treatments should be changed from oral to transdermal, intravenous route, or rectal (i.e., aspirin 300 mg). It is better to plan the change some days in advance, in order to assess its efficacy.

15.1.3 Pharmacological Interactions Between Cardiac and Antineoplastic Drugs

The pharmacological interactions may be due to both a metabolic interaction (drugs metabolized by inhibitors or substrates of Cytochrome p450 [CYP450]) or to a cumulative side effect.

Metabolic Interactions

The association of a drug metabolized by the CYP 450 and a substrate, inhibitor, or inducer of the same cytochrome may be dangerous and require dose adjustments).

- Almost all the tyrosine kinase inhibitors (TKI) are ***metabolized*** by **the CYP450 3A4**, as several cardiac drugs (amiodarone, apixaban, diltiazem, edoxaban, flecainide, losartan, prasugrel, ranolazine, rivaroxaban, most statins excluding pravastatin and rosuvastatin, verapamil).
- Verapamil, diltiazem, amiodarone, and imatinib are ***inhibitors*** of CYP 450 3A4
- Other oncologic drugs (docetaxel, paclitaxel, imatinib, irinotecan, ondansetron, sirolimus, tamoxifen, paclitaxel, vincristine) and cardiac drugs (all the calcium channel blockers, atorvastatin, lovastatin, simvastatin) are ***substrates*** of CYP450 3A4.

In ◘ Table 15.1, the major interaction between the most used oncologic and cardiovascular drugs are summarized. However, many other interactions—not considered in this text—may be possible. There are several regularly updated sites to check interactions, as: www.drugs.com/drug_interaction.php

In ◘ Table 15.2 , are described antineoplastic drugs with low risk of cardiac toxicity

Cumulative Effects

QT interval may be prolonged by drugs commonly used in oncology (TKI, arsenic trioxide, bortezomib, ondansetron, tamoxifen, tacrolimus) and by several cardiac drugs (amiodarone, dronedarone, flecainide, furosemide, indapamide, nicardipine, ranolazine, quinidine, sotalol).

- The use of two or more drugs prolonging the QT interval may lead to severe, even life-threatening ventricular arrhythmias, as torsade de pointes and ventricular fibrillation.
- However, some drugs (as octreotide and the antiemetics dolasetron and granisetron) prolong the QT interval without inducing arrhythmias; with some other drugs the arrhythmic risk is limited to the higher doses or to the presence of a genetic predisposition.

A frequently updated, useful site to check drugs which may prolong the QT interval and related the arrhythmic risk is: www.qtdrugs.org

- Some TKI, as Sunitinib and thalidomide, may cause **bradycardia**, which may be severe and symptomatic in combination with cardiac drugs with the same effect, as beta-blockers and transdermal clonidine
  - In case of severe bradycardia, consider reduction/changes of cardiovascular drugs. In extreme cases, a pacemaker implantation might be indicated in order to continue the therapy.
- Lenalidomide given together with statins may increase the risk of **rhabdomyolisis.**
- Clopidrogrel, commonly used in coronary artery disease, especially with drug-eluting stents, has hepatic metabolism but in cancer patients with liver failure the efficacy has not been well established.
- Prasugrel without the same problem has major risk of bleeding.

15.2 Practical Approach to the Patient with Cardiovascular Disease

Any cardiac disease may be adversely influenced by different antineoplastic treatment side effects (◘ Fig. 15.1). As a general rule, a patient with known heart disease, before starting an antineoplastic therapy, should have his cardiac problem reassessed, and his/her therapy optimized (◘ Table 15.3).

Table 15.1 Pharmacological Interactions Between Cardiac and Antineoplastic Drugs

	Drug	Sunitinib	Sorafenib	Axitinib	Regorafenib	Pazopanib	Imatinib	Nilotinib	Erlotinib	Dasatinib	Everolimus	Others
Diuretics	Furosemide	NO	NO	NO	NO	NO	NO	NO	NO	NO	NO	
	Torasemide	NO	NO				A+	A+		NO		
	Hydroclorotiazide	NO	NO	NO	NO	NO					NO	
	Spironolacton	NO	NO									
B-blockers	Metoprolol	AE*§	NO				***A+***	A+		***P+***		
	Bisoprolol	AE*§	NO				***A+***	A+		***A+***		
	Carvedilol	AE*§	NO				A+	A+		A+		
	Atenolol	AE*§	NO	NO	NO	NO	NO	NO		NO	NO	
	Nebivol	NO	NO	NO	NO	NO	II	NO		NO	NO	
	Sotalolol	AE#	AE#			AE#		***A+ AE#***				
Ace-inhibitors	Enalapril	NO	NO	NO	NO	NO	A+P+	A+		P+	NO	
	Ramipril	NO	NO	NO	NO	NO	NO	NO		NO	NO	
	Lisinopril	NO	NO	NO	NO	NO	A+			P+	NO	
	Quinapril	NO	NO	NO	NO	NO					NO	
Sartanes	Losartan	NO	A-	II	II	II	A-P+	A+		A+P+	II	
	Candesartan	NO	NO	NO	NO		NO	NO		NO	NO	
	Telmisartan	NO	NO	NO	NO						NO	
	Olmesartan	NO	NO	NO	NO						NO	
	Irbesartan	NO	NO	NO	NO	NO	NO	NO	NO	NO	NO	

(continued)

Table 15.1 (continued)

	Drug	Sunitinib	Sorafenib	Axitinib	Regorafenib	Pazopanib	Imatinib	Nilotinib	Erlotinib	Dasatinib	Everolimus	Others
Calcium-channel antagonists	Verapamil	***Ø AE*§***	II	II (P+)	II (P+)	***Ø P+***	***ØP+***	A+P+	***ØP+***	***A+P+***	***Ø P+***	**+ Ibrutinib:P+ Ø**
	Diltiazem	***Ø P+ AE*§***	II	II (P+)	II (P+)	***Ø P+***	***ØA+P+***	P+		***Ø P+AE§A+***	***Ø P+AE§***	**+ Ibrutinib:P+ Ø**
	Nifedipine	AE*	II	II (P+)	II	II	***A+***	A+		***A+***	II	
	Amlodipine	AE*	II	II (P+)	II	II	A+	A+		A+	II	
	Lacedipine	II	II	II (P+)	II	II					II	
	Nicardipine	II	II								Ø **P+**	
	Ranolazine	***AE#***	***AE#***	II (P+)	II	***AE#***		***AE#***		***AE#***	II	
Lipid-lowering drugs	Simvastatine	NO	A+				***A+P+***	***A+P+***	***Ø^^***	***A+P+***	**A+**	**+ Lenalidomide: rabdomyolysis**
	Atorvastatin	NO	A+				***A+***P+	A+	***Ø^^***	A+P+		**+ Lenalidomide: rabdomyolysis**
	Pravastatin	NO	NO	NO	NO	NO	NO	NO	***Ø^^***	NO	NO	**+ Lenalidomide: rabdomyolysis**
	Rosuvastatin	NO							***Ø^^***			**+ Lenalidomide: rabdomyolysis**
	Ezetimibe	NO	NO	NO	NO	NO					NO	
	Gemfibrozil	NO	NO	NO	NO	NO	NO	NO	NO	NO	NO	
	Fluvastatin	NO	NO	NO	NO	NO	NO	NO	NO	NO	NO	**+ Lenalidomide: rabdomyolysis**

Antiplatelets, anticoa-gulants	Aspirin	NO	A+				NO	NO	&			**+ Ibrutinib: AE &; + Sirolimus: renal failure**
	Clopidogrel	NO	NO	NO	NO		A+	A+		A+	NO	**+ Ibrutinib: AE** &
	Ticlopidine				**AE** &					**AE**		**+ Ibrutinib: AE** &
	Acenocumarol	NO	A+				A+	A+				**+ Ibrutinib: AE** &
	Ticagrelor				**AE** &							**+ Ibrutinib/ Cabozantinib: AE** &
	Prasugrel											**+ Ibrutinib/ Cabozantinib: AE** &
	Warfarin	II	II				A+	A+	&	A+		**+ Ibrutinib: AE** &
	Heparin	NO	NO				A+			P+		**+ Ibrutinib: AE** &
	Dabigatran	NO	NO	NO	**Ø AE** &	NO	NO	NO		**Ø AE** &	NO	**+ Ibrutinib: AE** &
	Rivaroxaban				**AE** &					**AE** &		**+ Ibrutinib: AE** &
	Apixaban									**AE** &		**+ Ibrutinib/ temsirolimus: AE**&
	Digoxin	EA#	A-				***A-***	**AE #**		***AE#***		

(continued)

Table 15.1 (continued)

	Drug	Sunitinib	Sorafenib	Axitinib	Regorafenib	Pazopanib	Imatinib	Nilotinib	Erlotinib	Dasatinib	Everolimus	Others
Anti-arrhythmics	Amiodarone	***AE# P+***	***AE# P+***	II	***AP+***	AE#	***A+P+***	***A+ AE #***		***A+ AE #***	II	
	Dronedarone	***Ø AE#***	***Ø AE#***			***Ø AE#***		**A+ AE #**			**Ø AE#**	**+ Ibrutinib:P+**
	Propafenone	***AE#***	***AE#***	II	II			**A+ AE #**			II	
	Flecainide	***AE#***	***AE#***	II	II			**A+ AE #**			II	

***A* active interactions** (the oncologic drug alters the cardiovascular drug metabolism), *AE* addictive effect, Hypothetic= possible interaction (according to pharmacokinetics) but never reported so far, *NO* no interaction, *P* passive interaction (the oncologic drug metabolism is altered by the cardiovascular drug).
+ increases the concentration or effect of the drug; – reduces the concentration or effect of the drug
* Increases PR interval at ECG (possible atrio-ventricula block)
§ Bradicardia
# Increases QT interval at ECG (possible ventricular arrhythmias)
& Hemorrhagic risk
In bold the most frequent or clinically relevant interactions
Ø = dangerous interaction (black box warning)

15

Table 15.2 Antineoplastic drugs with low risk of cardiac toxicity

Drug	Use in oncology	Cardiotoxicity	Warnings
Citarabine	AML and other lymphoproliferative diseases.	At the usual dosage, very rare cases of arrhythmias have been reported; cardiomyopathy with fatal consequences has been described only when cytarabine is used at high dosage, in autologous staminal cell transplant.	Hematological, pulmonary, CNS, gastrointestinal toxicities
Gemcitabine	Bladder, lung, pancreatic, breast, and ovarian cancer	Cardiac toxicity is described as not common or rare. It can be used for all patients except for those with severe heart failure.	Pulmonary, hepatobiliary, gastrointestinal, and hematological toxicity
Vinorelbine	NSCLC, breast cancer	Only few cases of angina, myocardial infarction, and ECG abnormalities have been reported. It may cause respiratory distress which can mimic heart failure.	Pulmonary, gastrointestinal, and hematological toxicity
Carboplatin	NSCLC, breast, ovarian, endometrial cancer	Cardiovascular events, such as heart attack, have been seldom reported	Hematological toxicity, neurotoxicity. It should not be administered in case of kidney injury or immunosuppression
Chlorambucil	CLL, follicular lymphoma.	Cardiac events never reported	Gastrointestinal and bone marrow toxicity
BCNU	Brain cancer, multiple myeloma, Hodgkin disease, Non-Hodgkin lymphoma	Rare cases of cardiac events	Pulmonary, gastrointestinal, hematological, hepatic, kidney, testicular toxicity.
DTIC	Melanoma, Hodgkin disease, sarcoma.	Cardiac events never reported	Hematological toxicity, hepatic veno-occlusive disease, and hepatic necrosis
Bleomycin	Testicular cancer, Hodgkin disease.	Moderately increased MI risk at young ages has been described, probably because it is used with other drugs.	Lung fibrosis.

(continued)

Table 15.2 (continued)

Drug	Use in oncology	Cardiotoxicity	Warnings
Etoposide	SCLC, testicular cancer, high grade neuroendocrine tumors	Arrhythmias and myocardial ischemia are not common. Congestive heart failure has been reported in high-dose therapies	Gastrointestinal and hematological toxicity
Fludarabine	CLL, follicular lymphoma	Arrhythmias and heart failure rarely reported	Hematological and gastrointestinal toxicity
Methotrexate	Breast cancer	Pericarditis and pericardial effusion are very rare; hypotension is rarely reported.	
Mitomycin C	Different types of cancer such as breast cancer or colon cancer	Cardiac events not reported	Hematological and gastrointestinal adverse events
Oxaliplatin	Colon and pancreatic cancer	Cardiac events not reported	Neurological and gastrointestinal toxicity
Topotecan	Ovarian and cervical cancer, SCLC	Cardiac events not reported	Hematological toxicity

AML acute myeloblastic leukemia, *CLL* chronic lymphocytic leukemia, *SCLC* small cell lung carcinoma
Very common ≥1/10
Common from ≥ 1/100 to <1/10
Not common from ≥ 1/1000 to <1/100
Rare from ≥1/10,000 to <1/1000

15

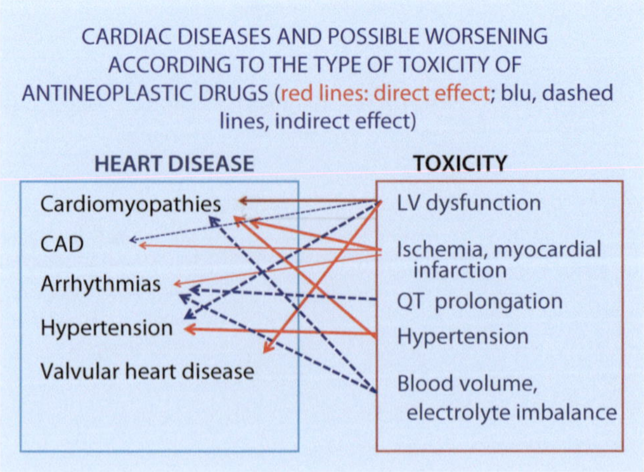

Fig. 15.1 Cardiac diseases (*left column*) at risk to be worsened/decompensated by some anticancer treatments' side effects (*right column*). *CAD* coronary artery disease, *LV* left ventricle

Table 15.3 General rules to be followed by the cardiologist in evaluating a patient undergoing anticancer therapy

1. Basal assessment of cardiologic problem
Severity (even second level tests)
Clinical impact (symptoms, mandatory drugs…)
Comorbidities (renal failure, diabetes, etc.)
Stratify the risk of progression
2. Optimize pharmacological therapy
Optimal blood pressure
Correct electrolyte imbalances
Check for drug interactions
Prefer potentially cardioprotective drugs
3. Consider possible non-pharmacological interventions
At short term
At medium term

15.2.1 Dilated and/or Hypokinetic Cardiomyopathies (CMP)

Cardiac function or symptoms may be worsened:

- By treatments which may impair left ventricular function (as anthracyclines, trastuzumab, tyrosine kinase inhibitors)
- By treatments requiring a large volume overload (as platinum)
- By any treatment which cause an increase in heart rate (either directly or causing severe anemia)

The oncologist may prevent/reduce the risk, when prescribing some antineoplastic therapies:

- Anthracyclines: the cardiac damage may be reduced by the association of prolonged infusions, dexrazoxane, of refracted reducing dose or use of liposomal formulations.
- TKI should be used—if possible—at lower dosage
- Anemia should be treated with erythropoietin

The cardiologist should check a baseline left ventricular function and optimize the cardiologic therapy before starting and follow up the patient frequently during the antineoplastic treatment.

- **Anthracyclines**: if at baseline echocardiogram shows any systolic or diastolic dysfunction, follow the suggestions above (CMP).
- **Anti-VEGF**: have a baseline and regular follow-up echocardiograms.

After an acute coronary syndrome or revascularization, the risk/benefit ratio of starting immediately or postpone for some weeks a required anti-VEGF therapy should be evaluated in the single patient; in either case, a close symptomatic monitoring should be done at least for the first 3 months if possible.

Table 15.4 Drugs preferred in the hypertensive patient undergoing anticancer treatments according to the possible side effects

Antineoplastic drug	Possible side effects	Cardiac drugs of choice
Anthracyclines, trastuzumab	Left ventricular dysfunction	ACE inhibitors or ARB, Beta-blockers
Fluoropyrimidines	Ischemia	Calcium channel blockers (amlodipine, nifedipine, diltiazem)
Bevacizumab	Hypertension, endothelial dysfunction, reduced NO production	Nebivolol, ACE inhibitors or ARB, Beta-blockers, Diuretics
Anti-VEGF TKI	Hypertension, Left ventricular dysfunction, CYP450 interaction	ACE or ARB inhibitors (no Losartan), Beta-blockers (Nebivolol and Atenolol preferred), Diuretics
Taxanes	Tachycardia, edema	Beta-blockers, Diuretics

ACE angiotensin converting enzyme, *ARB* angiotensin receptor blockers, *TKI* tyrosine kinase inhibitors, *VEGF* vascular endothelial growth factor

- **Fluoropyrimidines**: have a stress test before starting CT and adjust medical therapy (or consider revascularization) if positive; start first course at 50–75 % of regular dose; check side effects with ECG, visit and possibly stress test the last day of first course (see also Chap. 11, "Cardiac ischemia")

15.2.2 Hypertension

In patients with hypertension, a cardiologic evaluation and possibly some changes in chronic therapy should be planned before antineoplastic therapies, according to the possible side effects (Table 15.4).

- Before starting therapies with anti-VEGFR, the blood pressure should be optimized.
- If the antineoplastic treatments may cause bradycardia (as sunitinib, sorafenib, 5-fluorouracil) avoid verapamil, diltiazem (which may also interfere with the TKI), and strong beta-blockers.
- Have an echocardiogram before starting therapies with anthracyclines or trastuzumab: if hypertensive CMP is detected, follow the same rules above mentioned. Moreover, amongst the antihypertensive drugs, choose those with a protective effect on the myocardium (ACE-inhibitors, beta-blockers).

15.2.3 Coronary Artery Disease (CAD)

A baseline cardiologic evaluation should be planned before any possibly cardiotoxic antineoplastic therapy. Further interventions will be planned according to the possible cardiotoxicity of each antineoplastic agent.

Treatment Options for Chronic CAD

Treatment options for chronic CAD are: medical treatment in patients with stable angina; revascularization in patients with severe CAD and unstable or severe angina. The choice depends on the severity of cancer status [8].

- Revascularization with surgical coronary artery by-pass grafting (**CABG**) may be considered in patients with good cancer prognosis. Using of extracorporeal circulation considers the possibility of spread of the tumor, bleeding, and infections
- Percutaneous angioplasty (**PTCI**) may be preferred in patients with aggressive cancer. It may be performed with different techniques:
  - Dilatation without stenting (POBA). It is suitable in limited anatomic conditions only
  - Dilatation with implant of bare metal stent (BMS). It requires dual antiplatelet treatment for 4 weeks
  - Dilatation with implant of drug-eluting stent (DES). It requires dual antiplatelet treatment for one year. For the use of antiplatelets agents in cancer patients, see below the paragraph about acute coronary syndromes. Second and third generation DES appear to have comparable risk of stent thrombosis compared with bare metal stents with less restenosis and should be considered in the majority of the cancer patients.
- In case of **neoplasms requiring surgery and CAD requiring revascularization**, the timing of treatments should be planned on an individual basis, considering various options: staged approach (surgical treatment of neoplasm followed by revascularization or vice versa) or combined approach (cardiac and cancer surgery at the same session) [9].

Treatment Options for CAD with Acute Coronary Syndrome (ACS)

Treatment options for CAD with ACS are: medical treatment, thrombolysis, and catheter-based revascularization.

- Often the more aggressive strategy is not given to cancer patients, either because a concern about the cancer prognosis, cancer-related or unrelated comorbidities, including thrombocytopenia. Each decision should be taken on a individual basis, and poor cancer prognosis, renal or hepatic failure, or other severe comorbidities (like sepsis or cachexia) will trigger a more conservative approach.
- **A rather frequent condition which can be observed in cancer patients and should be discussed in detail is thrombocytopenia. It should be considered that:**
  - Thrombocytopenia does not protect from thrombosis, because platelets may be larger and more adhesive to the vascular surface.
  - Actually AMI has been reported in patients who have thrombocytopenia that is associated with various conditions and occurs in up to 39 % of patients who have both thrombocytopenia and cancer.
  - In a retrospective study of 2007, therapy with ASA was associated with a significantly improved 7-day survival after ACS in cancer patients, with or without thrombocytopenia, and not associated with more severe bleeding [10].
  - There are no large studies to assess the safety of antiplatelet or fibrinolytic agents in thrombocytopenic cancer patients, but several cases published in the literature report that their use may be relatively safe [11].

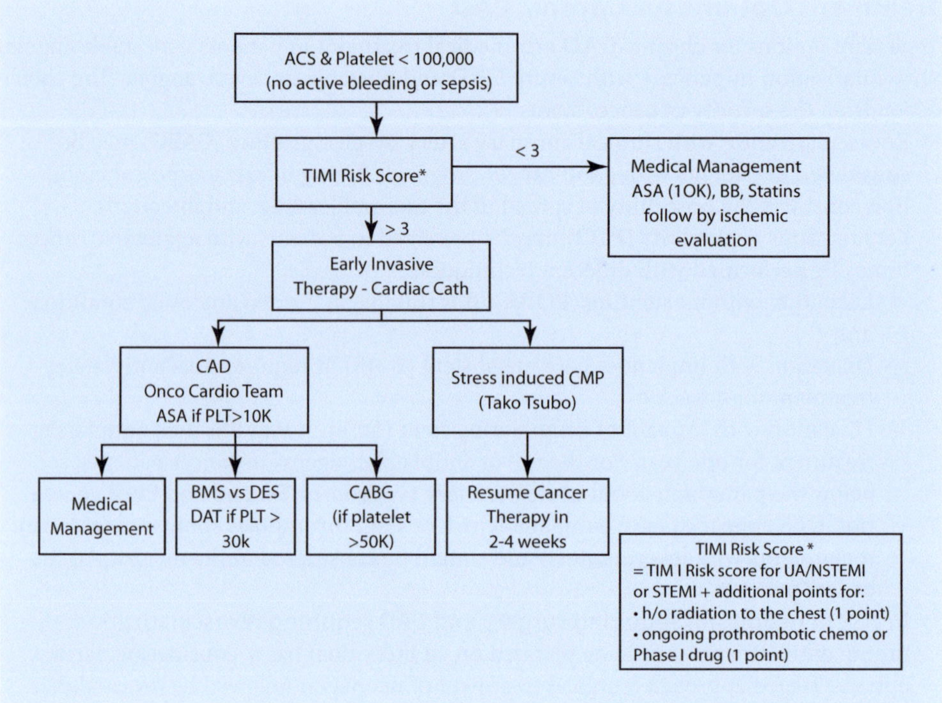

Fig. 15.2 Suggested operative flowchart in presence of Acute Coronary Syndrome (ACS) in thrombocytopenic patients. *ASA* acetylsalicylic acid, *BB* beta-blockers, *BMS* bare metal stent, *CABG* coronary artery by-pass graft, *CAD* coronary artery disease, *CMP* cardiomyopathy, *DAT* dual antiplatelet therapy, *DES* drug-eluting stent, *NSTEMI* non-ST elevation myocardial infarction, *STEMI* ST elevation myocardial infarction, *UA* unstable angina. Reproduced with permission from Iliescu CA, Iliescu GD, Marmagkiolis K. Myocardial Ischemia and Acute Coronary Syndrome in Cancer Patients. In: OncoCardiology, 2015.

- A retrospective study from MD Anderson Cancer Center published in 2012 showed that the patients treated with catheter-based reperfusion had a significantly better outcome; a significant advantage in survival was also given by beta-blockers, aspirin, and statins [12].
- Approaches to the treatment of AMI in thrombocytopenic patients might be better directed toward the evaluation of platelet function than toward platelet count, and the risk–benefit equation of invasive procedures and antithrombotic therapies may need to take this information into account [11].
- An operative flowchart for thrombocytopenic patients with ACS is reported in Fig. 15.2.

Patients with acute coronary syndrome and a cancer with medium-long term good prognosis should be treated according to the current guidelines for non-cancer patients. Changes in the treatment strategy may be necessary in particular cases, but thoughtfully weigh the risk and benefit.

In case of urgent surgery after PCI, intravenous tirofiban can be administered and clopidogrel restarted with dose of 300 mg.

- Cancer patients with bare metal stents (BMS) appear to have a sevenfold increase in risk of stent thrombosis compared to general population with the majority of events in patients on dual antiplatelet therapy (DAPT) [13].

- As cancer is a prothrombotic state, one might think that more potent antiplatelet therapies now available (Prasugrel, Ticagrelor) would be a better therapeutic option for this patient population. The advent of an oral reversible P2Y12 inhibitor (Ticagrelor), with rapid onset of action and offset of antiplatelet effect within 2–3 days, would allow better flexibility in the management of all types of patients with acute coronary syndromes.
  - The TRITON-TIMI 38 was a head-to-head trial to assess the efficacy and safety of the experimental antiplatelet agent prasugrel vs. standard care with clopidogrel on top of aspirin. Besides ischemic protection at expense of bleeding disadvantage, **prasugrel-treated patients experienced a three times higher rate of colonic neoplasms than with clopidogrel, and this difference was significant.** The gastrointestinal bleeding preceded the diagnosis of colonic neoplasms only in half of the patients.
  - More delicate platelet inhibition and shorter exposure to oral antiplatelet agents will prevail. We have used Ticagrelor in cancer patients with multivessel stenting, but larger clinical trials with different dual antiplatelet therapy combinations are needed to prove the superiority of one specific regimen [14].

15.2.4 Arrhythmias

- **Atrial fibrillation**: before starting therapies with drugs which could impair LV function, obtain a ventricular rate <80/m' and check regularly heart rate during chemotherapy; beta-blockers are the preferred drugs if anthracyclines are used. Thromboembolic prophylaxis and effective stroke prevention with oral anticoagulation should be prescribed, but the balance between thromboembolic and bleeding risk and the possible drug interactions must be evaluated (See Chaps. 6 and 7)
- **Bradycardia**: be careful when using fluoropyrimidines (mostly with 5-FU), sunitinib, and sorafenib. Obtain ECGs and possibly Holter monitoring during at least the first course of therapy, to assess the tolerability.
- **Ventricular arrhythmias**: check blood K+ and Mg++ (and correct with supplements if low) before starting CT and during the treatment in case of prolonged emesis; have regular ECG and possibly Holter monitoring when using fluoropyrimidines, platinum, or drugs which can prolong the QT interval. Consider also the possibility of underlying cardiac ischemia.

15.2.5 Valvular Heart Disease

The approach differs in patients with native valve disease and patients with prosthetic valves.

Native Valve Disease

Assess the entity of the dysfunction, the clinical impact, the possibility of progression.

- **Mild dysfunction** usually does not require any change in planned therapies
- **Moderate dysfunction** should be evaluated in prospect, considering the possible indication of cardiac surgery on the medium term, the planned time to be spent in antineoplastic treatments, and the prognosis of the tumor. The risk of an urgent cardiac surgery in a patient under chemotherapy may be very high. If CT is not urgent,

anticipating cardiac surgery, with insertion of a biologic valve which will not require lifelong anticoagulation, might be the best choice, mostly in patients with low grade tumors.
- **Severe dysfunction** usually requires cardiac surgery, which should be planned possibly before the antineoplastic treatment. In case of patients with severe aortic stenosis requiring urgent major abdominal or gynecological surgery for cancer, balloon aortic valvuloplasty may be used as bridge therapy [15]. In patients with expected survival more than 2 years, Transcatheter Aortic Valve Replacement (TAVR) can be considered.

There is a concern about the risk that cardiac surgery with extracorporeal circulation might favor the metastatic spread in solid tumors or worsen the prognosis in hematologic tumors [16, 17]. This risk has not been confirmed in the most recent studies [18–20].

A joint evaluation by the oncologist and the cardiologist (including careful assessment of severity, prognosis, and treatment options of each disease) is necessary to plan the best therapeutic approach in the individual patient.

Prosthetic Valves

- **Biologic valves** have no particular problem, beside the risk of bacterial endocarditis in case of severe depression of immunity defenses.
- **Mechanical valves** require chronic oral anticoagulation, which should be continued—if possible—even during chemotherapy. The ***oncologist*** should use—if possible—drugs less likely to induce thrombocytopenia, which do not interfere with oral anticoagulants and which do not cause emesis. If these drugs cannot be avoided, or if there is any risk of bleeding, LMWH may be used as an alternative.

LMWH must be prescribed at dose of 100 Units/kg twice a day. It should be taken in mind that the thrombosis of a mechanical prosthetic valve requires few days and is a life-threatening event. Proper and constant anticoagulation is mandatory. If blood platelets are reduced to <75,000/ml and there is a risk of bleeding, the dose of LMWH may be reduced but always given every 12 h.

15.2.6 Varicose Veins

Some antineoplastic treatments, as tamoxifen, fluoropirimidines, and anti-VEGFR, may increase the risk of deep vein thrombosis.
- Consider mechanical and/or pharmacological prophylaxis
- Suggest regular physical activity (walking, cycling)

15.2.7 Patients with Cardiac Implantable Electronic Devices (CIED) Who Need Radiotherapy

Radiotherapy may impair the function (signal interference, memory data loss or parameter reset) of these devices, even if they are not included in the radiation field, because of scatter radiation. The consequences may be asymptomatic or cause even severe symptoms:

- **Pacemakers (PM)** are generally implanted for advanced heart block and symptomatic bradycardia. If the patient is "***pacemaker dependent***," the loss of PM function may cause severe symptoms.
- **Internal Cardioverter Defibrillator (ICD)** are implanted in patients with an increased risk of life-threatening ventricular arrhythmias. If it detects tachyarrhythmias, it delivers an electric shock to revert the rhythm. A dysfunction of an ICD may cause both inappropriate (i.e., in absence of dangerous arrhythmias) shock deliveries and failure of shock delivery in presence of life-threatening arrhythmias.

The risk of clinically relevant complications depends mostly on:

1. Cumulative dose of radiation received by the device
2. Pacing-dependency of the patient

In a recently published study, proximity of the radiation treatment field to the device did not predict for malfunction (actually, the malfunction rates were higher with treatments to the abdomen and pelvis region), and the use of neutron-producing radiation (>10 MV) was the principal risk factor for device malfunction [21].

15.3 Practical Approach to the Patient with Cardiac Implantable Electronic Devices [22, 23]

15.3.1 Before Starting Radiotherapy

- Inform the treating cardiologist and inform the patient
- Evaluate if patients is pacing-dependent. If so, evaluate if there are medical approaches which can reduce this condition (i.e., reduce digitalis, beta-blockers, or other drugs causing bradycardia)
- If ICD, check if anti-tachycardia therapy can be switched off by magnet
- Plan a device check-up if the last one was done > 3 months before starting radiotherapy

15.3.2 During Radiotherapy

- *If the dose is <2 Gy:*
- *PM in patient not pacing dependent:* Monitor heart rate during radiotherapy
  - **ICD**: program tachycardia therapy off or use magnet
- *If the dose is 2 to 10 Gy and patients is pacing dependent:*
  - Crash cart present during RT
  - Weekly check-up of the device
  - Have an external pacing device (external defibrillator for patients with ICD) ready
  - Alert the cardiologist to be able to intervene within 10 min
- **If the dose is estimated to exceed 10 Gy** consider device relocation and discuss the indications for radiation therapy device-related risks. If the treatment is necessary:
  - Monitor ECG during each treatment session
  - Crash cart present during RT

- Have an external pacing device (external defibrillator for patients with ICD) ready
- Alert cardiology to be able to intervene within 10 min
- Check-up within 24 h of each treatment session by a pacemaker technician

15.3.3 After Radiotherapy

CIEDs need to be interrogated 1, 3, and 6 months after the last RT due to the risk of latent damage.

References

1. Mitrugno A, Tormoen GW, Kuhn P, McCarty OJ. The prothrombotic activity of cancer cells in the circulation. Blood Rev. 2016;30(1):11–9.
2. Franco AT, Corken A, Ware J. Platelets at the interface of thrombosis, inflammation, and cancer. Blood. 2015;126:582–8.
3. Donato J, Campigotto F, Uhlmann EJ, et al. Intracranial hemorrhage in patients with brain metastases treated with therapeutic enoxaparin: a matched cohort study. Blood. 2015;126:494–9.
4. Easaw JC, Shea-Budgell MA, Wu CM, et al. Canadian consensus recommendations on the management of venous thromboembolism in patients with cancer. Part 1: prophylaxis. Curr Oncol. 2015;22:133–43.
5. Easaw JC, Shea-Budgell MA, Wu CM, et al. Canadian consensus recommendations on the management of venous thromboembolism in patients with cancer. Part 2: treatment. Curr Oncol. 2015;22: 144–55.
6. Khorana AA, Francis CW, Culakova E, et al. Thromboembolism is a leading cause of death in cancer patients receiving outpatient chemotherapy. J Thromb Haemost. 2007;5:632–4.
7. Oppelt P, Betbadal A, Nayak L. Approach to chemotherapy-associated thrombosis. Vasc Med. 2015;20:153–61.
8. Mistiaen WP. Cancer in heart disease patients: what are the limitations in the treatment strategy? Future Cardiol. 2013;9:535–47.
9. Darwazah AK. Surgical management of coronary artery disease associated with malignancy. J Card Surg. 2012;27:581–8.
10. Sarkiss MG, Yusuf SW, Warneke CL, et al. Impact of aspirin therapy in cancer patients with thrombocytopenia and acute coronary syndromes. Cancer. 2007;109:621–7.
11. Yusuf SW, Iliescu C, Bathina JD, et al. Antiplatelet therapy and percutaneous coronary intervention in patients with acute coronary syndrome and thrombocytopenia. Tex Heart Inst J. 2010;37:336–40.
12. Yusuf SW, Daraban N, Abbasi N, et al. Treatment and outcomes of acute coronary syndrome in the cancer population. Clin Cardiol. 2012;35:443–50.
13. Gross CM, Posch MG, Geier C, et al. Subacute coronary stent thrombosis in cancer patients. J Am Coll Cardiol. 2008;51:1232–3.
14. Serebruany VL. Aggressive chronic platelet inhibition with prasugrel and increased cancer risks: revising oral antiplatelet regimens? Fundamental and Clinical Pharmacology. 2009;23:411–7.
15. Kogoj P, Devjak R, Bunc M. Balloon aortic valvuloplasty (BAV) as a bridge to aortic valve replacement in cancer patients who require urgent non-cardiac surgery. Radiol Oncol. 2014;48:62–6.
16. Bach DS, Cimino N, Deeb GM. Unoperated patients with severe aortic stenosis. J Am Coll Cardiol. 2007;50:2018–9.
17. Samuels LE, Kaufman MS, Morris RJ, et al. Open heart surgery in patients with chronic lymphocytic leukemia. Leuk Res. 1999;23:71–5.
18. Yusuf SW, Sarfaraz A, Durand JB, et al. Management and outcomes of severe aortic stenosis in cancer patients. Am Heart J. 2011;161:1125–32.
19. Guler A, Sahin MA, Cingoz F, et al. Can cardiac surgery be performed safely on patients with haematological malignancies. Cardiovasc J Afr. 2012;23:194–6.
20. Plumereau F, Pinaud F, Roch A, Baufreton C. Do patients with haematological malignancy who need cardiopulmonary bypass have a short-term higher mortality or a higher chance of disease progression? Interact Cardiovasc Thorac Surg. 2014;19:474–8.

21. Grant JD, Jensen GL, Tang C, et al. Radiotherapy-induced malfunction in contemporary cardiovascular implantable electronic devices: clinical incidence and predictors. JAMA Oncol. 2015;1:624–32.
22. Hurkmans CW, Knegjens JL, Oei BS, et al. Dutch Society of Radiotherapy and Oncology (NVRO). Management of radiation oncology patients with a pacemaker or ICD: a new comprehensive practical guideline in The Netherlands. Dutch Society of Radiotherapy and Oncology (NVRO). Radiat Oncol. 2012;7:198.
23. Gauter-Fleckenstein B, Israel CW, Dorenkamp M, et al. DEGRO/DGK. DEGRO/DGK guideline for radiotherapy in patients with cardiac implantable electronic devices. Strahlenther Onkol. 2015;191: 393–404.

Hematopoietic Stem Cell Transplantation and Cardiotoxicity

Annalisa Natale, Stella Santarone, and Paolo Di Bartolomeo

C. Lestuzzi et al. (eds.), *Manual of Cardio-oncology*, DOI 10.1007/978-3-319-40236-9_16

16.1 Introduction

Hematopoietic stem cell transplantation (HCT) is now used worldwide in the treatment of many malignant and nonmalignant hematologic disorders and in the treatment of various solid tumors [1]. Every year, many thousands of patients receive an autologous or allogeneic transplant procedure. The diseases most often treated with autologous and/or allogeneic HCT are listed in ◘ Table 16.1. Our current knowledge of HCT biology derives from a vast body of experimental and clinical applications extending back from more than 60 years. The original context of using HCT to permit the use of myeloablative doses of anticancer therapy is still relevant today in the treatment of malignant diseases. The biologic bases of autologous HCT are completely different as compared to those of allogeneic HCT.

Autologous HCT involves the infusion of a patient's own hematopoietic stem cells to rescue the patient from bone marrow injury caused by high-dose chemotherapy and/or radiotherapy (total body irradiation) as part of a treatment for a malignant disorder. This preparative therapy is also called conditioning regimen. Usually, the patient's hematopoietic stem cells have been previously collected either from bone marrow or peripheral blood, cryopreserved and then thawed before reinfusion. In this setting, acute complications of conditioning regimen are very limited and include some well-known regimen-related organ toxicities, including cardiotoxicity, in addition to a very short (7–10 days) period of pancytopenia and associated infections.

Allogeneic HCT refers to any procedure where hemopoietic stem cells of any healthy donor type (related or unrelated) and any HLA compatibility (identical or partially identical) are given to a recipient with the intention of repopulating and replacing the hemopoietic system in total or in part. Stem cells can be collected from bone marrow, peripheral blood, or cord blood. The objective of the conditioning regimen before allogeneic HCT is both to eradicate cancer and to induce the immunosuppression that permits engraftment of donor cells. The preparative regimen can also augment the antitumor immune response by causing a breakdown of tumor cells, which results in a flood of tumor antigens into antigen-presenting cells. This flooding can lead to the proliferation of T cells, which attack the surviving malignant cells (graft-versus-tumor effect) [2]. A better understanding of graft-versus-tumor biology led to the development of reduced-intensity regimens in the late 1990s. These regimens are usually applied in older patients (>50 years) and are primarily immunosuppressive. In any case, the conditioning regimen carries substantial risks for toxic effects to other organs leaving the patients vulnerable to a succession of acute complications as shown in ◘ Table 16.2. Graft-versus-host disease (GvHD) is the major complication following allogeneic HCT and is associated with considerable morbidity and mortality. In the human setting, we traditionally recognize two forms of GvHD, acute (aGvHD) and chronic (cGvHD). The major target organs of aGvHD are skin, liver, and intestinal tract, although other organs including the heart may be involved. The presentation in each organ is extremely variable ranging from a mild self-limiting condition to a serious and potentially fatal disorder. aGvHD occurs in approximately 40 % to 60 % of all recipients of allogeneic HCT. In the first classification scheme, the acute form was distinguished from a chronic form by the time of onset (less or more than 100 days from HCT). aGvHD remains, directly or indirectly, the major cause of short-term (day 100) mortality after allogeneic HCT. It is the result of an alloimmune attack of donor lymphocytes against host organ tissues [3]. Although the most important risk factor for the occurrence of aGvHD is the HLA disparity between donor and recipient, several risk factors have been recognized and include older patient age, the use of female donors for male recipients,

Table 16.1 Diseases commonly treated with hematopoietic stem cell transplantation

Autologous transplantation
Malignant disease
Multiple myeloma
Non-Hodgkin's lymphoma
Hodgkin's lymphoma
Acute myeloid leukemia
Neuroblastoma
Ovarian cancer
Germ cell tumors
Other diseases
Autoimmune disorders
Amyloidosis
Allogeneic transplantation
Malignant disease
Acute myeloid leukemia
Acute lymphoblastic leukemia
Chronic myeloid leukemia
Myelodysplastic syndromes
Myeloproliferative disorders
Non-Hodgkin's lymphoma
Hodgkin's disease
Chronic lymphocytic leukemia
Multiple myeloma
Juvenile chronic myeloid leukemia
Nonmalignant disease
Aplastic anemia
Thalassemia major
Sickle cell anemia
Paroxysmal nocturnal hemoglobinuria
Fanconi's anemia
Blackfan–Diamond anemia
Severe combined immunodeficiency
Wiskott–Aldrich syndrome
Inborn errors of metabolism

◘ Table 16.2 Acute complications of allogeneic hematopoietic stem cell transplantation
Pancytopenia
Oral mucositis
Nausea and emesis
Gastroenteritis and diarrhea
Acute graft-versus-host disease
Hemorrhagic cystitis
Renal toxicity
Hepatic damage including veno-occlusive disease of the liver
Cutaneous toxicity
Neurotoxicity
Bacterial, fungal, and viral infections
Cardiotoxicity
Fluid and electrolyte imbalance

prior alloimmunization of the donor, and the nature of GvHD prophylaxis. cGvHD is an immunoregulatory disorder occurring after allogeneic HCT and shares features of autoimmunity and immunodeficiency. Features of cGvHD resemble other autoimmune diseases such as Sjogren's syndrome, scleroderma, primary biliary cirrhosis, and immunocytopenias. Similarly to aGvHD, cGvHD is also thought to be induced by the immune cells of the donor, but the pathophysiology is even less well understood. Depending on a number of factors, cGvHD occurs in about half (ranging from 10 % to 80 %) of 3-month survivors after allogeneic HCT. Another main concern following allogeneic HCT is the profound and long-lasting immunodeficiency which follows this procedure. Many factors relating to the donor and/or to the recipient as well as the source of hemopoietic stem cells and their transplant manipulation can contribute to generate the posttransplant immunodeficiency and can affect the immune reconstitution. In the long-term follow-up of these patients, severe posttransplant infections, relapse, secondary malignancies, and organ damage, including cardiac complications, may be directly related to persistent immune defects. The most important delayed complications following allogeneic HCT are listed in ◘ Table 16.3.

Cardiac complications associated with HCT have been documented in several series, but the incidence of reported cardiotoxicity has varied largely among investigators, ranging from 2 % to 28 % [5–11] probably reflecting patient selection, differences in HCT conditioning regimens, and lack of universal grading system for cardiotoxic events. A retrospective study evaluated 2821 patients transplanted at the University of Minnesota and reported only 26 patients (0.9 %) suffering life-threatening or lethal cardiac toxicity during the first 100 days posttransplant [6]. This low incidence is comparable to previously

Table 16.3 Delayed complications following allogeneic hematopoietic stem cell transplantation

Chronic graft-versus-host disease
Marrow dysfunction
Immunodeficiency
Infection
Autoimmune disorders
Pulmonary disease
Neuroendocrine dysfunction
Impaired growth in children
Infertility
Cataracts
Aseptic necrosis
Secondary malignancies
Intellectual impairment
Psychological problems

reported smaller studies. Hertenstein et al. evaluated prospectively three of 170 patients (1.8 %) with clinically significant major cardiotoxicity associated with HCT conditioning regimen [7]. In several other series [8–10], no serious or fatal acute cardiac toxicity was observed, while a higher frequency (6 % and 9 %) of major cardiac events was reported by Bearman et al. [11] and by Cazin et al. [5], respectively.

In our personal experience, cardiac complication was the first cause of death in 12 out of 876 (1.4 %) patients who received an allogenic HCT between 1982 and 2014 (unpublished data). This complication included congestive heart failure (CHF) ($n=6$), infarction ($n=3$), myocardiopathy ($n=2$), and endocarditis ($n=1$). Cardiac complication was a serious contributing cause of death in other six patients (0.7 %), in all cases manifesting with congestive heart failure.

Clinical results following HCT vary according to the type and stage of disease, the age and functional level of the patient, the source of stem cells to be transplanted, and the degree of HLA compatibility. Many patients survive a lethal disease and reach the dream of a definitive cure of their disease due to the immense dedication knowing that a transplant team is the results of many individuals including physicians from different specialties, scientists, nurses, laboratory technicians, radiotherapists, blood banks, data managers, and many volunteers with their obscure work.

This chapter will focus on the cardiac complications occurring either in the early period following HCT or in the long-term phase.

16.2 Pretransplant Evaluation

16.2.1 Medical History

Risk factors for cardiac complications follow:

- Patient-related
  1. Age (>70 years old).
  2. Prior anthracycline therapy.
  3. Prior history of hypertension: adequate blood pressure control is important as posttransplant immunosuppressive therapy (cyclosporine, tacrolimus) can worsen hypertension.
  4. Prior history of conduction or rhythm abnormalities: increased risk of supraventricular tachyarrhythmias and less commonly ventricular arrhythmias.
  5. Obesity.

16.2.2 Twelve-Lead Electrocardiogram (ECG)

Risk factors for developing acute heart failure posttransplantation are as follows:

- QT-interval prolongation (normal QTc is 390–450 ms for men and 390–460 ms for women)
- QT-interval dispersion (difference between the maximum and minimum QT intervals, normal QT-interval dispersion is 40–50 ms)

16.2.3 Chest X-Ray

- Presence of cardiomegaly (increased cardiothoracic ratio) suggests cardiomyopathy.
- Pulmonary edema and pleural effusions suggest congestive heart failure (CHF).

16.2.4 Assessment of Left Ventricular Ejection Fraction (LVEF)

- LVEF ≥ 45–50 % is arbitrarily chosen as an eligibility criterion for HCT by most centers.
- Transthoracic echocardiography (TTE) is a commonly available and validated diagnostic modality, provides additional information such as valvular function, diastolic function, and global longitudinal strain (early indicator of myocardial dysfunction with the potential to predict future systolic dysfunction).

16.2.5 Noninvasive Stress Testing

- Routinely performed in some centers, even if conclusive data lacking to suggest improving ability to predict risk of posttransplant cardiac complications
- Should be performed only if pretransplant evaluation reveals abnormal findings suggestive of ischemic heart disease (e.g., newly diagnosed cardiomyopathy, valvular heart disease, arrhythmias, significant risks for coronary artery disease)

16.2.6 Cardiac Biomarkers

- Cardiac troponin (cTnT) reflects minimal myocyte damage or loss of cell membrane integrity, providing cardiac structural information. Natriuretic peptide (NT-proBNP) elevations reflect myocardial wall stress, providing cardiac functional information. Both these biomarkers were investigated as potential diagnostic tool to predict cardiac complications during and after HCT.
- Persistent elevations in both cardiac biomarkers may reflect the presence of an underlying reduced functional myocardial reserve or reduced cardiac tolerance to cardiac stressor and predict cardiotoxicity before its clinical manifestation.
- No clear evidence from data published but persisting simultaneous elevations in NT-proBNP and TnT concentrations for a period exceeding 14 days might identify patients at risk of developing cardiotoxicity and requiring further cardiological follow-up [12, 13].

16.3 Clinical Manifestation of Cardiac Complication

16.3.1 Early Manifestations

The conditioning regimen with high-dose chemotherapy and/or radiotherapy precedes stem cell reinfusion and is a critical element in the HCT procedure. Conditioning is a possible cause of early mortality related to toxicity (cardiac, renal, hepatic, pulmonary, and gastrointestinal) but also has the potentiality of long-term disease control. In the autologous setting, the aim of conditioning is to give higher dose of chemotherapy/radiotherapy to eradicate the disease for which the transplant is being performed. In addition in the allogenic setting, another purpose of the preparative regimen is to provide adequate immunosuppression to prevent rejection of the transplanted graft. Management of cardiac complications requires a multidisciplinary approach for the peculiar setting of HCT patients (e.g., management of cardiac ischemia or acute coronary syndrome in patients with severe thrombocytopenia after HCT conditioning requiring antithrombotic and/or anticoagulant therapy).

As a Consequence of High-Dose Chemotherapy

- **High-Dose Cyclophosphamide**

- Incidence up to 43 % in studies from 1970s and 1980s reduced in recent years after the adoption of multifractionated schedule of administration.
- Dose and schedule dependent, not related to cumulative drug dose, dose-related risk (>150 mg/kg and 1.5 g/m^2/day) [8, 10].
- Pathophysiology: toxic endothelial damage followed by extravasation of toxic metabolites with consequent myocyte damage, interstitial hemorrhage, and edema [4, 15].
- Clinical manifestation: acute or subacute congestive heart failure with pulmonary congestion, weight gain, and oliguria; pericarditis; pericardial effusion; and sometimes cardiac tamponade may be associated or may be the only clinical manifestation [14].
- Potentially reversible, but may be fatal within few weeks in patient who develop severe, progressive chronic heart failure.
- Occurs within 1–10 days after first dose administration.

- Associated risk factors: prior anthracycline therapy, total body and mediastinal irradiation, advanced age, obesity, underlying cardiac disease, and concomitant administration of cytarabine or mitoxantrone [15].

High-Dose Melphalan

- Cardiotoxicity is dose limiting at higher dose (>280 mg/m^2) [4].
- Most arrhythmogenic of all chemotherapeutic agents.
- Incidence from 6 % up to 20 % in the advanced age patients and/or concomitant cardiovascular comorbidities [16, 17].
- Pathophysiology: not well established, direct or indirect chemotherapy-mediated cardiac injury, and acting on an atrial substrate rendering more predisposed to develop atrial fibrillation. [17].

Etoposide

- Association with vasospastic angina and myocardial infarction.
- Association with atrial fibrillation [13].

High-Dose Corticosteroids

- Atrial fibrillation.
- Fluid retention [13].

As a Consequence of Radiotherapy

Accelerated Development of Coronary Artery Disease

- Pathophysiology: endovascular proliferation and accelerated atherosclerosis.
- Ostial lesions are common, frequently involved left anterior descending artery due to its location.
- Management similar to conventional treatment for ischemic heart disease, coronary bypass surgery may be more difficult than general population because of prior irradiation in surgery field.

Valvular Heart Disease

- Pathophysiology: fibrotic changes of the heart valves
- More common regurgitant lesions than stenotic lesions
- More common in left-sided valves

Pericardium Toxicity

- Acute pericarditis, subacute and chronic pericardial effusion, constrictive pericarditis and, rarely, cardiac tamponade
- More common in the right side of the heart

Restrictive Cardiomyopathy

- Pathophysiology: myocardial fibrosis and small-vessel ischemic disease
- Decreased myocardial compliance→increased end-diastolic pressure →increased systemic and pulmonary venous pressure
- Clinical signs: right-sided heart failure: peripheral edema, no significant dyspnea, and no significant clinical benefit from adequate diuresis

16.3.2 Infectious Complications

Infections remain a significant cause of morbidity and mortality in patients undergoing HCT. The occurrence of infections varies according to the phase of the transplant process and reflects the type of immune defects, underlying disease, endogenous host flora, previous exposure history, and past pretransplant infectious process. Mucosal damage after conditioning regimen, immunosuppressive therapy, use of corticosteroids, abnormal B- and T-lymphocyte function, hypogammaglobulinemia, and GvHD are some of the predisposing factors. Involvement of the cardiac system during the occurrence of an infectious process is quite rare but potentially fatal in transplanted patients.

Endocarditis

- Rare incidence reported in literature, probably underestimated due to difficulty in making the diagnosis in the antemortem period and the low reported autopsy rate. In one of the largest and more recent published series, Kuruvilla et al. reported 20 cases (1.3 %) in 1547 patients receiving either an allogeneic or autologous HCT. Martino et al. reported an incidence of 5 % (7 out of 141 patients) [18].
- Risk Factors: central venous catheter, sepsis, mucositis, immunosuppressive therapy, graft-versus-host disease.
- Etiology: bacterial and fungal.
- Clinical signs: nonspecific (fever, chills, cough).
- Management: in addition to infectious work-up (cultures, biochemical analyses, imaging techniques), EKG (conduction or rhythm disturbance, myocardial ischemic changes), and echocardiogram (vegetation, decreased ventricular function of heart valves).

Myocarditis and Pericarditis

- Incidence: mainly case reports described in literature, data from large series lacking [19, 20].
- Risk factors: infections, immunological, toxins, drugs, and physical agents such as radiation.
- Etiology: important in order to direct management strategies appropriately but in presence of multiple risk factors and comorbidities, definitive diagnosis is often difficult if not impossible. Viral infections are considered one of the important factors. In many cases it is not clear if these are associations or actual causations. The presence of virus either in peripheral blood or in cardiac myopericardium could be incidental, because of concomitant infection in other organs or from previous virus seeding from prior infection. Adenoviruses were the commonest viral pathogens identified from endomyocardial biopsy samples in patients with myocarditis and dilated cardiomyopathy. In immunocompromised patients where polymicrobial frequent infections are common, attributing etiology to a condition is not easy, and specific management decisions are more difficult because of lack of specific therapy or toxic side effects of therapeutic agents [19, 20].

16.3.3 As a Consequence of Hematopoietic Stem Cell Reinfusion

In the autologous transplant, the patient's hematopoietic stem cells collected from bone marrow or peripheral blood are cryopreserved in addition to dimethyl sulfoxide (DMSO), essential for the preservation of liquid nitrogen-frozen stem cells.

Dimethyl Sulfoxide (DMSO)

- Association with hypotension, bradycardia, hypertension, acute myocardial infarction, atrial fibrillation, and various cardiac arrhythmias including cardiac arrest [21, 22]

16.4 Cardiac Complications of GvHD

GvHD is a major cause of morbidity and mortality after HCT. aGvHD manifestations are predominantly limited to the skin, gastrointestinal tract, and liver. However, severe aGvHD is associated with a marked release of cytokines (cytokine storm) [23], that may result in more widespread organ involvement. Cardiac involvement during aGvHD or cGvHD has been reported to be infrequent, mild, and generally asymptomatic [24, 25].

The most accurate way to evaluate the cardiac effects of GvHD would be to obtain cardiac biopsy samples and subject them to histopathologic analysis. Unfortunately, it is not easy to perform cardiac biopsies because the invasive nature of the procedure could put patients at risk. In the majority of cases, the diagnosis of GvHD-linked cardiac complication is driven from clinical manifestations and exclusion of other possible causes. There are few published data, mostly in pediatric patients, regarding cardiac damage directly due to GvHD mainly [26–29].

In addition to direct cardiac damage as a consequence of GvHD, most of cardiac complications in association of GvHD are due to immunosuppressive drugs used both to prevent or to treat GvHD.

16.4.1 Immunosuppressive Therapy

Cyclosporine and Tacrolimus (Calcineurin Inhibitors)

- Inhibition of calcineurin results in a decreased production of interleukin-2 (IL-2), one of the major cytokines responsible for activation and proliferation of T cells.
- Cardiovascular side effects are as follows:
- Hypertension (common): calcium blocker therapy preferred, avoid angiotensin converting enzyme (ACE) inhibitors, and diuretics. They can exacerbate the already reduced renal blood flow due to afferent arteriole vasoconstriction. The aim is to maintain diastolic blood pressure <90 mm/Hg.
- Electrolyte abnormalities: hypomagnesemia and hyperkalemia.
- Diabetes.

Mycophenolate Mofetil

- Inhibition of T- and B-lymphocyte proliferation via inhibition of inosine monophosphate dehydrogenase (IMPDH)

- Cardiovascular side effects are as follows:
  - Hypertension
  - Edema

Sirolimus

- Inhibition T- and B-lymphocyte proliferation by binding to FK-binding protein 12, resulting in a complex that directly affects the function of mammalian target of rapamycin (mTOR), an enzyme responsible for growth of cells in the G phase.
- Cardiovascular side effects are as follows:
  - Hypertension
  - Edema
  - Hypercholesterolemia/hypertriglyceridemia
  - Electrolyte abnormalities: hypokalemia

16.5 Long-Term Complications

HCT survivors have a significantly increased risk for developing treatment-related complications that affect the quantity and quality of survival, even 10–15 years after their transplant procedure.

The Bone Marrow Transplant Survivor Study (BMTSS) followed 1022 patients who survived at least 2 years post-HCT and showed that the survival probability at 15 years after allogeneic HCT was 80 %, with mortality rates twice that of the general population after 15 years. Two of three HCT survivors will develop a chronic health condition, and >33 % will develop a condition that is severe life-threatening or fatal [30].

For autologous HCT recipients, the mortality rate is also higher for the first 10 years of survivorship before approaching that of the general population. The risk of death due to cardiac dysfunction is greater than 4-fold for female autologous HCT patients [31].

HCT survivors are twice as likely as the general population to die from cardiac conditions. Cardiovascular complications are not only more common in HCT survivors but often occur earlier than would be expected for the general population [32, 33].

Careful health surveillance, healthy lifestyle choices, and prompt management of medical conditions are essential to reduce non-relapse mortality and improve quality of life:

16.5.1 Risk Factors

- Previous anthracycline exposure
- Thoracic radiotherapy (heart in the radiation field), either before or after HCT
- Dyslipidemia
- Hypertension
- Diabetes:
  1. Data from BMTSS documenting allogeneic HCT recipients were 3.7 times more likely to report a diagnosis of diabetes than their matched sibling cohort.
  2. Risk factors: corticosteroid therapy, obesity, family history, and physical inactivity.

3. Follow-up: annual fasting blood glucose and Hb A1c levels, hypoglycemic agents if needed, dietary modification, and physical exercise.

- Metabolic syndrome (defined as the presence of three of these conditions: hypertension, insulin resistance, abdominal obesity, elevated triglycerides, reduced high-density lipoprotein (HDL)):
  1. Prevalence in HCT survivors is 2 –3 times that of the general population.
  2. 2–3 times higher risk of developing cardiovascular disease.
- Iron overload (consequence of multiple transfusions)

16.5.2 Follow-Up

- Screening for hypertension and cardiovascular risk annually
- Fasting lipid panel annually
- Electrocardiogram and/or echocardiogram as clinically indicated

16.5.3 Interventions

- Early intervention for identified risk factors
- Promote healthy lifestyle: healthy diet, physical activity, and smoking cessation
- Cardiology referral and evaluation when indicated
- Endocarditis prophylaxis

References

1. Copelan EA. Hematopoietic stem-cell transplantation. N Engl J Med. 2006;354(17):1813–26.
2. Lake RA, Robinson BW. Immunotherapy and chemotherapy—a practical partnership. Nat Rev Cancer. 2005;5(5):397–05.
3. Markey KA, MacDonald KP, Hill GR. The biology of graft-versus-host disease: experimental systems instructing clinical practice. Blood. 2014;124(3):354–62.
4. Bensinger W. High-dose preparatory regimens. In: Appelbaum FR, Forman SJ, Negrin RS, Blume KG, editors. Thomas hematopoietic cell transplantation. 4th ed. West Sussex: Wiley-Blackwell Ed; 2004. p. 316–32.
5. Cazin B, Gorin NC, Laporte JP, et al. Cardiac complications after bone marrow transplantation: a report on a series of 63 consecutive transplantations. Cancer. 1986;57(10):2061–9.
6. Murdych T, Weisdorf DJ. Serious cardiac complications during bone marrow transplantation at the University of Minnesota, 1977–1997. Bone Marrow Transplant. 2001;28(3):283–7.
7. Hertenstein B, Stefanic M, Schmeiser T, et al. Cardiac toxicity of bone marrow transplantation: predictive value of cardiologic evaluation before transplant. J Clin Oncol. 1994;12(5):998–1004.
8. Baello EB, Ensberg ME, Ferguson DW, et al. Effect of high dose cyclophosphamide and total-body irradiation of left ventricular function in adult patients with leukemia undergoing allogeneic bone marrow transplantation. Cancer Treat Rep. 1986;70(10):1187–93.
9. Jain B, Floreani AA, Anderson JR, et al. Cardiopulmonary function and autologous bone marrow transplantation: results and predictive value for respiratory failure and mortality. Bone Marrow Transplant. 1996;17(14):561–8.
10. Braverman AC, Antin JH, Plappert MT, et al. Cyclophosphamide cardiotoxicity in bone marrow transplantation: a prospective evaluation of new dosing regimens. J Clin Oncol. 1991;9(7):1215–23.
11. Bearman SI, Petersen FB, Schor RA, et al. Radionuclide ejection fractions in the evaluation of patients being considered for bone marrow transplantation: risk of cardiac toxicity. Bone Marrow Transplant. 1990;5(3):173–7.

12. Roziakova L, Bojtarova E, Mistrik M, et al. Serial measurements of cardiac biomarkers in patients after allogeneic hematopoietic stem cell transplantation. J Exp Clin Cancer Res. 2012;31:13.
13. Roziakova L, Mistrik M, Batorova A, et al. Can we predict clinical cardiotoxicity with cardiac biomarkers in patients after haematopoietic stem cell transplantation? Cardiovasc Toxicol. 2015;15(3):210–6.
14. Heitner S, Chou S. Cardiovascular complications. In: Maziarz R, Slater S, editors. Blood and marrow transplant handbook Comprehensive guide for patient care. 2nd ed. Heidelberg: Springer; 2015. p. 287–97.
15. Morandi P, Ruffini PA, Benvenuto GM, et al. Cardiac toxicity of high-dose chemotherapy. Bone Marrow Transplant. 2005;35(4):323–34.
16. Shaw PJ, Nath CE, Lazarus HM. Not too little, not too much—just right! (Better ways to give high dose melphalan). Bone Marrow Transplant. 2014;49(12):1457–65.
17. Feliz V, Saiyad S, Ramarao SM, Khan H, et al. Melphalan-induced supraventricular tachycardia: incidence and risk factors. Clin Cardiol. 2011;34(6):356–9.
18. Kuruvilla J, Forrest DL, Lavoie JC, et al. Characteristics and outcome of patients developing endocarditis following hematopoietic stem cell transplantation. Bone Marrow Transplant. 2004;34(11): 969–73.
19. Bhattacharya S, Paneesha S, Chaganti S, et al. Viral myocarditis in a patient following allogenic stem cell transplant: diagnostic dilemma and management considerations. J Clin Virol. 2009;45(3):262–4.
20. El-Asmar J, Kharfan-Dabaja MA, Ayala E. Acute pericarditis and tamponade from Coxsackie B3 in an adult Hematopoietic-Cell-Allograft recipient: a rare but potentially serious complication. Hematol Oncol Stem Cell Ther. 2016;9(2):82–5. pii: S1658-3876(15)00056-4. doi: 10.1016/j.hemonc.2015.06.004.
21. Morris C, de Wreede L, Scholten M, et al. Chronic Malignancies and Lymphoma Working Parties of EBMT. Should the standard dimethyl sulfoxide concentration be reduced? Results of European Group for Blood and Marrow Transplantation prospective non interventional study on usage and side effect of dimethyl sulfoxide. Transfusion. 2014;54(10):2514–22.
22. Zenhäusern R, Tobler A, Leoncini L, et al. Fatal cardiac arrhythmia after infusion of dimethyl sulfoxide-cryopreserved hematopoietic stem cells in a patient with severe primary cardiac amyloidosis and end-stage renal failure. Ann Hematol. 2000;79(9):523–6.
23. Antin JH, Ferrara JL. Cytokine dysregulation and acute graft versus-host disease. Blood. 1992;80(12): 2964–68.
24. Moir D, Turner J, Ma D, et al. Autopsy findings in bone marrow transplantation. Pathology. 1982;14(2): 197–204.
25. Shulman HM, Sullivan KM, Weiden PL, et al. Chronic graft versus-host disease: a long term clinicopathologic study of 20 Seattle patients. Am J Med. 1980;69(2):204–17.
26. Roberts S, Leeborg N, Loriaux M, et al. Acute graft-versus-host disease of the heart. Pediatr Blood Cancer. 2006;47(5):624–8.
27. Rackley C, Schultz K, Goldman F, et al. Cardiac manifestations of graft-versus-host disease. Biol Blood Marrow Transplant. 2005;11(10):773–80.
28. Norkin M, Ratanatharathorn V, Ayash L, et al. Large pericardial effusion as a complication in adults undergoing SCT. Bone Marrow Transplant. 2011;46(10):1353–6.
29. Gilman AL, Kooy NW, Atkins DL, et al. Complete heart block in association with graft-versus-host disease. Bone Marrow Transplant. 1998;21(1):85–8.
30. Sun CL, Francisco L, Kawashima T, et al. Prevalence and predictors of chronic health conditions after hematopoietic cell transplantation: a report from the Bone Marrow Transplant Survivor Study. Blood. 2010;116(17):3129–39.
31. Bhatia S, Robison LL, Francisco L, et al. Late mortality in survivors of autologous hematopoietic cell transplantation. Blood. 2005;105(11):4215–22.
32. Tichelli A, Passweg J, Wojcik D, et al. Late cardiovascular events after allogeneic hematopoietic stem cell transplantation: a retrospective multicenter study of the Late Effects Working Party of the European Group for Blood and Marrow Transplantation. Haematologica. 2008;93(8):1203–10.
33. Armenian SH, Chow EJ. Cardiovascular disease in survivors of hematopoietic cell transplantation. Cancer. 2014;120(4):469–79.

Cardiotoxicity in Long-Term Survivors

Paolo Tralongo, Sebastiano Bordonaro, Antonino Carmelo Tralongo, and Massimiliano Berretta

C. Lestuzzi et al. (eds.), *Manual of Cardio-oncology*, DOI 10.1007/978-3-319-40236-9_17

17.1 General Consideration of Cancer Survivorship

Survivorship represents a new season of cancer with an increasing number of patients [1]. In Italy, there are 2.8 million patients diagnosed with cancer, twice as many as 15 years ago as a result of improved screening programs, therapeutic advances, and an aging society.

It is estimated that in the next few years, the incidence will tend to further increase by a rate of 3 % annually. Identify survivors is relevant because it provides the opportunity to use a common language and to plan care-specific models [2]. It is necessary to emphasize that cancer disease definition refers to a biologically uncontrolled cell replication and, clinically, is revealed with different pathologies. This requires the identification of survivors through the natural history of cancer.

If, therefore, we want to categorize the patients, we must evaluate the natural history of each cancer disease and the epidemiological data. We can distinguish:

- Cancer patients with early locoregional disease or distant metastasis with the same tendency over the years.
- Cancer patients with little tendency to relapse and often who do not fall over several years.
- Cancer patients with also advanced disease that can secure a remission with integrated treatments.
- Cancer patients with disease that tends to recur early and infrequently.
- Cancer patients with metastatic disease and great impacting symptoms [1].

The first three groups could be defined as "chronic" cancer patients, the fourth group patients with "curable" disease, and finally, patients with "acute" disease.

More recently a proper categorization of patients with cancer has been suggested [3] (◘ Fig. 17.1). However, to date, all patients with a prior diagnosis of cancer are called cancer survivors [4], and survivorship refers to a distinct phase in the cancer course between primary treatment and cancer recurrence or end of life [5, 6].

Category	Description
Acute	Patients/survivors ar first diagnosis or relapse, who require acute intervention
Chronic	Patients/surviors with cancer that slowly progresses or alternates between phases of remission and relapse, often accompanied by acceptable quality of life
Long term	Patients/surviors in clinical remission for long periods of time or for their entire life, who remain at risk for distant relapse or second tumors and who potentially can experience late treatment-related medical and psychosocial sequelae
Cured	Disease-free patients/survivors whose cancer-specific mortality and life expetancy years after years diagnosis equals that of sex-and age-matched members of the general population

◘ **Fig. 17.1** Categories of patients with and survivors of cancer [3]

By new diagnostic and therapeutic approaches, it is now possible to live long after cancer diagnosis; it could mean either living free from oncological disease or with "chronic" disease. Some patients, for example, are disease free after surgical resection of a small tumor, or after prolonged and integrated treatments (surgery, radiotherapy, chemotherapy, high-dose chemotherapy, bone marrow transplantation, endocrine or target treatments). However, the characteristics of these patients are different. After the diagnosis of lymphoma, breast cancer, or colon cancer, for example, the late side effects and the quality of life (QoL) are not comparable to those of a patient suffering from lung or kidney cancer [7]. Moreover, the disease and the patient characteristics (age, gender, ethnicity, culture, religion, education and social status) may contribute to the different experience during the treatment and follow-up.

Cancer disease is, therefore, a complex and evolving path. The patient in different stages should be always driven and educated on the variability, the disease, and the treatments.

As with other chronic diseases (diabetes, hypertensive heart disease, chronic renal failure), the patient should be monitored after treatment for related side effects, and exacerbation of these effects that may require a different therapeutic approach depends on the severity of the same effect. However, we are met with a not indifferent cultural barrier, because despite the diagnostic and therapeutic innovations, even today cancer is considered an insurmountable obstacle and the term is only a synonym of an exclusively negative experience .

17.2 Cardiotoxicity and Cancer Treatment

The chemotherapy treatments are designed to induce rapid apoptosis and/or necrosis of proliferating cancer cells, with inhibition of cell growth, suppression of angiogenesis, or both. When these mechanisms are transferred to the heart muscle, the result may be a limitation of the proliferation and differentiation of the limited body, with cell death and organ dysfunction. The latter occurs when there is a cumulative myocardial damage and impairment in the formation of an endogenous capacity for cardiac repair, predisposing to heart failure induced by treatment. Many classes of chemotherapy drugs can alter the cardiovascular homeostasis and promote cardiovascular disorders. This is most evident in long-living patients: as survival increases, the greater is the probability that cardiovascular consequences of cancer treatments represent a serious health problem caused after healing of the tumor. The side effects most commonly encountered after a cancer treatment include vasospastic ischemia or thromboembolism, hypertension, arrhythmias, and cardiac dysfunction to heart failure [8, 9]. This last long-term complication of chemotherapy is considered with particular fear, because it remains a condition which eventually can also lead to a heart transplant.

17.2.1 Definition

The Cardiac Review and Evaluation Committee (CROSS) established the following criteria for the diagnosis of cardiac dysfunction related to chemotherapy (CRCD):

1. Cardiomyopathy, characterized by a decrease in left ventricular ejection fraction (LVEF), either global or worse in the septum;
2. Symptoms of heart failure (HF);

3. Signs associated with HF, including but not limited to, in S3 gallop, tachycardia, or both;
4. Decline in LVEF between 10 % and 55 %, without accompanying signs or symptoms.

The presence of any of the four criteria is sufficient to confirm a diagnosis of CRCD [10].

17.2.2 Classification

The CRCD can be subclassified into two types.

- **CRCD Type I** exemplified by a cardiac dysfunction related to treatments with *anthracyclines*, with a mechanism of action not yet well understood. The damage to the myocytes could be attributed to the production of free radicals with a consequent increase in oxidative stress [11]. The iron homeostasis could play a role in myocardial injury and anthracyclines could affect iron metabolism with its subsequent accumulation in cardiomyocytes [12]. The cumulative anthracycline dose [13] is strongly associated with cardiotoxicity; however, a different kind of response to different doses of anthracyclines has been seen [14]. Even the mode of administration, the concomitant use of other cardiotoxic drugs, age, and female gender may contribute to the progression of cardiomyopathy [15]. Myocardial damage induced by anthracyclines and other chemotherapeutic agents (alkylating agents, taxanes), specifically in relation to its pathogenic mechanism, is irreversible and is maintained even after cessation of chemotherapy.
- **CRCD Type II** exemplified by *trastuzumab*-induced cardiomyopathy. The mechanism of cardiomyopathy related to trastuzumab is not well defined, but the signal path epidermal growth (HER2) in cardiac muscle suggests that the related cardiotoxicity with trastuzumab is linked to the blocking of HER2 [16, 17]. Unlike the anthracycline-induced cardiotoxicity, heart damage induced by trastuzumab is not related to cumulative dose and is often reversible after cessation of treatment [18]. The risk of developing a trastuzumab-induced cardiotoxicity in patients receiving concomitant therapy with anthracyclines occurs especially if the cumulative dose of doxorubicin is > 300 mg/m^2. Other risk factors include age over 50 years, a preexisting cardiac dysfunction, and a high body mass index. Cardiotoxicity type II is usually asymptomatic and often occurs with a decrease in LVEF and less often with overt cardiac failure [18]. Within this subgroup also falls the cardiotoxicity induced by other biomolecular target drugs (anti-angiogenic, TKI) [19–21], of which frequency and pathogenesis will be exposed subsequently.

17.2.3 Pathogenesis

The most studied chemotherapeutic agents associated with adverse cardiac events are the anthracyclines (*doxorubicin, epirubicin*), used in adults for the treatment of various malignancies such as breast cancer, sarcoma, lymphoma, or gynecological tumors, and also in a number of childhood tumors, which, in combination with other chemotherapy regimens, have contributed to achieving overall survival rates exceeding 75 % [22]. Other cytostatics most frequently correlated with cardiotoxic effects are taxanes (paclitaxel, docetaxel), alkylating agents (carboplatin, cisplatin, cyclophosphamide), small molecule tyrosine kinase inhibitors (lapatinib, imatinib, sorafenib, sunitinib), the antibodies VEFG (Bevacizumab, Aflibercept), and Herceptin, a monoclonal antibody directed against the receptor for human epidermal growth factor type 2 (HER2), used primarily in the treatment of breast cancer. The pathogenesis of cardiotoxicity Types I and II has been widely described in the Chap. 8 to which we refer.

17.2.4 Diagnosis

In Chap. 8 to which we refer, the diagnostic criteria of CRCD are widely exposed. It nevertheless reiterates the concept that the echocardiogram is the test for making a diagnosis of cardiomyopathy with impaired contractile induced by chemotherapy drugs. LVEF should be evaluated in cancer patients undergoing chemotherapy, although there is no consensus regarding frequency and mode. A baseline LVEF should always be carried out for comparison with subsequent echocardiographic controls. The cardiac biomarkers such as troponin I and atrial natriuretic peptide have been investigated with promising results [23, 24]. Although the endomyocardial biopsy remains the gold standard for the diagnosis of type I cardiomyopathy induced by chemotherapy, data on type II are still lacking. Unfortunately, the invasive nature of this procedure limits its use.

17.3 Antineoplastic Drugs Associated With Chronic Cardiotoxicity

17.3.1 Anthracyclines and Other Agents Associated with Type 1 Cardiotoxicity

Anthracyclines are antibiotics belonging to the family of rodomicine, originally isolated from *Streptomyces peucetius*, with potent antineoplastic activity [25]. *Doxorubicin and epirubicin* are currently the most widely used drugs in many cancers, including breast cancer, lymphomas, and sarcomas. It has been estimated that approximately 10 % of patients treated with doxorubicin or its derivatives will develop cardiac complications, even up to 10 years after completion of chemotherapy [26]. In addition, early deterioration and subclinical systolic function can be observed by Doppler ultrasound or echocardiographic monitoring in the majority of patients exposed to anthracyclines [27]. The delay between the cardiac injury and its clinical expression may be explained by the fact that the anthracycline cardiotoxicity is temporarily compensated by the activation of routes of protection and the presence of a functional myocardial reserve [28]. The likelihood of developing anthracycline cardiomyopathy is mainly dose dependent [29]. Contributing factors are genetic predisposition, age, very young or very old age, female gender, intravenous bolus, hypertension, diabetes mellitus, preexisting heart disease, a previous or concomitant radiotherapy to the mediastinum, and the eventual combination with alkylating or microtubule inhibitors [30, 31]. The mechanisms of type I cardiotoxicity induced by chemotherapy have been widely expressed in the Chaps. 8 and 13, to which reference is made for every detail.

17.3.2 Cardiotoxicity of Type II Agents

The advent of monoclonal antibodies and of tyrosine kinase inhibitors has profoundly changed the survival of many malignancies, allowing them to become chronic, and in some cases even healing. The mechanisms by which these drugs can induce cardiotoxicity are a useful tool for the identification of long-term effects in survivors.

- **Anti-ErbB2 Agents.** The first and most common drug with type II cardiotoxicity is trastuzumab, a humanized monoclonal antibody directed against the extracellular domain of HER IV/ErbB2 [32]. ErbB2 is overexpressed in about 30 % of breast cancers, in which it spontaneously interacts with the other ErbBs independent of ligand stimulation and triggers a signaling cascade that promotes the growth and survival of tumor [33]. Herceptin is highly effective in the treatment of breast cancer and also in ErbB2-positive gastric cancer. However, it causes cardiac dysfunction in a substantial proportion of patients, up to 28 % when administered in combination with anthracyclines [34]. Cardiac dysfunction induced by trastuzumab seems to result from a failure of contractility rather than by the loss of myocytes, and the release of troponin shown in sequential treatment with anthracyclines + trastuzumab seems mainly due to previous chemotherapy [35]. The ejection fraction (EF) may, in fact, be recovered, and there is evidence that re-administering trastuzumab is relatively safe, after it has been previously stopped, when the contractile function returns to baseline levels [36].

  Pertuzumab is another recent anti-HER2 antibody that binds to domain II of the receptor, but while trastuzumab inhibits only the signals HER2 ligand-independent, pertuzumab also interferes with the formation of HER2 heterodimers induced by the ligand. Data on the toxicity of pertuzumab are limited. A Phase II study designed to evaluate tumor response and cardiac safety when trastuzumab and pertuzumab are combined has been limited to 11 patients (37 planned) due to an excessive rate of cardiotoxicity [37]. All patients have been previously treated with anthracyclines and trastuzumab, and 54 % of them reported a decrease in LVEF (one patient had symptomatic HF) by combining pertuzumab-trastuzumab. Considering the survival results obtained with the CLEOPATRA study (median OS of 56.5 months compared to 40.8 months with placebo, HR: 0.68) [38] and the successes seen in clinical practice, it is important to evaluate the induced cardiotoxicity in breast cancer patients when the disease has become chronic.

  A third anti-HER2 agent is *lapatinib*, a small molecule inhibitor of the intracellular tyrosine kinase domain of HER2. The effect of lapatinib regards both the signals triggered by ligand and the signals HER2 ligand-independent [32]. Interestingly lapatinib seems to be less cardiotoxic than trastuzumab [39]. The results of three Phase III studies evaluating the addition of lapatinib to chemotherapy or hormonal therapy have not shown any significant increase in adverse cardiac events [39–41]. The cardiotoxic action of anti-HER2 drugs has been shown in Chap. "8" to which reference is made for every detail.

- **Anti-angiogenic Agents.** Among the drugs that induce type II cardiotoxicity, the anti-angiogenic agents, in particular, bevacizumab, sorafenib, and sunitinib, are the most used in oncology. More recently, pazopanib and vandetanib have received approval from the FDA [32, 42, 43]. All these drugs interfere with the signals of the vascular endothelial growth factor (VEGF). VEGF contributes to both the function of cardiomyocytes' growth and expansion and the integrity of the coronary and systemic circulation [44–46]; therefore, its antagonism may lead to cardiovascular side effects, mainly hypertension, thrombo-embolism, left ventricular dysfunction, and HF [47, 48]. In fact, like cancer, the heart is highly dependent on adequate perfusion for its normal functions [43, 44, 46, 49]. The inhibition of HIF-1 by p53 causes cardiac dysfunction in case of chronic pressure overload [50], and the altered expression of VEGF causes rarefaction of micro-vessels and slow-down infarction lasting for months even after turning off the signal receptor [51]. These data suggest that the heart is particularly sensitive to treatment with anti-angiogenic, and the mode of pressure overload is related to hypertension.

Avastin is an antibody that specifically binds to the VEGF-A assets (which activates signals in endothelial cells) and is currently approved for the treatment of carcinoma of the lung, breast, colorectal, and advanced ovarian cancers [52–54]. Avastin is responsible for left ventricular dysfunction in 1 % of chemotherapy-naïve patients and in 3 % of patients who have previously received chemotherapy [55]. A recent meta-analysis of five randomized trials with a total of 3784 patients with MBC has studied the incidence of HF when using chemotherapy with or without bevacizumab. The incidence of high-grade HF has been 1.6 % in patients treated with Avastin and 0.4 % in patients who have not received the drug. In addition, patients treated with bevacizumab have shown a higher relative risk (4.74, $p = 0.001$) of developing HF than the control/placebo group [56].

Sunitinib and sorafenib, which are used in metastatic kidney cancer, HCC, and gastrointestinal stromal tumors resistant to imatinib [57, 58], belong to the class of small molecule inhibitors of tyrosine kinase. They are not very selective also blocking the signal cascades of different types of VEGF [59]. Several studies [60, 61] have shown the importance of these routes in cardiovascular homeostasis. The highest incidence of cardiotoxicity with sunitinib has also been explained by the inhibition of kinases such as the ribosomal S6 kinase (RSK), resulting in the activation of the intrinsic apoptotic pathway, and 5'AMP-activated kinase (AMPK important for the stress response of energy), with worsening of the exhaustion of ATP [62]. The alteration of myocytes then determines left ventricular dysfunction. The rate of cardiotoxicity associated with sorafenib is not yet clear [63]. Significant hypertension has been observed with all three main anti-angiogenic agents [64]. Surprisingly, it has been suggested that hypertension induced by these drugs may be a biomarker of antitumor efficacy and patients who developed hypertension survived longer than those who had not [65]. In the work of Scartozzi et al [66] in patients with metastatic colorectal cancer, 20 % of patients have developed grade 2–3 hypertension. Partial remission has been observed in 75 % of patients with hypertension related to bevacizumab and in only 32 % of those without hypertension. Moreover, in patients who developed hypertension grade 2–3, PFS has been significantly longer than in patients without hypertension [66]. ◘ Figure 17.2 illustrates the cardiotoxic action of the main chemotherapeutic agents.

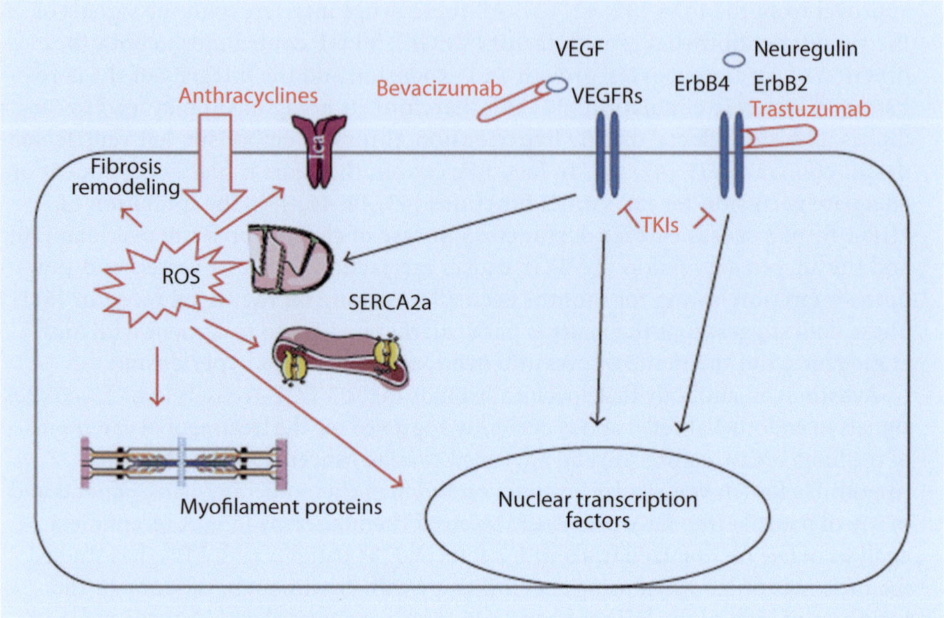

Fig. 17.2 Schematic representation of the main mechanisms by which cardiomyocytes are damaged by anticancer effect cardiotoxic agents [67]

17.4 Cardiac Toxicity in Cancer Survivors

Over the past 15 years, the cardiac complications resulting from cancer treatments have been increasingly recognized as a major cause of morbidity and ultimately mortality in cancer survivors [68–70]. In view of the successes achieved in the management of cancer and the complexity of treatment regimens that are increasingly used to control chronicity of the disease, patients may develop different heart conditions that must be taken in consideration in cancer survivors. Although the term "cardiotoxicity" generally refers to heart damage as a result of treatment, this term is most commonly used to describe the systolic dysfunction of the left ventricle (LV) and heart failure (HF) related to certain types of chemotherapy [71, 72]. It is, however, important to recognize that other components of the cardiovascular system (e.g., valves, vasculature, and pericardium) may also suffer from the effects of radiotherapy, with consequent effects on cardiac function [73–76]. Recognizing the cardiological problems of long-living cancer patients and implementing the strategies for the prevention, diagnosis, and treatment of cardiac toxicity induced by anticancer drugs are innovative aspects widely discussed and debated among healthcare workers, both European and Americans. The goal of much research in this field is precisely to find common guidelines, capable of directing the scientific community toward a common program for the prevention and management of these aspects.

17.4.1 Definitions of "Cardiotoxicity" in Cancer Survivors

The *Common Terminology Criteria for Adverse Events* (CTCAE) formulated by the *US National Cancer Institute for clinical research* defines "cardiotoxicity" exclusively as symptomatic left ventricular systolic dysfunction that manifests itself with an ejection fraction (LVEF) <50 % or congestive HF [77]. In the major phase 3 studies, often only grade 3 cardiac toxicity (severe reduction in systolic symptomatic with an LVEF <20 %) is subject to disclosure, and, therefore, the cases of more moderate left ventricular dysfunction are not recorded. Furthermore, cancer survivors would be excluded from clinical cardiological research, and those who have been enrolled in a study due to cardiac toxicity generally do not pursue a systematic follow-up. This means that no safe epidemiological studies on the true incidence of cardiotoxicity in cancer survivors can be prepared. Given the potential long range (up to 2 or 3 years in some cases) between exposure to cancer therapies (chemotherapy and/or radiotherapy) and demonstration of next measurable adverse event affecting heart's health, these may represent the delayed effect affecting the prognosis of long-term cancer survivors [70, 72, 78, 79]. In addition, although the LVEF remains a major index commonly used to monitor the performance of myocardial systolic LV, a reduction in LVEF is often discovered very late [80]. Currently, cardiotoxicity is commonly defined as either LVEF decrease of more than 10 percentage points with a final LVEF <50 % or a reduction in LVEF of more than 15 percentage points, with a final LVEF > 50 % [81]. It is clear that if there is a minimum reduction of 5 percentage points with accompanying symptoms of an HF, it is sufficient for a diagnosis of cardiotoxicity [82].

17.4.2 Risk Factors of Cardiotoxicity

The relationship between anthracyclines or radiation doses and consequent cardiotoxicity has been extensively studied [79, 83, 84]. In a prospective study of European young cancer survivors, the most important predictor of worsening cardiac performance was the total dose of anthracyclines [85]. Patients treated with anthracyclines continue to experience an increased risk of developing chronic diseases, usually dilated cardiomyopathy, which could not be detected until years or even decades after exposure, especially in patients who received cumulative doses greater than 250 or 300 mg/m^2 [85, 86]. A retrospective Swedish study in young patients, including children, who had received chemotherapy and radiation therapy for Hodgkin lymphoma showed that the age at diagnosis (<40 years) and family history of HF are both predictive for subsequent development of HF and stroke at a median follow-up of 20 years [87]. If young age is a risk for childhood cancers, the same way, very old age may be a significant risk factor for older women with breast cancer who are receiving Herceptin in the adjuvant treatment [88] to a greater extent for all patients who had previously received anthracyclines [89].

Similarly to chemotherapy, radiation therapy-related late effects can usually take years to manifest in the form of coronary syndrome or other vascular disease, such as valvular dysfunction, pericardial disease, and, at times, left ventricular dysfunction with restrictive cardiomyopathy [90–92]. Although there is also a clear dose–response relationship, especially in patients with breast cancer to the left side, some studies suggest that the risk may be increased with doses <5Gy [79]. For the deepening cardiotoxic action of radiation treatments, see Chap. 12.

Although cardiac complications associated with anthracyclines and radiotherapy have been mostly studied, other agents have been associated with cardiac toxicity, with different mechanisms, as previously described (anti-HER2, in particular trastuzumab, anti-VEGF, TKI, etc.), and therefore, prolonged exposure to these antitumor agents is a risk factor for the development of HF [93–95]. Finally, even if the exposure to cancer therapy is the most important factor linked to cardiotoxic effect, many studies have shown that conventional risk factors, such as smoking, hypertension [96], and diabetes [97, 98], remain important independent risk factors.

17.4.3 Early Diagnosis of Cardiac Toxicity

Considering that the cardiotoxicity is a limit in the survival of patients with cancer, early detection of such event is a primary objective for both cardiologists and oncologists. Currently, the most used method to detect cardiotoxicity is the periodic measurement of LV systolic function by the two-dimensional echocardiography (2D ECHO) or the multiple gates acquisition scan (MUGA) [99]. At the moment, however, there are no common guidelines for evidence-based monitoring of cardiotoxicity during and after cancer treatments in adults [100, 101]. The recently published ESMO guidelines [102] recommend to evaluate cardiac function 4 years and 10 years after anthracycline therapy in patients who have been treated before the age of 15 years (level of evidence, III [with the level I considered to be more rigorous]; grade of recommendation, B [with A considered superior]) or even after the age of 15 years, but with a cumulative dose of doxorubicin > 240 mg/m^2 or epirubicin > 360 mg/m^2 (level of evidence III B). There are also recommendations for patients receiving trastuzumab who should undergo a serial evaluation of LVEF every 3 months [103, 104]. In fact, the measurement of LVEF represents a relatively insensitive tool for the detection of cardiotoxicity in an initial phase, mostly because no considerable change in LVEF occurs until a critical amount of myocardial damage has occurred and this manifests only after all compensatory mechanisms are exhausted. Serial measurements of troponin can provide additional information in this setting but are not regularly recommended [105, 106]. Therefore, evidence of a decrease in LVEF excludes any possibility of preventing the development of cardiotoxicity [107], while a normal value of the LVEF does not exclude the possibility of a subsequent cardiac deterioration. In addition, the measurement of LVEF is often operator dependent. New ultrasound imaging techniques, such as echocardiography with contrast, real-time, and three-dimensional echocardiography, have emerged allowing an improvement in the accuracy of calculation of LVEF [108]. Alternative methods of imaging and serum biomarkers may be necessary for early detection. Currently, the measurement of cardiac biomarkers (troponin 1 and troponin T, B-type natriuretic peptide [BNP] and N-terminal pro-BNP) is becoming more widely used to detect cardiac toxicity in patients receiving active treatment for cancer, as well as for the survivors in the short term [109]. MUGA or cardiac imaging with magnetic resonance imaging (MRI) has been used, especially in the USA, to detect the cardiac toxicity. However, currently, there is no international consensus on recommendations regarding the expected range or for the tests required in adult patients, because data are more predominant in long-living children/young patients [110, 111].

17.4.4 Treatment of Cardiotoxicity in Cancer Patient Survivors

The treatment of cardiac toxicity is greatly influenced by comorbidities existing in a given patient and the context in which the damage is detected. For example, a patient with an acute stage of cancer may suffer from a transient left ventricular dysfunction related to several causes and, after a period of stabilization, the patient may resume the cardiotoxic chemotherapy if it is necessary for an optimal cancer. Alternatively, a patient with no previous heart disease, who has received an anthracycline-based therapy 4 years previously developing a severe left ventricular dysfunction, may not currently be considered for a cardiotoxic chemotherapy even if it is necessary. The following general principles that apply to the treatment of left ventricular dysfunction in all patients are equally important in cancer survivors:

1. Dietary adjustments, in particular sodium restriction (See Chap. 3)
2. Careful monitoring of exercise and weight management restriction (See Chap. 3)
3. Maximum tolerated dose of inhibitors of the renin-angiotensin system (ACE-Is, ARBs, and beta-blockers)
4. Selective use of aldosterone antagonists
5. Appropriate use of implantable cardiac defibrillators or bi-ventricular pacemakers
6. Other therapies as preventive measures (aspirin, statins, abolition of alcohol/smoke) [112].

However, data supporting the efficacy of these interventions are limited, in particular among adult cancer survivors, and there are no effective recommendations for the treatment of cancer patients who develop HF as a result of an anticancer treatment. One of problems of this form of cardiac dysfunction is that it usually remains asymptomatic for a very long time [113]. Many cancer patients who develop cardiac dysfunction do not seem to be receiving optimal treatment and are treated only if symptomatic [114], probably because they are considered fragile and unsuitable to aggressive therapies (ACE-Is, beta blockers, etc.). A prospective study recently published that included the largest population of patients with anthracycline-induced cardiomyopathy (N 5201, including many still in active cancer therapy) has shown that the time elapsed since the end of chemotherapy and the start of therapy for HF with ACE-I and / or beta-blockers is a crucial variable for the recovery of cardiac dysfunction [115]. In fact, the chances of getting a full recovery of LVEF are greater for patients who started treatment within 2 months after the end of chemotherapy, then this percentage decreased gradually, and no full recovery in LVEF has been observed in patients who had begun therapy after 6 months. In particular, in this study, the clinical benefit was more evident in asymptomatic patients compared to those symptomatic. These results underline the crucial importance of early detection of cardiotoxicity and suggest that an aggressive pharmacological approach, with ACE-Is, possibly in combination with beta-blockers, should always be considered in all cases of cardiomyopathy related to anthracyclines [116]. The duration of treatment of HF related to chemotherapy remains uncertain, even if some data suggest that it should be long term [117]. As regards the management of the cardiotoxicity of type II, the beginning of the standard treatment of heart failure as well as the suspension of the cardiotoxic agent will increase the probability of recovery of left ventricular function. These patients are likely to be treated again with cardiotoxic drugs (trastuzumab, bevacizumab, sunitinib), also with close cardiac monitoring [118].

17.4.5 Prevention of Chemotherapy-Related Cardiac Dysfunction (CRCD)

Effective prevention to delay cardiotoxicity in cancer patients begins even before the administration of chemotherapy: a cardiovascular basic evaluation and effective control of cardiovascular risk factors are necessary to avoid late cardiac toxicity. Aspirin, control of hypertension and dyslipidemia, and tobacco cessation are all actions that should be pursued when necessary [119–121]. Improvements in the protocols of chemotherapy and radiotherapy have led to decreased rates of cardiovascular disease in cancer survivors followed over time [122]. The continuous improvements in technology (e.g., the advent of the intensity-modulated and the proton radiation therapy) have potentially reduced the dispersion of the radiation to critical organs [123]. As well as reducing the cumulative dose of anthracyclines, other approaches that can reduce the risk of developing Type I CRCD are the infusion of anthracycline rather than bolus administration [124], the structural change of doxorubicin [125], and the liposomal formulation of doxorubicin [126]. These are all measures that can help to reduce the degree of cardiac toxicity. Dexrazoxane, as an EDTA chelation, can reduce the risk of cardiac toxicity when administered in combination with doxorubicin or epirubicin [125]. However, its use has been limited to patients receiving a cumulative dose of doxorubicin > 300 mg/m^2 because of its potential impact on the antitumor efficacy [127]. Carvedilol, a beta-blocker with antioxidant properties [128], may reduce the risk of anthracycline-induced cardiomyopathy, as well.

17.4.6 Follow-Up of Chemotherapy-Related Cardiac Dysfunction (CRCD) in Cancer Survivors

The prevention of cardiotoxicity induced by cancer therapy, already begun before the start of the same, must be continued even after the end of the specific care, through a joint effort of cancer specialist and cardiologist, by a careful evaluation of the patient, for both the treatment of cancer and cardiotoxicity prevention and the continuous monitoring of cardiovascular parameters and cardiac function. Blood chemistry parameters, along with blood pressure, electrocardiogram, an echo-Doppler to assess the volume and thickness of the heart chambers, the LVEF, the ST interval, rhythm disturbances, and the presence of any valve dysfunction, must, therefore, be periodically evaluated. The long-term monitoring in cancer survivors is thus indicated, although there are no true cardio-monitoring programs and guidelines shared on the follow-up. Some examples have, however, emerged for the prevention or treatment of cardiac damage and their management in childhood cancer survivors [129]. For example, a Swedish retrospective study on long-term risk of cardiovascular disease in young survivors of Hodgkin's lymphoma [130] has shown an increased risk of being hospitalized for cardiovascular disease extending even more than 20 years after their diagnosis of lymphoma than the general Swedish population. It is, therefore, essential that the oncology community continue working to develop appropriate guidelines for early cardiac risk assessment, through a follow-up program that can identify and treat cardiotoxicity in cancer survivors. On the basis of the risk factors, several strategies have been proposed for the early diagnosis of cardiomyopathy induced by chemotherapy. These include the endocardial biopsy, measuring levels of BNP or troponin, MUGA, exercise testing, and echocardiography [131, 132]. At this time, none of these strategies has become a standard and most of the published studies describe that the monitoring of long-term survivors treated with cardiotoxic drugs is based on data deriving from studies with echocardiography and Doppler [133, 134]. The frequency with which these diagnostic procedures should be performed in cancer survivors remains unknown and is a cause for debate. Further clinical studies are, therefore, needed to define these approaches and their application.

17.5 Conclusions

The chemotherapy-related cardiac dysfunction is a serious late complication related to the treatment of cancer, and the early identification of patients at high risk is the key to reduce this risk. An acceptable and unified definition of cardiomyopathy induced by chemotherapy should be shared and adopted by both cardiologists and oncologists, who must work together according to shared guidelines for the health of cancer survivors. To facilitate this collaboration, new companies based in Europe and the United States, such as the Italian Association of Cardio-Oncology (AICO) (www.aicocardiologia.) and the International CardiOncology Society (ICOS) [135], have been formed gathering together researchers and clinicians from both fields. In conclusion, further research on adult cancer survivors should be developed separately from research in childhood cancer survivors.

References

1. De Angelis R, Sant M, Coleman MP, on behalf of the eurocare-5 Working Group, et al. Cancer survival in Europe 1999–2007 by country and age: results of eurocare-5—a population-based study. Lancet Oncol. 2014;15:23–34.
2. Oeffinger KC, McCabe MS. Models for delivering survivorship care. J Clin Oncol. 2006;24:5117–24.
3. Surbone A, Tralongo P. Categorization of cancer survivors: why we need it. J Clin Oncol. 2016 Jul 25. pii: JCO683870. [Epub ahead of print]
4. Leigh S. Cancer survivorship: today and tomorrow, 2007. Chapter 2, Ed Ganz P, Springer, New York, NY, pp 8–13
5. Institute of Medicine and the National Research Council. From cancer patient to cancer survivor: lost in transition. Washington, DC: National Academies Press; 2006.
6. Rowland JH, Hewitt M, Ganz PA. Cancer survivorship: a new challenge in delivering quality cancer care. J Clin Oncol. 2006;24(32):5101–4.
7. Wu HS, Harden JK. Symptom burden and quality of life in survivorship: a review of the literature. Cancer Nurs. 2015;38(1):E29–54.
8. Suter TM, Ewer MS. Cancer drugs and the heart: importance and management. Eur Heart J. 2013;34(15):1102–11.
9. Ky B, Vejpongsa P, Yeh ETH, Force T, Moslehi JJ. Emerging paradigms in cardiomyopathies associated with cancer therapies. Circ Res. 2013;113(6):754–64.
10. Albini A, Pennesi G, Donatelli F, et al. Cardiotoxicity of anticancer drugs: the need for cardio-oncology and cardio-oncological prevention. J Natl Cancer Inst. 2010;102(1):14–25.
11. Singal PK, Deally CM, Weinberg LE. Subcellular effects of adriamycin in the heart: a concise review. J Mol Cell Cardiol. 1987;19(8):817–28.
12. Kwok JC, Richardson DR. Anthracyclines induce accumulation of iron in ferritin in myocardial and neoplastic cells: inhibition of the ferritin iron mobilization pathway. Mol Pharmacol. 2003;63(4):849–61.
13. Yeh E, Tong A, Lenihan D, et al. Cardiovascular complcations of cancer therapy: diagnosis, pathogenesis, and management. Circulation. 2004;109:3122–31.
14. Shan K, Lincoff AM, Young JB. Anthracycline-induced cardiotoxicity. Ann Untern Med. 1996;125(1):47–58.
15. Yeh E, Bickford C. Cardiovascular complications of cancer therapy: incidence, pathogenesis, diagnosis, and management. J Am Coll Cardiol. 2009;53:2231–47.
16. Perik PJ, de Vries EG, Gietema JA, van der Graaf WT, Smilde TD, Sleijfer DT, van Veldhuisen DJ. Serum HER2 levels are increased in patients with chronic heart failure. Eur J Heart Fail. 2007;9(2):173–7. Epub 2006 Jul 24.
17. Chien KR. Herceptin and the heart – a molecular modifier of cardiacfailure. N Engl J Med. 2006;354(8):789–90.
18. Ewer M, Lippman S. Type II chemotherapy-related cardiac dysfunction: time to recognize a new entity. J Clin Oncol. 2005;23(13):2900–2.

19. Izumiya Y, Shiojima I, Sato K, Sawyer DB, Colucci WS, Walsh K. Vascular endothelial growth factor blockade promotes the transition from compensatory cardiac hypertrophy to failure in response to pressure overload. Hypertension. 2006;47:887–93.
20. Force T, Krause DS, van Etten RA. Molecular mechanisms of cardiotoxicity of tyrosine kinase inhibition. Nat Rev Cancer. 2007;7(5):332–44.
21. Cheng H, Force T. Molecular mechanisms of cardiovascula r toxicity of targeted cancer therapeutics. Circ Res. 2010;106:21–34.
22. Smith LA, Cornelius VR, Plummer CJ, Levitt G, Verrill M, Canney P, et al. Cardiotoxicity of anthracycline agents for the treatment of cancer: systematic review and meta-analysis of randomised controlled trials. BMC Cancer. 2010;10:337.
23. Cardinale D, Sandri MT, Martinoni A, Borghini E, Civelli M, Lamantia G, Cinieri S, Martinelli G, Fiorentini C, Cipolla CM. Myocardial injury revealed by plasma troponin I in breast cancer treated with high-dose chemotherapy. Ann Oncol. 2002;13(5):710–5.
24. Nousiainen T, Vanninen E, Jantunen E, et al. Natriuretic peptides during the development of doxorubicin-induced left ventricular diastolic dysfunction. J Intern Med. 2002;251(3):228–34.
25. Octavia Y, Tocchetti CG, Gabrielson KL, Janssens S, Crijns HJ, Moens AL. Doxorubicin-induced cardiomyopathy: from molecular mechanisms to therapeutic strategies. J Mol Cell Cardiol. 2012;52(6): 1213–25.
26. Suter TM, Ewer MS. Cancer drugs and the heart: importance and management. Eur Heart J. 2013;34(15):1102–11.
27. Mavinkurve-Groothuis AMC, Marcus KA, Pourier M, et al. Myocardial 2D strain echocardiography and cardiac biomarkers in children during and shortly after anthracycline therapy for acute lymphoblastic leukaemia (ALL): a prospective study. Eur Heart J Cardiovasc Imaging. 2013;14(6):562–9.
28. Cardinale D, Sandri MT, Martinoni A, et al. Myocardial injury revealed by plasma troponin I in breast cancer treated with high-dose chemotherapy. Ann Oncol. 2002;13(5):710–5.
29. Allen A. The cardiotoxicity of chemotherapeutic drugs. Semin Oncol. 1992;19(5):529–42.
30. von Hoff DD, Layard MW, Basa P, et al. Risk factors for doxorubicin-induced congestive heart failure. Ann Intern Med. 1979;91(5):710–7.
31. Lipshultz SE, Lipsitz SR, Mone SM, et al. Female sex and higher drug dose as risk factors for late cardiotoxic effects of doxorubicin therapy for childhood cancer. N Engl J Med. 1995;332(26):1738–43.
32. De Keulenaer GW, Doggen K, Lemmens K. The vulnerability of the heart as a pluricellular paracrine organ: lessons from unexpected triggers of heart failure in targeted ErbB2 anticancer therapy. Circ Res. 2010;106(1):35–46.
33. Slamon DJ, Clark GM, Wong SG, Levin WJ, Ullrich A, McGuire WL. Human breast cancer: correlation of relapse and survival with amplification of the HER-2/neu oncogene. Science. 1987;235(4785):182–91.
34. Slamon DJ, Leyland-Jones B, Shak S, et al. Use of chemotherapy plus a monoclonal antibody against her2 for metastatic breast cancer that overexpresses HER2. N Engl J Med. 2001;344(11):783–92.
35. Ewer MS, Ewer SM. Troponin I provides insight into cardiotoxicity and the anthracycline-trastuzumab interaction. J Clin Oncol. 2010;28(25):3901–4.
36. Ewer MS, Vooletich MT, Durand J-B, et al. Reversibility of trastuzumab-related cardiotoxicity: new insights based on clinical course and response to medical treatment. J Clin Oncol. 2005;23(31): 7820–6.
37. Portera CC, Walshe JM, Rosing DR, et al. Cardiac toxicity and efficacy of trastuzumab combined with pertuzumab in patients with human epidermal growth factor receptor 2-positive metastatic breast cancer. Clin Cancer Res. 2008;14:2710–6.
38. Baselga J, Cortes J, Kim SB, et al. Pertuzumab plus trastuzumab plus docetaxel for metastatic breast cancer. N Engl J Med. 2012;366:109–19.
39. Geyer CE, Forster J, Lindquist D, et al. Lapatinib plus capecitabine for HER2-positive advanced breast cancer. N Engl J Med. 2006;355:2733–43.
40. Di Leo A, Gomez HL, Aziz Z, et al. Phase III, double-blind, randomized study comparing lapatinib plus paclitaxel with placebo plus paclitaxel as fi rst-line treatment for metastatic breast cancer. J Clin Oncol. 2008;26:5544–52.
41. Johnston S, Pippen Jr J, Pivot X, et al. Lapatinib combined with letrozole versus letrozole and placebo as fi rst-line therapy for postmenopausal hormone receptor-positive metastatic breast cancer. J Clin Oncol. 2009;27:5538–46.
42. Steingart RM, Bakris GL, Chen HX et al. Management of cardiac toxicity in patients receiving vascular endothelial growth factor signaling pathway inhibitors. Am Heart J. 2012; 163(2): 156–63

43. Tocchetti CG, Gallucci G, Coppola C, et al. The emerging issue of cardiac dysfunction induced by antineoplastic angiogenesis inhibitors. Eur J Heart Fail. 2013;15(5):482–9.
44. Force T, Krause DS, van Etten RA. Molecular mechanisms of cardiotoxicity of tyrosine kinase inhibition. Nat Rev Cancer. 2007;7(5):332–44.
45. Curigliano G, Cardinale D, Suter T, et al. Cardiovascular toxicity induced by chemotherapy, targeted agents and radiotherapy: ESMOclinical practice guidelines. Ann Oncol. 2012;23 Suppl 7:vii155–66.
46. Marone G, Granata F. Angiogenesis, lymphangiogenesis and clinical implications. Preface. Chem Immunol Allergy. 2014;99:11–2.
47. Schmidinger M, Zielinski CC, Vogl UM, et al. Cardiac toxicity of sunitinib and sorafenib in patients with metastatic renal cell carcinoma. J Clin Oncol. 2008;26(32):5204–12.
48. Gressett SM, Shah SR. Intricacies of bevacizumabinduced toxicities and their management. Ann Pharmacother. 2009;43(3):490–501.
49. Eschenhagen T, Force T, Ewer MS, et al. Cardiovascular side effects of cancer therapies: a position statement from the Heart Failure Association of the European Society of Cardiology. Eur J Heart Fail. 2011;13(1):1–10.
50. Sano M, Minamino T, Toko H, et al. p53-induced inhibition of Hif-1 causes cardiac dysfunction during pressure overload. Nature. 2007;446(7134):444–8.
51. Walsh K, Shiojima I. Cardiac growth and angiogenesis coordinated by intertissue interactions. J Clin Invest. 2007;117(11):3176–9.
52. Hurwitz H, Fehrenbacher L, Novotny W, et al. Bevacizumab plus irinotecan, fluorouracil, and leucovorin for metastatic colorectal cancer. N Engl J Med. 2004;350(23):2335–42.
53. Sandler A, Gray R, Perry MC, et al. Paclitaxel-carboplatin alone or with bevacizumab for non-small-cell lung cancer. N Engl J Med. 2006;355(24):2542–50.
54. Perren TJ, Swart AM, Pfisterer J, et al. A phase 3 trial of bevacizumab in ovarian cancer. N Engl J Med. 2011;365(26):2484–96.
55. Miller KD, Chap LI, Holmes FA, et al. Randomized phase III trial of capecitabine compared with bevacizumab plus capecitabine in patients with previously treated metastatic breast cancer. J Clin Oncol. 2005;23(4):792–9.
56. Choueiri TK, Mayer EL, Je Y, et al. Congestive heart failure risk in patients with breast cancer treated with bevacizumab. J Clin Oncol. 2011;29:632–8.
57. Gressett SM, Shah SR. Intricacies of bevacizumab induced toxicities and their management. Ann Pharmacother. 2009;43(3):490–501.
58. Chintalgattu V, Ai D, Langley RR, et al. Cardiomyocyte PDGFR-β signaling is an essential component of the mouse cardiac response to load-induced stress. J Clin Investig. 2010;120(2):472–84.
59. Cheng H, Force T. Molecular mechanisms of cardiovascular toxicity of targeted cancer therapeutics. Circ Res. 2010;106(1):21–34.
60. Anisimov A, Alitalo A, Korpisalo P, et al. Activated forms of VEGF-C and VEGF-D provide improved vascular function in skeletal muscle. Circ Res. 2009;104(11):1302–12.
61. De Boer RA, Pinto YM, Van Veldhuisen DJ. The imbalance between oxygen demand and supply as a potential mechanism in the pathophysiology of heart failure: the role of microvascular growth and abnormalities. Microcirculation. 2003;10(2):113–26.
62. Kerkela R, Woulfe KC, Durand J-B, et al. Sunitinib-induced cardiotoxicity is mediated by off-target inhibition of AMPactivated protein kinase. Clin Transl Sci. 2009;2(1):15–25.
63. Di Lorenzo G, Autorino R, Bruni G, et al. Cardiovascular toxicity following sunitinib therapy in metastatic renal cell carcinoma: a multicenter analysis. Ann Oncol. 2009;20(9):1535–42.
64. Mourad J, Levy BI. Mechanisms of antiangiogenicinduced arterial hypertension. Curr Hypertens Rep. 2011;13(4):289–93.
65. Goodwin R, Ding K, Seymour L, et al. Treatment-emergent hypertension and outcomes in patients with advanced nonsmall-cell lung cancer receiving chemotherapy with or without the vascular endothelial growth factor receptor inhibitor cediranib: NCIC Clinical Trials Group Study BR24. Ann Oncol. 2010;21(11):2220–6.
66. Scartozzi M, Galizia E, Chiorrini S, et al. Arterial hypertension correlates with clinical outcome in colorectal cancer patients treated with first-line bevacizumab. Ann Oncol. 2009;20(2):227–30.
67. Molinaro M, Ameri P, Marone G, et al. Recent advances on pathophysiology diagnostic and therapeutic insights in cardiac dysfunction induced by antineoplastic. Drugs Biomed Res Int. 2015;2015:138148.
68. Oeffinger KC, Mertens AC, Sklar CA, et al. Chronic health conditions in adult survivors of childhood cancer. N Engl J Med. 2006;355:1572–82.

69. Reulen RC, Winter DL, Frobisher C, et al. Long-term cause-specific mortality among survivors of childhood cancer. JAMA. 2010;304:172–9.
70. Meinardi MT, Gietema JA, van der Graaf WT, et al. Cardiovascular morbidity in long-term survivors of metastatic testicular cancer. J Clin Oncol. 2000;18:1725–32.
71. Lenihan DJ, Cardinale D, Cipolla CM. The compelling need for a cardiology and oncology partnership and the birth of the International CardiOncology Society. Prog Cardiovasc Dis. 2010;53:88–93.
72. van der Pal HJ, van Dalen EC, Hauptmann M, et al. Cardiac function in 5-year survivors of childhood cancer: a long-term follow-up study. Arch Intern Med. 2010;170:1247–55.
73. Hull MC, Morris CG, Pepine CJ, et al. Valvular dysfunction and carotid, subclavian, and coronary artery disease in survivors of Hodgkin lymphoma treated with radiation therapy. JAMA. 2003;290:2831–7.
74. Heidenreich PA, Hancock SL, Lee BK, et al. Asymptomatic cardiac disease following mediastinal irradiation. J Am Coll Cardiol. 2003;42:743–9.
75. Carver JR, Shapiro CL, Ng A, et al. American Society of Clinical Oncology clinical evidence review on the ongoing care of adult cancer survivors: cardiac and pulmonary late effects. J Clin Oncol. 2007;25:3991–4008.
76. Chen MH, Colan SD, Diller L. Cardiovascular disease: cause of morbidity and mortality in adult survivors of childhood cancers. Circ Res. 2011;108:619–28.
77. US Department of Health and Human Services, National Institutes of Health, National Cancer Institute. Common Terminology Criteria for Adverse Events (CTCAE), version 4.0. Available at: http:// evs.nci.nih.gov/ftp1/CTCAE/CTCAE_4.03_2010-06-14_QuickReference_ 5x7.pdf. Accessed May 28, 2009.
78. Cardinale D, Sandri MT, Colombo A, et al. Prognostic value of troponin I in cardiac risk stratification of cancer patients undergoing high-dose chemotherapy. Circulation. 2004;109:2749–54.
79. Schultz-Hector S, Trott KR. Radiation-induced cardiovascular diseases: is the epidemiologic evidence compatible with the radiobiologic data? Int J Radiat Oncol Biol Phys. 2007;67:10–8.
80. Ewer MS, Lenihan DJ. Left ventricular ejection fraction and cardiotoxicity: is our ear really to the ground? J Clin Oncol. 2008;26:1201–3.
81. Bird BR, Swain SM. Cardiac toxicity in breast cancer survivors: review of potential cardiac problems. Clin Cancer Res. 2009;14:14–24.
82. Martin M, Esteva FJ, Alba E, et al. Minimizing cardiotoxicity while optimizing treatment efficacy with trastuzumab: review and expert recommendations. Oncologist. 2009;14:1–11.
83. Gianni L, Herman EH, Lipshultz SE, et al. Anthracycline cardiotoxicity: from bench to bedside. J Clin Oncol. 2008;26:3777–84.
84. Sawyer DB, Peng X, Chen B, et al. Mechanisms of anthracycline cardiac injury: can we identify strategies for cardioprotection? Prog Cardiovasc Dis. 2010;53:105–13.
85. Sorensen K, Levitt GA, Bull C, et al. Late anthracycline cardiotoxicity after childhood cancer: a prospective longitudinal study. Cancer. 2003;97:1991–8.
86. Pinder MC, Duan Z, Goodwin JS, et al. Congestive heart failure in older women treated with adjuvant anthracycline chemotherapy for breast cancer. J Clin Oncol. 2007;25:3808–15.
87. Andersson A, Naslund U, Tavelin B, et al. Long-term risk of cardiovascular disease in Hodgkin lymphoma survivors—retrospective cohort analyses and a concept for prospective intervention. Int J Cancer. 2009;124:1914–7.
88. Tarantini L, Cioffi G, Gori S, et al. Trastuzumab adjuvant chemotherapy and cardiotoxicity in real-world women with breast cancer. J Card Fail. 2012;18:113–9.
89. Du XL, Xia R, Liu CC, et al. Cardiac toxicity associated with anthracycline-containing chemotherapy in older women with breast cancer. Cancer. 2009;115:5296–308.
90. Hull MC, Morris CG, Pepine CJ, et al. Valvular dysfunction and carotid, subclavian, and coronary artery disease in survivors of Hodgkin lymphoma treated with radiation therapy. JAMA. 2003;290:2831–7.
91. Travis LB, Ng AK, Allan JM, et al. Second malignant neoplasms and cardiovascular disease following radiotherapy. J Natl Cancer Inst. 2012;104:357–70.
92. Hooning MJ, Botma A, Aleman BM, et al. Long-term risk of cardiovascular disease in 10-year survivors of breast cancer. J Natl Cancer Inst. 2007;99:365–75.
93. Telli ML, Witteles RM. Trastuzumab-related cardiac dysfunction. J Natl Compr Canc Netw. 2011;9:243–9.
94. Escudier B, Eisen T, Stadler WM, et al. Sorafenib in advanced clearcell renal-cell carcinoma. N Engl J Med. 2008;356:125–34.
95. Richards CJ, Je Y, Schutz FA, et al. Incidence and risk of congestive heart failure in patients with renal and nonrenal cell carcinoma treated with sunitinib. J Clin Oncol. 2011;29:3450–6.

96. Piccart-Gebhart MJ, Procter M, Leyland-Jones B, et al. Trastuzumab after adjuvant chemotherapy in HER2-positive breast cancer. N Engl J Med. 2005;353:1659–72.
97. Zhang S, Liu X, Bawa-Khalfe T, et al. Identification of the molecular basis of doxorubicin-induced cardiotoxicity. Nat Med. 2012;18:1639–42.
98. Sorensen K, Levitt GA, Bull C, et al. Late anthracycline cardiotoxicity after childhood cancer: a prospective longitudinal study. Cancer. 2003;97:1991–8.
99. Geiger S, Lange V, Suhl P, et al. Anticancer therapy induced cardiotoxicity: review of the literature. Anticancer Drugs. 2010;21:578–90.
100. Eschenhagen T, Force T, Ewer MS, et al. Cardiovascular side effects of cancer therapies: a position statement from the Heart Failure Association of the European Society of Cardiology. Eur J Heart Fail. 2011;13:1–10.
101. Hunt SA, Abraham WT, Chin MH, et al. 2009 Focused update incorporated into the ACC/AHA 2005 Guidelines for the Diagnosis and Management of Heart Failure in Adults. A Report of the American College of Cardiology Foundation/American Heart Association Task Force on Practice Guidelines Developed in Collaboration with the International Society for Heart and Lung Transplantation [serial online]. J Am Coll Cardiol. 2009;53:e1–e90.
102. Curigliano G, Cardinale D, Suter T, et al. Cardiovascular toxicity induced by chemotherapy, targeted agents and radiotherapy: ESMO Clinical Practice Guidelines. Ann Oncol. 2012;23 suppl 7:vii155–66.
103. Martin M, Esteva FJ, Alba E, et al. Minimizing cardiotoxicity while optimizing treatment efficacy with trastuzumab: review and expert recommendations. Oncologist. 2009;14:1–11.
104. Jones AL, Barlow M, Barrett-Lee PJ, et al. Management of cardiac health in trastuzumab-treated patients with breast cancer: updated United Kingdom National Cancer Research Institute recommendations for monitoring. Br J Cancer. 2009;100:684–92.
105. Ewer MS, Lenihan DJ. Left ventricular ejection fraction and cardiotoxicity: is our ear really to the ground? J Clin Oncol. 2008;26:1201–3.
106. Cardinale D, Colombo A, Torrisi R, et al. Trastuzumab-induced cardiotoxicity: clinical and prognostic implications of troponin I evaluation. J Clin Oncol. 2010;28:3910–6.
107. Altena R, Perik PJ, van Veldhuisen DJ, et al. Cardiovascular toxicity caused by cancer treatment: strategies for early detection. Lancet Oncol. 2009;10:391–9.
108. Jenkins C, Leano R, Chan J, et al. Reconstructed versus real-time 3-dimensional echocardiography: comparison with magnetic resonance imaging. J Am Soc Echocardiogr. 2008;20:862–8.
109. Cardinale D, Sandri MT. Role of biomarkers in chemotherapyinduced cardiotoxicity. Prog Cardiovasc Dis. 2010;53:121–129. Lenihan D MM, Baysinger KB, et al. Superior detection of cardiotoxicity during chemotherapy using biomarkers [abstract]. J Card Fail. 2007;S151. Abstract 265.
110. Landier W, Bhatia S, Eshelman DA, et al. Development of riskbased guidelines for pediatric cancer survivors: the Children's Oncology Group Long-Term Follow-Up Guidelines from the Children's Oncology Group Late Effects Committee and Nursing Discipline. J Clin Oncol. 2004;22:4979–90.
111. Skinner R, Wallace WH, Levitt GA. Long-term follow-up of people who have survived cancer during childhood. Lancet Oncol. 2006;7:489–98.
112. Lenihan DJ. Statins in preparation for chemotherapy: "do these medications help your fitness for battle?". J Am Coll Cardiol. 2012;60:2391–2.
113. Silber JH, Cnaan A, Clark BJ, et al. Enalapril to prevent cardiac function decline in long-term survivors of pediatric cancer exposed to anthracyclines. J Clin Oncol. 2004;22:820–8.
114. Yoon GJ, Telli ML, Kao DP, et al. Left ventricular dysfunction in patients receiving cardiotoxic cancer therapies are clinicians responding optimally? J Am Coll Cardiol. 2010;56:1644–50.
115. Cardinale D, Colombo A, Lamantia G, et al. Anthracycline-induced cardiomyopathy: clinical relevance and response to pharmacologic therapy. J Am Coll Cardiol. 2010;55:213–20.
116. Cardinale D. Chapter 90: cardiovascular complication of cancer therapeutic agents. In: Bonow RO, Zipes DP, Libby P, editors. Braunwald's heart disease: a textbook of cardiovascular medicine. 9th ed. Philadelphia, PA: Saunders Elsevier; 2012.
117. Shukla A, Yusuf SW, Daher I, Lenihan D, Durand JB. High mortality rates are associated with withdrawal of beta blockers and ACE inhibitors in chemotherapy-induced heart failure [abstract]. Circulation. 2008;118:S797. Abstract 2942.
118. Ewer M, Lippman S. Type II Chemotherapy-related cardiac dysfunction: time to recognize a new entity. J Clin Oncol. 2005;23(13):2900–2.
119. Pinder MC, Duan Z, Goodwin JS, et al. Congestive heart failure in older women treated with adjuvant anthracycline chemotherapy for breast cancer. J Clin Oncol. 2007;25:3808–15.

120. Hooning MJ, Botma A, Aleman BM, et al. Long-term risk of cardiovascular disease in 10-year survivors of breast cancer. J Natl Cancer Inst. 2007;99:365–75.
121. Meacham LR, Chow EJ, Ness KK, et al. Cardiovascular risk factors in adult survivors of pediatric cancer—a report from the Childhood Cancer Survivor Study. Cancer Epidemiol Biomarkers Prev. 2010;19: 170–81.
122. Giordano SH, Kuo YF, Freeman JL, et al. Risk of cardiac death after adjuvant radiotherapy for breast cancer. J Natl Cancer Inst. 2005;97:419–24.
123. Travis LB, Ng AK, Allan JM, et al. Second malignant neoplasms and cardiovascular disease following radiotherapy. J Natl Cancer Inst. 2012;104:357–70.
124. Casper ES, Gaynor JJ, Hajdu SI, et al. A prospective randomized trial of adjuvant chemotherapy with bolus versus continuous infusion of doxorubicin in patients with high-grade extremity soft tissue sarcoma and an analysis of prognostic factors. Cancer. 1991;68(6):1221–9.
125. Smith LA, Cornelius VR, Plummer CJ, et al. Cardiotoxicity of anthracycline agents for the treatment of cancer: systematic review and meta-analysis of randomised controlled trials. BMC Cancer. 2010;10:337.
126. Young AM, Dhillon T, Bower M. Cardiotoxicity after liposomal anthracyclines. Lancet Oncol. 2004;5(11):654.
127. Hensley ML, Hagerty KL, Kewalramani T, et al. American Society of Clinical Oncology 2008 clinical practice guideline update: use of chemotherapy and radiation therapy protectants. Clin Oncol. 2009;127(1): 127–45.
128. Dulin B, Abraham WT. Pharmacology of carvedilol. Am J Cardiol. 2004;93(9A):3B–6B.
129. Bryant J, Picot J, Levitt G, et al. Cardioprotection against the toxic effects of anthracyclines given to children with cancer: a systematic review . Health Technol Assess. 2007; 11(27): iii, ix–x, 1–84.
130. Andersson A, Naslund U, Tavelin B, Enblad G, Gustavsson A, Malmer B. Long-term risk of cardiovascular disease in Hodgkin lymphoma survivors – retrospective cohort analyses and a concept for prospective intervention. Int J Cancer. 2009;124(8):1914–7.
131. Steinherz LJ, Graham T, Hurwitz R, et al. Guidelines for cardiac monitoring of children during and after anthracycline therapy: report of the cardiology committee of the childrens cancer study group. Pediatrics. 1992;89:942–9.
132. Ganz WI, Sridhar KS, Ganz SS, et al. Review of tests for monitoring doxorubicin-induced cardiomyopathy. Oncology. 1996;53:461–70.
133. Kapusta L, Thijssen JM, Groot-Loonen J, et al. Discriminative ability of conventional echocardiography and tissue Doppler imaging techniques for the detection of subclinical cardiotoxic effects of treatment with anthracyclines. Ultrasound Med Biol. 2001;27:1605–14.
134. Kapusta L, Thijssen JM, Groot-Loonen J, et al. Tissue Doppler imaging in detection of myocardial dysfunction in survivors of childhood cancer treated with anthracyclines. Ultrasound Med Biol. 2000;26:1099–108.
135. www.cardioncology.com [accessed 22 January 2013].

Cardiac Tumors

Contents

Cardiac Malignancies: Clinical Aspects

Paolo Giuseppe Pino and Chiara Lestuzzi

C. Lestuzzi et al. (eds.), *Manual of Cardio-oncology*, DOI 10.1007/978-3-319-40236-9_18

18.1 Symptoms

Most cardiac tumors are clinically silent and are diagnosed only postmortem. If present, symptoms that are nonspecific can be distinguished with difficulty from other causes of cardiovascular disease and are known to be "great mimickers" [1]. One of the most important problems concerning to the diagnosis of cardiac tumors is the lack of specific signs and symptoms. The clinical manifestations of cardiac metastases mainly depend on the size and anatomical location of the tumor, rather than on its histological type. The symptoms of cardiac metastases can be grouped into the following major categories [2–7]:

- **Mechanical (obstructive)** cardiac symptoms:
  - Large pericardial effusion with cardiac tamponade, or tumor encasement of the heart with cardiac constriction.
  - Obstruction of veins (i.e., superior or inferior vena cava syndrome) or valves.
  - A primary tumor of the pulmonary artery may mimic pulmonary embolism.
- **Systemic embolization:**
  - Pulmonary embolism.
  - Cerebral or peripheral embolism (stroke, transient ischemic attack, myocardial infarction, retinal artery embolism, embolism of the arteries of the lower or upper extremities) due to the embolism of tumor cells or thrombi formed on the tumor surface. Predisposition to embolic episodes depends mainly on the type of the tumor, its location (intramural or intracardial), and the fragility of its surface.
- **Infiltrative cardiac symptoms:**
  - Atrial or ventricular arrhythmias (atrial fibrillation, ventricular fibrillation)
  - Atrioventricular blocks (including complete atrioventricular block) by infiltration of the myocardium and cardiac conduction system
- **Symptoms mimicking acute coronary syndromes** (even in the absence of coronary artery involvement): chest pain, elevated cardiac biomarkers, ST- and T-wave abnormalities. They may be secondary to myocardial or pericardial metastases [8].
- **Congestive heart failure due to** replacement of the myocardium by tumor cells (Figs. 18.1 and 18.2) or to obstruction of valvular orifice (large intracavitary and prolapsing masses) (Fig. 18.3).

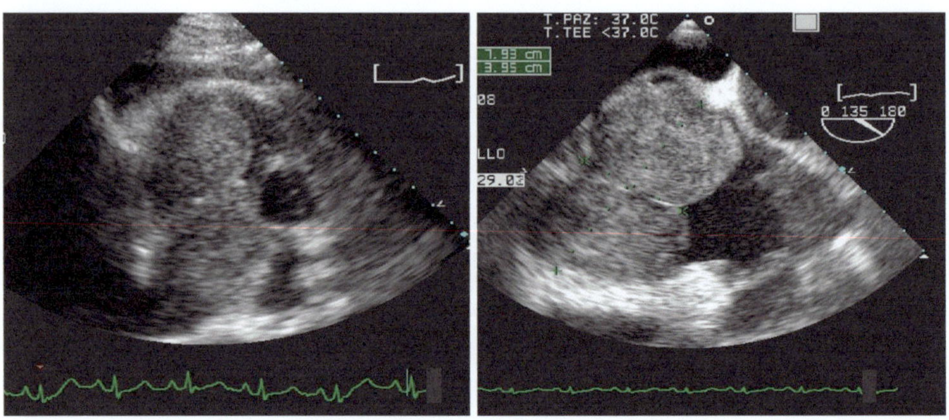

Fig. 18.1 Patient presenting with signs of *right* heart failure (distended jugular veins, peripheral edema, liver enlargement). At transthoracic (*left*) and transesophageal (*right*) echocardiogram, the *right* chambers are occupied and infiltrated by a huge mass. Final diagnosis: pulmonary sarcoma

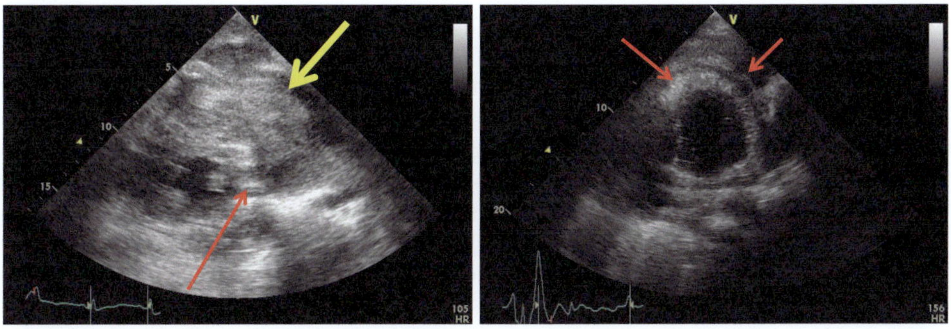

Fig. 18.2 Patient with mediastinal lymphoma (*yellow arrow*) and infiltration of the myocardium (*left*) and the pericardium (*right*) (*red arrows*)

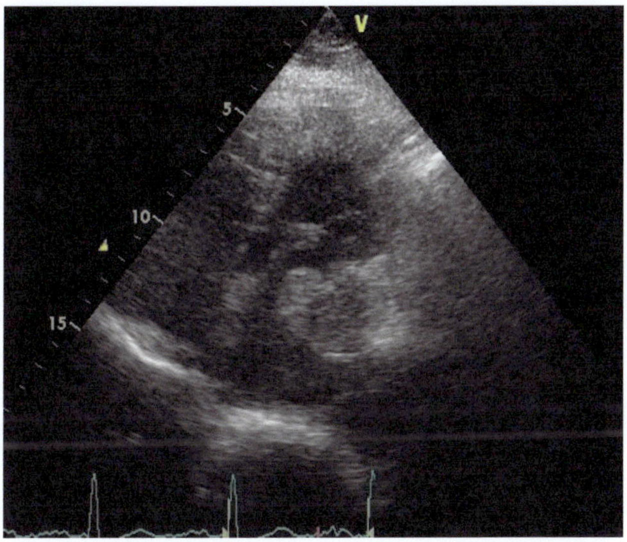

Fig. 18.3 Patient complaining of dizziness and dyspnoea. In diastole a huge left atrial mass prolapses in the left ventricle through the mitral valve orifice

The most frequent clinical symptoms leading the patient to the medical observation are:

- **Dyspnea.** Differential diagnosis includes other cardiac diseases (cardiomyopathies, valvular heart disease, etc.) and pleural and lung diseases [9]:
  - In the presence of tachycardia and engorged jugular veins, without pulmonary rales a pericardial pathology, right heart disease, obstruction of superior vena cava, or pulmonary artery pathology should be considered.
  - **Chest X-ray** usually can orient the diagnosis: look at the cardiac shadow (normal/enlarged), pleural effusion, lung abnormalities, and mediastinum.
  - **Transthoracic echocardiography** is the second diagnostic step.
- **Tachycardia** is a common finding in many clinical conditions, including fever and anemia. In a patient with already diagnosed cancer, consider these options first. However, in the presence of engorged jugular veins, consider the possibility of a superior vena cava obstruction.
- **Dizziness and syncope** may be the first symptoms of an intracavitary tumor, mostly of highly mobile masses.

18.2 Physical Examination

The physical examination is often negative. However, there are some signs which should alert the physician:

- **Engorged jugular veins** are typical of large pericardial effusion, superior vena cava obstruction (by a thrombus, a tumor, or by a compressive mediastinal mass), right heart masses, and possibly pulmonary embolism [10].
- **Pulsus paradoxus** (an exaggerated reduction of the systolic blood pressure during quiet respiration) may be suggestive of cardiac tamponade:
  - **Pitfalls:** also severe obstructive lung disease and the presence of a mediastinal mass may cause pulsus paradoxus. See Chap. 21 for further details.

18.3 ECG Abnormalities

Some ECG abnormalities may be observed in primary and secondary cardiac tumors:

- **Atrial flutter/fibrillation** may be the first sign of an atrial tumor in young people with low probability of arrhythmia. A careful evaluation of the atria is mandatory in patients with unexplained recurrent atrial arrhythmias (◘ Figs. 18.4 and 18.5).
- **ECG signs of ischemia** may be the sign of a myocardial infiltration by a primary or secondary tumor (◘ Fig. 18.6). The finding is much suspect if the patient is at low risk for a cardiac event and does not refer chest pain or other symptoms suggesting an acute coronary syndrome [10–13].
- **Low voltages** are common in large neoplastic pericardial effusion, mostly in the presence of cardiac tamponade. However, low voltages may be observed also in the presence of pleural effusion, large mediastinal masses, and diffuse edema. The association of *electrical alternans* and *sinus tachycardia* are also suggestive of cardiac tamponade; the presence of all three ECG abnormalities is highly suggestive of tamponade (100 % specificity) [14].

Even large primary or secondary cardiac tumors may be silent from the clinical and physical point of view. However, some signs and symptoms may rise the suspicion and should be considered together. See the ◘ Table 18.1 for a summary.

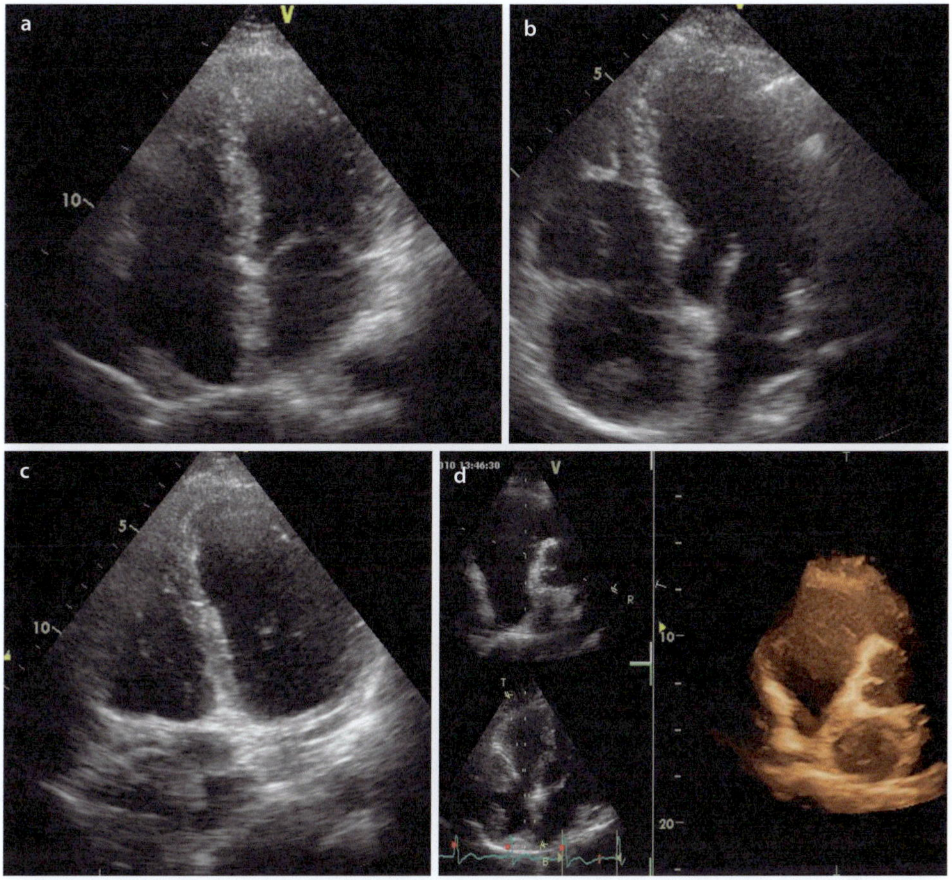

Fig. 18.4 Young patient with recurrent supraventricular tachyarrhythmias. **a** At transthoracic echocardiography the standard apical four-chamber view seems almost normal, only with a thickened interatrial septum. **b**, **c** Using different angulations of the transducer, a mass arising from the *right* atrial roof and posterior wall is evident. **d** At 3D echo a mass infiltrating the lateral wall is also evident

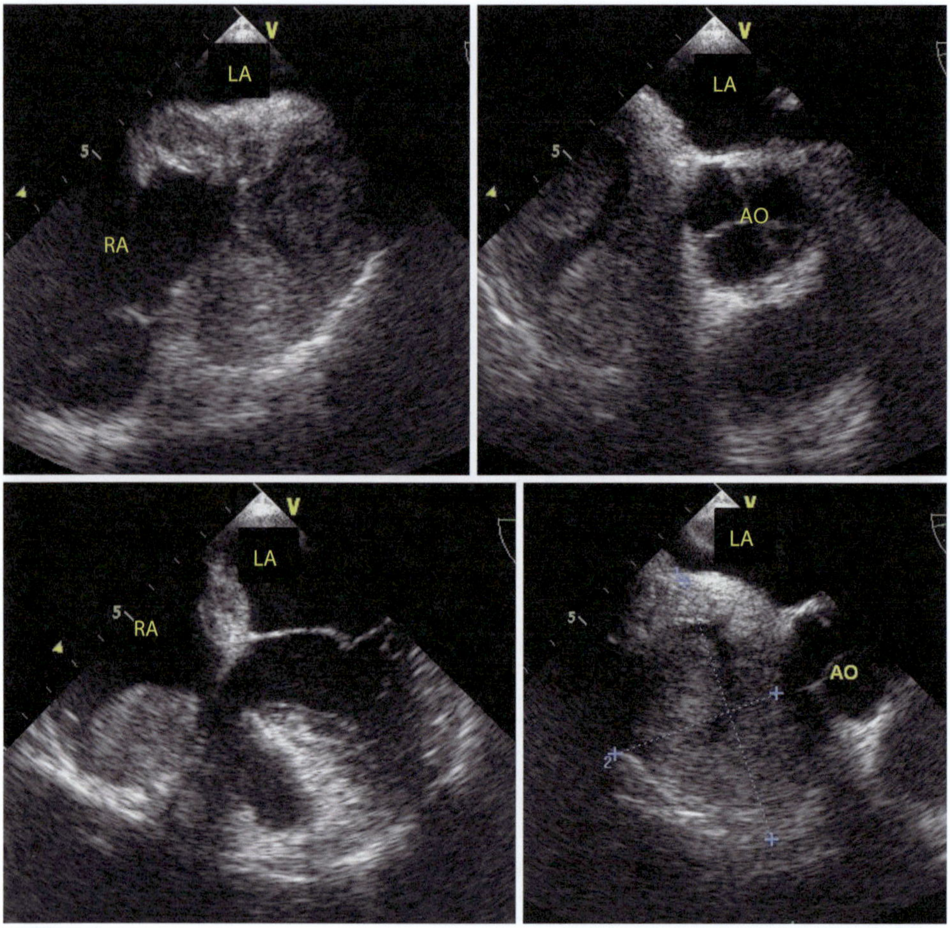

Fig. 18.5 Same patient as in Fig. 18.4. From the transesophageal approach, a huge, polilobated *right* atrial mass is evident. The mass infiltrates the interatrial septum, the posterior and lateral wall, and the tricuspid annulus

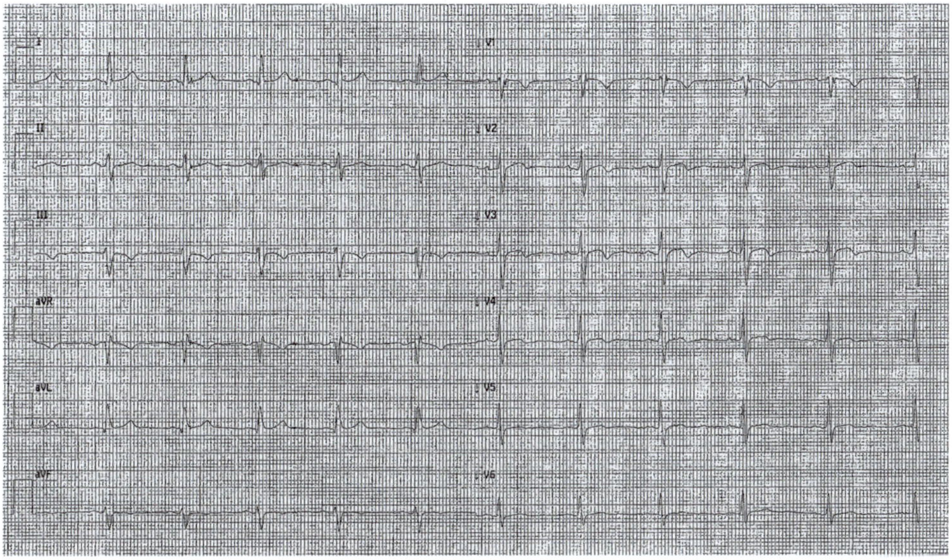

Fig. 18.6 ECG abnormalities mimicking an acute ischemia in an asymptomatic patient with angiosarcoma metastasis to the cardiac apex

Table 18.1 Frequency of signs and symptoms as regards he site of the mass

	Pericardial tumors	Atrial tumors	Ventricular tumors	Venous obstruction	Differential diagnosis
Dyspnea	Frequent	Rare	Rare	Rare	Pleural effusion, lung diseases, mediastinal syndrome, pulmonary embolism
Tachycardia	Frequent	Possible	Possible	Rare	Anemia, fever, pulmonary embolism
Chest pain	Possible	Rare	Possible	Rare	Bone metastases, pleural pathology, pulmonary embolism
Hypotension	Frequent	Rare	Possible	Frequent	Severe anemia, fever, cachexia, mediastinal syndrome
Syncope, Dizziness	Unusual	Possible	Possible	Unusual	Severe anemia, fever, cachexia, mediastinal syndrome

(continued)

Table 18.1 (Continued)

	Pericardial tumors	Atrial tumors	Ventricular tumors	Venous obstruction	Differential diagnosis
Distended jugular veins	Frequent	Possible	Unusual	Frequent	Mediastinal syndrome
Peripheral edema	Frequent	Unusual	Unusual	Frequent	Lymph node enlargement, hypoproteinemia
Atrial flutter/ fibrillation	Rare	Frequent	Unusual	Unusual	Lung cancer, hypoxia, chemotherapy side effect
ECG signs of ischemia	Possible	Unusual	Unusual	Unusual	Coronary artery disease, chemotherapy side effect
Conduction defects	Unusual	Possible	Possible	Unusual	Coronary artery disease, age-related cardiac disease

References

1. Butany J, Nair V, Naseemuddin A, Nair GM, Catton C, Yau T. Cardiac tumours: diagnosis and management. Lancet Oncol. 2005;6:219–28.
2. Goldberg AD, Blankstein R, Padera RF. Tumour metastatic to the heart. Circulation. 2013;128:1790–4.
3. Neragi-Miandoab S, Kim J, Vlahakes GJ. Malignant tumours of the heart: a review of tumour type, diagnosis and therapy. Clin Oncol (R Coll Radiol). 2007;19:748–56.
4. Hudzik B, Miszalski-Jamka K, Glowacki J, Lekston A, Gierlotka M. Malignant tumors of the heart. Cancer Epidemiol. 2015;39:665–72.
5. Perazzolo Marra M, Thiene G, De Lazzari M, et al. Concealed metastatic lung carcinoma presenting as acute coronary syndrome with progressive conduction abnormalities. Circulation. 2012;125:e499–502.
6. Bussani R, De-Giorgio F, Abbate A, Silvestri F. Cardiac metastases. J Clin Pathol. 2007;60:27–34.
7. Reynen K, Köckeritz U, Strasser RH. Metastases to the heart. Ann Oncol. 2004;15:375–81.
8. Di Michele S, Mirabelli F, Galzerano D, Mankad S. An unusual myocardial infarction. Echo Res Prac. 2014; 1:K9–12.
9. Angeli D, Angeli SJ. Respiratory failure in an adolescent with primary cardiac sarcoma. Case Rep Cardiol. 2015;2015, 592385.
10. Huang G, Shu L, Xu J. Heart failure and main pulmonary artery obstruction caused by right ventricular metastatic adult hepatoblastoma: a case report. Medicine (Baltimore). 2015;94, e1535.
11. Lestuzzi C, Nicolosi GL, Biasi S, Piotti P, Zanuttini D. Sensitivity and specificity of electrocardiographic ST-T changes as markers of neoplastic myocardial infiltration. Echocardiographic correlation. Chest. 1989;95:980–5.
12. Abe S, Watanabe N, Ogura S, et al. Myocardial metastasis from primary lung cancer: myocardial infarction-like ECG changes and pathologic findings. Jpn J Med. 1991;30:213–8.
13. Pan KL, Wu LS, Chung CM, et al. Misdiagnosis: cardiac metastasis presented as a pseudo-infarction on electrocardiography. Int Heart J. 2007;48:399–405.
14. Argula RG, Negi SI, Banchs J, Yusuf SW. Role of a 12-lead electrocardiogram in the diagnosis of cardiac tamponade as diagnosed by transthoracic echocardiography in patients with malignant pericardial effusion. Clin Cardiol. 2015;38:139–44.

Secondary Cardiac Tumors

Chiara Lestuzzi and Carlos A. Roldan

C. Lestuzzi et al. (eds.), *Manual of Cardio-oncology*, DOI 10.1007/978-3-319-40236-9_19

19.1 Introduction

- Secondary cardiac tumors are tumors originating in other organs/tissues that extend to the heart.
- The primary tumor may be localized within the thorax (lung and mediastinal tumors), below the diaphragm (renal carcinoma), or be extrathoracic (breast carcinoma).
- In autopsy studies the prevalence of secondary cardiac tumors is about 10–15 % [1].
- The incidence of secondary cardiac tumors in living patients is unknown. In our experience, it is rare and varies according to the type of the primary cancer. For example, in a tertiary care hospital with many patients with lung cancer or lymphoma, about 5–10 cases/year involving the heart are diagnosed.
- The most common malignancies extending to the heart are lung carcinomas (35–40 %), hematologic malignancies (10–20 %), and breast carcinomas (10 %) [2]. Other various types constitute about 30 %.
- The most common endocavitary metastases are due to renal, hepatic, or gynecologic carcinomas, which reach the heart through the inferior vena cava.
  - These endocavitary metastases often have superimposed thrombus [3].
- Cardiac metastases may be diagnosed because of the appearance of nonspecific symptoms (mostly dyspnea) or incidentally detected during a routine imaging test [chest X-ray, electrocardiography (ECG), echocardiography, computed tomography (CT), or magnetic resonance imaging (MRI)].

19.2 Pathophysiology

- Cardiac metastases reach the heart through the inferior or superior vena cava, the coronary arteries, and the lymphatic vessels or by continuity [4].
- The cardiac involvement may be either limited to the pericardium, myocardium, and endocardium or affect more than one structure:
  - The parietal and/or visceral pericardium is the most commonly involved site (65–70 % of cases) and is usually secondary to a retrograde lymphatic spread from mediastinal lymph nodes, less commonly by direct infiltration of a thoracic tumor:
    - Among patients with pericardial involvement, the epicardium is the metastatic site in 30 % of cases, and it is involved through retrograde lymphatic spread and hematogenous spread or by extension from pericardial or myocardial metastases.
  - Myocardial metastases (25–30 % of cases) are usually secondary to dissemination through the coronary vessels or through the lymphatic channels that run along the vessels from the epicardium into the myocardium, less commonly from extension from pericardial or intracavitary metastases.
  - Endocardial and intracavitary metastases are rare (3.5 % of cases) and reach the heart through the bloodstream.

19.3 Neoplastic Pericardial Disease

19.3.1 General Considerations

- A pericardial effusion is a rather frequent finding in patients with cancer and may be secondary to pericardial metastases, lymphatic obstruction, or cancer treatment (mostly radiation therapy) [5].

About 65–70 % of pericardial effusions in cancer patients are due to metastases.

- The most frequent tumors causing a pericardial effusion are lung and breast carcinomas and lymphomas:

Less frequent causes are renal or gastrointestinal carcinomas.

- In neoplastic pericarditis, the associated pericardial effusion is usually slowly progressive, but infrequently may increase rapidly and lead to cardiac tamponade:

Large pericardial effusion and cardiac tamponade are more frequent in neoplastic pericardial disease than any other cause of pericarditis.

- Clinically manifested neoplastic pericardial disease can also be caused by solid masses, with only minimal pericardial effusion. The masses may be isolated, multiple, or in advanced cases, an encasing tumor of the heart.

19.3.2 Clinical Manifestations

Typical Cardiac Tamponade

- It is characterized by distended jugular veins, pulsus paradoxus (a decrease in systolic blood pressure of >10 mmHg during quiet inspiration), tachycardia and-in severe cases-hypotension, oliguria, or shock.
- However, the clinical manifestations of cardiac tamponade are dependent of the size and rate of accumulation of the pericardial effusion, underlying intracardiac pressures and volume status. Therefore, the clinical manifestations of cardiac tamponade may be highly variable [6, 7].

Atypical Cardiac Tamponade

- This syndrome does not present with the characteristic manifestations of cardiac tamponade (i.e., pulsus paradoxus).
- It is observed in patient with underlying high right or left ventricular end-diastolic pressures or in those patients with solid pericardial masses without or with minimal pericardial effusion causing isolated compression of a cardiac chamber (including the left heart chambers).
- Occurs more frequently in patients with neoplastic pericardial disease than in viral or idiopathic pericarditis.

Constrictive or Effusive Constrictive Pericarditis

- Occurs in those cases of encasing pericardial tumors, infiltrative pericardial tumors, or postradiation therapy

Asymptomatic Pericardial Effusions

- They are incidentally diagnosed during routine echocardiographic or radiologic investigations.

They are rather frequent, 5–10 % in our experience, and usually mild to moderate and in most cases do not require any therapeutic intervention. However, they do require close clinical and echocardiographic follow-up.

Pitfalls of the Clinical Diagnosis of Malignant Pericardial Disease

- Anemia and hypovolemia may exacerbate some signs and symptoms (tachycardia, dyspnea, hypotension) and masquerade others (absent jugular vein distension) of cardiac tamponade or constriction.
- Common pulmonary parenchymal, pleural, and/or mediastinal involvement leading to pulmonary hypertension and/or cor pulmonale in these patients can cause symptoms and signs mimicking (dyspnea, tachycardia, jugular venous distension) or masquerading (absent pulsus paradoxus) cardiac tamponade or constriction:
- Rarely, a large pleural effusion can cause cardiac compression and clinical manifestations of tamponade.
- Neoplastic pericarditis with tumor encasement of the heart may cause an effusive constrictive pattern which may also mimic clinically cardiac tamponade.

Caveat

In patients with malignant pericardial disease, the diagnosis of typical or atypical cardiac tamponade or constriction requires the integration of a thorough history and physical examination with Doppler echocardiography and commonly with CT or MRI and in few selected cases with invasive hemodynamic assessment with or without intravenous volume loading of 300–500 ml of saline.

19.3.3 Diagnosis of Neoplastic Pericardial Diseases

Echocardiography

- The most commonly used imaging modality
- The most commonly observed echocardiographic findings in neoplastic pericardial disease are [7, 8]:
  - **Moderate to large pericardial effusion** (circumferential effusion with >10 mm separation between the pericardial layers) without evidence of tamponade
  - Cardiac tamponade:
    - The most frequent and relevant echocardiographic findings in cardiac tamponade are right atrial and right ventricular diastolic compression (◘ Table 19.1, ◘ Fig. 19.1a–c).
    - Variability of the tricuspid and mitral inflow Doppler velocities during inspiration (increase in tricuspid inflow velocities >30 % with simultaneous >30 % decrease in mitral inflow velocities) is of complementary diagnostic value (◘ Fig. 19.1d).
    - In patients with atypical cardiac tamponade, right heart chamber compression may be absent, or compression of an isolated chamber (including the left heart chambers) may occur. Also, in these cases the respiratory variability of the tricuspid and mitral inflows may be absent.
  - Intrapericardial solid metastatic masses (◘ Figs. 19.1c and 19.2)
  - The most relevant echocardiographic findings of these masses are:
    - Large dimensions
    - Moderate to high echogenicity
    - Echogenicity similar to other intrathoracic masses known to be neoplastic

◘ **Table 19.1** Right atrial and right ventricular diastolic compression in cardiac tamponade

Right atrium	Right ventricle
Occurs with intrapericardial pressure >4 mmHg	Occurs with intrapericardial pressure >6–8 mmHg
Earliest finding (most common)	Late finding (after right atrial collapse)
High sensitivity, but low specificity	Lower sensitivity, but higher specificity
Low positive predictive value	High positive predictive value
Occurs during late diastole/early systole, worsens during expiration or apnea	Occurs during early diastole, may be transient or last through early and mid-diastole and disappear after atrial contraction
More specific if lasting ≥one third of the cardiac cycle	Its degree and duration do not correlate with the severity of tamponade
Best noted on the midportion of the lateral or posterolateral walls	Best noted on the anterior and posterolateral wall
Best seen from apical and subcostal views	Best seen from parasternal and subcostal views

Adapted with permission from Roldan CA. The Ultimate Echo Guide. Lippincott Williams & Wilkins, Philadelphia 2012

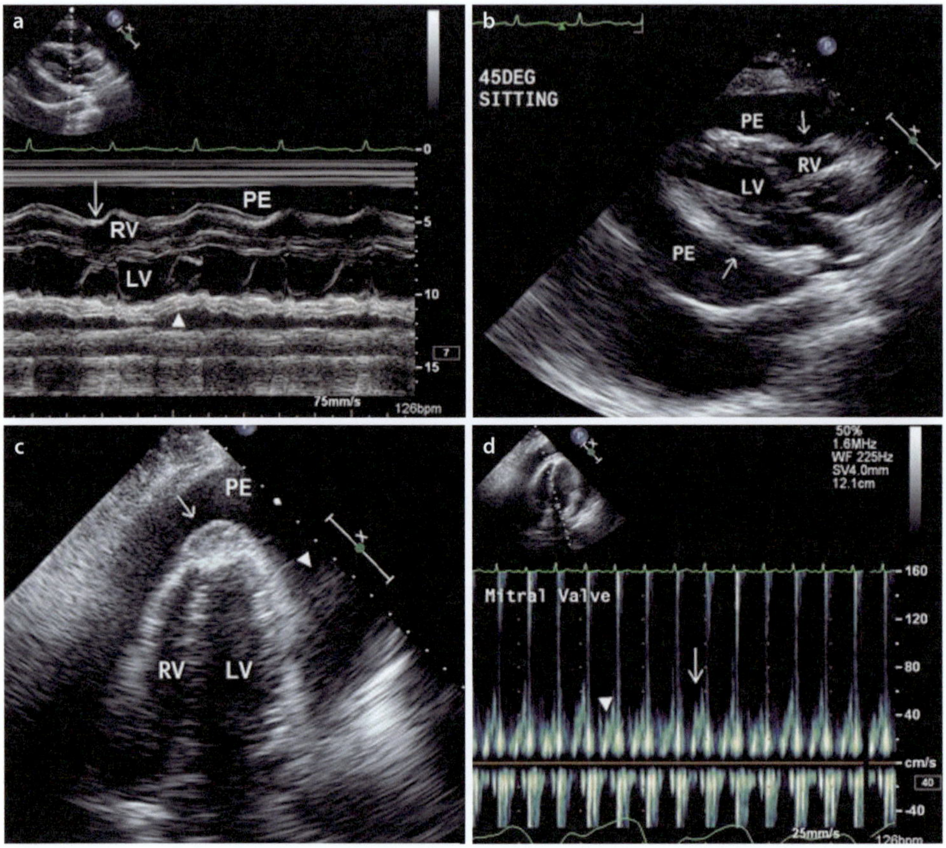

Fig. 19.1 Metastatic breast cancer complicated with a large malignant pericardial effusion and cardiac tamponade. **a** This two-dimensional (2D) guided parasternal long-axis M-mode echocardiogram demonstrates a large pericardial effusion causing diastolic compression of the right ventricle (RV) anterior (*arrow*) and posterior left ventricular (LV) (*arrowhead*) walls. **b** This 2D parasternal long-axis view demonstrates a circumferential pericardial effusion with visceral pericardial thickening and diastolic compression of the RV anterior and LV inferolateral walls (*arrows*). **c** This **2D** apical four-chamber view demonstrates a large and circumferential pericardial effusion (PE) associated with severe visceral pericardial thickening and a visceral pericardial mass at the cardiac apex (*arrow*) and fibrin strands (*arrowhead*). **d** Pulse wave Doppler echocardiogram of the mitral inflow demonstrates a significant (≥30 %) decrease during inspiration (*arrowhead*) and increase during expiration (*arrow*) of early diastolic inflow velocities. Adapted with permission from Roldan CA. The Ultimate Echo Guide. Lippincott Williams & Wilkins, Philadelphia 2012

  - Increased echogenicity after injection of contrast medium
  - Common infiltration of the underlying myocardium and associated with pericardial effusion (Fig. 19.1c).
- Encasing tumors causing pericardial constriction (Table 19.2 and Fig. 19.2):
  - Diffuse thickening (≥2 cm) of the epicardium (with or without pericardial effusion)
  - Inspiratory leftward displacement of the interventricular septum
  - Mitral E peak velocity reduction of >30 % during inspiration and a reciprocal ≥30 % increase in the tricuspid E peak velocity
  - Dilated inferior vena cava

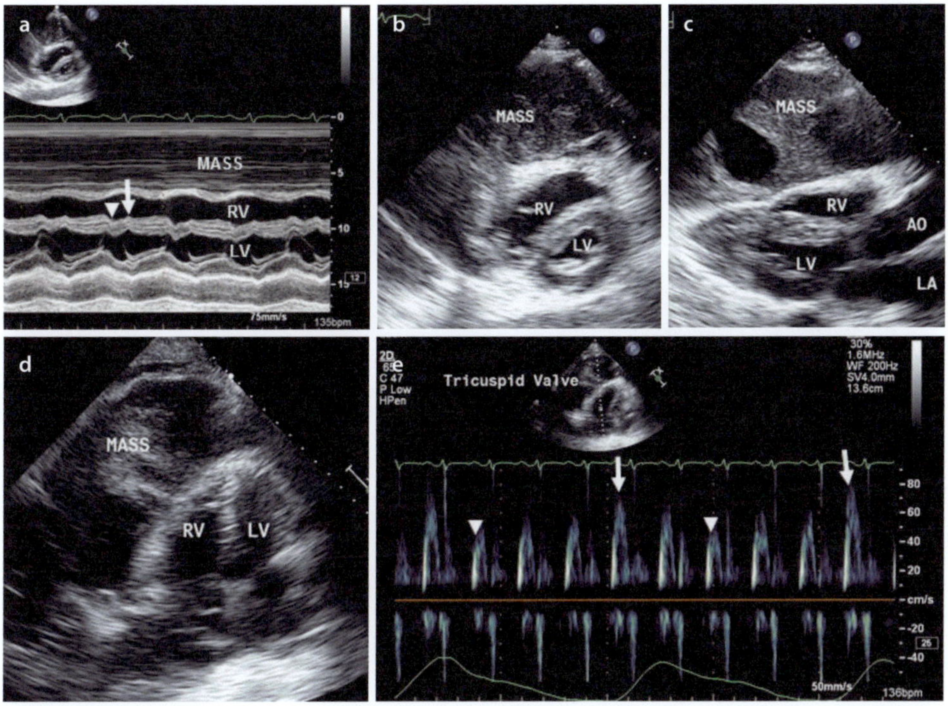

Fig. 19.2 Large mediastinal germ cell tumor causing cardiac tamponade or constriction-like echocardiographic findings. **a** This two-dimensional (2D) guided parasternal short-axis M-mode echocardiogram demonstrates a large retrosternal germ cell tumor (*mass*) extending to the pericardium and compressing the entire heart, predominantly the right ventricle (RV). Limited systolic and diastolic excursion of both ventricles with small cavities and the consequent abnormal double dip (posterior and then anterior) septal motion (*arrowhead* and *arrow*). **b**, **c**, **d** These 2D parasternal short- **b** and long-axis **c** views and apical four-chamber view **d** define better the large soft tissue echoreflectant mass with cystic transformation extending to the anterolateral pericardium and compressing the entire heart with consequent compromised filling leading to small ventricles. **e** Pulse wave Doppler echocardiography of the tricuspid inflow demonstrates a significant increase (>30 %) from expiration (*arrowheads*) to inspiration (*arrows*) of early inflow velocities indicative of hemodynamically significant cardiac compression. Adapted with permission from Roldan CA. The Ultimate Echo Guide. Lippincott Williams & Wilkins, Philadelphia 2012

Pitfalls of Echocardiography

- Loculated effusions (even those of hemodynamic significance) may be missed in technically difficult studies.
- In patients who had undergone pneumonectomy or thoracic irradiation, a complete visualization of the heart and pericardium may be limited.
- Epicardial fat (low echogenic and more commonly seen over the right ventricle epicardium or right atrioventricular groove), intrapericardial fibrin strands, or clots in bloody effusion may mimic metastatic masses.

Caveat

Since echocardiography has some limitations and up to 30 % of pericardial effusions or masses in cancer patients are not neoplastic, the diagnosis of neoplastic pericardial disease must be confirmed by more than one diagnostic method.

Table 19.2 Echocardiographic findings in constrictive pericarditis in neoplastic pericarditis

Finding	Frequency
Pericardial and/or epicardial thickening	>95 %
Pericardial effusion (often effusive constrictive pericarditis)	50 %
Enlarged atria	75 %
Abnormal septal diastolic motion	≥70 %
Left atrial hypertension	>90 %
Plethoric inferior vena cava	≥70 %
Constrictive or restrictive Doppler pattern of the mitral or tricuspid valve inflow (E/A ratio >1.5)	≥90
Mitral annulus reversus by tissue Doppler (lateral E′ velocity < septal E′ velocity)	

Adapted with permission from Roldan CA. The Ultimate Echo Guide. Lippincott Williams & Wilkins, Philadelphia 2012

Computed Tomography

- Allows quantification and location of pericardial effusions
- Provides better imaging in cases of technically difficult echocardiograms (in patients with obesity, with emphysema, or with displaced heart by mediastinal masses or after pneumonectomy)
- Differentiates better than echocardiography intrapericardial masses as tumors from thrombi, fibrin, or fat
- May identify other causes of pericardial effusion (i.e., aortic dissection) or other associated pathology (pulmonary or mediastinal masses, pleural effusions, pulmonary embolism)

Pitfalls of Computed Tomography

- It is less helpful than echocardiography in defining the hemodynamic impact of pericardial effusion, thickening, or masses.
- It is not available at all or not easily available.
- It is not possible to perform in an emergency room or at bedside.

Magnetic Resonance Imaging (MRI)

- Allows quantification and location of pericardial effusions.
- Provides better imaging as compared to technically limited echocardiography.
- With the use of gadolinium contrast, has high specificity in the differential diagnosis of intrapericardial masses.
- May identify other possible causes of pericardial effusion (i.e., aortic dissection) or other associated pathologies (pulmonary or mediastinal masses, pleural effusions, pulmonary embolism).
- With real-time cine MRI, it can provide hemodynamic information.

Pitfalls of MRI

- Limited availability.
- As for CT scan, it cannot be performed in the emergency room.
- Requires long acquisition time and therefore it is not appropriate for unstable or very sick patients.

Positron Emission Tomography (PET) with 18-Fluorodeoxiglucose (^{18}FDG)

- Provides improved specificity for a malignant tumor when it detects a mass with high FDG uptake (◘ Fig. 19.3)
- Provides the possibility of scanning the whole body in one exam (useful if the primary tumor and other metastatic sites are still unknown)

Pitfalls of PET

- High cost and high radiation burden.
- Its specificity may be compromised because the normal myocardium and inflamed pericardium can show FDG uptake.

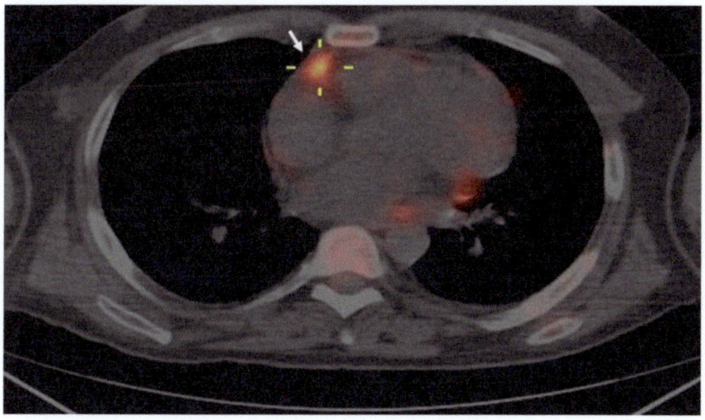

◘ **Fig. 19.3** Pericardial metastasis by lymphoma detected by PET. This PET in a patient with lymphoma demonstrates a well-defined mass with high FDG uptake (*arrow*) located at the right atrioventricular groove.

Cytology of the Pericardial Fluid [9]

- The gold standard is the finding of neoplastic cells in the pericardial fluid:
  - Its sensitivity and specificity varies according to tumor type and pathology procedures from 30 % to >90 %
- The diagnostic yield is highest (>90 % of diagnostic samples in our experience):
  - When all drained fluid is sent immediately to the pathologist.
  - When the pathologist centrifuges the fluid as soon as possible and performs various analyses (morphologic exam, immunohistochemistry, cell block analysis).

If the pathologic analysis is delayed (in the case of emergency pericardiocentesis during the weekend or in a hospital without pathology laboratory), the drained fluid is refrigerated at 4° and examined within 48 h.

Pitfalls of Cytology

- If the fluid sample is limited or not well preserved, the cytologic diagnosis may be difficult.
- The specificity of the pericardial fluid cytology for mesothelioma is limited because hyperplastic or reactive mesothelial cells may mimic malignant mesothelioma.
- Its sensitivity is very low in Hodgkin lymphoma.

Neoplastic Markers in the Pericardial Fluid

- The detection of Claudine4 is highly sensitive, but does not provide information about the histologic type of a tumor:
  - It is most useful in patients with already known neoplasm.
  - Has high sensitivity and specificity in distinguishing reactive mesothelium from metastatic carcinoma (85–99 % and 100 %, respectively).
- Other markers include the carcinoembryonic antigen (CEA) and serum cytokeratin 19 fragments (CYFRA 21-1):
  - The diagnosis may be considered very likely if these markers in the pericardial fluid are very high (CEA > 90 ng/ml, CYFRA 21-1 > 500 ng/ml).
  - A CEA > 10 ng/ml and/or CYFRA 21-1 > 100 ng/ml are highly suggestive of neoplastic pericarditis.
  - A high value of CYFRA 21-1 with low CEA in the pleural fluid can identify patients with mesothelioma.

Pitfalls of Neoplastic Markers in the Pericardial Fluid

- No single tumor marker is highly sensitive or specific.
- Mild to moderate elevations are nonspecific.

19.4 Practical Diagnostic Imaging Approach in Neoplastic Pericardial Disease

- Echocardiography is the routine initial imaging technique:
  - Intrapericardial masses should be further evaluated with ultrasound contrast medium.
- If intrapericardial masses of possible neoplastic nature are observed on echocardiography, CT and/or PET if available should be performed for further determination of the etiology of pericardial masses.
  - If the diagnosis needs to be defined because of clinical relevance from the oncologic point of view (i.e., if it would change the prognosis or the therapeutic approach):
  - Pericardial drainage should be performed if a moderate effusion is present and a drainage is safely feasible
  - If pericardial drainage is not possible, MRI with gadolinium or high-speed CT could help in defining the diagnosis.
  - PET is useful if a pericardial mass is >5 mm in size.

19.4.1 Treatment of Neoplastic Pericardial Disease

Treatment of Cardiac Tamponade

- Percutaneous drainage:
  - It is performed using the Seldinger technique and usually by an experienced cardiologist [10].
  - It is the preferred technique in hospitals without cardiac or thoracic surgery.
  - Echocardiographic guidance is commonly used to choose the most feasible and safe approach (subcostal, apical, parasternal) according to the localization of the pericardial fluid and largest visceral and parietal pericardial separations (>1.5 cm) [7, 11, 12]:

    The injection of a small amount of saline solution after pericardial puncture helps to verify the correct intrapericardial position of the catheter [7, 12].
  - CT may also be used to guide pericardiocentesis when expert echocardiographic guidance is not available [13, 14].
- Surgical drainage:
  - May be used if percutaneous drainage is not safely feasible or pericardial effusion is recurrent.
  - It is a reasonable approach in centers with cardiac or thoracic surgery.

Prevention of Recurring Tamponade

- Extended drainage:
  - It is obtained by leaving the pericardial catheter open and draining in a sterile sac:

    This approach is generally not recommended since it may be uncomfortable for the patient and increases the risk of catheter displacement, occlusion, and infection.
- Pericardial sclerosis:
  - It is performed by instilling bleomycin and thiotepa (antineoplastic agents with sclerosing properties), into the pericardial space with lower rate of side effects as compared to tetracycline.

  - A risk of pericardial sclerosis is the evolution to adhesive pericarditis and to loculated effusion requiring redo surgery in the case of relapse.
- Pericardial window:
  - It may be done through a surgical approach or percutaneously with a balloon catheter [15, 16].
  - In a study comparing cases treated by systemic chemotherapy alone versus combining it with pericardiocentesis or pericardial window, patients treated with pericardial window had better outcome [17].
  - The surgical approach, however, has a higher rate of complications compared to percutaneous pericardial drainage [18].

Treatment of Pericardial Metastases

- Intrapericardial chemotherapy:
  - *Alone or in combination with systemic chemotherapy seems to be effective mainly in* tumors that spread through the retrograde lymphatic way, such as lung and breast carcinomas.
  - In a study of 119 lung cancer patients, combined systemic and local chemotherapy as compared to intrapericardial therapy alone yielded the highest rate of long-term control of neoplastic pericarditis [19].

19.5 Myocardial Metastases

19.5.1 General Considerations

- The most common tumors causing myocardial metastasis are hematologic malignancies, breast carcinoma, and sarcomas.

19.5.2 Clinical Manifestations

- Myocardial metastases are commonly asymptomatic and therefore commonly incidentally diagnosed.
- However, they can manifest clinically with angina, heart failure, or ventricular arrhythmias.

19.5.3 Diagnostic Imaging (See Also ▶ Chap. 24 for Further Details)

Electrocardiography (ECG)

- The ECG is often abnormal and may show pseudo-ischemic changes [20].
- The most typical change is ST segment elevation in cases of large metastases or transmural infiltration (◘ Fig. 19.4).
- When the infiltration is limited within the ventricular wall thickness, negative T waves may be evident.

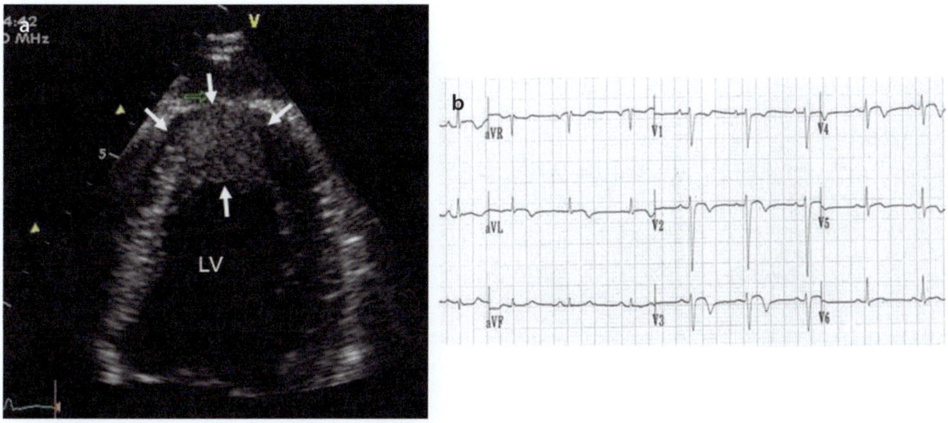

Fig. 19.4 Myocardial metastasis from a breast carcinoma causing electrographic ischemic changes. **a** This two-dimensional apical close-up view of the left ventricle (LV) demonstrates an oval and soft tissue echoreflectant mass (*arrows*) located at the LV apex. **b** This 12-lead ECG demonstrates ST elevation with T wave inversion in the precordial (V1–V6) and lateral (I, AVL) leads mimicking acute anterolateral myocardial injury ischemia.

Pitfalls of ECG

- It is nonspecific since ischemic-like ECG changes may be caused by ischemic heart disease, acute pericarditis, severe anemia, electrolyte imbalances, or chemotherapy-related cardiotoxicity.
- Detection of new ST segment elevation in a cancer patient with no symptom or signs of cardiac ischemia or pericarditis should prompt echocardiography to define better the diagnosis.

Echocardiography (Fig. 19.5)

- Myocardial metastases appear as noncontractile masses with different echogenicity from the surrounding normal myocardium (Fig. 19.5a, b).
- When the myocardium is diffusely infiltrated, the ventricular walls appear thickened with irregular echogenicity and reduced contractile thickening.

After the injection of echocardiographic contrast medium, the echogenicity of the infiltrated myocardium appears reduced or echolucent as compared to the surrounding normal myocardium—in the early phase—(Fig. 19.5c, d), but after few minutes appears as an irregularly enhanced mass (Fig. 19.5e, f).

Pitfalls of Echocardiography

- It may not differentiate tumor from other focal infiltrative diseases such as sarcoid.
- With poor acoustic windows or in particular sites (as near the mitral or tricuspid annulus), the sensitivity of echocardiography is low.

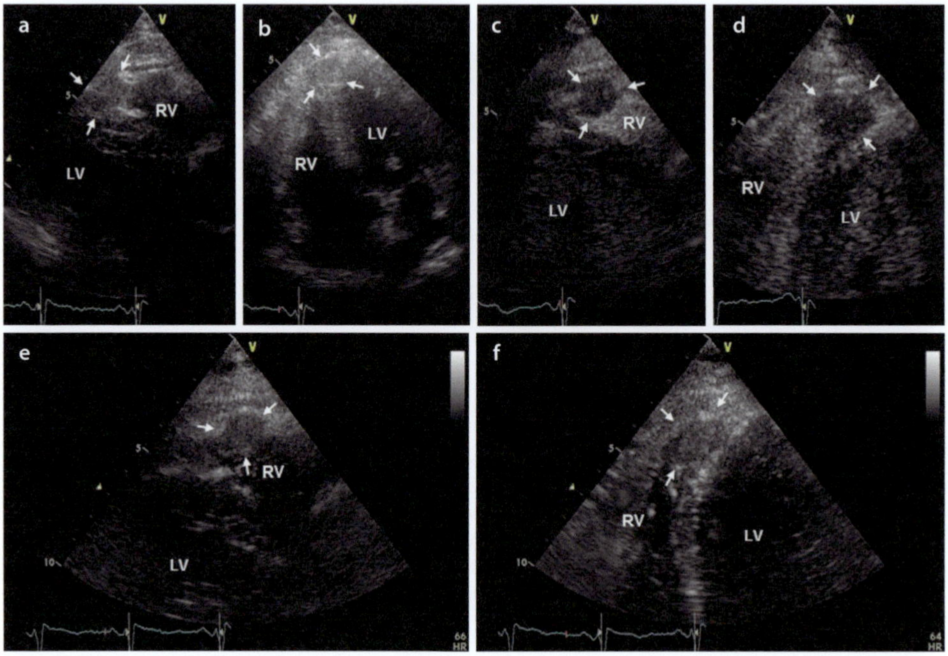

Fig. 19.5 Myocardial metastasis assessed by contrast echocardiography. Technically difficult two-dimensional (2D) long parasternal **a** and apical four-chamber **b** views demonstrating an ill defined oval and soft tissue echoreflectant mass (*arrows*) located within the apical anterior and apical lateral RV wall. **c**, **d** Corresponding close-up 2D views to **a** and **b** after echocardiographic contrast injection demonstrating early ventricular cavities and normal myocardial opacification leading to the demonstration of a well-defined, oval, and echolucent mass located within the RV wall (*arrows*). **e**, **f** Similar corresponding close-up 2D views after 5 min of echocardiographic contrast injection demonstrating increased contrast uptake and therefore enhanced echoreflectance of the well-defined RV wall mass (*arrows*).

Computed Tomography and Magnetic Resonance Imaging (Fig. 19.6)

- These techniques are indicated for better definition of the size and number of metastases. (See also Chap. 14 for further information.)
- Myocardial metastases appear as enhanced masses after several minutes of contrast injection.
- The advantage of CT and MRI is the possibility of obtaining a good quality image of the whole heart and to identify other intrathoracic tumors.

Pitfalls of CT and MRI

- Limited ECG synchronization in patients with tachycardia or irregular rhythm significantly compromises image quality.
- Small masses can be missed with CT.
- CT or routine MRI may not provide information on the hemodynamic impact of masses on ventricular systolic or diastolic function or the degree of intracardiac inflow or outflow obstruction.

19

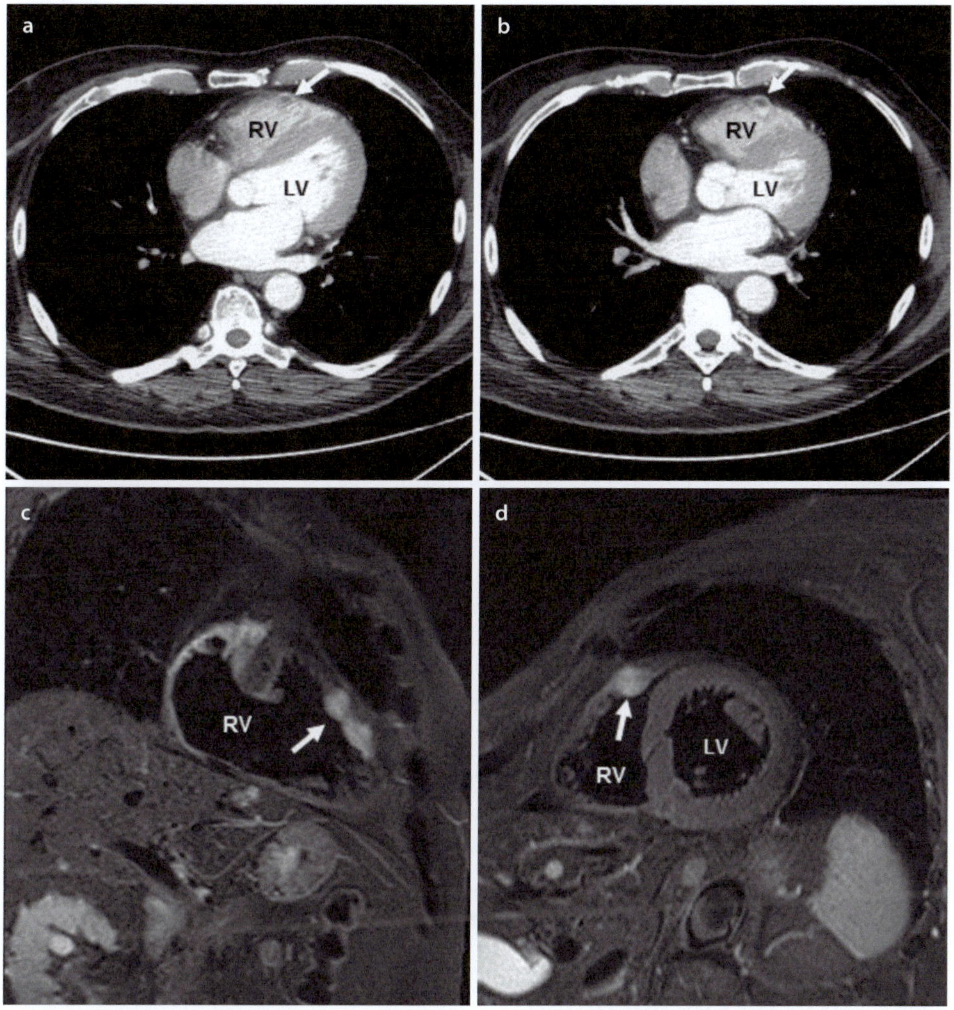

Fig. 19.6 Myocardial metastasis assessed by computed tomography and magnetic resonance imaging. These four-chamber computed tomographic views during diastole **a** and systole **b** demonstrate a well-defined and walled oval mass located within the RV apical lateral wall (*arrows*). These magnetic resonance images **c**, **d** confirm a well-defined and oval mass located within the apical anterior/apical lateral RV wall (*arrows*).

PET

- A useful complementary diagnostic imaging technique when the diagnosis is still undefined by the combination of echocardiography and CT and/or MRI:
  - To improve the diagnostic ability of PET, the patient should be fasting for at least 10 h before the exam, and the last meal should be fat rich and carbohydrate poor (this will shift the myocardial metabolism toward the fatty acids and reduce FDG uptake of the normal myocardium).

Pitfall of PET

- Less useful for the assessment of intramyocardial metastases, because of the highly variable uptake of ^{18}FDG by the normal myocardium

Biopsy

- For large masses protruding into the ventricular cavity or infiltrating the ventricular wall, a biopsy through a transvenous access for right-sided masses or through a mini-thoracotomy for left-sided masses may be useful if technically feasible.

19.5.4 Treatment of Myocardial Metastases

- Treatment should be planned according to the histology of the primary tumor, the size of the metastases, and the degree of hemodynamic impairment.
- Systemic chemotherapy is usually effective, mostly in lymphomas.
- An alternative treatment is local radiation therapy.
- Surgery should be limited to patients with single metastases that interfere with cardiac function, to those with contraindications to chemo- or radiotherapy, or to those with unknown primary tumor.

  Any therapeutic decision should be made by the caring oncologist.

Caveat

The role of the cardiologist is to suggest the most appropriate diagnostic imaging work-up, provide expert opinion on the hemodynamic impact of the tumor, and suggest available therapeutic interventions.

19.6 Endocavitary Metastases

19.6.1 General Considerations

- The most common endocavitary metastases are due to renal, hepatic, or gynecologic carcinomas.
- Endocavitary tumors reach the heart more commonly through the inferior vena cava:
  - Often these metastases are a mix of tumor and thrombus.
- These metastases are more frequently localized in the right heart chambers and may appear both as solid masses and elongated and highly mobile masses (a typical aspect of tumor-associated thrombosis).

19.6.2 Clinical Manifestations

- They are frequently asymptomatic.
- The presence of symptoms is generally related to obstruction to inflow or outflow (shortness of breath, dyspnea, dizziness, near syncope, or syncope) caused by larger masses.
- Pulmonary or systemic embolism may also be their initial manifestation.

19.6.3 Cardiac Imaging (See Also ▸ Chap. 24 for Further Details)

- Large masses are easily detected by conventional 2D transthoracic echocardiography (◘ Figs. 19.7a–d and 19.8a–b).

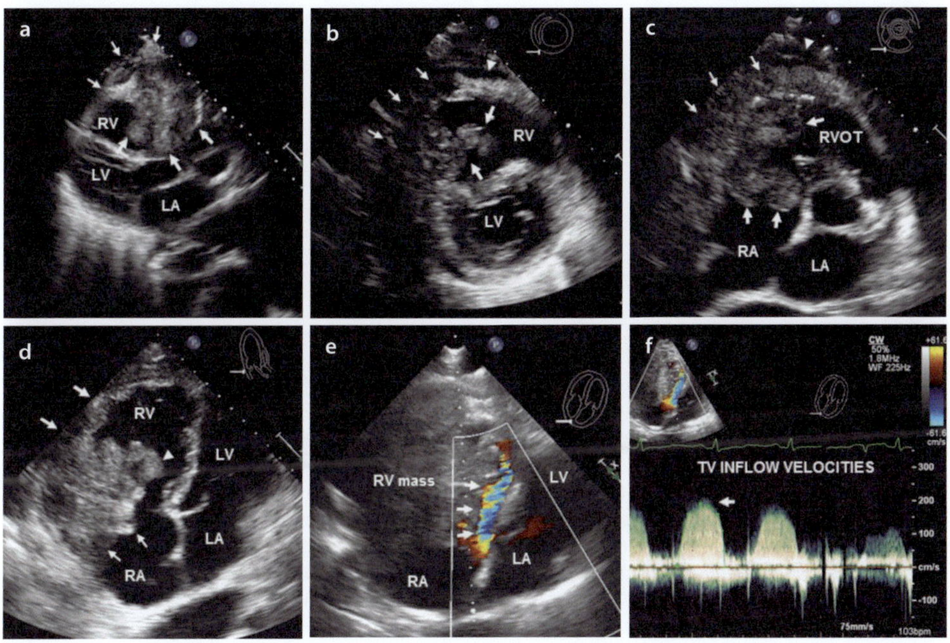

◘ **Fig. 19.7** Large B cell lymphoma complicated with endocavitary, myocardial, and pericardial metastases. **a** This 2D parasternal long-axis view demonstrates a severely enlarged right ventricle (RV) with a large, multilobed, heterogeneously echoreflectant and with irregular border endocavitary mass (*arrows*) extending into the RV anterior wall, epicardium, and visceral pericardium (*small arrows*). **b**, **c** These 2D parasternal short-axis views at the mid-cavity **b** and basal level **c** demonstrate the large endocavitary mass (*arrows*) extending into the right atrium (*upward pointing arrows in* **c**), RV anterolateral wall and epicardium (*small arrows*), and visceral pericardium with a very small anteriorly located effusion (*arrowheads*). **d** This 2D four-chamber view demonstrates a severely enlarged RV with a large endocavitary mass extending into the RV lateral wall (*arrows*), tricuspid annulus, anterior tricuspid leaflet (*arrowhead*), and right atrium (*small arrows*). **e** This 2D four-chamber view with color Doppler demonstrates the large RV mass occupying nearly the entire RV cavity and extending into the tricuspid annulus and valve causing severe obstruction as noted by the narrow inflow color Doppler jet (*arrows*). **f** This 2D four-chamber view with color Doppler-guided continuous wave Doppler demonstrates severe tricuspid valve stenosis with an inflow peak velocity up to 2 m/s (*arrow*), which is equivalent to a diastolic peak gradient of 16 mmHg.

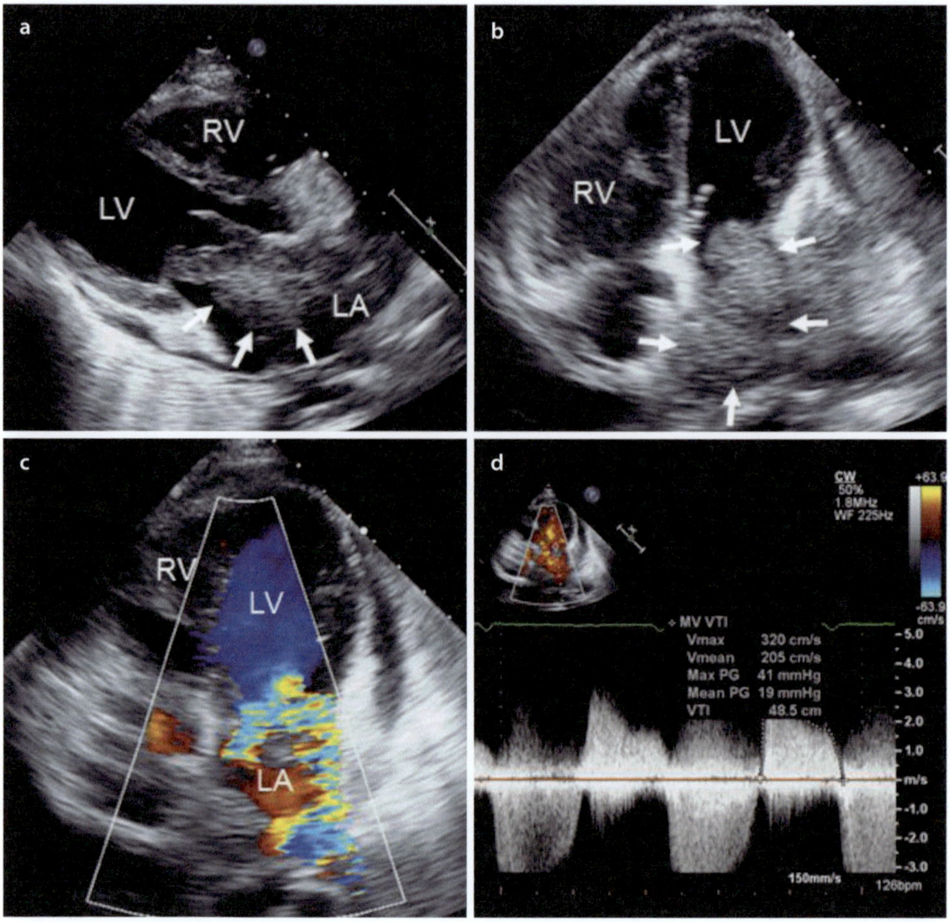

Fig. 19.8 Endocavitary cardiac fibromyosarcoma. These two-dimensional (2D) parasternal long **a** and apical four-chamber **b** views demonstrate a large, multilobed, irregular, and soft tissue echoreflectant mass nearly occupying the entire left atrial (LA) cavity and prolapsing into the mitral valve causing both severe mitral regurgitation **c** and mitral stenosis **d** with a peak and mean gradients of 41 mmHg and 19 mmHg, respectively. Associated severe pulmonary hypertension and right heart enlargement and dysfunction were present. The histopathologic diagnosis of this mass was of a fibromyosarcoma. Adapted with permission from Roldan CA. The Ultimate Echo Guide. Lippincott Williams & Wilkins, Philadelphia 2012

- Clinically relevant information on the presence and severity of cardiac inflow or outflow obstruction is accurately provided by color and continuous wave Doppler echocardiography (Figs. 19.7e, f and 19.8c, d).
- Ventricular masses are better identified using an echocardiographic contrast medium:
  - Soon after injection they appear as an echolucent image within the opacified ventricle.
  - After a few minutes, their echogenicity may be enhanced as the contrast is taken by the tumor.
- Atrial masses may be missed or poorly defined on routine transthoracic echocardiography:

  - Transesophageal echocardiography may be indicated for better definition of the size, shape, mobility, and location of atrial metastases.
  - Real-time 3D echocardiography is particularly useful in further characterizing the size, location, extent, and mobility of these masses.
- Abdominal echo is useful in right-sided masses for more complete evaluation of the inferior vena cava.
- CT with contrast and/or MRI are usually necessary to assess the extracardiac extension of masses originating in the systemic or pulmonary vein system:
  - CT scan and MRI are also useful in defining the site and dimensions of the primary tumor
  - MRI is particularly helpful in differentiating tumors from thrombi.
- PET is useful in differentiating between thrombi and malignant tumors: a high FDG uptake is highly suggestive of malignant tumor.

Pitfalls of Imaging of Endocavitary Masses
- The main limitation of echocardiography is the inability to differentiate between thrombi, benign tumors, or metastases.
- The diagnostic power of both CT scan and MRI is limited in small or highly mobile masses.
- The main limitation of PET is its spatial resolution since masses <5 mm in diameter can be missed.

Caveat
CT, MRI, and/or PET are routinely used during the staging and follow-up of primary cancer and metastases. The information obtained by these imaging modalities (even if they were not primarily focused on the heart) must be integrated with a thorough history and physical examination and Doppler echocardiography.

19.6.4 Treatment of Endocavitary Metastases

- The most appropriate therapy depends on the primary tumor, the size of the masses, and the tumor embolic risk:
  - Tumor thrombosis is better treated with the combination of systemic chemotherapy and low molecular weight heparin.
  - Large masses, with impending embolic risk, may require surgery if feasible [21].
- Surgery of metastases from the inferior vena cava usually requires a team including a cardiac and abdominal surgeon or urologist since they require a complex approach, require a long operating time, and pose a high risk of pulmonary embolism [22, 23].
- Surgery of metastases from the superior vena cava or pulmonary veins requires a cardiothoracic surgeon or a team of a cardiac surgeon and a thoracic surgeon.

References

1. Bussani R, De-Giorgio F, Abbate A, Silvestri F. Cardiac metastases. J Clin Pathol. 2007;60:27–34.
2. Goldberg AD, Blankstein R, Padera RF. Tumor metastatic to the heart. Circulation. 2013;128:1790–4.
3. Kraft C, Schuettfort G, Weil Y, et al. Thrombosis of the inferior vena cava and malignant disease. Thromb Res. 2014;134(3):668–73.
4. Debourdeau P, Gligorov J, Teixeira L, Aletti M, Zammit C. Tumeurs cardiaques malignes (Malignant cardiac tumors). Bull Cancer. 2004;91:S136–46.
5. Lestuzzi C. Neoplastic pericardial disease: old and current strategies for diagnosis and management. World J Cardiol. 2010;2:270–9.
6. Jacob S, Sebastian JC, Cherian PK, Abraham A, John SK. Pericardial effusion impending tamponade: a look beyond Beck's triad. Am J Emerg Med. 2009;27(2):216–9.
7. Roldan CA. Pericardial diseases. In: Roldan CA, editor. The ultimate echo guide. Lippincott: Philadelphia; 2012. p. 320–39.
8. Lestuzzi C. Epidemiology, diagnosis and therapy of neoplastic pericarditis. J Cardiovasc Echogr. 2011;21(2):86–91.
9. Pawlak Cieślik A, Szturmowicz M, Fijałkowska A, et al. Diagnosis of malignant pericarditis: a single centre experience. Kardiol Pol. 2012;70:1147–53.
10. L'italien AJ. Critical cardiovascular skills and procedures in the emergency department. Emerg Med Clin North Am. 2013;31:151–206.
11. Loukas M, Walters A, Boon JM, Welch TP, Meiring JH, Abrahams PH. Pericardiocentesis: a clinical anatomy review. Clin Anat. 2012;25:872–81. Review.
12. Pepi M, Muratori M. Echocardiography in the diagnosis and management of pericardial disease. J Cardiovasc Med (Hagerstown). 2006;7:533–44. Review.
13. Klein SV, Afridi H, Agarwal D, Coughlin BF, Schielke LH. CT directed diagnostic and therapeutic pericardiocentesis: 8-year experience at a single institution. Emerg Radiol. 2005;11:353–63.
14. Hoey ET, Mankad K. Computed tomography-guided pericardiocentesis: utility in the management of malignant pericardial effusion. Am J Emerg Med. 2010;28:388.e1–3.
15. Jeon HW, Cho DG, Park JK, et al. Prognostic factors affecting survival of patients with cancer-related pericardial effusion managed by surgery. World J Surg Oncol. 2014;12:249.
16. Ruiz-García J, Jiménez-Valero S, Moreno R, et al. Percutaneous balloon pericardiotomy as the initial and definitive treatment for malignant pericardial effusion. Rev Esp Cardiol (Engl Ed). 2013;66:357–63.
17. Celik S, Lestuzzi C, Cervesato E, et al. Systemic chemotherapy in combination with pericardial window has better outcomes in malignant pericardial effusions. J Thorac Cardiovasc Surg. 2014;148:2288–93.
18. Patel N, Rafique AM, Eshaghian S, et al. Retrospective comparison of outcomes, diagnostic value, and complications of percutaneous prolonged drainage versus surgical pericardiotomy of pericardial effusion associated with malignancy. Am J Cardiol. 2013;112:1235–9.
19. Lestuzzi C, Bearz A, Lafaras C, et al. Neoplastic pericardial disease in lung cancer: impact on outcomes of different treatment strategies. A multicenter study. Lung Cancer. 2011;72:340–7.
20. Lestuzzi C, Nicolosi GL, Biasi S, Piotti P, Zanuttini D. Sensitivity and specificity of electrocardiographic ST-T changes as markers of neoplastic myocardial infiltration. Echocardiographic correlation. Chest. 1989;95:980–5.
21. Kokudo T, Hasegawa K, Yamamoto S, et al. Surgical treatment of hepatocellular carcinoma associated with hepatic vein tumor thrombosis. J Hepatol. 2014;61:583–8.
22. Goto H, Hashimoto M, Akamatsu D, et al. Surgical resection and inferior vena cava reconstruction for treatment of the malignant tumor: technical success and outcomes. Ann Vasc Dis. 2014;7:120–6.
23. George J, Grebenik K, Patel N, Cranston D, Westaby S. The importance of intraoperative transoesophageal monitoring when operating on renal cancers that involve the right atrium. Ann R Coll Surg Engl. 2014;96:e18–9.

Primary Cardiac Malignancies: Epidemiology and Pathology

Stefania Rizzo, Gaetano Thiene, Marialuisa Valente, and Cristina Basso

C. Lestuzzi et al. (eds.), *Manual of Cardio-oncology*, DOI 10.1007/978-3-319-40236-9_20

20.1 Epidemiology

Primary tumors are uncommon in the heart and malignancies are even more uncommon and mostly metastatic. Therefore, before making a diagnosis of primary cardiac malignancies, the metastasis from extracardiac origin must be excluded through extensive clinical and imaging investigations.

One must remember, however, that at the level of the heart, even benign cardiac tumors may lead to significant morbidity and mortality by affecting blood flow and causing arrhythmias and embolism (hemodynamic malignancy).

If in the past virtually all cardiac tumors were diagnosed after death, nowadays these tumors are detected frequently in vivo and have become often surgically curable thanks to recent advances in diagnostic imaging modalities and cardiac surgical techniques.

The exact incidence and prevalence of cardiac tumors are unknown. Knowledge of the prevalence of cardiac tumors is still based on postmortem studies. The prevalence of primary cardiac tumors is estimated on 0.001–0.3 % in autopsy reports [1–7]. In a 20-year study (1972–1991) of 12,485 autopsy cases, there was a 0.056 % incidence of primary tumors and a 1.23 % incidence of secondary tumors [8]. Based upon the data of 22 large autopsy series reported by McAllister et al., the frequency of primary cardiac tumors is approximately 0.02 % [9]. In a study carried out in the Institute of Pathology of the University of Padua in time year interval 1967–1976, among 7460 autopsies the cause of death was due to malignancies in 1181, in 74 of which cardiac metastases occurred (1 % of all the autopsies and 6 % of those with any malignancy). Thus, we can approximately say that autopsy prevalence of primary cardiac tumor is 1 out of 2000 and that of secondary cardiac tumors is 1 out of 100 autopsies, with a secondary/primary ratio of 20:1 [10]. A review of 3314 autopsies found a 2.9 % frequency of metastatic tumors involving the heart, arising by direct extension of adjacent organs or spreading via hematogenous, lymphatic, or intracavitary routes [11]. The most common primary sites are the lung, breast, and cutaneous melanoma [12, 13]. Available data from single-center studies vary with a reported prevalence between 3 and 28.7 % [14–16]. However these data may have a high referral bias and may not reflect population-based incidence rates. The rate of malignant cardiac tumors is frequently erroneously reported up to 30 % among all primary cardiac tumors, when based upon data derived from pathology tertiary centers, where the most difficult cases are sent for consultancy [17]. Surgical pathology data certainly underestimate tumors that do not require surgery (e.g., rhabdomyomas and metastases), as well as tumors possibly revealed by sudden death.

In 2015, the World Health Organization (WHO) updated the classification of cardiac tumors as reported in ◘ Table 20.1 [1]. The WHO classifies tumors of the heart into three types: benign tumors and tumorlike lesions, malignant tumors, and pericardial tumors. The major changes in malignant tumors of the heart have been: the removal of the term "malignant fibrous histiocytoma" as synonymous with undifferentiated pleomorphic sarcoma, incorporation of epithelioid hemangioendothelioma as an angiosarcoma with low-grade malignance, remarkable expansion of the cytogenetic and molecular genetic characterization of many cardiac tumors, and reintroduction of the primary cardiac osteosarcoma and myxofibrosarcoma subtypes. Intimal sarcoma has been recently reported in the heart as the most frequent sarcoma histotype and, as in large vessels, is characterized by overexpression of MDM2 as well as alterations in genes like PDGFRA and EGFR that could be targets for novel therapeutic approaches [18]. However this

Table 20.1 WHO classification 2015 of cardiac tumors [1]

Benign tumors and tumorlike lesions	
Histiocytoid cardiomyopathy	
Hamartoma of mature cardiac myocytes	
Rhabdomyoma	8900/0
Adult cellular rhabdomyoma	8904/0
Cardiac myxoma	8840/0
Papillary fibroelastoma	
Hemangioma, NOS	9120/0
Capillary hemangioma	9131/0
Cavernous hemangioma	9121/0
Cardiac fibroma	8810/0
Lipoma	8850/0
Cystic tumor of the atrioventricular node	8454/0
Inflammatory myofibroblastic tumor	8825/1
Granular cell tumor	9580/0
Schwannoma	9560/0
Germ cell tumors	
Mature teratoma	9080/0
Immature teratoma	9080/3
Yolk sac tumor	9071/3
Paraganglioma	8680/1
Malignant tumors	
Angiosarcoma	9120/3
Undifferentiated pleomorphic sarcoma	8830/3
Osteosarcoma	9180/3
Myxofibrosarcoma	8811/3
Leiomyosarcoma	8890/3
Rhabdomyosarcoma	8900/3
Synovial sarcoma	9040/3
Miscellaneous sarcomas	
Cardiac lymphomas	
Metastatic tumors	

Table 20.1 (continued)

Tumors of the pericardium	
Solitary fibrous tumor	8815/1
Malignant	8815/3
Angiosarcoma	9120/3
Synovial sarcoma	9040/3
Malignant mesothelioma	9050/3
Germ cell tumors	
Teratoma mature	9080/0
Teratoma immature	9080/3
Mixed germ cell tumor	9085/3

clinical–pathological entity has been not included in the new WHO classification since it requires further investigation.

Up to 90 % of primary tumors are benign and 10 % malignant, with the majority of these being sarcomas (90 %) arising from the parenchymal or mesenchymal cells of the structural elements of the heart such as the blood vessels, muscle, connective tissue, fat, and even bone. Lymphoma and primary pericardial mesothelioma represent most of the remaining cases.

Concerning the epidemiology and prevalence of various histotypes, we refer to the experience of the University of Padua [6, 10]. In the time interval 1970–2010, 267 consecutive primary cardiac neoplasms were studied, 213 (89.5 %) of which were benign and 26 (10.5 %) malignant. This is mostly a biopsy-based experience (89.5 % of cases), just to emphasize that nowadays cardiac tumors are rarely fatal, with exception of primary malignancies. Among the benign cardiac tumors, the majority (66 %) were myxomas, followed by papillary fibroelastomas (9.5 %). There was a female predominance (88, 62.5 %), mean age 54 years. As far as malignant primary cardiac tumors, leiomyosarcoma and angiosarcoma ranked first (19 % each). There was a male predominance, mean age 50 years. As far as metastatic cardiac tumors, lung carcinoma was by far the leading one in our experience (32.5 %), especially as pericardial carcinosis with effusion, followed by lymphoma and leukemia (16 %), breast carcinoma (5 %), hepatic carcinoma (5 %), and kidney carcinoma (4 %).

More important than the cell type is the proximity of the tumor to vital intracardiac structures. Two different types of growth are found:

- Intramural, producing conduction abnormalities and arrhythmias as well as heart failure due to systolic and diastolic dysfunction
- Intracavitary, with obstruction to blood flow or embolization of thrombi or tumor cells

20.2 Clinical Features

Patients with cardiac tumors may present with cardiovascular-related or constitutional symptoms, through any of the four mechanisms:

- Mass effect: they can obstruct intracardiac blood flow or interfere with valve function.
- Local invasion: leading to arrhythmias or pericardial effusions with tamponade.
- Embolization: parts of tumor or thrombi can embolize, causing systemic or pulmonary infarctions (if on the left or right side of the heart respectively).
- The tumors may cause constitutional symptoms or hematologic abnormalities.

Moreover, cardiac malignant tumors may also present with problems related to metastatic disease. In rare cases, the first manifestation of a cardiac tumor is sudden cardiac death. Some tumors produce no symptoms and are incidental findings during an imaging investigation performed for an unrelated indication.

20.3 Surgical Pathology

Histopathology is mandatory in any resected cardiac mass, to establish the benign or malignant nature and the precise histotype. This information may be crucial in the case of malignancy for the choice of therapy and prognosis. Masses may be neoplastic, but even thrombotic, calcific, septic, and infective. The employment of traditional histological and histochemical stainings should be accompanied by immunohistochemistry with a large panel of antibodies, for establishing the histotype of tumor cell proliferations, particularly in the setting of malignant unresectable masses that require histological characterization before starting chemotherapy [1]. In rare cases of cardiac sarcoma, electron microscopy may also be of help. Consultancy in tertiary referral centers of cardiovascular or soft tissue tumor pathology is advisable. Before surgery, tissue diagnosis can be achieved through percutaneous endomyocardial biopsy, particularly in the setting of right-sided cardiac masses. Moreover, endomyocardial biopsy can be useful for unresectable tumors requiring histological characterisation before chemotherapy.

20.4 Tumor Grading and Staging

Due to the low frequency of malignant cardiac tumors, as far as histologic grading of malignancy, there are no specific parameters, and we have to refer to soft tissue neoplasms [19]. A histologic grading system has been put forward by the French Federation Nationale des Centre de Lutte Contre le Cancer (FFNCLCC) [20], which is based upon a cumulative score deriving from three parameters, i.e., (a) tumor differentiation (score 1, sarcomas closely resembling normal adult mesenchymal tissue; score 2, sarcomas for which histological typing is certain; score 3, undifferentiated sarcoma, angiosarcoma), (b) mitotic count (score 1, 0–9 mitoses per 10 high-power field, HPF, measuring 0.1734 mm2; score 2, 10–19 mitoses per 10 HPF; > or =20 mitoses per 10 HPF), and (c) tumor necrosis (score 0, no necrosis; score 1, <50% tumor necrosis; score 2, > or = 50% tumor necrosis). Three grades of malignancy are thus recognize: G1, low grade (total score 2, 3); G2, intermediate grade (total score 4, 5); G3, high grade (total score 6, 7, 8),

20.5 Treatment and Prognosis

The prognosis of patients with primary malignant cardiac tumors is very poor even if complete resection is attempted. Adjuvant chemotherapy and irradiation are usually also given, but these are not effective in most cases, with the exception of primary cardiac lymphoma which shows a better survival compared with sarcomas. Favorable results of heart transplantation for primary malignant cardiac tumors have been reported. Cardiac autotransplantation (cardiac explantation, ex vivo tumor resection, reconstruction, and reimplantation) may represent an option in many primary malignant cardiac tumors [21].

20.6 Key Points

- Cardiac tumors are rare with a frequency that varies in postmortem studies between 0.0017 % and 0.33 %.
- Consist of both primary and secondary tumors.
- Secondary cardiac tumors (metastases) are 20 times more common than primary cardiac tumors.
- The majority of primary cardiac tumors are benign, most being myxomas, accounting for up to 90 % of all cardiac tumors.
- The most common malignant primary cardiac tumor is sarcoma.
- Primary lymphoma of the heart is exceedingly rare, but with a better survival.
- Symptoms are nonspecific and can mimic many other heart diseases.
- The clinical presentation depends on the size, location of the cardiac tumor, and type of growth (intramural or intracavitary).
- "Histological examination of any resected cardiac mass is mandatory to achieve a certain diagnosis and to plan the proper treatment".

20.7 Cardiac Sarcomas

Sarcomas are mesenchymal tumors of various histologic morphologies and constitute most of primary malignant cardiac tumors [1, 6, 7, 10, 17, 22, 23]. By definition, they are confined to the heart or pericardium at the time of diagnosis without any evidence of extracardiac primary neoplasm. They occur in adults and have no predilection for either sex.

Primary cardiac sarcomas may occur in any chamber of the heart, although the right heart is the most frequent site of origin. Histologic type shows no consistent relation to the location within the heart, except for angiosarcoma, which has a predilection for the right atrium. Although arising from the endocardium or pericardium more often than from the myocardium, malignant tumors rapidly infiltrate all layers of the heart, invade adjacent mediastinal structures, and metastasize. Systemic metastases, particularly to the lungs and mediastinal lymph nodes, are present in 80 % of cases when first diagnosed. This growth pattern makes cardiac sarcomas often unresectable and thus the prognosis is poor. Survival is measured in weeks or months.

20.7.1 Angiosarcoma

Definition

20.7.1.1 Angiosarcoma is a malignant tumor with endothelial differentiation. According to the new WHO classification [1], there are two types, with distinctive histological and genetic features: angiosarcoma (high-grade sarcomas) and epithelioid hemangioendothelioma (low-grade sarcomas).

Epidemiology

20.7.1.2 Angiosarcomas are the most common primary malignant cardiac neoplasms, accounting for 40 % of primary cardiac malignancies. The peak incidence is in the fourth decade with slight male predilection.

Localization

It most often arises in the right atrium, close to the atrioventricular groove (80 %) [4, 24, 25], but has been reported in the other heart three chambers as well as in the pericardium. Cardiac epithelioid hemangioendothelioma typically occurs in the atria and may present as an incidental mass or embolism.

Clinical Features

Symptoms tend to develop late in the course of the disease and are often nonspecific. Clinical symptoms usually relate to cardiac tamponade or right heart failure secondary to intracavitary obstruction. Affecting the right heart, angiosarcoma often produces right-sided heart failure, superior vena cava obstruction, and pericardial effusion. Presentation with lung metastases is not uncommon. The predominant right-sided location allows for diagnosis by endomyocardial biopsy [26] (◘ Fig. 20.1).

Pathology

Macroscopically, it is a large mural, lobulated, and brown-reddish mass with a necrotic or hemorrhagic appearance, that widely infiltrates the wall and the pericardium and protrudes in right cardiac cavities, with invasion of the inferior vena cava and the tricuspid orifice. Histologically, two thirds of angiosarcoma are moderately to well differentiated and are composed of irregular vascular spaces with papillary intraluminal tufting lined by pleomorphic and atypical cells. Mitoses are frequent. In one third of cases, the tumor is poorly differentiated, without discrete vascular structures, and consists of anaplastic spindle cells within a hyaline stroma, containing focally extravascular red cells. No definite Weibel-Palade bodies are identified with electron microscopy. However, pynocytotic vesicles, abundant intermediate filaments, and a moderate amount of rough endoplasmic reticulum and Golgi apparatus may be found.

Epithelioid hemangioendothelioma is composed of epithelioid cells arranged in short strands or solid nests. The constituent endothelial cells are round or oval, contain small intracellular lumina, and frequently infiltrate the vessels.

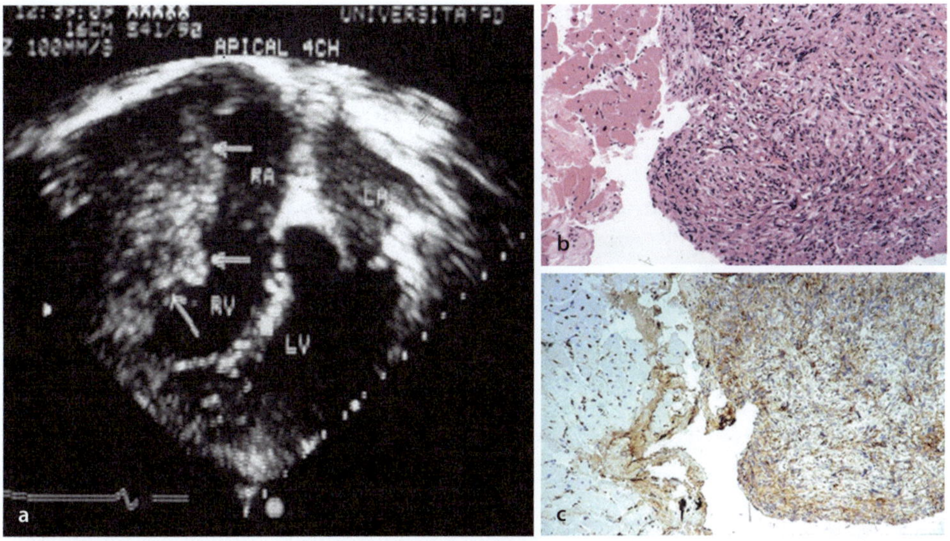

Fig. 20.1 Angiosarcoma in a 36-year-old woman, suffering from dyspnea and fever (Modified from Poletti et al. [26]). **a** Two-dimensional echocardiogram, four-chamber view, showing an endocavitary and intramural large mass in the right atrium extending into the right ventricle, measuring 6 × 8 cm. **b** Photomicrograph of transvenous biopsied tumor: the myocardium was infiltrated by pleomorphic spindle cells with hyperchromatic nuclei forming vascular spaces. **c** Tumor cells arranged in vascular channels were positive for factor VIII

Immunohistochemistry

Angiosarcomas typically express endothelial markers, including von Willebrand factor, CD34, CD31, and VEGF.

Differential Diagnosis

Differential diagnosis includes fibrosarcoma, undifferentiated pleomorphic sarcomas, and Kaposi sarcoma. The detection of endothelial vacuoles or papillary structures is helpful. Immunohistochemistry plays a crucial role in diagnosis, especially in undifferentiated forms. Kaposi sarcoma generally forms small nodules involving the pericardium with minimal invasion of the myocardium. Pericardial angiosarcomas can be mistaken for mesotheliomas. Stains for cytokeratin, calretinin, cytokeratin 5/6, and CD31 can help to differentiate the two populations of cells. The intracellular lumina of epithelioid hemangioendothelioma may mimic the vacuoles of adenocarcinoma, which should be initially considered in the microscopic differential diagnosis.

Genetics

Molecular analyses on tumor tissues have focused on genetic alterations of TP53 and K-ras [27].

Prognosis

Prognosis is poor, usually because of delayed diagnosis and metastases, with a median survival of less than 1 year, even after surgical exeresis and adjuvant therapy.

Key Points: Angiosarcoma

- Angiosarcoma (high-grade sarcoma) is the most common primary cardiac malignant tumor.
- Epithelioid hemangioendothelioma is a subtype with low-grade malignancy.
- Male predominance and a peak incidence in the fourth decade.
- Right atrial free wall and atrioventrentricular groove are involved in 80 % of cases, allowing diagnosis by endomyocardial biopsy.
- Hemorrhagic mass composed by multiple, irregular vascular channels lined by pleomorphic and atypical cells, CD31, von Willebrand factor, and CD34 positive.

20.7.2 Undifferentiated Pleomorphic Sarcomas

Definition

High-grade malignant cardiac sarcomas showing fibroblastic or myofibroblastic differentiation and areas of marked cellular pleomorphism, with no specific histologic and immunohistochemical markers [1]. Malignant fibrous histiocytoma is a synonym.

Epidemiology

Undifferentiated pleomorphic sarcoma is the second most common malignant cardiac sarcoma in adults with a reported prevalence of 24–37.5 %. There is no gender predilection and the mean age is around 45 years (range, 20–80 years).

Localization

Undifferentiated pleomorphic sarcomas tend to be intracavitary, located in the left atrium of the heart, where they most often present like cardiac myxomas, but most commonly arise along the posterior wall in comparison to the septum.

Clinical Features

Most occur on the left side of the heart and cause signs and symptoms related to pulmonary congestion, mitral stenosis, and pulmonary vein obstruction. Constitutional signs and symptoms may precede symptoms referable to the heart. They may also present with metastases and the lungs, lymph nodes, kidney, and skin are common sites.

Pathology

Undifferentiated pleomorphic sarcoma typically presents as a soft or firm polypoid endocardial-based tumor. It may be sessile or pedunculated, simulating myxoma, but unlike myxoma, may form multiple masses. The mass may distend the atrium and impinge upon the mitral valve. Extension into the pulmonary veins and lung parenchyma may be

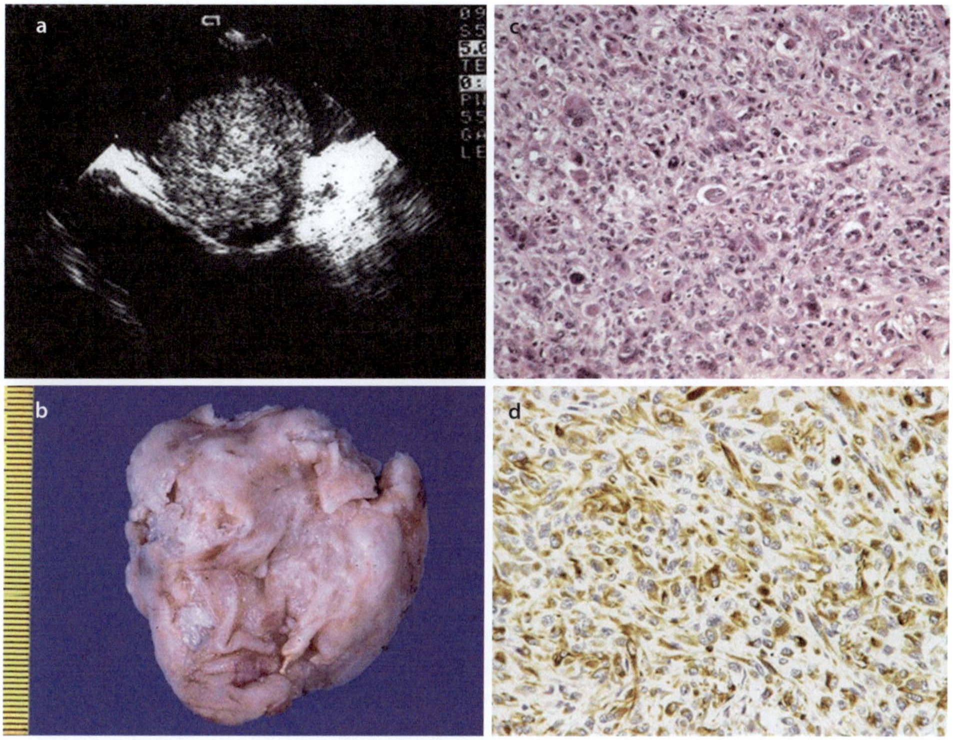

Fig. 20.2 Left atrial undifferentiated pleomorphic sarcoma in a 68-year-old man, presenting with fever and increased serum level of flogistic markers. **a** Echocardiogram: endoluminal round mass in the left atrium, simulating a myxoma. **b** Grossly, the surgical resected mass showed a rough and irregular surface. **c** At histology, bizarre cells with pleomorphic nuclei admixed to giant cells and spindle-shaped cells, with high mitotic rate, are seen. **d** At immunohistochemistry, tumor cells are positive for vimentin

present. They may be uniform whitish or variegated due to hemorrhage and necrosis, with hard consistency. Calcification is uncommon. The diagnosis of Undifferentiated pleomorphic sarcoma is achieved by exclusion, when the use of a large panel of immunohistochemical stains fails to give evidence of myogenic or other specific differentiations (endothelial, cardiomyocyte, smooth muscle cells, fibroblast, adipose, nerves, epithelial). Microscopically, the proliferation consists of bizarre, pleomorphic cells, frequently giant multinuclear, with high mitotic activity (Fig. 20.2).

Prognosis

The prognosis of undifferentiated pleomorphic sarcoma is very poor, because surgical resection is often incomplete. Chemiotherapy and radiotherapy give only temporary improvement. Survival patients ranges from 5 to 18 months. Most patients die of metastasis or local recurrence.

Key Points: Undifferentiated Pleomorphic Sarcomas

- Undifferentiated pleomorphic sarcomas are malignant neoplasms with fibroblastic or myofibroblastic differentiation and areas of marked cellular pleomorphism, with no specific histologic and immunohistochemical markers.
- The second most common primary malignant cardiac sarcoma in adults with a prevalence of 24–37.5 %.
- No gender predilection, mean age 45 years.
- The left atrium is frequently involved with an intracavitary growth.
- Proliferation of bizarre, pleomorphic cells, frequently giant multinuclear, with high mitotic activity.
- Diagnosis is achieved by exclusion, when immunohistochemical stains fail to give evidence of specific differentiation.

20.7.3 Osteosarcoma

Definition

Primary cardiac osteosarcoma originates in the heart and produces the osteoid or bone, occasionally with chondroblastic differentiation. These have been grouped in the past WHO classification within malignant pleomorphic fibrous histiocytomas/undifferentiated pleomorphic sarcomas with osteosarcomatous differentiation, but nowadays they represent a distinct subtype [1]. Osteogenic sarcoma, osteoblastic osteosarcoma and extraskeletal osteosarcoma are synonyms.

Epidemiology

Osteosarcomas are quite rare, making up approximately 10 % of primary cardiac sarcomas. Cardiac osteosarcomas occur most commonly between the second and fifth decades of life, with a mean patient age of 40 years, and do not show any gender predominance.

Localization

Primary osteosarcomas are more frequently left sided and may be mistaken for atrial myxomas. The second most common location is the right atrium, with extension into the vena cava.

Clinical Features

Due to the left atrial location, initial symptoms are most frequently related to mitral valve obstruction. Dyspnea, chest pain, palpitations, dizziness, murmurs, and congestive heart failure have been reported.

Pathology

Cardiac osteosarcomas usually present as nodular masses with infiltrative margins. The cut surface is heterogeneous, firm, and white, with areas of hemorrhage and necrosis. They may have osteo-, chondro-, or fibroblastic differentiation. The bone-forming areas range from well-differentiated trabeculated osteosarcoma to poorly differentiated sarcomas with stromal osteoid. Chondrosarcomatous areas are also present in about half of all cases.

Immunohistochemistry

Most tumors express smooth muscle actin; S100 protein is expressed in chondroid areas. Epithelial membrane antigen can be focally positive in epithelioid areas.

Differential Diagnosis

Atrial myxomas, given the left-sided location and presence of calcification.

Prognosis

Prognosis of cardiac osteosarcoma is poor, with survival rarely beyond 1 year due to early metastases to lungs, skin, and skeleton.

Key Points: Osteosarcoma

- Malignant tumor that produces the osteoid or bone, occasionally with chondroblastic differentiation
- 10 % of primary cardiac sarcomas
- No gender predominance, mean age 40 years
- Left-sided tumor with intracavitary growth
- Osteo-, chondro-, or fibroblastic differentiation

20.7.4 Myxofibrosarcoma

Definition

Myxofibrosarcoma is a low-grade cardiac sarcoma composed of spindle cells in a myxoid matrix [1, 28] Myxoid malignant fibrous histiocytoma, fibromyxosarcoma and myxoid fibrosarcoma are synonyms. It should be not considered a malignant variant of myxoma, the latter basically being a benign tumor.

Epidemiology

Because of the various terms that have been used for this tumor, the precise incidence rate is uncertain, but myxofibrosarcoma probably accounts for about 10 % of cardiac sarcomas, making it the fourth most common cardiac sarcoma (after angiosarcoma, undifferentiated pleomorphic sarcoma, and osteosarcoma).

Localization

The most common location for cardiac myxofibrosarcoma is in the atria (particularly the left), followed by the right ventricle, and the ventricular septum.

Clinical Features

Cardiac myxofibrosarcomas have been described most frequently in the left atrium with both intracavitary and mural growth, typically causing obstruction and symptoms of mitral stenosis.

Pathology

Myxofibrosarcoma is typically an endocardial-based tumor with little necrosis or hemorrhage, with intracavitary growth. Histologically, myxofibrosarcomas show spindle or rounded cells often within a myxoid matrix, without significant pleomorphism (■ Fig. 20.3).

Immunohistochemistry

Immunohistochemical staining is not helpful in the diagnosis, except to exclude other tumors, being positive only vimentin.

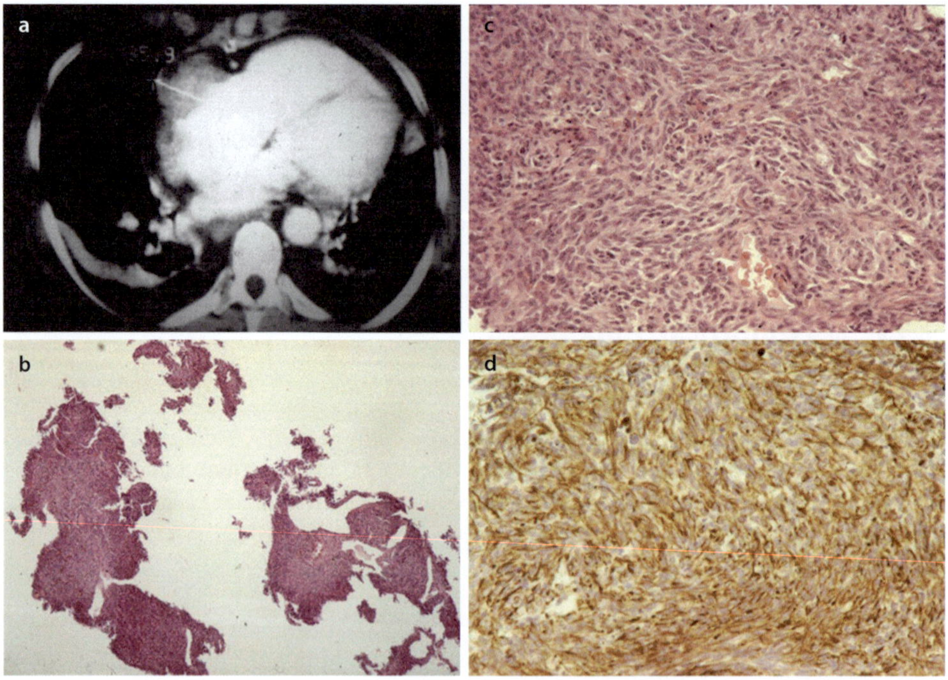

■ **Fig. 20.3** Fibrosarcoma of the right atrium in a 62-year-old woman, suffering from weakness and effort dyspnea. **a** CT showing a mass infiltrating right atrial free wall. **b** Transvenous endomyocardial biopsy: note the elevated number of bioptic specimens. **c** At higher magnification, note atypical spindle cells within fibrous stroma. **d** Tumor cells are immunoreactive to vimentin

Differential Diagnosis

Myxoma may be confused with myxofibrosarcoma because of the proteoglycan-rich matrix. Because myxofibrosarcoma may be histologically bland, the absence of pleomorphism is not a distinguishing feature between myxoma and myxofibrosarcoma.

Prognosis

In spite of surgery is often possible, survival is poor, but slightly better than angiosarcoma of the heart.

Key Points: Myxofibrosarcoma
- Low-grade cardiac sarcoma composed of spindle cells in a myxoid matrix.
- About 10 % of cardiac sarcomas.
- The left and right atrium are the main location with intracavitary and mural growth.

20.7.5 Leiomyosarcoma

Definition

Leiomyosarcoma is a malignant tumor with smooth muscle cell differentiation [1, 29, 30].

Epidemiology

Cardiac leiomyosarcoma is rare, representing less than 10 % of primary cardiac sarcomas. There is no sex predilection, and most occur in patients between 40 and 50 years of age.

Localization

It has a predilection for the left atrium and pulmonary infundibulum.

Clinical Features

The commonest manifestation is dyspnea and cardiac failure from mitral obstructive symptoms. Pulmonary embolism may occur in case of right-sided tumors.

Pathology

The tumors appear firm, fleshy, gray, and sessile. They may present as multiple intracavitary nodules. Leiomyosarcoma consists of compact bundles of spindle cells with blunt-ended nuclei, glycogen, and perinuclear vacuoles, often oriented at sharp angle or 90° to one another. Zones of necrosis and mitotic figures are frequent.

Immunohistochemistry

The spindle cells show reactivity for alpha smooth muscle actin and desmin (◘ Fig. 20.4).

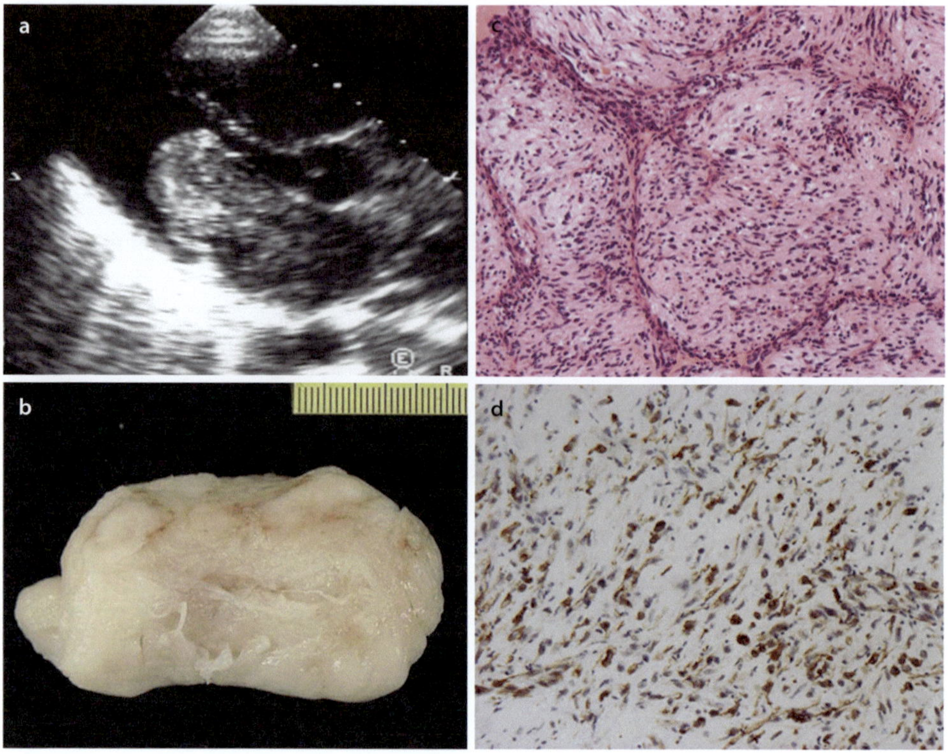

Fig. 20.4 Leiomyosarcoma of the left atrium in a 21-year-old woman with acute pulmonary edema and preoperative diagnosis of left atrial myxoma. **a** Echocardiogram: endoluminal mass in the left atrium prolapsing in the left ventricular cavity during diastole, simulating a myxoma. **b** Gross features of the cardiac mass resected at the surgery, showing rough and irregular surface. **c** Pleomorphic cells arranged in a storiform pattern within a myxoid background. **d** Immunohistochemical staining showing tumor cell positivity for desmin

Prognosis

Surgical resection is usually palliative in association with adjuvant chemotherapy and radiotherapy. The reported mean survival time is about 1 year.

Key Points: Leiomyosarcoma

- Malignant tumor with smooth muscle cell differentiation
- No sex predilection, 40 and 50 years of age
- Predilection for the left atrium and pulmonary infundibulum
- Bundles of spindle cells with blunt-ended nuclei, often oriented at sharp angle or 90° to one another, and alpha smooth muscle actin and desmin positive

20.7.6 Rhabdomyosarcoma

Definition

Rhabdomyosarcoma is a malignant tumor with striated muscle differentiation [1]. Rhabdomyosarcomas arise de novo, not from malignant degeneration of a rhabdomyoma.

Epidemiology

Rhabdomyosarcoma is a rare subtype of cardiac sarcoma (less than 5 %) [31], but remains the most common pediatric cardiac malignancy. In the past, before immunohistochemical analysis, a large proportion of cardiac sarcomas were wrongly considered rhabdomyosarcomas.

Localization

Rhabdomyosarcomas may arise from any location in the heart, but ventricular involvement is greater than other cardiac sarcomas. They are usually mural tumors.

Clinical Features

The clinical presentation, as with other cardiac tumors, depends on the cardiac location. Pericardial effusion, dyspnea, conduction disturbances and extracardiac metastases are the usual presentation.

Pathology

Cardiac rhabdomyosarcomas are large, bulky, infiltrative tumors that may be grossly mucoid or gelatinous, similar to cardiac myxoma, or soft and necrotic, highly heterogeneous. In the heart there are two distinct histologic types: embryonal, which occur mainly in children and adults, and a pleomorphic, which are much less frequent and occur in adults. Embryonal rhabdomyosarcoma is a small-cell neoplasm with variable numbers of PAS-positive rhabdomyoblasts (tadpole or strap cells). Alveolar rhabdomyosarcoma has been described in the heart as a metastatic lesion. Sarcoma botryoides, with characteristic grape-like structures, has also been described in the heart [32] At electron microscopy, the diagnostic features are thick and thin filaments and Z-bands.

Immunohistochemistry

Immunohistochemical staining shows positivity for desmin and myogenin.

Differential Diagnosis

The differential diagnosis includes other cardiac sarcomas, especially undifferentiated lesions and metastatic small round cell tumors in children and young adults. Immunohistochemical stains are vital in identifying rhabdomyoblasts.

Somatic Genetics

Cytogenetic analysis shows mutation at exon 1 of K-ras.

Prognosis

Surgical rection is palliative due to local and distant metastases. Response to adjuvant chemotherapy and radiation is poor. In selected cases, cardiac transplantation is considered.

> **Key Points: Rhabdomyosarcoma**
> - Malignant tumor with striated muscle differentiation that involves the myocardium.
> - The most common cardiac malignancy in pediatric population.
> - Embryonal rhabdomyosarcoma is the most frequent variant in the heart, characterized by small cells and variable numbers of PAS-positive rhabdomyoblasts (tadpole or strap cells), with positivity for desmin and myogenin.

20.7.7 Synovial Sarcoma

Definition

Synovial sarcoma is a biphasic tumor composed of spindle and epithelioid cells, characterized by X;18 chromosomal translocations.

Epidemiology

Synovial sarcomas account for approximately 5 % of all primary cardiac sarcomas. The male-to-female ratio is 3:1. The mean patient age at diagnosis is 37 years, ranging from 13 to 70 years.

Localization

Most common site for synovial sarcoma is the lower limb. Synovial sarcoma of the heart is extremely rare. There is a predilection for the atria and pericardial surfaces. Right side synovial sarcoma is twice more common than the left side [33, 34].

Clinical Features

The clinical presentation is nonspecific, so the diagnosis is almost always at advanced stage in most of the cases. Left-sided tumor manifests earlier than right-sided tumor due to their mass effect and obstruction to pulmonary veins.

Pathology

On macroscopic examination synovial sarcomas are firm, whitish, infiltrative tumors with areas of necrosis and hemorrhage. The size of tumor varies from 2.9 to 15 cm. Left-sided tumors are comparatively small. Cardiac synovial sarcoma may be biphasic or monophasic.

The latter is the most common form in the heart. The classical biphasic synovial sarcoma has epithelial and spindle cell components in varying proportion. The classical monophasic variant contains only spindle cell component.

Immunohistochemistry

Immunohistochemically, cytokeratin and epithelial membrane antigen are strongly expressed in the epithelioid cells. Spindle cells express vimentin and focally smooth muscle actin. The cells do not express CD34.

Differential Diagnosis

Differential diagnosis includes sarcomatoid mesothelioma, solitary fibrous tumor, and fibrosarcoma. Distinction of synovial sarcoma from mesothelioma, another biphasic tumor, can usually be made on the basis of tumor location (mesotheliomas do not occur within the atria) and growth pattern (synovial sarcoma is usually a solitary mass, while mesothelioma tends to grow diffusely over the pericardium). Additionally, the spindle cell component of synovial sarcoma tends to be relatively uniform. The SS18/SSX transcripts are specific markers of synovial sarcoma and can be detected by the reverse transcriptase–polymerase chain reaction (RT-PCR) [35].

Genetics

Cytogenetically the reciprocal translocation *t*(X;18) (p11.2;q11.2) between SYT gene on chromosome 18 and SSX1 or SSX2 gene on chromosome X is seen in more than 90 % of soft tissue synovial sarcomas.

Prognosis

Primary cardiac synovial sarcoma is an extremely rare malignancy, with a very poor prognosis due to high local recurrence and metastasis rate. Chemotherapy with or without radiotherapy seems to improve survival.

Key Points: Synovial Sarcoma

- Synovial sarcoma is an extremely rare and highly aggressive tumor composed of epithelial and spindle cells.
- Male-to-female ratio is 3:1, mean age 37 years.
- Right side synovial sarcoma is twice more common than the left side.
- Cardiac synovial sarcoma may be biphasic (epithelial and spindle cell components) or monophasic (only spindle cell component), the latter being the most common form in the heart. The epithelioid cells express cytokeratin and epithelial membrane antigen, while spindle cells vimentin and smooth muscle actin.
- X;18 chromosomal translocations is seen in more than 90 % of soft tissue synovial sarcomas.

20.7.8 Miscellaneous Sarcomas

Definition

Miscellaneous sarcomas include rare primary cardiac sarcomas: malignant peripheral nerve sheath tumor (MPNST), liposarcoma, extraskeletal Ewing sarcoma/primitive neuroectodermal tumor/the Ewing family of tumors (EFTs), carcinosarcoma, desmoplastic small round cell tumor (DSRCT), extrarenal rhabdoid tumor/malignant extrarenal rhabdoid tumor (MERT), and chondrosarcoma [1].

20.8 Primary Cardiac Lymphoma

20.8.1 Definition

Primary cardiac lymphoma is defined as an extranodal non-Hodgkin lymphoma that involves only the heart and/or the pericardium.

20.8.2 Epidemiology

Primary cardiac lymphomas represent about 1% of all primary cardiac tumors. The median age is 60 years, with male/female ratio approximately 3:1, and it occurs not necessarily in immune-deficient people [36].

20.8.3 Location

Primary cardiac lymphomas may arise in any cardiac chamber, but in two thirds of cases, the right atrium is the site of involvement with an intramural, whitish infiltrating mass extended to the pericardium with massive effusion.

20.8.4 Clinical Features

The clinical presentation has usually an acute onset, with chest pain, pericardial effusion, congestive heart failure, arrhythmias, syncope, and even complete AV block.

20.8.5 Pathology

Usually the tumor is large, infiltrating myocardium and forming multiple intracavitary polypoid nodules, which may eventually obliterate the cavities. The pericardium is usually thickened by white–grayish tumor infiltration with massive pericardial effusion.

20.8.6 Immunohistochemistry

Histopathologically, the subtype most frequently observed (80 % of cases) is diffuse large B-cell lymphoma with CD20-positive cells, whereas the remaining 20 % are CD3-positive T-cell lymphomas. Immunocytochemical staining, cytogenetic studies, and polymerase chain reaction are necessary to differentiate B- and T-cell lymphomas from reactive lymphocyte hyperplasia, detecting the presence of a monoclonal population.

20.8.7 Differential Diagnoses

The differential diagnoses include secondary cardiac involvement by a primary mediastinal large B-cell lymphoma and primary cardiac sarcomas.

20.8.8 Prognosis

The prognosis is poor, with a mean survival of 7 months. Chemotherapy can often improve the patient's survival (◘ Fig. 20.5).

20.8.9 Key Points: Primary Cardiac Lymphoma

- Defined as an extranodal non-Hodgkin lymphoma involving primarily and only the heart and pericardium.
- Secondary cardiac involvement by lymphoma is more common than primary cardiac lymphoma.
- Primary cardiac lymphoma typically involves the right heart and more than one cardiac chamber.
- Diffuse large B-cell lymphoma with CD20-positive cells is the most frequent subtype.
- Chemotherapy is the main treatment.

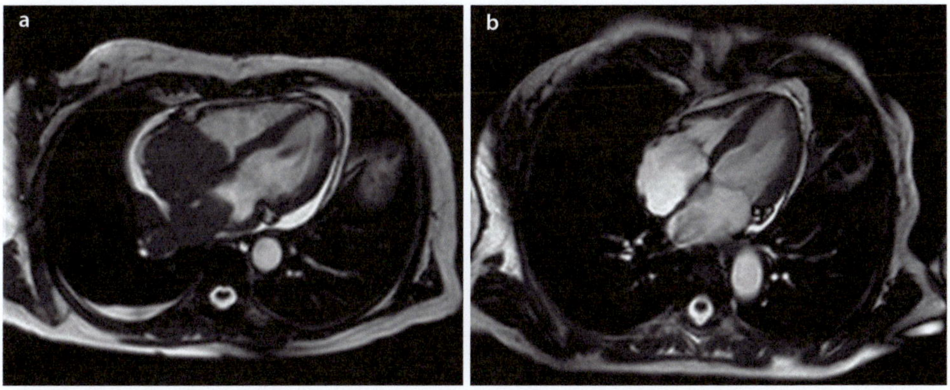

◘ **Fig. 20.5** Magnetic resonance imaging in a case of primary cardiac non-Hodgkin lymphoma. **a** At diagnosis the mass occupied both atria, extending to pulmonary veins. **b** After R-CHOP chemotherapy there was complete remission

20.9 Tumors of the Pericardium

Pericardial tumors in WHO classification [1] include solitary fibrous tumor, malignant mesotheliomas, germ cell tumors, sarcomas (angiosarcomas and synovial sarcoma), and metastatic pericardial tumors.

Pericardial tumors are most likely to be metastatic in nature or an extension of primary tumors from the surrounding structures, in most cases from lung and breast tumors, melanoma, or hematologic malignancies.

Pericardial teratomas and malignant mesotheliomas are the most common primary pericardial tumors.

Pericardial tumors often cause symptoms related to pericardial effusion.

The combination of cytologic fluid analysis and histologic pericardial biopsy is necessary to making the final diagnosis.

20.9.1 Solitary Fibrous Tumor

Definition

A spindle cell tumor with a hemangiopericytoma-like vascular pattern. Localized fibrous tumor and haemangiopericytoma are synonyms.

Localization

Solitary fibrous tumors usually arise from the pleura, but also in various sites. Rare examples have been reported in the pericardium and within the heart [37].

Clinical Features

Clinical features are related to pericardial mass effect, including pericarditis and pericardial effusion.

Pathology

Macroscopically, solitary fibrous tumor is firm and well circumscribed. Histopathologic examination shows spindle cell proliferation with often a hemangiopericytoma-like vascular pattern. Areas of hypercellularity typically alternate with myxoid or fibrous areas.

Immunohistochemistry

Solitary fibrous tumors are CD34 positive. STAT6 nuclear expression is a specific and sensitive marker for solitary fibrous tumor.

Differential Diagnosis

Malignant mesotheliomas of the pericardium show diffuse growth pattern and keratin and calretinin reactivity. Fibrosarcoma tends to be more monomorphic and negative for CD34. Monophasic synovial sarcoma has higher-grade cytology and focal keratin reactivity.

Prognosis

The prognosis is good, although recurrences after surgical resection and local spread have been reported.

Key Points: Solitary Fibrous Tumor

- Spindle cell tumor showing alternating hypercellular and hypocellular areas, with hemangiopericytoma-like patterns.
- Diffuse positivity for CD34 and STAT6.
- Prognosis is good.

20.9.2 Malignant Mesothelioma

Definition

A malignant tumor derived from mesenchymal tissue showing a mesothelial differentiation. The definition of primary pericardial mesothelioma requires that there is no tumor present outside the pericardium, with the exception of lymph node metastases.

Epidemiology

Pericardial mesotheliomas represent less than 1 % of all malignant mesotheliomas, but they are the most common primary pericardial tumor, with a higher incidence among men than women and a mean age of 45 years. Risk factors for malignant mesothelioma include asbestos exposure, therapeutic radiation, and pericardial dusting as a treatment for angina pectoris.

Clinical Features

Symptoms usually result from constriction of the heart and diastolic impairment or compression of surrounding structures either from hemorrhagic pericardial effusion or direct infiltration. Cytological examination is a poor method for detection of mesothelioma. Although clinical data and imaging are very helpful for the diagnosis of pericardial mesothelioma, a definite diagnosis still relies on pericardial biopsy or postmortem examination [38].

Pathology

Macroscopically, malignant mesotheliomas of the pericardium may present as localized nodules that fill the pericardial cavity or may spread diffusely over the pericardial surface encasing the heart and the great vessels. At histology, the majority are of the epithelioid type, forming tubules and papillary structures. The sarcomatous variant is also common. Ultrastructurally, mesothelioma cells contain microvilli.

Immunohistochemistry

Expressions of mesothelial antigens, such as calretinin and cytokeratins 5/6, are helpful in the diagnosis. Negative are the reactions for adenocarcinoma markers, such as carcinoembryonic antigen.

Differential Diagnosis

The distinction between mesothelioma and metastatic adenocarcinoma can be difficult and is generally based on immunohistochemical findings. Distinction from reactive mesothelial cell proliferations may also be difficult. Malignancies that may be confused with mesothelioma include pericardial angiosarcoma, which may elicit a prominent mesothelial response, malignant solitary fibrous tumor, and synovial sarcoma. Mesothelioma lacks the X;18 translocation of synovial sarcoma.

Prognosis

The median survival of patients with pericardial mesothelioma is approximately 6 months [39].

Key Points: Malignant Mesothelioma

- Primary malignant pericardial mesothelioma is extremely rare; however, it is the most common primary malignancy of the pericardium.
- No constant relationship between the asbestos exposure and the development of pericardial mesothelioma.
- Male-to-female ratio of 3:1, mean age 45 years.
- Progressive encasement of the heart causing breathlessness and chest pain, often with clinical signs of pericardial constriction and/or tamponade.
- Prognosis is poor.

20.9.3 Germ Cell Tumors

Definition

Tumors of germ cell origin arising within the myocardium or pericardial cavity.

Epidemiology

The great majority of germ cell tumors are benign teratomas and the remainders are yolk sac tumors. Teratomas typically affect infants and children. Its occurrence in adults is very rare, <1 % [40, 41], with a peak incidence in the second and third decades of life and a male predominance.

Localization

Approximately 90 % of the cardiac teratomas involve the pericardium [1].

Clinical Features

The main clinical findings relate to pericardial effusion. Intramyocardial teratoma often manifests with congestive heart failure or arrhythmias.

Pathology

Macroscopically they have a multicystic and lobulated appearance, with intervening solid areas. The size goes from a few millimeters up to 15 cm.

Histologically, teratomas contain elements derived from the three embryonic layers (endodermal, ectodermal, and mesodermal) in varying degrees. If more than 50 % of the tumor is comprised of well-differentiated elements, then the tumor is referred to as a mature teratoma. The immature teratoma is less well differentiated, with components resembling fetal-type tissues. Malignant areas may be observed within a benign teratoma, with features of yolk sac tumor.

Immunohistochemistry

Immunohistochemical staining positive for alpha-fetoprotein suggests the diagnosis of a germ cell tumor.

Differential Diagnosis

The differential diagnosis of intra cardiac teratomas is cystic tumor of the atrioventricular node; however, the latter does not contain mesodermal or ectodermal structures.

Prognosis

Recurrence or malignant degeneration is rare. The prognosis depends upon the extension of malignant areas. Yolk sac tumors metastasize at an early stage and invade the surrounding structures and organs.

Key Points: Germ Cell Tumors

- Tumors of germ cell origin that contain endodermal, mesodermal, and ectodermal elements.
- Strong predilection toward pediatric population.
- Most of them are intrapericardial benign teratomas.
- Areas of malignant degeneration ("yolk sac tumor") secreting alpha-fetoprotein may be present.
- Prognosis depends on these malignant areas.

References

1. Travis WD, Brambilla E, Burke AP, Marx A, Nicholson AG. WHO classification of tumours of the lung, thymus and heart. Pleura: IARC Press; 2015.
2. Reynen K. Frequency of primary tumors of the heart. Am J Cardiol. 1996;77:107.
3. Roberts WC. Primary and secondary neoplasms of the heart. Am J Cardiol. 1997;80:671–82.
4. Burke AP, Virmani R. Tumours of the heart and great vessels. 3rd ed. Washington, DC: Armed Forces Institute of Pathology; 1996.
5. Burke A, Jeudy Jr J, Virmani R. Cardiac tumours: an update. Heart. 2008;94:117–23.
6. Basso C, Valente M, Thiene G. Cardiac tumor pathology. New York: Springer Humana Press; 2013.
7. Basso C, Rizzo S, Valente M, Thiene G. Cardiac masses and tumours. Heart 2016; 102:1230-45.
8. Lam KY, Dickens P, Chan AC. Tumors of the heart. A 20-year experience with a review of 12,485 consecutive autopsies. Arch Pathol Lab Med. 1993;117:1027–31.
9. McAllister HA, Hall RJ, Cooley DA. Tumors of the heart and pericardium. Curr Probl Cardiol. 1999;24:57–116.
10. Basso C, Valente M, Thiene G. Tumori del cuore. Monografie di Cardiologia. Società Italiana di Cardiologia. Novate-Milan: Arti Grafiche Color Black; 2005.

11. Abraham KP, Reddy V, Gattuso P. Neoplasms metastatic to the heart: review of 3314 consecutive autopsies. Am J Cardiovasc Pathol. 1990;3:195–8.
12. Goldberg AD, Blankstein R, Padera RF. Tumors metastatic to the heart. Circulation. 2013;128:1790–4.
13. Bussani R, De-Giorgio F, Abbate A, Silvestri F. Cardiac metastases. J Clin Pathol. 2007;60:27–34.
14. Bossert T, Gummert JF, Battellini R, Richter M, Barten M, Walther T, Falk V, Mohr FW. Surgical experience with 77 primary cardiac tumors. Interact Cardiovasc Thorac Surg. 2005;4:311–5.
15. Centofanti P, Di Rosa E, Deorsola L, Dato GM, Patanè F, La Torre M, Barbato L, Verzini A, Fortunato G, di Summa M. Primary cardiac neoplasms: early and late results of surgical treatment in 91 patients. Ann Thorac Surg. 1999;68:1236–41.
16. Burazor I, Aviel-Ronen S, Imazio M, Markel G, Grossman Y, Yosepovich A, Adler Y. Primary malignancies of the heart and pericardium. Clin Cardiol. 2014;37:582–8.
17. Basso C, Valente M, Poletti A, Casarotto D, Thiene G. Surgical pathology of primary cardiac and pericardial tumours. Eur J Cardiothorac Surg. 1997;12:730–7.
18. Neuville A, Collin F, Bruneval P, Parrens M, Thivolet F, Gomez-Brouchet A, Terrier P, de Montpreville VT, Le Gall F, Hostein I, Lagarde P, Chibon F, Coindre JM. Intimal sarcoma is the most frequent primary cardiac sarcoma: clinicopathologic and molecular retrospective analysis of 100 primary cardiac sarcomas. Am J Surg Pathol. 2014;38:461–9.
19. Fletcher CDM, Unni KK, Mertens F. World health organization classification of tumours. Pathology and genetics of tumours of soft tissue and bone. Lyon: IARC Press; 2002.
20. Trojani M, Contesso G, Coindre JM, Rouesse J, Bui NB, de Mascarel A, Goussot JF, David M, Bonichon F, Lagarde C. Soft-tissue sarcomas of adults: study of pathological prognostic variables and definition of a histopathological grading system. Int J Cancer. 1984;33:37–42.
21. Reardon MJ, Walkes JC, Benjamin R. Therapy insight: malignant primary cardiac tumors. Nat Rev Cardiol. 2006;3:548–53.
22. Burke AP, Cowan D, Virmani R. Primary sarcomas of the heart. Cancer. 1992;69:387–95.
23. Donsbeck AV, Ranchere D, Coindre JM, Le Gall F, Cordier JF, Loire R. Primary cardiac sarcomas: an immunohistochemical and grading study with long-term follow-up of 24 cases. Histopathology. 1999;34:295–304.
24. Rao U, Curtin J, Ryding A. Primary angiosarcoma of the heart. Heart. 2013;99:1878–9.
25. Hermann MA, Shankerman RA, Edwards WD, Shub C, Schass HV. Primary cardiac angiosarcoma: a clinicopathologic study of six cases. J Thorac Cardiovasc Surg. 1992;103:655–64.
26. Poletti A, Cocco P, Valente M, Fasoli G, Chioin R, Thiene G. In vivo diagnosis of cardiac angiosarcoma by endomyocardial biopsy. Cardiovasc Pathol. 1993;2:89–91.
27. Garcia JM, Gonzalez R, Jm S, Dominguez G, Vegazo IS, Gamallo C, Provencio M, España P, Bonilla F. Mutational status of K-ras and TP53 genes in primary sarcomas of the heart. Br J Cancer. 2000;82:1183–5.
28. Basso C, Stefani A, Calabrese F, Fasoli G, Valente M. Primary right atrial fibrosarcoma diagnosed by endocardial biopsy. Am Heart J. 1996;131:399–402.
29. Mazzola A, Spano JP, Valente M, Gregorini R, Villani C, Di Eusanio M, Ciocca M, Minuti U, Giancola R, Basso C, Thiene G. Leiomyosarcoma of the left atrium mimicking a left atrial myxoma. J Thorac Cardiovasc Surg. 2006;131:224–6.
30. Pessotto R, Silvestre G, Luciani GB, Anselmi M, Pasini F, Santini F, Mazzucco A. Primary cardiac leiomyosarcoma: seven-year survival with combined surgical and adjuvant therapy. Int J Cardiol. 1997;60:91–4.
31. Hui KS, Green LK, Schmidt WA. Primary cardiac rhabdomyosarcoma: definition of a rare entity. Am J Cardiovasc Pathol. 1988;2:19–29.
32. Hajar R, Roberts WC, Folger Jr GM. Embryonal botryoid rhabdomyosarcoma of the mitral valve. Am J Cardiol. 1986;57:376.
33. Nicholson AG, Rigby M, Lincoln C, Meller S, Fisher C. Synovial sarcoma of the heart. Histopathology. 1997;30:349–52.
34. Varma T, Adegboyega P. Primary cardiac synovial sarcoma. Arch Pathol Lab Med. 2012;136:454–8.
35. Hazelbag HM, Szuhai K, Tanke HJ, Rosenberg C, Hogendoorn PC. Primary synovial sarcoma of the heart: a cytogenetic and molecular genetic analysis combining RT-PCR and COBRA-FISH of a case with a complex karyotype. Mod Pathol. 2004;17:1434–9.
36. Petrich A, Cho SI, Billett H. Primary cardiac lymphoma: an analysis of presentation, treatment and outcome patterns. Cancer 2011; 117: 581–9.

37. Bortolotti U, Calabro F, Loy M, Fasoli G, Altavilla G, Marchese D. Giant intrapericardial solitary fibrous tumor. Ann Thorac Surg. 1992;54:1219–20.
38. Nilsson A, Rasmuson T. Primary pericardial mesothelioma: report of a patient and literature review. Case Rep Oncol. 2009;2:125–32.
39. Sardar MR, Kuntz C, Patel T, Saeed W, Gnall E, Imaizumi S, Lande L. Primary pericardial mesothelioma unique case and literature review. Tex Heart Inst J. 2012;39:261–4.
40. Luk A, Ahn E, Vaideeswar P, Butany JW. Pericardial tumors. Semin Diagn Pathol. 2008;25:47–53.
41. Bruce CJ. Cardiac tumours: diagnosis and management. Heart. 2011;97:151–60.

Diagnosis of Primary Cardiac Malignancies: Echocardiography

Paolo Pino and Chiara Lestuzzi

C. Lestuzzi et al. (eds.), *Manual of Cardio-oncology*, DOI 10.1007/978-3-319-40236-9_21

21.1 Echocardiography

21.1.1 Transthoracic Echocardiography

Cardiac malignancies are often detected at transthoracic echocardiography, either done for the presence of symptoms or during a routine screening [1–5]. Echocardiography for its spatial and temporal resolution can define precise anatomic details and pathology: location, morphologic appearance (size, shape), mobility, and relation to adjacent cardiac structures so that the embolic potential and hemodynamic consequences of the tumors are well determined [6, 7].

- In most cases the cardiac tumor appears as an abnormal intracardiac mass. The sensitivity of echocardiography is greatest for endocavitary lesions, where the contrast between the tumor and the blood of cardiac chamber is greatest, permitting detection of the mass. Intramyocardial lesions and pericardial tumors without pericardial effusion are less well appreciated because of the lack of contrast between the mass and cardiac structures.
- When an intracardiac mass is observed at echocardiography, a systematic approach is essential, and the differential diagnosis includes artifacts and normal structures or variants, thrombi, vegetations, benign, and metastatic tumors [8]. The clinical context may suggest the diagnosis of a thrombus (for instance, in patients with atrial fibrillation, enlarged atrium, ventricular aneurysm) or of a vegetation (in patients with fever): it is important to interpret echo findings in light of the clinical setting.
- Echocardiography provides limited information about tissue characterization, and identification of the nature of the mass at echocardiography might be challenging even for the most experienced examiners. A diagnostic approach has been proposed to determine etiology of the mass with a consideration of four factors [9]:
  1. The histology-based likelihood (after surgery, only about 10 % of primary cardiac tumors are diagnosed as malignant; among them, the great majority are sarcomas, only 10 % are lymphomas)
  2. The age of the patient at time of presentation (rhabdomyomas and fibromas are the most common tumors in children)
  3. The tumor location (see below and ◘ Box 1)
  4. Noninvasive tissue characterization might be based on the echogenicity and calcification of the mass or on its vascularity, assessed with color Doppler and echocardiographic contrast agents
- Some tumors are usually observed in specific sites (◘ Box 1):
  - Angiosarcomas grow usually in the right chambers and the pericardium is often involved.

Box 1 Presumptive Diagnosis of Malignant Cardiac Tumors According to MASS SITE

- **Right Atrium:** Angiosarcoma; Liposarcoma; Lymphoma
- **Left Atrium:** Hystiocitoma, leiomyosarcoma, osteosarcoma
- **Ventricles:** Rabdomyosarcoma, lymphoma
- **Pumonary artery:** Leiomyosarcoma
- **Pericardium:** Angiosarcoma; mesothelioma.

Box 2 Echocardiographic characteristics suggesting malignant nature of the mass

- The mass is large and broad-based
- A stalk is often non present
- Extension beyond anatomic boundaries
- Infiltration of cardiac walls and extension within cardiac chambers or pericardium
- Morphology: masses are multiple, with irregular shape and irregular texture
- Motion: infiltrating and broad-based masses exhibit a slowdowned motion
- Pericardial effusion with intrapericardial masses.

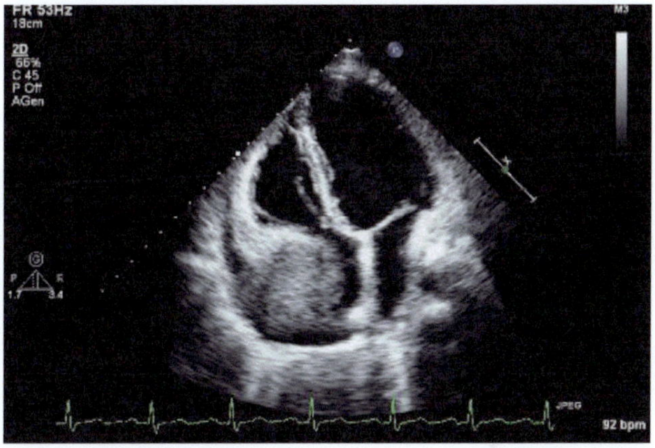

Fig. 21.1 Right atrial mass. Transthoracic echocardiography: apical four chambers in systole. A large mass with irregular texture is seen infiltrating the right atrium lateral wall. The mass invades the right atrium cavity and pericardium (pericardial effusion). These echocardiographic characteristics suggest a malignant nature of the mass. A pathological exam showed high-grade sarcoma, consistent with angiosarcoma

  - Pleomorphic sarcomas are most often observed in the left atrium (usually arising from the roof or from the lateral wall).
  - Leiomyosarcomas are usually found in the pulmonary artery and in the left atrium.
  - Lymphomas are more common in the right chambers with the aspect of an intracavitary mass or of masses infiltrating the cardiac walls.
- Echocardiographic characteristics of primary malignant tumors are not specific and do not permit a reliable "noninvasive histologic diagnosis." Nevertheless, some echocardiographic characteristics can suggest a malignant nature of the mass (Box 2, Figs. 21.1, 21.2, and 21.3).
- The mass is large and broad-based, without a stalk, extending beyond anatomic boundaries: for instance, right atrium sarcoma extends through the tricuspid valve into the right ventricle.
- Direct infiltration of cardiac walls, extension within cardiac chambers, and pericardium or outside the heart are often detected.

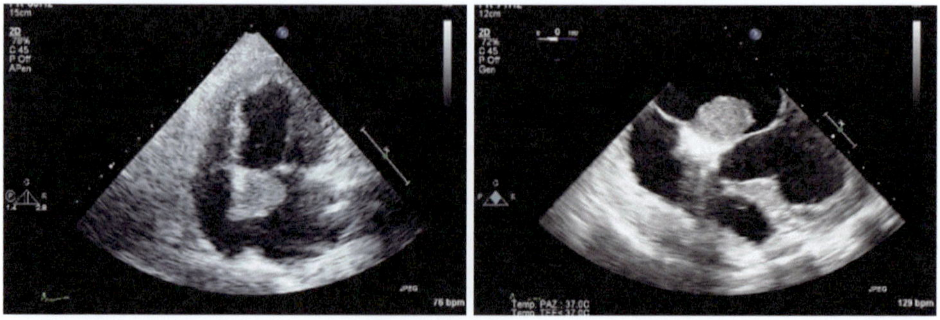

Fig. 21.2 Left atrial mass. Transthoracic echocardiography: apical four chambers in systole (*left*). Transesophageal echocardiography: mid-esophageal four chambers in systole (*right*). A large mass is seen on the interatrial septum; the fossa ovalis is free and the mass is close to the mitral valve. The mass is broad-based and no stalk is recognizable. These echocardiographic characteristics suggest a malignant nature of the mass. A pathological exam showed a myxoma

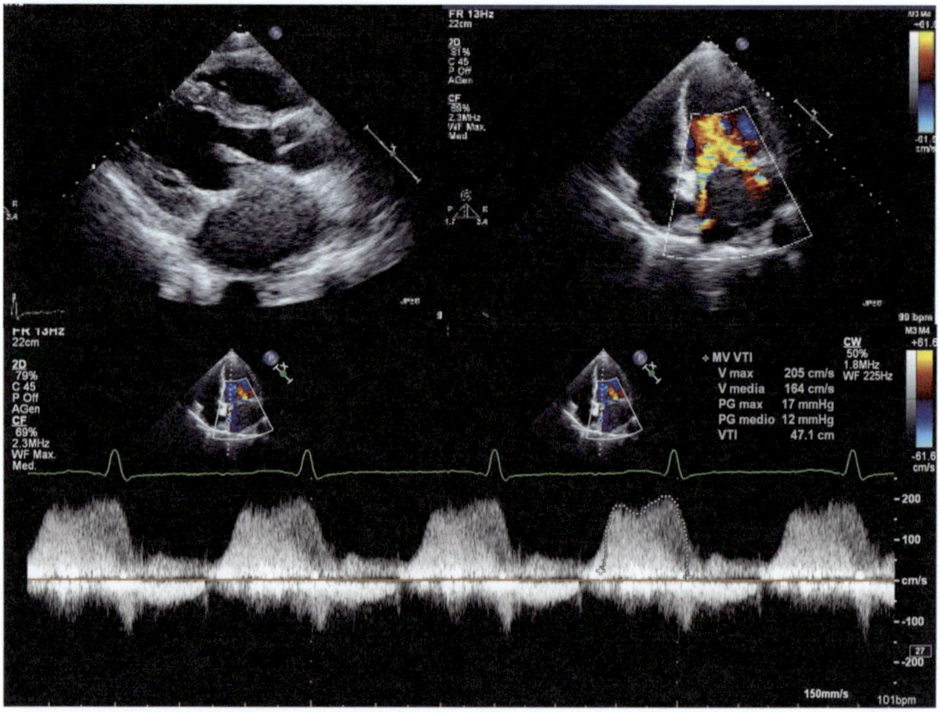

Fig. 21.3 Left atrial mass (sarcoma). Transthoracic echocardiography: long axis and color Doppler four chamber in diastole. A large mass invades the left atrium protruding in the left ventricle cavity through mitral valve. Color and spectral echocardiography suggest an obstructive lesion mimicking mitral stenosis (mean gradient 12 mmHg)

- Masses are multiple with irregular shape and irregular texture characterized by mixed echogenicity, predominantly cystic with fluid consistent with a vascular tumor.
- Their slowdowned motion in real-time imaging suggests stiffness, clue of malignant nature of the masses.
- If the venae cavae and pulmonary veins are free from mass, the probability of a primary tumor of the atria is very high.
- Pericardial involvement with pericardial effusion is a common manifestation of malignant tumors.

Unexplained pericardial effusion should raise a high index of suspicion of malignancy [10].

21.2 Echocardiographic Contrast Agents

Echocardiographic contrast agents that traverse the pulmonary circulation are enhancing the vascularized masses and may be used to enhance the echogenicity of neoplastic masses (Figs. 21.4, 21.5, 21.6, and 21.7).

The quantification of echocardiographic perfusion imaging of cardiac masses with gray-scale power modulation improves the chances of echocardiography in recognizing the cardiac masses.

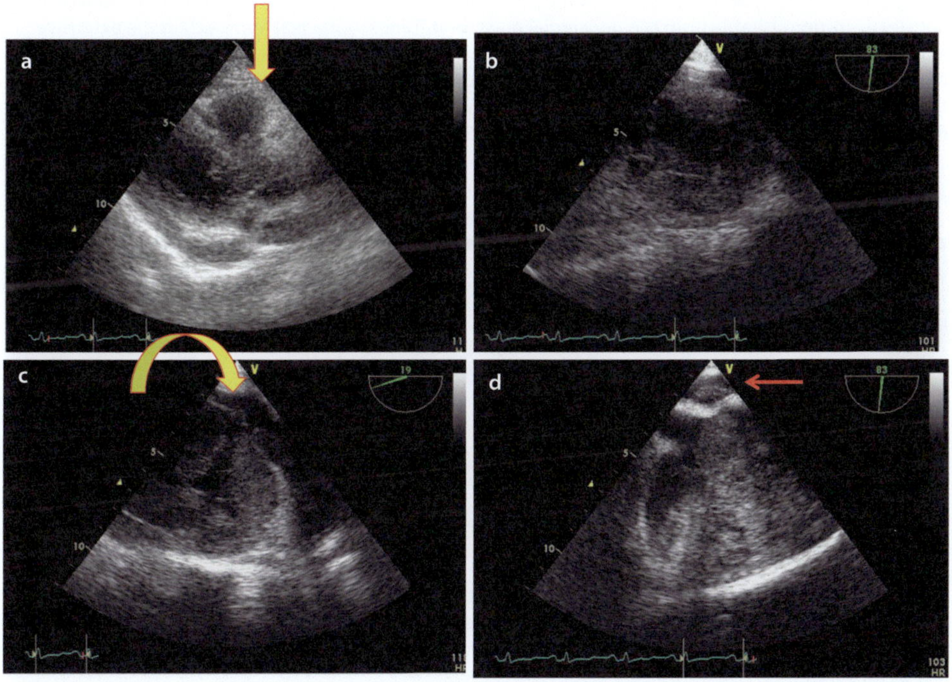

Fig. 21.4 Cardiac mass (angiosarcoma) with intracardiac and pericardial extension. **a** From the subcostal approach, the mass is low echogenic. **b** After injection of SonoVue®, the echogenicity of the mass is increased. **c** The vessels of the mass are opacified by SonoVue®. **d** Color Doppler signal of the tumor vessels is enhanced by SonoVue® (reproduced, with permission, from Lestuzzi C, in Ecocardiografia clinica, Piccin, Padova 2014)

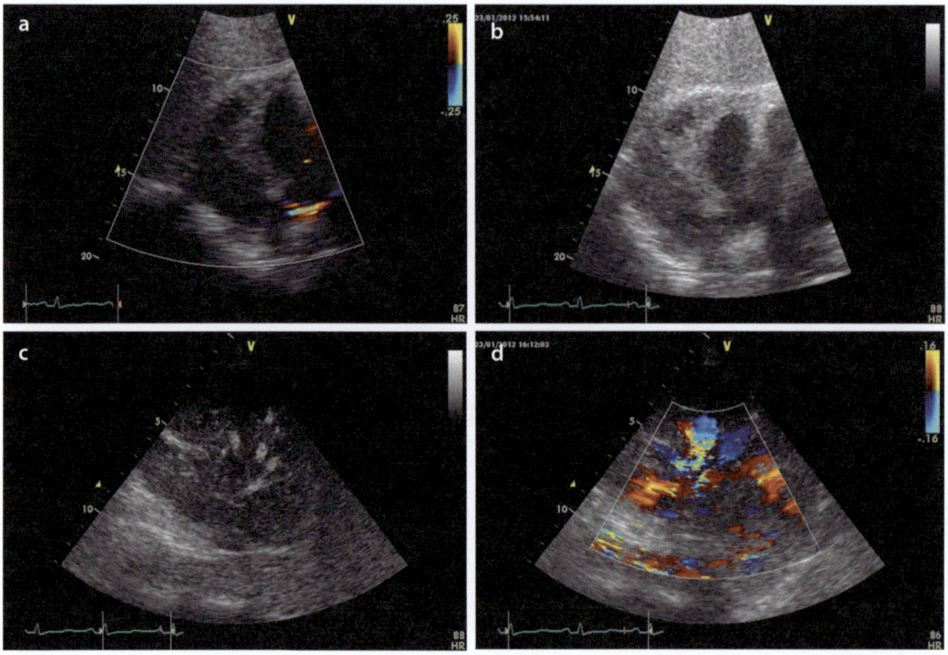

Fig. 21.5 Same case of Fig. 21.1. **a** Transthoracic long axis view. The intracardiac mass (*arrow*) is not clearly distinguishable from the pericardial mass. **b–d** Transesophageal approach: **b** the extensive infiltration of the right atrial wall is evident; **c** the point where the pericardial mass continues through the atrial wall prolapsing into the right ventricle is shown by the curved arrow; **d** from the right atrium, the mass extends to the left atrium (*thin, red arrow*) (reproduced, with permission, from Lestuzzi et al. Future Cardiology 2015, Volume 11, Issue 4, pp. 485–500)

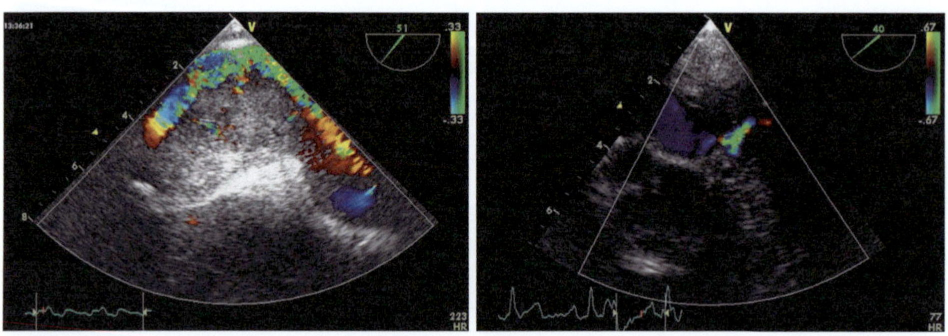

Fig. 21.6 Transesophageal visualization of a right atrial mass (low-grade angiosarcoma) extending to the inferior vena, which is sub-occluded and infiltrated (*left*) and of a left atrial mass (leiomyosarcoma) infiltrating a left pulmonary vein (*right*) (reproduced, with permission, from Lestuzzi et al. Future Cardiology 2015, Volume 11, Issue 4, pp. 485–500)

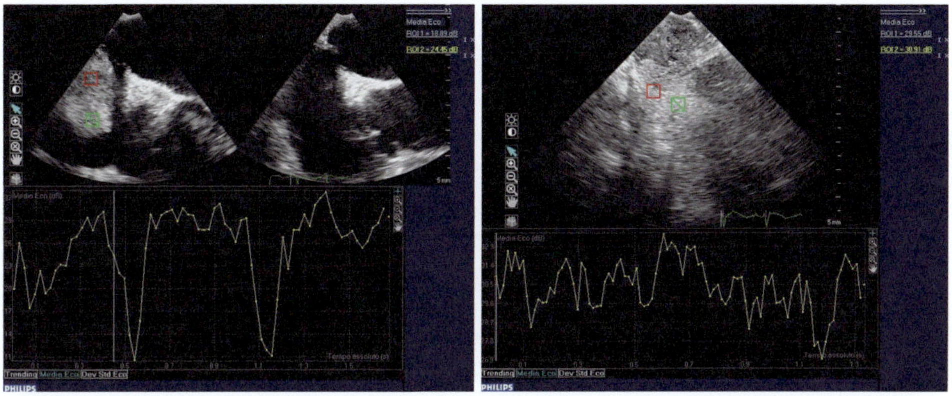

Fig. 21.7 Right atrial mass. Transesophageal echocardiography. Quantitative analysis of time-intensity curve obtained by quantification software with estimation of myocardial blood volume in two regions of interest (*red* and *green*) during contrast enhancement. The increase of decibel depends on rich vascularization of the mass (myxoma)

- Malignant and highly vascular tumors become hyper-enhanced and when analyzed quantitatively demonstrate more perfusion than the adjacent myocardium.
- Stromal tumors show a lesser enhancement compared to the adjacent myocardium.
- Thrombi show no enhancement.
- Contrast agents can be used both in the diagnostic phase and in the follow-up after antineoplastic treatments, mostly when anti-neoangiogenis or angiotoxic therapies have been used [11–20].
- Only a few case reports about the use of this agents applied to the study of cardiac tumors have been published so far; in our personal experience, its use may be helpful to better identify low echogenic masses in the atria and to enhance the Doppler signal in highly vascularized lesions.
- The use of contrast media in the study of cardiac tumors is slightly different from the method commonly used in cardiology to detect thrombi or to evaluate the myocardial perfusion.
  - A small quantity (0.5 ml) of contrast medium should be injected intravenously, followed by a rapid bolus of 5 ml of saline.
  - After a few seconds, the right cardiac chambers are opacified, and within a couple of minutes the left chambers are opacified as well; at this stage, the intracardiac mass appears as a minus (dark) image.
  - After 3 min or more, the contrast medium in the cardiac chambers is less visible, and the neoplastic mass becomes more echogenic. The enhancement depends both on the number of vessels and on the presence of necrotic areas within the tumor.
  - The washout of contrast medium from the mass is usually slow, so the enhancement of the mass can be examined for several minutes.
  - Should the mass echogenicity decrease, a new bolus can be injected.
  - The most relevant use of contrast is to better visualize an atrial tumor at transthoracic echocardiography and to help the differential diagnosis between a thrombus and tumor. However, both benign and malignant tumor may have the same aspects even using a contrast medium.

- Cardiac masses can be qualitatively analyzed by visual assessment of mass contrast or quantitatively by analysis of time-intensity curve obtained by quantification software with estimation of myocardial blood volume during optimal cavity contrast enhancement [20].

21.3 Transesophageal Echocardiography (TEE)

Transthoracic imaging in patients with poor echocardiographic window has improved with the advent of tissue harmonic imaging. However, small tumors can still be missed.

- TEE is more sensitive than transthoracic echocardiography in detecting abnormalities that involve the posterior cardiac structures, particularly the atria, interatrial septum, and pulmonary veins.
- It allows a more precise assessment of the size, the shape, the mobility of the mass, and its relationship with other cardiac structures.
  - This is mandatory to evaluate the feasibility of surgery and to plan the possible intervention in solid tumors.
- Satellite masses within the heart can also be detected [21].
- In the presence of atrial masses, TEE allows to assess if the tumor extends to the venae cave or to pulmonary veins.
- TEE is commonly used to plan and monitor a transvenous biopsy.
- After antineoplastic treatments of atrial tumors, TEE should be used in the follow-up, for the evaluation of size changes, and for early detection in case of a local relapse.

21.4 Three-Dimensional Echocardiography (3D-ECHO)

In recent years, 3D transthoracic and transesophageal echocardiography that uses 3DE matrix-array transducers, composed of nearly 3000 piezoelectric elements, has evolved into a new clinical diagnostic tool in cardiac imaging.

- Currently, with the use of this technique, morphologic, volume, and spatial assessment of masses can be appreciated without having to perform "mental reconstruction."
- Cropping permits noninvasive "sectioning" of the mass to better evaluate its morphologic characteristics as necrotic areas within the mass and relationship with cardiac structures.
- Although 3D reconstruction can be obtained from both transthoracic and transesophageal studies, transthoracic imaging yields poor quality images in patients with poor acoustic windows, thus three-dimensional transesophageal echocardiography is preferred [21–28].
- However, currently transthoracic 3D image resolution and quality are suboptimal for the detection of small tumors and of intramyocardial mass.

> **Therefore, standard 2D imaging techniques, both transthoracic and transesophageal, should still be used to identify cardiac tumors.**

21.5 Pitfall

Many normal variants (usually defined as **pseudo-masses**) can be misinterpreted as pathologic abnormalities.

A lot of normal intracardiac structures can be difficult to distinguish from cardiac tumors: the eustachian valve, the Chiari network, the crista terminalis, the ridge of tissue between the upper pulmonary vein and left atrial appendage (so-called Coumadin ridge), and the fatty infiltrate of the atrial septum, known as lipomatous atrial septal hypertrophy.

The *crista terminalis* is a fibromuscular ridge extending along the posterolateral right atrial wall. A prominent and thickened crista terminalis mimicking a right atrial mass can be correctly interpreted using transesophageal or three-dimensional echocardiography [29–31].

The *transverse sinus* consists of a pericardial reflection at the base of the heart that echocardiographically appears as a small, echo-free space between the pulmonary artery, the ascending aorta, and the left atrium. Infiltration of pericardial fat is detected as mass.

The most common misdiagnosis is between malignant and benign tumors (◘ Figs. 21.8 and 21.9).

- The most common benign tumors (myxomas) in the majority of cases are pedunculated and are attached to the interatrial septum within the left atrium. Thus, any mass which appears to be broad-based and/or is localized on a different site (right chambers, left atrial roof, or lateral wall) should be considered likely to be malignant even though this is not always true [1–5, 32, 33].
- Additional imaging techniques as computed tomography, magnetic resonance imaging, and positron emission tomography are usually required to define the differential diagnosis (benign versus malignant masses) and the extension of malignant tumors. Unlike echocardiography, computed tomography and magnetic resonance can differentiate tissue composition, for better identification of solid, liquid, hemorrhagic, and fatty space-occupying tumors [8, 34–36].

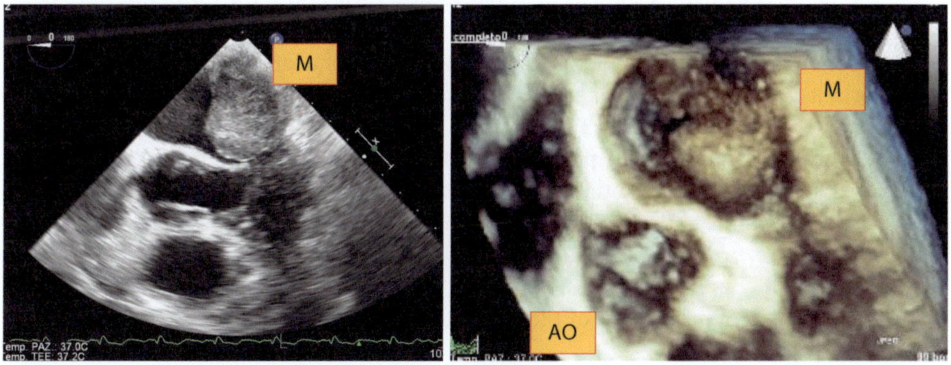

◘ **Fig. 21.8** Left atrial mass. Transesophageal echocardiography. Upper esophageal position of the probe (*left*). Three-dimensional reconstruction (*right*). A large mass (M) is seen on the left atrium lateral wall. The mass is broad-based and no stalk is recognizable. These echocardiographic characteristics suggest a malignant nature of the mass. A pathological exam showed a myxosarcoma

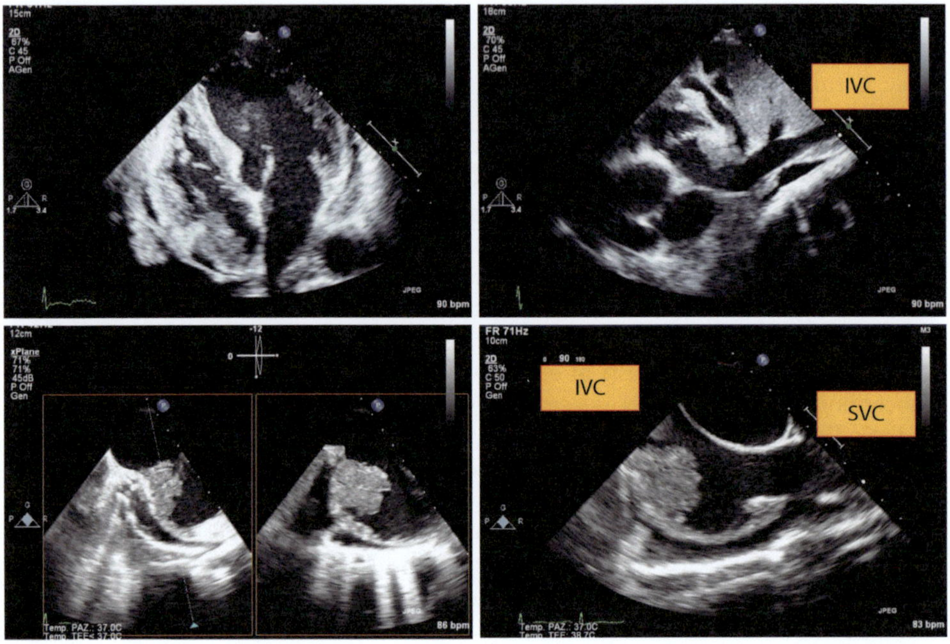

Fig. 21.9 Right atrial mass. Transthoracic (*upper panels*) and transesophageal (*lower panels*) echocardiography of a mass (M) with irregular shape and texture infiltrating the right lateral wall (well seen in the dual-plane imaging, *lower panel, left*). Inferior vena cava (IVC) and superior vena cava (SVC) are free (bicaval section, *lower panel right*)

- In malignant tumors, obtaining a pathologic diagnosis is of paramount importance in planning the therapeutic strategy.
  - In tumors which appears to be unresectable because of their extension, a biopsy should be obtained as soon as possible, in order to choose the most appropriate antineoplastic therapy.
- Transesophageal echocardiography and intracardiac echocardiography have an important role in invasive procedures related to diagnostic biopsy of cardiac masses, guiding percutaneous biopsy [37–40].
- Real-time visualization of the procedure enhances safety, minimizing risk of damage to surrounding structures and increasing diagnostic yield by directing the bioptome to the tumor (tumoral tissue and not overimposed thrombus). Clot related to bioptome damage is promptly detected and treated (Fig. 21.10).
- A diagnosis of lymphoma may be obtained through a transvenous biopsy or analyzing the cytology of pericardial or pleural effusion; bone marrow biopsy is usually negative [2].
- Histopathology analysis requires a period of some days (usually 7 to 10) to fixation and tissue preparation. Sarcomas are rather rare tumors: thus, the identification of the specific tumor histology and malignancy grading requires special expertise, and the revision by a referral center may be useful [41].

In the presence of large masses with significant obstruction to the cardiovascular circulation, surgery may be needed urgently. In such a case, a radical excision should be attempted.

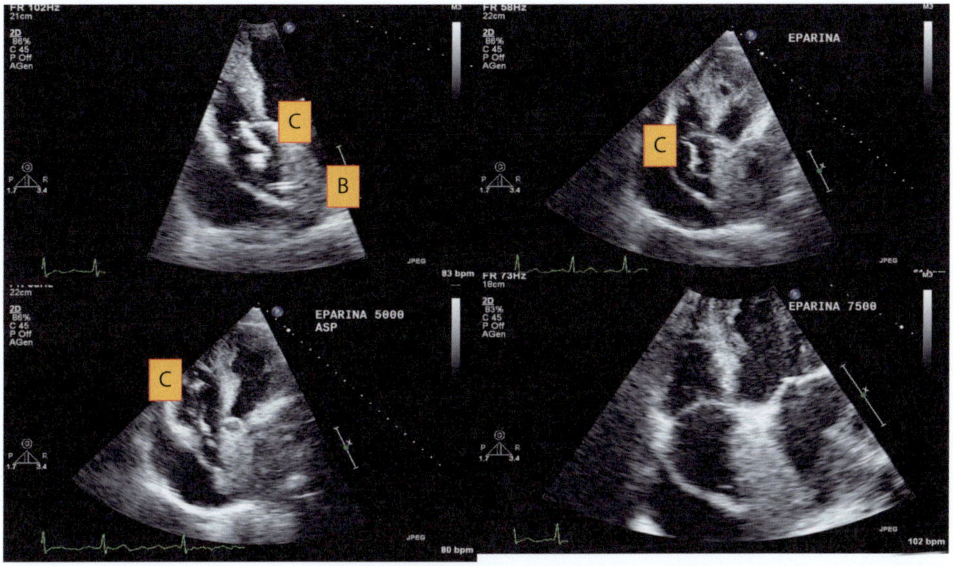

Fig. 21.10 Bi-atrial mass (angiosarcoma). Transthoracic echocardiography during biopsy. A very mobile clot **c** related to bioptome **b** damage is promptly detected and treated with unfractionated heparin (EPARINA) and thrombus aspiration (ASP). In the *right-lower panel* clot is not recognizable

If it is not feasible, almost all the mass should be resected, obtaining a large sample for pathology analysis.

In the presence of small masses, a biopsy is usually impossible and complete resection easy. In this case, the surgeon should resect en bloc the mass, leaving a margin of normal tissue around, and apply some markers to allow the orientation of the mass by the pathologist. The pathologist should examine not only the mass but also its margins, in order to assess if they are infiltrated by the tumor.

References

1. Valente ML, Rizzo S, Leone O, Basso C. Primary malignant tumors of the heart. In: Basso C, Valente ML, Thiene G, editors. Cardiac tumor pathology. New York: Springer (Humana Press); 2013. p. 73–89.
2. Miguel CE, Bestetti RB. Primary cardiac lymphoma. Int J Cardiol. 2011;149:358–63.
3. Jain D, Maleszewski JJ, Halushka MK. Benign cardiac tumors and tumorlike conditions. Ann Diagn Pathol. 2010;14:215–30.
4. Goswami KC, Shrivastava S, Bahl VK, Saxena A, Manchanda SC, Wasir HS. Cardiac myxomas: clinical and echocardiographic profile. Int J Cardiol. 1998;63:251–9.
5. Mazzola A, Spano JP, Valente M, et al. Leiomyosarcoma of the left atrium mimicking a left atrial myxoma. J Thorac Cardiovasc Surg. 2006;131:224–6.
6. Elbardissi AW, Dearani JA, Daly RC. Embolic potential of cardiac tumors and outcome after resection: a case–control study. Stroke. 2009;40:156–62.
7. Parissis JT, Zezas S, Sfiras N. An atypical left atrial myxoma causing intracavitary pressure gradient and typical diastolic transmitral flow of severe mitral stenosis. Int J Cardiol. 2005;102:165–7.
8. Tao TY, Yahyavi-Firouz-Abadi N, Singh GK, Bhalla S. Pediatric cardiac tumors: clinical and imaging features. Radiographics. 2014;34:1031–46.
9. Bruce CJ, Otto CM. The practice of clinical echocardiography. 4th ed. Amsterdam: Elseiver; 2012. p. 902–4.

10. Lee CH, Chan GS, Chan WM. Unexplained recurrent pericardial effusion: a lethal warning? Heart. 2003;89, e11.
11. Lassau N, Chami L, Chebil M, et al. Dynamic contrast- enhanced ultrasonography (DCE-US) and anti-angiogenic treatments. Discov Med. 2011;11(56):18–24.
12. Lepper W, Shivalkar B, Rinkevich D, Belcik T, Wei K. Assessment of the vascularity of a left ventricular mass using myocardial contrast echocardiography. J Am Soc Echocardiogr. 2002;15:1419–22.
13. Kirkpatrick JN, Wong T, Bednarz JE, Spencer KT, Sugeng L, Ward RP. Differential diagnosis of cardiac masses using contrast echocardiographic perfusion imaging. J Am Coll Cardiol. 2004;43:1412–9.
14. Haverkamp MC, Scholte AJ, Holman ER, Jongbloed MR, Schippers EF, de Roos A. Contrast echocardiography as a useful additional diagnostic tool in evaluating a primary cardiac tumor. Eur J Echocardiogr. 2005;6:388–91.
15. Jang JJ, Danik S, Goldman M. Primary cardiac lymphoma: diagnosis and treatment guided by trans-esophageal echocardiogram perfusion imaging. J Am Soc Echocardiogr. 2006;19:1073.e7–9.
16. Moustafa SE, Sauve C, Amyot R. Assessment of a right ventricular metastasis using contrast echocardiography perfusion imaging. Eur J Echocardiogr. 2008;9:326–8.
17. Trost B, Croft L, Nair A, Henzlova M. Primary cardiac lymphoma detected by myocardial perfusion imaging: case report. J Nucl Cardiol. 2007;14:e6–10.
18. Uenishi EK, Caldas MA, Saroute AN, Tsutsui JM, Piotto GH, Falcão SN. Contrast echocardiography for the evaluation of tumors and thrombi. Arq Bras Cardiol. 2008;91:e48–52.
19. Lestuzzi C, De Paoli A, Baresic T, et al. Malignant cardiac tumors: diagnosis and treatment. Future Cardiol. 2015;11:485–500.
20. Uenishi EK, Caldas MA, Tsutsui JM, Abduch MCD, Sbano JCN. Evaluation of cardiac masses by real-time perfusion imaging echocardiography. Cardiovasc Ultrasound. 2015;13:23.
21. Peters PJ, Reinhardt S. The echocardiographic evaluation of intracardiac masses: a review. J Am Soc Echocardiogr. 2006;19:230–40.
22. Borges AC, Witt C, Bartel T, et al. Preoperative two- and three-dimensional transesophageal echocardiographic assessment of heart tumors. Ann Thorac Surg. 1996;61:1163–7.
23. Espinola-Zavaleta N, Morales GH, Vargas-Barron J, et al. Three-dimensional transesophageal echocardiography in tumors of the heart. J Am Soc Echocardiogr. 2002;15:972–9.
24. Lokhandwala J, Liu Z, Jundi M, et al. Three-dimensional echocardiography of intracardiac masses. Echocardiography. 2004;21:159–63.
25. Mehmood F, Nanda NC, Vengala S, et al. Live three-dimensional transthoracic echocardiographic assessment of left atrial tumors. Echocardiography. 2005;22:137–43.
26. Asch FM, Bieganski SP, Panza JA, Weissman NJ. Real-Time 3-Dimensional Echocardiography Evaluation of Intracardiac Masses. Echocardiography. 2006;23:218–24.
27. Zaragoza-Macias E, Chen MA, Gill EA. Real time three-dimensional echocardiography evaluation of intracardiac masses. Echocardiography. 2012;29:207–19.
28. Plana JC. Three-dimensional echocardiography in the assessment of cardiac tumors: the added value of the extra dimension. Methodist Debakey Cardiovasc J. 2010;6:12–9.
29. Pharr JR, West MB, Kusumoto FM, Figueredo VM. Prominent crista terminalis appearing as a right atrial mass on transthoracic echocardiogram. J Am Soc Echocardiogr. 2002;15:753–5.
30. McKay T, Thomas L. Prominent crista terminalis and Eustachian ridge in the right atrium: Two dimensional (2D) and three dimensional (3D) imaging. Eur J Echocardiogr. 2007;8(4):288–91.
31. Akcay M, Bilen ES, Bilge M, Durmaz T. Prominent crista terminalis: as an anatomic structure leading to atrial arrhythmias and mimicking right atrial mass. J Am Soc Echocardiogr. 2007;20:197.e9–e10.
32. Butany J, Nair V, Naseemuddin A. Cardiac tumors: diagnosis and management. Lancet Oncol. 2005;6: 219–28.
33. Patil HR, Singh D, Hajdu N. Cardiac sarcoma presenting as heart failure and diagnosed as recurrent myxoma by echocardiogram. Eur J Echocardiogr. 2010;11:E12.
34. Masui T, Takahashi M, Miura K. Cardiac myxoma: identification of intratumoral hemorrhage and calcification on MR images. Am J Roentgenol. 1995;164:850–2.
35. Lie JT. Petrified cardiac myxoma masquerading as organized atrial mural thrombus. Arch Pathol Lab Med. 1989;113:742–5.
36. Restrepo CS, Largoza A, Lemos DF. CT and MR imaging findings of malignant cardiac tumors. Curr Probl Diagn Radiol. 2005;34:1–11.
37. Burling F, Devlin G, Heald S. Primary cardiac lymphoma diagnosed with transesophageal echocardiography-guided endomyocardial biopsy. Circulation. 2000;101:E179–81.

38. Jurkovich D, de Marchena E, Bilsker M. Primary cardiac lymphoma diagnosed by percutaneous intracardiac biopsy with combined fluoroscopic and transesophageal echocardiographic imaging. Catheter Cardiovasc Interv. 2000;50:226–33.
39. Segar DS, Bourdillon PD, Elsner G. Intracardiac echocardiography-guided biopsy of intracardiac masses. J Am Soc Echocardiogr. 1995;8:927–9.
40. Bruce CJ, Nishimura RA, Rihal CS. Intracardiac echocardiography in the interventional catheterization laboratory: preliminary experience with a novel, phased-array transducer. Am J Cardiol. 2002;89:635–40.
41. Ray-Coquard I, Montesco MC, Coindre JM. Conticanet group. Sarcoma: concordance between initial diagnosis and centralized expert review in a population-based study within three European regions. Ann Oncol. 2012;23:2442–9.

Diagnosis of Primary Cardiac Malignancies: Magnetic Resonance

Giovanni Donato Aquaro

C. Lestuzzi et al. (eds.), *Manual of Cardio-oncology*, DOI 10.1007/978-3-319-40236-9_22

22

22.1 Introduction

- Magnetic resonance (MRI) is a multiparametric imaging technique permitting to evaluate the signal properties, morphological characteristics (location, size, infiltrative nature, presence of pleural/pericardial effusions), and contrast enhancement of cardiac tumors [1].
- MRI is considered the gold-standard imaging technique for the characterization of soft tissue by the assessment of signal properties on T1-weighted, T2-weighted, and proton density (PD) images and after the injection of gadolinium-based contrast agents [2].
- The main features of MRI are:
  - The ability to distinguish between mass and pseudomass
  - High accuracy to predict the likely malignancy of a cardiac mass
  - Follow-up after therapy
- The main limitations of MRI are:
  - Contraindications to strong magnetic fields
  - Arrhythmias limiting imaging quality
  - Severe chronic kidney disease

MRI may not provide valid tissue characterization in high mobile mass smaller than 5 mm.

22.2 MRI Technique and Protocol

MRI protocols for mass evaluation should include functional and morphological evaluation with cine-imaging and static black-blood sequence and tissue characterization with T1- and T2-weighted pulse sequence and post-contrast imaging [3]. Example of the MRI protocol is shown in Fig. 22.1. A summary of MRI diagnostic algorithm is reported in Table 22.1.

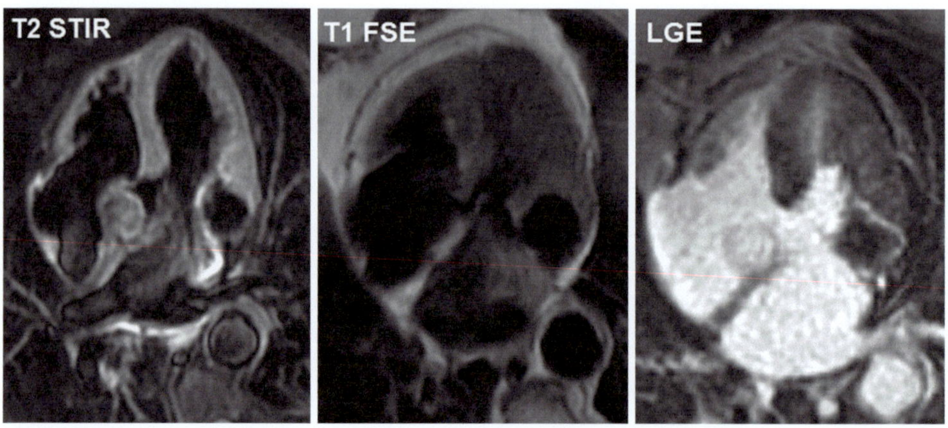

Fig. 22.1 Calcific necrosis or "caseous" calcification of posterior leaflet of mitral valve. The solid mass is hypointense in T1- and T2-weighted images indicating calcification. After gadolinium injection, on LGE image, the mass is hypointense with a hyperintense margin

Table 22.1 Summary of the MRI findings of cardiac tumors

Tumors	Prevalent site	Number	Dimensions (cm)	Margin	Infiltration	SSFP	T1w	T2w	First pass	LGE
Myxoma	Left atrium	Single/multiple	<5	Well-defined	No	Hyper	Iso	Hyper	enh	enh
Fibroma	Interventricular septum	Single	<5	Well-defined	No	Iso-hypo	iso	Hypo	No enh	enh
Lipoma	Every site	Single	<5	Well-defined	No	Hyper + India ink	Hyper[a]	Hypo[a]	No enh	no enh
Hemangioma	Epicardium, pericardium, myocardium	Single	<5	Well-defined	No	Hyper	Iso-vessel lumen	Hyper	enh	enh
Rhabdomyoma	Left ventricle	Multiple	<5	Well-defined	No	Iso-hyper	Iso	Hyper	No enh	enh
Fibroelastoma	Valves	Single	<1	Well-defined	No	Hypo	Hypo	Hypo	No enh	–
Angiosarcoma	Right atrium	Single	>5	Irregular	Yes	Iso-hyper	Heterogeneous	Hyper	enh	enh
Rhabdomyo-sarcoma	Every site/ valves	Multiple	>5	Irregular	Yes	Iso-hyper	Heterogeneous	Hyper	enh	enh
Other sarcomas	Left heart	Single	>5	Irregular	Yes	Iso-hyper	Heterogeneous	Hyper	enh	enh
Lymphoma	Every site	Single/multiple	–	Irregular	Yes	Iso-hyper	Heterogeneous	Hyper	enh	enh
Metastasis	Right heart	Single/multiple	–	Irregular	Yes	Iso-hyper	Heterogeneous	Hyper	enh	enh
Melanoma metastasis	Right heart	Single/multiple	–	Irregular	Yes	Iso-hyper	Hyper	Hyper	enh	enh

Hyper hyperintensity, *Hypo* hypointensity, *enh* enhancement, *iso* isointense to myocardium
[a]hyperintensity in T2-weighted FSE, hypointensity in T2-STIR

22.2.1 Morphological and Functional Evaluation

- The morphological evaluation of cardiac mass by MRI includes [2]:
  - Identification and localization of the mass
  - Dimensions
  - Anatomical relation with normal myocardium, epicardial fat, pericardium, and paracardiac structures
  - Assessment of local invasivity
  - Effect of mass on valvular and myocardial function, obstruction of cardiac chambers, flow turbulences
- For the morphological assessment, cine-SSFP (steady-state free precession) images are now preferred to the traditional static black-blood pulse sequences [4].
- Cine-SSFPs are bright-blood images, characterized by high contrast between myocardium and blood, with high temporal resolution, providing accurate morphological details of cardiac mass [5].
- Cine images are used to confirm the location and morphology of a cardiac mass and allow an assessment of the mobility of a mass and any functional consequences such as contractile impairment or obstruction to flow [3].
- To localize the mass and to ascertain multiple localization, cine images should be acquired covering the entire heart in long axis view (from diaphragm to the great vessels) and in short axis views covering both the atria and ventricles.
- After the localization, the anatomical relations of the mass are evaluated by the acquisition of other planes centered on the mass (at least three orthogonal planes).

22.2.2 Tissue Characterization

- In MRI the relative signal intensity from a particular tissue depends principally on its proton density (PD) and the T1 and T2 relaxation times [6].
- MRI exploits these tissue differences of PD, T1, and T2 to help differentiate normal from abnormal and benign from malignant lesions.

Normal myocardium has intermediate intensity in all weighting, while calcifications and gas are hypo-/anintense in all pulse sequences.

- Neoplastic cells tend to be larger than normal cells, contain more free intracellular water, and are usually associated with an inflammatory reaction and increased interstitial fluid (edema). Then, malignant cells usually have longer T2 and shorter T1 relaxation times compared with benign pathology.
- Malignant tissue is also associated with a greater degree of neo-angiogenesis and hence first pass contrast enhancement. Necrotic tumor tissue is associated with slow wash-in during first pass of gadolinium (perfusion defect) and with a delayed washout of gadolinium-based contrast agents.

22.2.3 MRI Pulse Sequences

T1-Weighted Pulse Sequence

Black-blood T1-weighted fast spin echo (FSE) pulse sequence are used to help localize a suspected cardiac or paracardiac mass and to characterize its tissue composition [7].

- The T1 weighting is obtained using a short repetition time (TR < 1000) and echo time (TE < 10 msec).
- In T1-weighted FSE images, fluids filled mass as pericardial cysts with poor protein concentration are markedly hypointense, while bronchogenic cysts, due to higher concentration of proteins, have higher signal [8].
- Thrombus and hemorrhagic lesions are hyperintense in acute phase and afterwards become hypointense.
- Fat is hyperintense in both PD and T1-weighted FSE. The suspicion may be confirmed using a fat-saturation or a short-tau inversion recovery (STIR) pulse which nulls selectively signal from fat. This feature permits to make diagnosis of lipoma, while liposarcoma is generally undifferentiated and usually lose the signal characteristics of fat [7].
- The other cardiac masses are generally isointense to myocardium in T1-weighted FSE images.

Heterogeneous signal may be found in malignancies, myxoma, and hemangioma due to the presence of hemorrhage, calcifications, or vascular lacunae.

Metastasis and high vascularized mass may have lower signal intensity than normal myocardium.

Melanoma metastasis is hyperintense by the paramagnetic effect of melanin.

T2-Weighted Pulse Sequence

T2-weighted images are acquired using a FSE or a STIR FSE pulse sequence [9].
- The STIR FSE pulse sequence has the advantage of fat nulling and is generally preferred.
- The T2 weighting is obtained using a long repetition time (TR > 1800) and echo time (TE 60–70 msec).
- On T2-weighted images, slow flow is hyperintense and then all fluids-containing mass, as cysts, are hyperintense regardless of protein concentration.

Myocardial edema is hyperintense as well as high vascularized and myxomatous masses.

The presence of hemorrhage, old necrosis, and calcifications produces heterogeneous, generally low, signal in T2-weighted images.

Fibroma is characteristically hypointense in T2-weighted images with a hyperintense peripheral margin.

T2*-Weighted Pulse Sequence

Gradient echo (GRE) T2* images are used to evaluate the presence of iron overload, hemorrhage, and calcifications.

SSFP Images

In cine-SSFP images, both slow and fast moving fluids are hyperintense:
- With SSFP sequences, tissue contrast is dependent on the T2/T1 ratio of the tissue [10].
- Intracavitary tumors with similar T2/T1 ratios to blood can be poorly visualized with this technique [5].
- Fat is hyperintense and surrounded by a black boundary, called “India Ink” artifact [11].

Myxoma with no calcifications or hemorragy rarely may be undetected by cine-SSFP or identified only indirectly by the flow turbulence.

The interruption of the black boundary of epicardial fat may be a direct sign of local invasion, suggesting the infiltrative nature of the mass.

First Pass Perfusion

In cardiac applications of magnetic resonance, perfusion is obtained by the acquisition of a set of cardiac images repeated for 60 consecutive beats, starting from the injection of gadolinium-based contrast agents.

- The signal of high vascularized mass as malignancies, myxoma, and hemangioma increased during the first pass of gadolinium (with perfusion defects for necrosis, hemorrhage, or calcifications) [2].
- Less-vascularized mass as fibroma and rhabdomyoma usually don't exhibit a first pass perfusion but may uptake gadolinium after few minutes following the injection [6].

Early Enhancement

The acquisition of T1-weighted images are generally repeated early (at 1–3 min) after gadolinium injection.

Late Gadolinium Enhancement (LGE)

A progressive washout of gadolinium is found in normal myocardium, while fibrosis and tumors present a persistent enhancement for 20 min after gadolinium (late gadolinium enhancement) [12]. Intracavitary thrombi are not perfused during the first pass of gadolinium and exhibit neither early nor late enhancement.

22.3 Benign Tumors and Pseudomass

One of the main features of MRI is to distinguish between mass and pseudomass. MRI ability of soft tissue characterization and cine-imaging allows to make this diagnosis in almost all the cases.

MRI characteristics of cardiac masses are summarized in Table 22.1.

22.3.1 Pseudomass

- **Chiari network and other embryological remnants** are easily diagnosed by the identification of morphological features by MRI. However, MRI may be not able to identify and characterize small and highly mobile masses [2].
- **Pericardial and bronchogenic cysts** are easily identified by MRI for the specific localization and for the signal characteristics of fluids (hyperintense in SSFP and T2-STIR) and variable signal on T1 (markedly hypointense for pericardial cysts, iso-high intensity for bronchogenic cysts) and for the absence of contrast uptake [13].
- **Intracavitary thrombi** are usually located in the left ventricle overlying an ischemic scar or in the left atrial appendage. T1 and T2 signal is related to the age of thrombi, but the more specific feature is the absence of signal enhancement during the first pass perfusion, early post-contrast images, and LGE [14].
- **"Caseous calcification" or "calcific necrosis" of the mitral valve** is predominantly found in older women presenting as a mass-like calcification located between the

ventricular side posterior mitral leaflet and the inferolateral wall [15]. It has the signal characteristics of calcification, with hypointensity in T1, T2, and SSFP images. In LGE images, calcific necrosis is hypointense; hyperenhancement is usually limited to the peripheral margin (Fig. 22.1). However, in early stage, the entire mass may appear hyperintense in LGE images [16].

- **Giant aneurysm of coronary artery** is a rare pseudomass, characterized by extreme dilatation of coronary artery, filled by thrombotic stratification. The diagnosis is performed by the localization along the course of one coronary artery and thanks to the identification of coronary lumen.

22.3.2 Lipoma

Lipomas are well-defined, homogeneous, encapsulated tumors. Diagnosis by MRI is often straightforward because fat is hyperintense in T1-weighted FSE and nulled using a STIR or a fat-saturation pre-pulse [17]. On SSFP cine images lipoma is hyperintense and surrounded by the black boundary of India ink artifact [11]. Lipoma is avascular and doesn't enhance after gadolinium injection.

22.3.3 Myxoma

Myxomas are the most common primary cardiac tumors. They are generally well defined, smooth, lobular, oval or pedunculated, mobile mass, within the left atrium (and less frequently in the right atrium), often flopping through the mitral valve orifice in diastole [1–3]. They usually appear slightly hypointense to the blood pool on cine-SSFP sequences, even if they may remain undetected in these sequences showing similar signal of water. They appear isointense on T1-weighted images and have higher signal intensity on T2-weighted images owing to the high extracellular water content. In the majority of case, the mass is heterogeneous because of the presence of necrotic elements, hemorrhage, and calcification (Fig. 22.2). At first, pass perfusion myxoma presents usually a good enhancement and in LGE images, the enhancement is often multifocal and patchy although may sometimes be homogeneous [13].

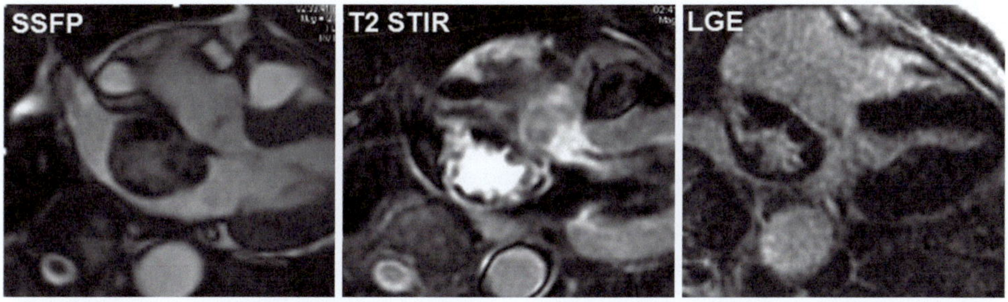

Fig. 22.2 A large *left* atrial myxoma. On SSFP and T2-STIR images, the well-defined, round mass is hyperintense with some regions of hypointensity due to necrosis or calcifications. At LGE image, a diffuse enhancement of the mass is shown with areas of hypointensity

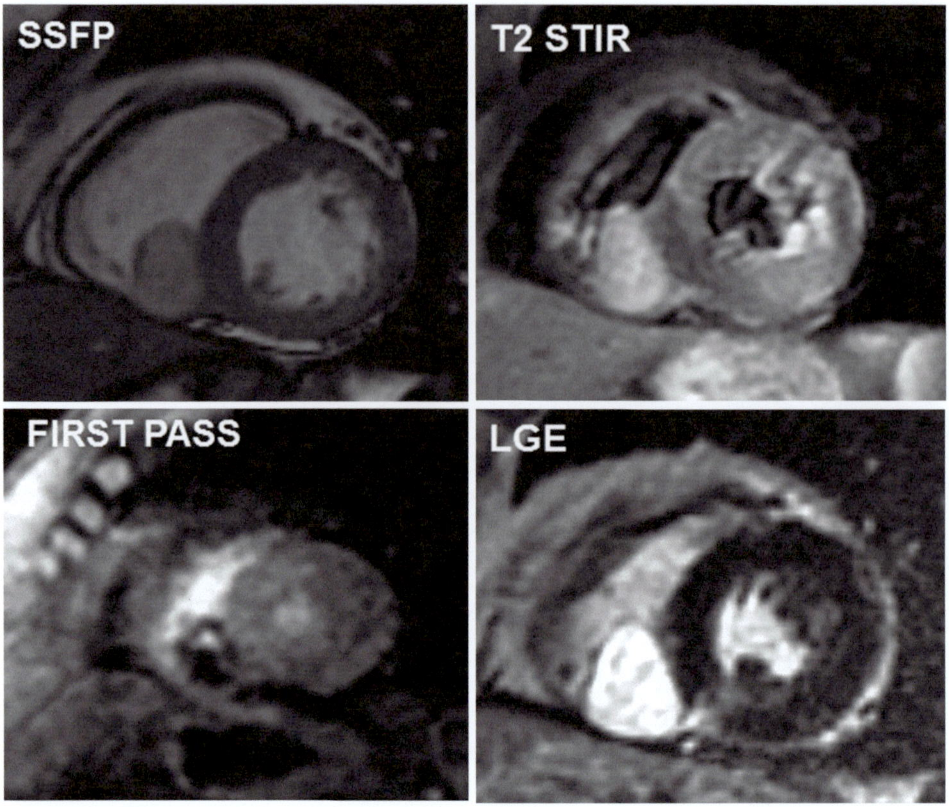

Fig. 22.3 A well-defined, *round-shaped right* ventricular mass characterized by hyperintensity on SSFP and T2-STIR images, a partial enhancement during first pass perfusion, and a homogeneous hyperintensity on LGE. These features suggested the diagnosis of hemangioma

22.3.4 Cardiac Hemangioma

Cardiac hemangiomas are vascular tumors that may involve the epicardium, myocardium, and pericardial space, originating from a coronary vessel. They are detected by MRI as a solid mass with heterogeneous isointense signal in T1-weighted pulse sequence and hyperintense in T2-STIR and SSFP images. It is frequent to detect vascular structures inside the solid mass [18]. During the first pass of gadolinium, the hemangioma usually manifests a significant enhancement which persists in LGE images (Fig. 22.3) [19].

Large hemangioma may exhibit only partial enhancement due to extensive necrosis and fibrosis. In these cases, the differential diagnosis between hemangioma and malignancies may be difficult and achieved only through morphological features.

22.3.5 Fibroma

Fibromas are most often located intramurally in the ventricles, involving the interventricular septum, and sometimes requiring differential diagnosis with hypertrophic cardiomyopathy. Fibromas are usually isointense to myocardium in T1 and SSFP images, and, unlike

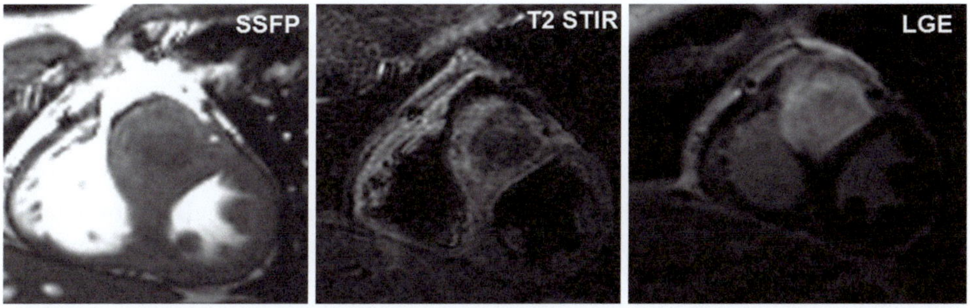

Fig. 22.4 Interventricular septal fibroma with the characteristic hypointensity on T2-STIR with peripheral hyperintensity. Diffuse enhancement on LGE image suggests fibrotic tissue

other masses, they are characteristically hypointense on T2-weighted images (often with a hyperintense peripheral margin) [20]. They are avascular tumors presenting with absent enhancement during the first pass of gadolinium (Fig. 22.4). However, fibromas are hyperintense in LGE image due to the interstitial collagen deposit and poor cellularity [13].

22.3.6 Rhabdomyoma

Rhabdomyomas are the most common primary cardiac tumors in infants and children. With cardiac MR imaging, they appear isointense to normal myocardium on T1-weighted images and hyperintense on T2-weighted images [21]. Rhabdomyomas may show absent or mild enhancement on first pass images and heterogeneous enhancement in LGE.

Rhabdomyoma with absent enhancement of fist pass may have similar MRI presentation to fibroma. In this case, it is indicated to repeat MRI over time because, differently from fibroma, rhabdomyomas disappear with age.

Yet, rhabdomyomas are multiple in 90 % of cases, and accurate imaging of the whole heart is mandatory.

22.3.7 Fibroelastoma

Fibroelastomas on cine-SSFP MR fibroelastomas are small, hypointense, highly mobile valvular mass with associated turbulent flow (which may be the unique finding). When mass dimensions allow tissue characterization, fibroelastomas appear isointense in T1 and hyperintense T2-weighted images [20].

Pitfalls: Fibroelastomas are characterized by small size and high mobility and may be missed by MRI. For this reason, they are usually best diagnosed by echocardiography.

22.3.8 Cystic Tumor of the Atrioventricular Node

It is one of the rarest cardiac tumor but is associated to sudden cardiac death due to lethal arrhythmias. On MRI this tumor is characterized by a well-defined nodule in the atrioventricular nodal region of basal septum. Signal is hyperintense in T1- and T2-weighted pulse sequence and with homogeneous hyperintensity in LGE images [20].

22.3.9 Paraganglioma

It originates from neuroendocrine ganglia cells within the atrioventricular grooves and at the root of the great vessel origins. Histologically benign, but it may produce symptoms due to catecholamine secretion. Resection is often difficult due to extensive vascularity and complex relationship with the adjacent coronary arteries. On MRI these lesions are isointense to myocardium on T1 and of intensely high signal on T2-weighted images ("lightbulb bright"). On first pass and LGE images, paraganglioma shows usually intense and uniform signal [13].

22.4 Malignant Tumors

- The most important MRI feature is the ability to predict the likely malignancy of a cardiac mass. Hoffman and colleagues found a diagnostic accuracy of 0.92 of MRI to distinguish between benign and malign masses [6].
- The suspicion of malignancy by MRI is given by different criteria, summarized in ◘ Table 22.2. Briefly, a malignancy should be suspected for broad mass (often >5 cm) with ill-defined margins and infiltrative aspect (loss of continuity of tissue interfaces as for loss of India ink boundary of epicardial fat in SSFP images). Pericardial effu-

◘ **Table 22.2** MRI criteria of malignancy

Criterion	
Location	Masses in the right heart are more frequently malign as well as when involve multiple cardiac chamber
Number	Multiple masses are more likely to be malign
Margins	Malignancies usually are irregular masses with ill-defined margins
Attachment	Broad-based attachment is typical of malignancies
Invasion	Direct invasion of different cardiac structures as myocardium, valve, epicardial fat, and pericardial layers
Effusion	The presence of unexplained pericardial effusion in the presence of a cardiac mass is associated to malignancy. High T1 signal suggests hemorrhagic effusion
Signal	Heterogeneous[a] signal on T1- and T2-weighted images but with a predominantly hyperintensity in T2
Perfusion	Malignant mass are generally well perfused during first pass of gadolinium-chelates, with heterogeneous[a] signal
LGE	Heterogeneous[a] late gadolinium enhancement

[a]Heterogeneous signal due to hemorrhage, necrosis and calcifications

sion, particularly with hemorrhagic signal (high T1 signal), is often associated to malign tumors. For tissue characteristics, malignant tumors are hyperintense in T2-weighted pulse sequence and have signal enhancement during first pass perfusion and a positive LGE [2, 22].
- However, the heterogeneity of pre- and post-contrast signal, for hemorrhage, calcifications, and necrosis, is one of the most important features of malignancies [23].

> **Because of the loss of specific tissue characteristics, undifferentiated malign tumors may be hard to be characterized by MRI. A liposarcoma, for example, may present hyperintense in STIR or fat-saturated pulse sequence because of loss of characteristics of fat. Then, in majority of case, the identification of malignancy is the final goal of MRI.**

- The most frequent malign cardiac tumors are metastasis. Sarcomas account for 95 % of primary cardiac malign tumors, and the remainder are prevalently lymphomas and primary pericardial mesotheliomas [22].

22.4.1 Sarcoma

Among the primary cardiac sarcomas, the most prevalent are angiosarcomas in adults and rhabdomyosarcomas in pediatric patients. Undifferentiated sarcomas account for a third of cases, while sarcomas with myofibroblastic differentiation as liposarcoma, leiomyosarcoma, osteosarcoma, and fibrosarcoma are extremely rare [24].
- **Angiosarcoma**, unlike the other sarcomas, is usually located in the right atrium (75 %) presenting often with obstruction of this chamber and infiltration of adjacent structures as tricuspidal valve, right coronary artery, pericardium, and right ventricle [25]. Hemorrhagic pericardial effusion is very frequent, and cardiac tamponade as well as signs of right heart failure may be the initial manifestations. MRI angiosarcoma appears as a large heterogeneous right atrial mass with or without pericardial involvement and with signs of infiltration of cardiac structures [2]. On T1-weighted images, angiosarcoma is predominantly isointense to myocardium with areas of high T1 signal change, reflecting intratumoral hemorrhage and areas of signal void reflecting blood flow within vascular lacunae. On T2-weighted images, angiosarcomas are predominantly hyperintense (■ Fig. 22.5). Because of the vascular origin, angiosarcomas have a good first pass perfusion and a positive LGE with hypointense region due to necrosis and hemorragy [13].
- **Rhabdomyosarcomas** have usually multiple sites of origin, may involve all the cardiac chambers, and, unlikely to the other sarcomas, may originate from the cardiac valve [26]. Signal characteristics of MRI are similar to other malignancies but with less inhomogeneity of signal in pre- and post-contrast images than other tumors. On first pass perfusion rhabdomyosarcomas have homogeneous enhancement, sometimes with central necrosis.
- **Other sarcomas**, as undifferentiated sarcomas and those with myofibroblastic differentiation, have no specific features but origin generally from the left chambers (■ Fig. 22.6) [2].

> **Sarcomas originating from the left atrium may present pre- and post-contrast tissue characteristics similar to atrial myxoma. In this case, local infiltration, broad attachment, and a poor mobility may be the only features permitting differential diagnosis.**

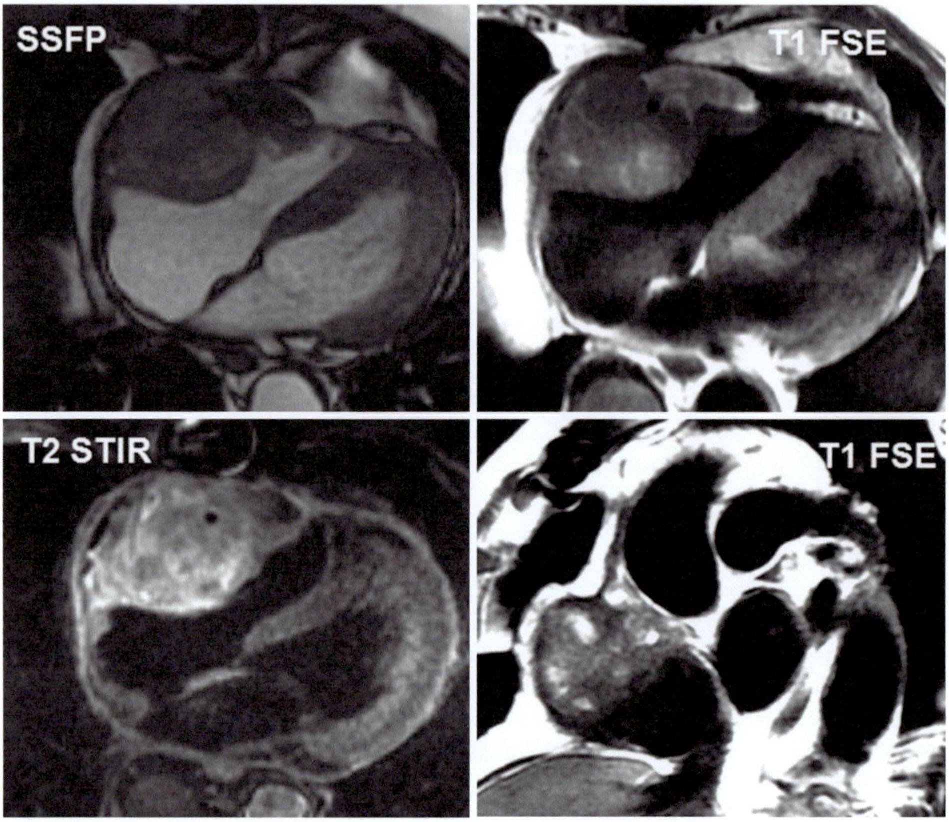

Fig. 22.5 The *right* atrial angiosarcoma infiltrating the atrioventricular groove, *right* ventricle, epicardial fat, and pericardium. Heterogeneous signal is shown on T1- and T2-weighted images. On T2-STIR the signal is prevalently hyperintense

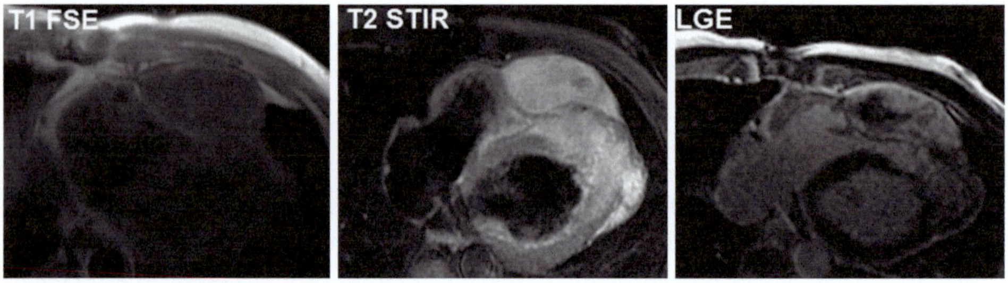

Fig. 22.6 A *left* ventricular liposarcoma infiltrating epicardial fat and pericardium and compressing the *right* ventricle. Noteworthy, the signal of the mass is not nulled in T2-STIR image, demonstrating the poor differentiation of the mass

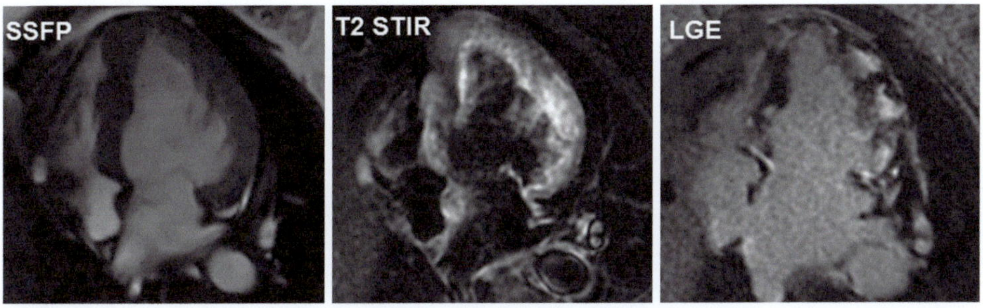

Fig. 22.7 A cardiac lymphoma involving all the *left* ventricular walls and causing pseudo-hypertrophy in a 40-year-old female presenting with fever and chest pain. In this case, the initial clinical suspicion was myocarditis and endomyocardial biopsy was necessary to make differential diagnosis

22.4.2 Lymphoma

- Primary cardiac lymphoma may involve all the cardiac chambers, despite a slight prevalence of right heart involvement, with frequent invasion of pericardium [27]. Two different patterns of lymphoma were reported by MRI:
  - The first is of multiple solid masses, mostly originated from the right ventricular myocardium, isointense on T1, and mildly hyperintense on T2-weighted images (Fig. 22.7).
  - The second is manifest as a diffuse pericardial soft tissue infiltration with a hemorrhagic effusion [22].
  - Unlike sarcomas, lymphoma generally lacks regions of central necrosis and often displays heterogeneous LGE.

22.4.3 Cardiac Metastasis

- Cardiac metastases are 40–500 times more frequent than primary cardiac tumors.
- Pericardial invasion is the most frequent structure involved through lymphatic and hematogenous diffusion. The right chambers are mostly involved through cava veins [28].
- The left ventricular involvement may be present in case of direct invasion of pulmonary vein by a bronchogenic cancer (Fig. 22.8).
- With the exception of melanoma metastasis, signal characteristics of MRI are similar to other malignancies: low signal on T1- and high signal on T2-weighted images and variable amount of signal heterogeneity due to necrosis, hemorrhage, and calcifications [29].
- After gadolinium, metastasis usually shows a significant enhancement on first pass images and LGE.

Melanoma metastasis has a specific MRI presentation because of the melanin that owns some paramagnetic effect. Melanoma is hyperintense in T1-weighted images and hypointense in T2.

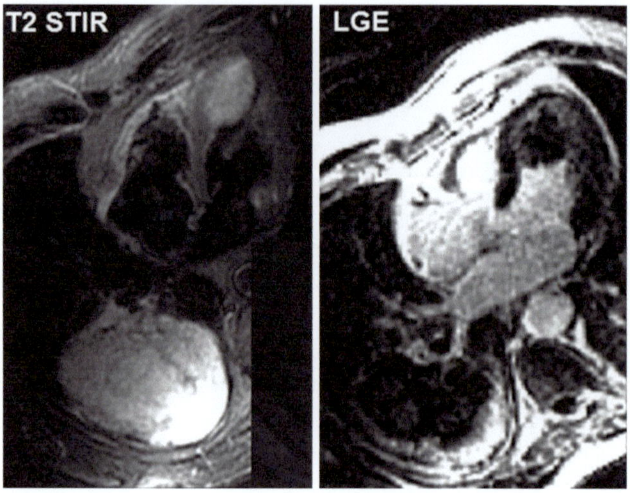

Fig. 22.8 A case of metastasis of the *left* ventricular apex. The images allowed identification of the primary mass, in the basal segments of the *right* lung. Metastasis of the *left* ventricle was caused by direct invasion of a *right* pulmonary vein. Of note, both the primary and the metastatic mass had the same signal characteristics

22.5 Future Perspectives

Cardiac MRI is an imaging technique in continued development, and new pulse sequence that are currently under investigations for other cardiac disease may have a role for the characterization of cardiac tumor in the next future.

- The direct measurement of tissue T1 and T2 by the new T1 and T2 mapping technique might strengthen the ability of tissue characterization by MRI.
- The combination of pre- and post-contrast T1 mapping allows the measurement of the extracellular and cellular volumes that might furnish important information for tumor characterizations.
- The additive role of combined machine as PET/MRI for the diagnosis of cardiac tumors has to be investigated in the near future.

References

1. Pennell DJ, Sechtem UP, Higgins CB, et al. Clinical indications for cardiovascular magnetic resonance (CMR): consensus panel report. Eur Heart J. 2004;25(21):1940–65.
2. Motwani M, Kidambi A, Herzog BA, Uddin A, Greenwood JP, Plein S. MR imaging of cardiac tumors and masses: a review of methods and clinical applications. Radiology. 2013;268(1):26–43.
3. O'Donnell DH, Abbara S, Chaithiraphan V, et al. Cardiac tumors: optimal cardiac MR sequences and spectrum of imaging appearances. AJR Am J Roentgenol. 2009;19(2):377–87.
4. Kramer CM, Barkhausen J, Flamm SD, Kim RJ, Nagel E. Society for cardiovascular magnetic resonance board of trustees task force on standardized protocols. Standardized cardiovascular magnetic resonance imaging (CMR) protocols, society for cardiovascular magnetic resonance: board of trustees task force on standardized protocols. J Cardiovasc Magn Reson. 2008;10:35.
5. Thiele H, Nagel E, Paetsch I, et al. Functional cardiac MR imaging with steady-state free precession (SSFP) significantly improves endocardial border delineation without contrast agents. J Magn Reson Imaging. 2001;14(4):362–7.
6. Hoffmann U, Globits S, Schima W, et al. Usefulness of magnetic resonance imaging of cardiac and paracardiac masses. Am J Cardiol. 2003;92(7):890–5.
7. Stehling MK, Holzknecht NG, Laub G, Böhm D, von Smekal A, Reiser M. Singleshot T1- and T2-weighted magnetic resonance imaging of the heart with black blood: preliminary experience. MAGMA. 1996;4(3–4):231–40.

8. Sparrow PJ, Kurian JB, Jones TR, Sivananthan MU. MR imaging of cardiac tumors. RadioGraphics. 2005;25(5):1255–76.
9. Simonetti OP, Finn JP, White RD, Laub G, Henry DA. "Black blood" T2-weighted inversion- recovery MR imaging of the heart. Radiology. 1996;199(1):49–57.
10. Plein S, Bloomer TN, Ridgway JP, Jones TR, Bainbridge GJ, Sivananthan MU. Steady-state free precession magneticresonance imaging of the heart: comparison with segmented k-space gradientecho imaging. J Magn Reson Imaging. 2001;14(3):230–6.
11. Aquaro GD, Todiere G, Strata E, Barison A, Di Bella G, Lombardi M. Usefulness of India ink artifact in steady-state free precession pulse sequences for detection and quantification of intramyocardial fat. J Magn Reson Imaging. 2013 Oct.
12. Kim RJ, Wu E, Rafael A, et al. The use of contrast-enhanced magnetic resonance imaging to identify reversible myocardial dysfunction. N Engl J Med. 2000;343(20):1445–53.
13. Hoey ET, Shahid M, Ganeshan A, Baijal S, Simpson H, Watkin RW. MRI assessment of cardiac tumours: part 1, multiparametric imaging protocols and spectrum of appearances of histologically benign lesions. Quant Imaging Med Surg. 2014;4(6):478–88.
14. Mollet NR, Dymarkowski S, Volders W, et al. Visualization of ventricular thrombi with contrast-enhanced magnetic resonance imaging in patients with ischemic heart disease. Circulation. 2002;106(23):2873–6.
15. Harpaz D, Auerbach I, Vered Z, Motro M, Tobar A, Rosenblatt S. Caseous calcification of the mitral annulus: a neglected, unrecognized diagnosis. J Am Soc Echocardiogr. 2001;14(8):825–31.
16. Gargani L, Pasanisi E, Aquaro GD, Masci P, Neglia D, Rovai D. The mysterious case of an intracardiac mass. Recenti Prog Med. 2009;100(1):22–6.
17. Hananouchi GI, Goff 2nd WB. Cardiac lipoma: six-year follow-up with MRI characteristics, and a review of the literature. Magn Reson Imaging. 1990;8(6):825–8.
18. Salerni S, Barison A, Masci PG, Aquaro GD. Rare presentation of asymptomatic pericardial effusion: Hemangioma of the atrioventricular groove in cardiac magnetic resonance imaging. Circulation. 2014;130:e15–7.
19. Bianchi G, Ferrarini M, Matteucci M, Monteleone A, Aquaro GD, Passino C, Pucci A, Glauber M. Giant solitary fibrous tumor of the epicardium causing reversible heart failure. Ann Thorac Surg. 2013;96(2):e49–51.
20. Araoz PA, Mulvagh SL, Tazelaar HD, Julsrud PR, Breen JF. CT and MR imaging of benign primary cardiac neoplasms with echocardiographic correlation. Radio-Graphics. 2000;20(5):1303–19.
21. Kiaffas MG, Powell AJ, Geva T. Magnetic resonance imaging evaluation of cardiactumor characteristics in infants and children. Am J Cardiol. 2002;89(10):1229–33.
22. Hoey ET, Shahid M, Ganeshan A, Baijal S, Simpson H, Watkin RW. MRI assessment of cardiac tumours: part 2, spectrum of appearances of histologically malignant lesions and tumour mimics. Quant Imaging Med Surg. 2014;4(6):489–97.
23. Fieno DS, Saouaf R, Thomson LE, Abidov A, Friedman JD, Berman DS. Cardiovascular magnetic resonance of primary tumors of the heart: a review. J Cardiovasc Magn Reson. 2006;8(6):839–53.
24. Hamidi M, Moody JS, Weigel TL, Kozak KR. Primary cardiac sarcoma. Ann Thorac Surg. 2010;90(1): 176–81.
25. Bruna J, Lockwood M. Primary heart angiosarcoma detected by computed tomography and magnetic resonance imaging. Eur Radiol. 1998;8(1):66–8.
26. Beghetti M, Gow RM, Haney I, Mawson J, Williams WG, Freedom RM. Pediatric primary benign cardiac tumors: a 15-year review. Am Heart J. 1997;134(6):1107–14.
27. Dorsay TA, Ho VB, Rovira MJ, Armstrong MA, Brissette MD. Primary cardiac lymphoma: CT and MR findings. J Comput Assist Tomogr. 1993;17(6):978–81.
28. Abraham KP, Reddy V, Gattuso P. Neoplasms metastatic to the heart: review of 3314 consecutive autopsies. Am J Cardiovasc Pathol. 1990;3(3):195–8.
29. Mousseaux E, Meunier P, Azancott S, Dubayle P, Gaux JC. Cardiac metastatic melanoma investigated by magnetic resonance imaging. Magn Reson Imaging. 1998;16(1):91–5.

Other Imaging Techniques: Computed Tomography and Positron Emission Tomography

Martina Urbani, Eugenio Borsatti, and Tanja Baresic

C. Lestuzzi et al. (eds.), *Manual of Cardio-oncology*, DOI 10.1007/978-3-319-40236-9_23

23.1 Introduction

The most used methods to study cardiac tumors are echocardiography (preferred first-step imaging technique: the cheapest, safest, and most widely available) and magnetic resonance (MR) imaging (preferred second-step imaging technique: the most sensitive and specific). However, both computed tomography and positron emission tomography may be useful in selected cases [1].

23.2 Computed Tomography

- Cardiac CT is routinely used in oncology to detect intrathoracic (mediastinal, lung) tumors
- As regards the cardiac masses, it is used as an alternative imaging modality in patients who cannot undergo MR because it is contraindicated or in patients already examined with other noninvasive methods without obtaining adequate images [2, 3].
- *Compared to echocardiography*, CT:
  - May better assess the size of huge masses and the infiltration or compression of the mediastinal and of the thoracic structures
  - Provides a more accurate tissue characterization, mostly useful for the evaluation of calcified masses
  - May exclude an obstructive coronary artery disease
  - May detect other intrathoracic masses
- *Compared to MRI*, CT:
  - Is more widely available and cheaper.
  - May be used with patients with pacemakers, obese, and very claustrophobic patients who cannot be examined by MRI.
  - In patients with severe renal insufficiency, gadolinium is contraindicated; on the other hand, iodinated contrast material may be used in patients treated by dialysis.
  - May be used to guide transthoracic biopsy of large masses.
- High-speed equipments with electrocardiographic (ECG) gating (in order to reduce motion artifacts) can provide images with resolution <1 mm; multiplanar and tridimensional reconstructions are also possible [4, 5].
  - Retrospective ECG gating allows a dynamic reconstruction and to assess the mass mobility, but carries a high radiation burden. It is preferred to evaluate mobile masses (for instance, pedunculated or prolapsing masses, masses attached to a cardiac valve).
  - Prospective ECG gating (data acquired at a single cardiac cycle point) exposes to a much lower radiation burden. It may be preferred when the mobility of the mass is minimal or not relevant (which is the case in most malignant tumors).
  - Larger masses may be visualized by CT scan, even without ECG gating.

23.2.1 Limits

- It uses ionizing radiations.
- The information obtained without the use of a contrast medium is limited.

- ECG gating is not available in all the equipments.
- Specific CT protocols (different from those commonly utilized for coronary imaging) should be used in cardiac tumors imaging, and a special expertise is necessary.
  - CT scan is not the preferred diagnostic tool, in the study of cardiac tumors; it may be considered as a complement to echocardiography in selected cases.

23.3 Positron Emission Tomography (PET)

This technique is based on the detection of metabolic activity after injection of radionuclides. The most commonly used tracing in oncology is fluorodeoxyglucose (^{18}F-FDG), which concentrates in tissue with high glucose metabolism and high lactic acid production (the so-called Warburg effect), such as malignant neoplasms. PET is usually performed together to computed tomography (PET/CT) or, less frequently, with MRI (PET/MRI) to improve the diagnostic power of the technique. The advantage of PET is the ability to detect also distant metastases [6] (◘ Figs. 23.1, 23.2, and 23.3).

- To quantify the glucose metabolism, the maximum standardized uptake value (SUV) is used. Malignant tumors have usually a high SUV, which may increase with the proliferative index [7].
  - A maximum SUV <3.5 is more probably due to a benignant lesion. On the other hand, a value >10 is highly suggestive of malignancy (lymphoma or poorly differentiated sarcoma). The SUV cutoff of 3.5 showed a sensitivity of 100 %, specificity of 86 %, and negative predictive value of 100 % [8, 9] (◘ Fig. 23.4).

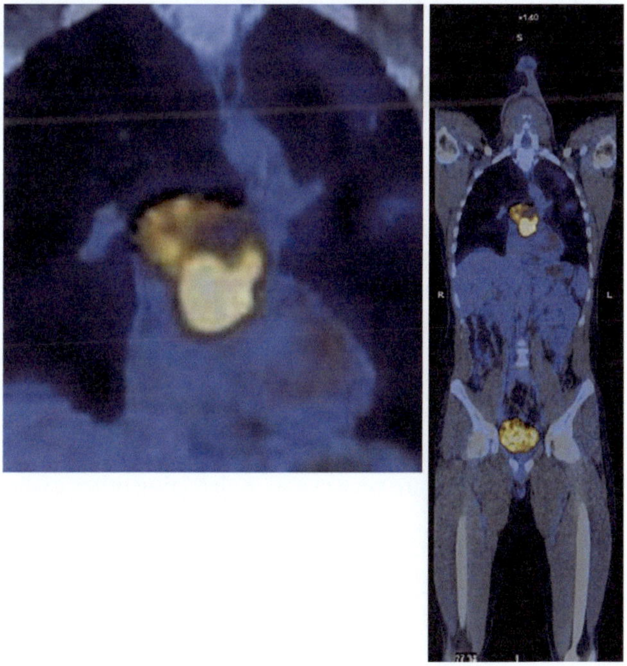

◘ **Fig. 23.1** Huge *left* atrial sarcoma. High uptake at FDG-PET (image *left*). There are no distant metastases at the whole body image (*right*). The bladder uptake is physiological

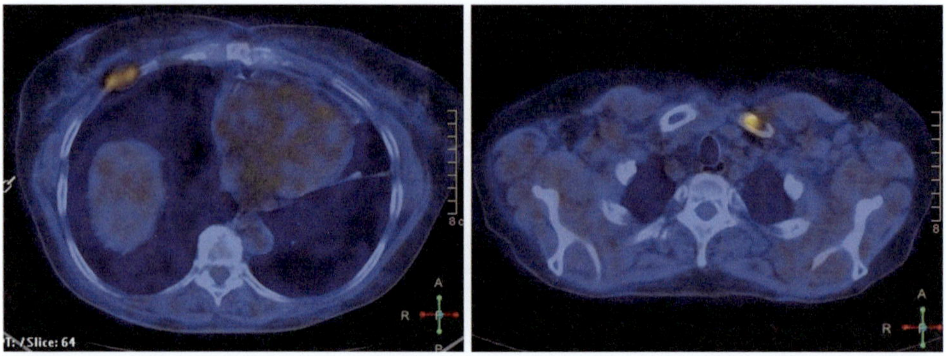

■ **Fig. 23.2** PET in a patient with relapsing cardiac sarcoma. There are metastases of the ribs (*left*) and bone (*right*). Cardiac surgery is NOT indicated in this case

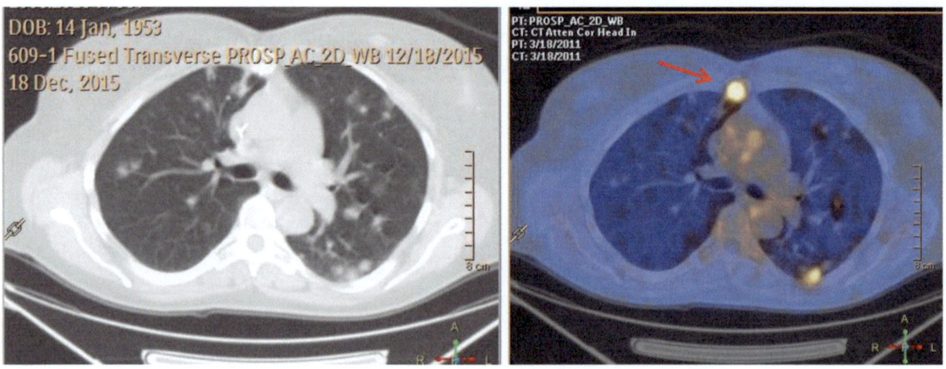

■ **Fig. 23.3** PET/CT of patients with cardiac angiosarcoma. There are multiple pulmonary nodules (metastases) at CT (*left*); some of them (the largest ones) have uptake of FDG (*right*). There is an area of increased uptake at sternal level (*red arrow*) due to flogosis after sternotomy

- ^{18}FDG PET has high sensitivity and specificity in assessing the differential diagnosis between neurofibroma and the malignant peripheral sheath nerve tumor.
- Normally, within the pericardium, no FDG activity is detectable. Diffuse pericardial FDG activity is rare, but may be observed in the presence of inflammation (■ Fig. 23.5).
- Among primary cardiac sarcomas, maximum SUV seems to be proportional to the grade of malignancy, while this is not always true for metastatic tumors.
- PET studies are very useful in detecting other malignant masses in the whole body at one time.
- ^{18}FDG PET may also be used in the follow-up, to assess the response to therapy.

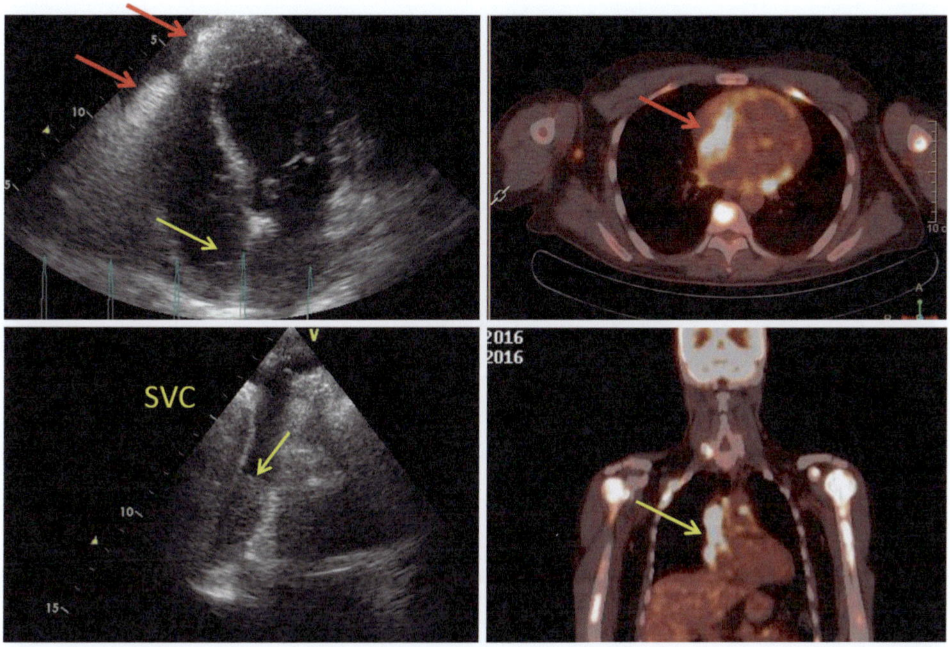

Fig. 23.4 Patient with lymphoma. *Left*: echocardiogram showing a pericardial effusion with intrapericardial masses (*red arrows*: Fat? Fibrin? Tumor?) and a solid mass in the *right* atrium and superior vena cava (SVC; *bottom*, from the supraclavicular approach) (*yellow arrows*). *Right*: The same masses show an evident uptake at PET and can be classified as neoplastic

23.3.1 Pitfalls [10]

- Some organs have a physiologically high glucose uptake: the brain, bladder, kidneys.
  - Some other organs, such as the liver and heart, may have variable uptake according with different metabolic conditions
  - Inflammation causes an increased FDG uptake (Fig. 23.3).
- Uptake time, blood glucose levels, insulin medication, and equipment affect SUV measurements. Thus, results may be different in different institutions and in different patients.
  - The follow-up studies should be made always in the same institution.
- The resolution power of PET is limited to 0.5 cm: smaller masses are not visualized (Fig. 23.6).
- The myocardial ^{18}FDG uptake may vary widely between different patients and – in the same patient – between different exams. In fact, sex, age, body weight, fasting state, and blood glucose, fat, and insulin levels may influence the myocardial uptake, which may be low or (diffusely or locally) increased [11].

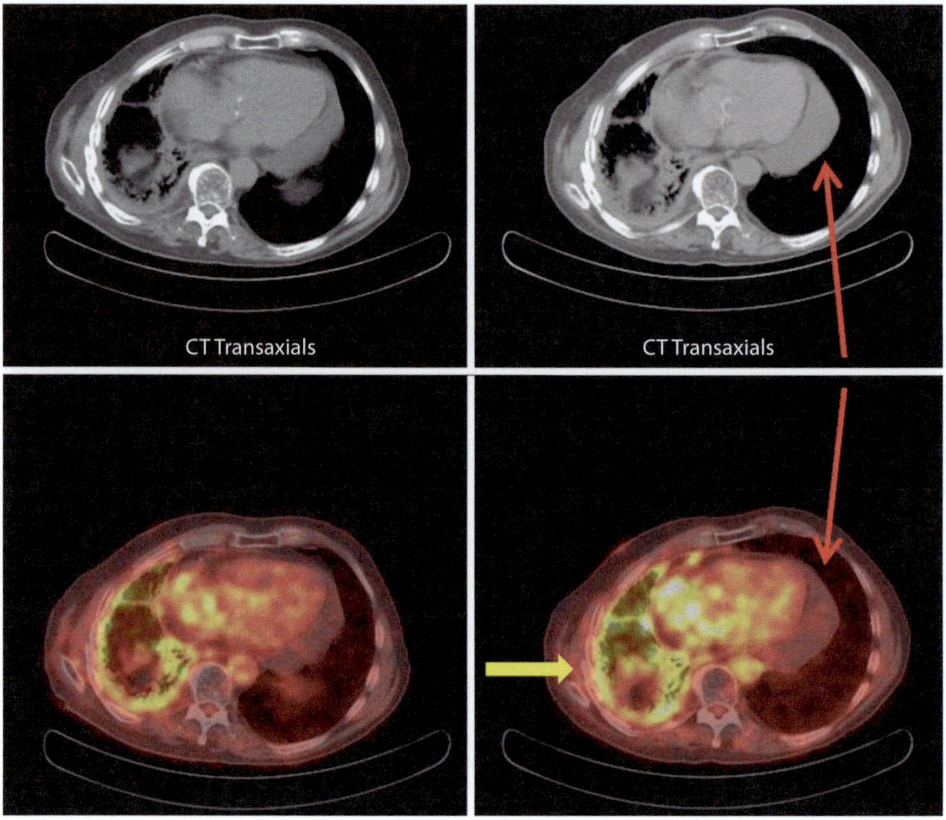

Fig. 23.5 PET/CT of a patient with pleural mesothelioma and pericardial effusion. There is a significant uptake at the *right* internal chest wall (*yellow arrow*), scattered uptake within the heart (without masses: physiological uptake), and no uptake within the pericardium. This finding rules out pericardial metastases

- Myocardial FDG metabolism is insulin-dependent (this is a main difference compared with tumors), and in the fasting state, the heart metabolism is shifted toward fats rather than glucose. Administration of insulin or ingestion of food close to the time of FDG injection will cause a diffuse increase in muscle FDG activity.
- In order to improve the accuracy of ^{18}FDG-PET in cardiac tumor imaging, a carbohydrate- poor and fat-rich meal followed by a fasting period of 12–18 h is suggested before the exam [12, 13]. The administration of unfractioned heparin (50 units/Kg of body weight in intravenous infusion) shortly before the injection of ^{18}FDG further reduces the physiological myocardial uptake, increasing the specificity of the exam; the uptake due to inflammation, however, is not affected [14, 15] (Figs. 23.7a, b).
- Several cardiac diseases, such as systemic and pulmonary hypertension, valvular heart disease, and cardiomyopathies, may show an enlargement of the left and right ventricles with a diffuse increase in FDG myocardial activity and should not be misinterpreted as a malignancy.

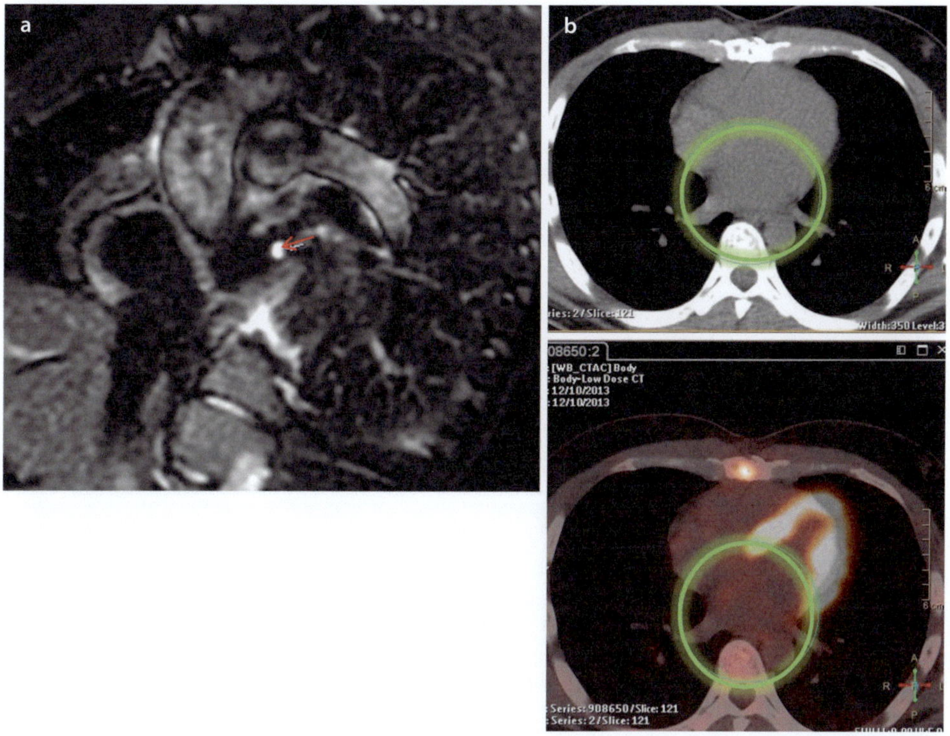

Fig. 23.6 False-negative and false-positive imaging at PET: a patient with a small *left* atrial malignant tumor (*arrow* in RM imaging, *left*) not evident at PET/CT (*right*; the *left* atrium is marked by a green *circle*), because of the small dimension of the mass. On the other hand, there is a strong FDG uptake by the *left* ventricular myocardium (*bottom right*)

- Cardiac FDG uptake is nonuniform and variable; regional FDG activity in normal fasted subjects showed a significant decrease in activity in the septum and anterior walls of the left ventricle (20 %) compared with the lateral and posterior walls. A posterolateral increase in cardiac FDG activity is a common normal physiologic pattern.
- Focally increased atrial uptake may be observed in subjects with atrial fibrillation.
- Lipomas do not show any FDG activity, but focal-increased FDG activity may be seen in lipomatous hypertrophy of the interatrial septum.
- Myocardial ischemia shifts cardiac metabolism from fatty acid to glucose utilization. Thus, patients with chronic myocardial ischemia may show an increased left ventricular FDG even when fasting. If the FDG activity follows a typical coronary artery distribution, the possibility of ischemia or hibernation should be considered.
- The combined PET/CT is useful in the differential diagnosis between benignant and malignant masses. A promising technique is PET/MRI, but there is still very limited experience in the field of cardiac tumors [16, 17]. This allows to assess the presence or absence of metastases in cardiac sarcomas and of other masses where a diagnostic biopsy may be easier than in the heart.

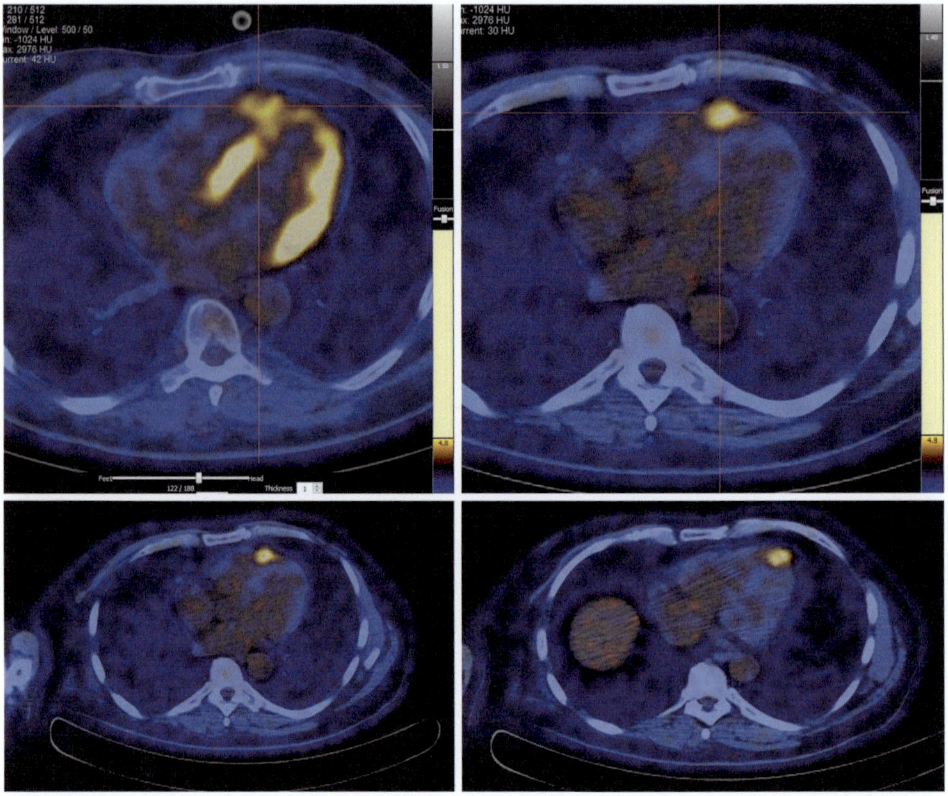

Fig. 23.7 **a** PET heart images in a patient with *right* ventricular sarcoma. *Left*: after carbohydrate-rich and followed by a 10-h fasting period, there is a diffuse uptake of the *left* ventricular myocardium, and the apical mass is hardly recognizable. *Right*: after a carbohydrate poor meal, followed by an 18-h fasting period and infusion of heparin, the myocardial uptake is abolished and the apical tumor is evident. **b** Same patient of Fig. 23.7a. After abolishing the physiologic myocardial uptake, it is possible to indentify two different masses: one in the *right* ventricular wall (*left*) and one at the apex (*right*)

References

1. Buckley O, Madan R, Kwong R, et al. Cardiac masses, part 1: imaging strategies and technical considerations. AJR Am J Roentgenol. 2011;197:W837–41.
2. Chu LC, Johnson PT, Halushka MK, Fishman EK. Multidetector CT of the heart: spectrum of benign and malignant cardiac masses. Emerg Radiol. 2012;19:415–28.
3. Rajiah P, Kanne JP, Kalahasti V, Schoenhagen P. Computed tomography of cardiac and pericardiac masses. J Cardiovasc Comput Tomogr. 2011;5:16–29.
4. Kassop D, Donovan MS, Cheezum MK, et al. Cardiac masses on cardiac CT: a review. Curr Cardiovasc Imaging Rep. 2014;7:9281. Review.
5. Hoey E, Ganeshan A, Nader K, et al. Cardiac neoplasms and pseudotumors: imaging findings on multidetector CT angiography. Diagn Interv Radiol. 2012;18:67–77.
6. Tokmak H, Demir N, Demirkol MO. Cardiac angiosarcoma: utility of [(18)F]fluorodeoxyglucose positron emission tomography-computed tomography in evaluation of residue, metastases, and treatment response. Vasc Health Risk Manag. 2014;10:399–401.
7. Maurer AH, Burshteyn M, Adler LP, Steiner RM. How to differentiate benign versus malignant cardiac and paracardiac 18F FDG uptake at oncologic PET/CT. Radiographics. 2011;31:1287–305.

8. Rahbar K, Seifarth H, Schäfers M, et al. Differentiation of malignant and benign cardiac tumors using 18F-FDG PET/CT. J Nucl Med. 2012;53:856–63.
9. Benz MR, Dry SM, Eilber FC, Allen-Auerbach MS, Tap WD, Elashoff D, Phelps ME, Czernin J. Correlation between glycolytic phenotype and tumor grade in soft-tissue sarcomas by 18F-FDG PET. J Nucl Med. 2010;51:1174–81.
10. Korn RL, Coates A, Millstine J. The role of glucose and FDG metabolism in the interpretation of PET studies. In: Lin EC, Alavi A, editors. PET and PET/CT. A clinical guide. 2nd ed. New York: Thieme; 2009.
11. Lin EC, Alavi A. Normal variants and benign findings. In: Lin EC, Alavi A, editors. PET and PET/CT. A clinical guide. 2nd ed. New York: Thieme; 2009.
12. Watanabe R, Tomita N, Takeuchi K, et al. SUVmax in FDG-PET and the biopsy site correlates with the proliferation potential of tumor cells in non-Hodgkin lymphoma. Leuk Lymphoma. 2010;51:279–83.
13. Kobayashi Y, Kumita S, Fukushima Y, et al. Significant suppression of myocardial (18) F-fluorodeoxyglucose uptake using 24-h carbohydrate restriction and a low-carbohydrate, high-fat diet. J Cardiol. 2013;62:314–9.
14. Manabe O, Yoshinaga K, Ohira H, et al. The effects of 18-h fasting with low-carbohydrate diet preparation on suppressed physiological myocardial (18)F-fluorodeoxyglucose (FDG) uptake and possible minimal effects of unfractionated heparin use in patients with suspected cardiac involvement sarcoidosis. J Nucl Cardiol. 2015 Aug 5.
15. Masuda A, Naya M, Manabe O, et al. Administration of unfractionated heparin with prolonged fasting could reduce physiological 18F-fluorodeoxyglucose uptake in the heart. Acta Radiol. 2015 Sep.
16. Loft A, Jensen KE, Löfgren J, Daugaard S, Petersen MM. PET/MRI for Preoperative Planning in Patients with Soft Tissue Sarcoma: A Technical Report of Two Patients. Case Rep Med. 2013;2013, 791078.
17. Nensa F, Beiderwellen K, Heusch P, Wetter A. Clinical applications of PET/MRI: current status and future perspectives. Diagn Interv Radiol. 2014;20:438–47.

Surgical Treatment of Primary Cardiac Malignancies

Francesco Santini, Gaia Viganò, Antonio Salsano, and Loris Salvador

C. Lestuzzi et al. (eds.), *Manual of Cardio-oncology*, DOI 10.1007/978-3-319-40236-9_24

24.1 Background

Primary tumors of the heart and pericardium are very uncommon, and most of them are benignant. Excluding large referral centers, only a few cases of primary malignant tumors are observed in single hospitals over years, challenging clinicians' diagnostic ability and surgical skills [1–4]:

- Literature data consists mostly of case reports, small series or larger series collected in multicenter studies or reviewing cases over decades.
- There are no established rules to approach a malignant tumor, and the surgical approach must be tailored on the single patient.

The first step when a cardiac tumor is identified is to assess if it is benignant or malignant and if surgery may represent a therapeutic option:

- Nowadays the vast majority of *benign cardiac tumors* are effectively treated by surgical resection.
- On the other hand, primary malignant tumors continue to represent a challenge because of the often delayed diagnosis and the technical difficulties involved in providing an extensive resection.
- The role and actual efficacy of chemo- and radiotherapy remain to be clarified.
- *Malignant cardiac tumors* should be treated by a multidisciplinary team. It is important for cardiologists, oncologists, radiotherapists, and heart surgeons to cooperate closely.

24.2 Clinical Scenarios

24.2.1 Background

Primary cardiac tumors are rare; the autopsy incidence is 0.0001–0.0003 % or, in practical terms, about 1 in every 500 surgical cardiac cases. Seventy-five percent of these primary cardiac tumors are benign and 25 % are malignant [5].

24.2.2 Clinical Features

- The majority of primary malignant cardiac tumors remain long asymptomatic.
- Symptoms usually appear when the tumor mass is large, possibly involving neighboring structures.
- They may evolve rapidly to heart failure or become abruptly life-threatening [6]:

An urgent surgical approach may be necessary in some cases.

24.2.3 Malignant Tumor Types and Cardiac Chamber Involvement: Surgeon's Tips

Cardiac Sarcomas

- Sarcoma accounts for 75 % of primary malignancies of the heart [5, 7] and occurs mostly within the fifth decade of life (range, 15–87 years) [5] and with no gender prevalence.

- Many patients present with high-grade tumors and distant metastases, especially in the lungs (35.7 %), lymph nodes (14.2 %), and liver (7.14 %) [8].
- Tumor spread to the bone is very rare and has a poor prognosis.
- Without treatment, patients have a life expectancy of few months.
- Histologically, sarcomas are classified into subgroups: angiosarcoma, sarcomas of various lines of differentiation, and rhabdomyosarcoma.

Angiosarcoma

- Angiosarcomas represent approximately 30–45 % of the malignant sarcomas.
- This is an aggressive primary malignancy that usually occurs over a wide age range with peak incidence at middle age.
- They originate from vascular endothelium and are more often found in the right side of the heart (80 % in the right atrium). They often replace the atrial wall and fill the entire atrium.
- Angiosarcomas may rapidly invade adjacent structures, such as the tricuspid valve, right ventricular free wall, ventricular septum, venae cavae, and, in some cases, even the right coronary artery. In rare instances, angiosarcomas may develop within the wall of the pulmonary artery or the vena cava. They may also arise from the epicardial surface of the heart and penetrate into the pericardial space.
- The majority are associated with signs of right-sided heart failure and/or pericardial disease with pericardial effusion and occasionally cardiac tamponade.
- By the time of diagnosis, most patients have metastases (47–89 %), most commonly to the lung, liver, brain, and bone.

Sarcomas of Various Lines of Differentiation

- This subgroup includes undifferentiated sarcoma, leiomyosarcoma, fibrosarcoma, liposarcoma, osteosarcoma, and cardiac Ewing sarcoma. These usually originate along the posterior wall and tend to exhibit slow, infiltrative growth.
- *Undifferentiated sarcoma* accounts for about 24 % of primary heart malignancies [9]. Most are found in the left atrium and have poor prognosis.
- *Osteosarcoma* of the heart has an incidence of 3–9 % and is approximately twice as common in men [10]. Predominantly it is attached to the wall of the left atrium, causing respiratory symptoms and left-sided heart failure.
- *Leiomyosarcomas* are very rare (8 % of cardiac sarcomas) but highly aggressive invasive tumors, most often diagnosed in adults within the fourth decade [10]. They are often located in the posterior wall of the left atrium and tend to invade the pulmonary veins and/or the mitral valve. Rarely, a right atrial location has been reported [11]. Patients usually present with signs and symptoms of right-sided heart failure or, alternatively, rhythm disturbance, hemopericardium, and sudden death.
- *Fibrosarcomas* and pleomorphic undifferentiated sarcoma (*histiocytomas*) constitute about 5 % of primary malignant cardiac tumors in surgical series [9].
- *Primary liposarcomas* are extremely rare, accounting for <1 % of cardiac sarcomas, and may occur in any cardiac chamber [9].

Rhabdomyosarcoma

- Rhabdomyosarcomas are malignant tumors that present striated muscle differentiation and account for about 5 % of all adult cardiac tumors. The patients range in age from 3 months to 80 years. It can arise in any cardiac chambers without specific predilection.

The pericardium is usually involved by direct extension from the myocardium. These bulky (>10 cm in diameter) tumors can also extend to valve leaflets [3].

Lymphoma

- Lymphoma accounts for 1–2 % of primary malignant cardiac tumors. The patients range in age from 18 to 77 years, with no specific differences in incidence among males and females. Incidence of lymphomas is increasing.
- Up to 20 % of patients with non-Hodgkin lymphoma will have evidence of cardiac lymphoma at autopsy [12].
- There has been an increased connection to acquired immune deficiency syndrome (AIDS) and transplant patients (i.e., cardiac transplantation).
- The elective therapy for lymphomas is based on steroids and on chemotherapy. Surgery is *not* indicated.

It is of utmost importance to exclude a lymphoma before planning cardiac surgery.

Primary Malignancy of the Pericardium

- Malignant mesothelioma is a neoplasm that can arise from the pericardial mesothelial cell layer and accounts for 50 % of primary pericardial tumors.
- Patients range in age from 2 to 78 years with a mean age of 46 years and a male-to-female ratio of 2:1.
- Most of the pericardial mesotheliomas are diffuse, cover visceral and parietal surfaces, and grow by direct extension into surrounding surfaces.
- Combined pleural and pericardial surgery is often necessary.
- Epicardial myocardium may be focally involved, but the tumor does not extend to the endocardial surface.
- Distant metastases are extremely unusual.
- Prognosis is poor, with few patients surviving beyond 12 months from the time of diagnosis.
- An association with asbestos exposure is assumed but not yet confirmed because of the rarity of this tumor.
- Pericardial synovial sarcomas are very aggressive tumors.

24.3 Surgery

Cardiac tumors present a particular challenge for heart surgeons, and great versatility is required. The treating cardiac center must have experience over the whole spectrum of heart surgery, including adult, pediatric, and rhythm surgery as well as transplantation and artificial heart implantation.

A surgical algorithm to help in the decision-making process when dealing with primary malignant cardiac tumors is reported in Fig. 24.1.

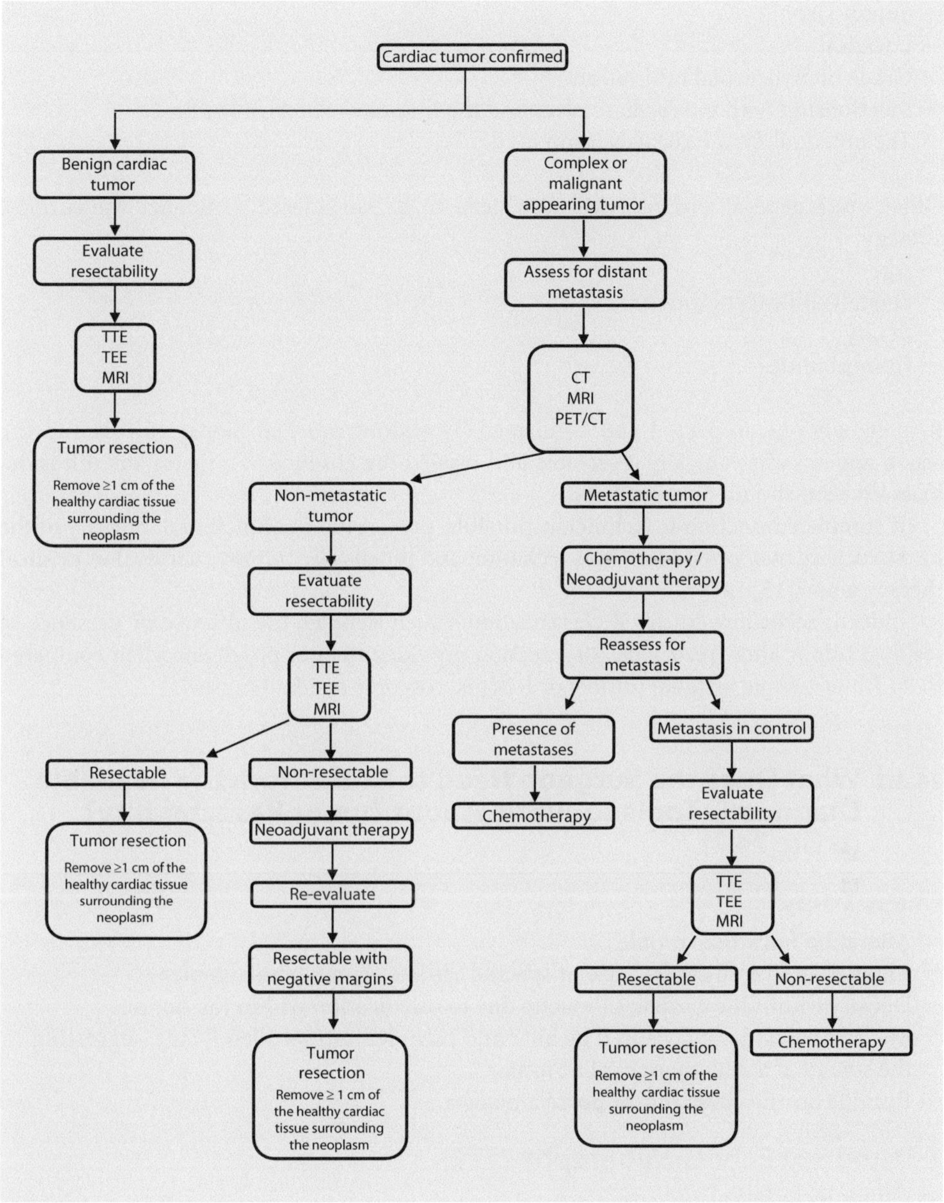

Fig. 24.1 Surgical algorithm to help in the decision-making process when dealing with primary malignant cardiac tumors

24.3.1 Resectability

The decision to resect a primary malignant cardiac tumor is based on several variables, including:

- Histology
- The absence of metastatic spread

- Tumor size
- Location
- Grade of myocardial infiltration
- Relationship with the cardiac valves and the fibrous skeleton of the heart
- The potential for a radical excision

Other more general variables will also need to be considered to finalize the surgical strategy:

- Age
- Overall clinical conditions
- Frailty
- Comorbidities

If malignancy is suspected and confirmed by endomyocardial biopsy (EMB) and the lesion appears anatomically resectable and proved the absence of a metastatic diffusion, mass excision should be considered.

If complete resection is technically possible, preserving the functional integrity of the heart, surgery may provide a better palliation and potentially improve survival vs medical therapy alone [13, 14].

Indeed, according to the R classification which denotes the absence or presence of residual tumor after treatment, R0 resection provides a better prognosis when compared to R1 (microscopic residual tumor) or R2 (macroscopic residual tumor).

24.3.2 What Does the Surgeon Need to Know from the Available Diagnostic Tools to Judge About Tumor Resectability? (■ Fig. 24.1)

Chest X-Ray

- Alteration in cardiac profile.
- Changes in overall cardiac size or specific cardiac chamber enlargement.
- Density within the cardiac silhouette due to calcification within the tumor.
- Mediastinal widening, caused by hilar and paramediastinal adenopathy, suggesting the spread of a malignant cardiac tumor.
- Exclude hostile chest and/or porcelain aorta.

2-D and 3-D Echocardiography (TTE)

- Tumor localization and size
- Site of attachment and modality (sessile or pedunculated)
- Mobility
- Valvular obstruction and/or incompetence and inflow/outflow impairment caused by the cardiac tumor (continuous-mode Doppler)

Transesophageal echocardiography (TEE) provides an unimpeded view of the cardiac chambers and atrioventricular septa and may prove superior in many patients. Its potential advantages include:

- Better resolution of the tumor and its attachment
- Ability to detect small masses not visualized by TEE (<3 mm)

TEE is also routinely used to guide percutaneous biopsy of right-sided cardiac masses favoring successful sampling of the target tissue for preliminary histologic evaluation.

Computed Tomography (CT)

- Excellent spatial resolution
- Ability to characterize fatty content and calcifications
- Tumor vascularity (intravenous contrast)
- May exclude an obstructive coronary artery disease (ECG gated/CT)
- May detect other intrathoracic masses
- May exclude hostile chest and/or porcelain or severely atherosclerotic aorta

Gated Cardiac Magnetic Resonance Imaging (MRI)

- Large field of view
- Superior tissue contrast
- Versatility in image planes
- Discrimination of different tissue characteristics (water and fat content, vascularity, and fibrosis [contrast material–enhanced MR])
- Mass relationship to other cardiac and extracardiac structures (tumor infiltration) [15]

Positron Emission Tomography (PET)/CT

- Molecular imaging methods with 18F-fluorodeoxyglucose (^{18}F-FDG) can visualize tumor metabolism and thereby assess metabolic activity (there is a correlation between the glucose accumulation in tumor tissue and the presence of malignancy).
- Quantification of ^{18}F-FDG uptake can support the noninvasive, pretreatment differentiation between benign and malignant cardiac tumors.
- It may be helpful in detecting metastases of malignant cardiac tumors.

Cardiac Catheterization

This is seldom required for diagnosis of cardiac tumors, but may be performed in adults to exclude coronary artery disease. Moreover, a tumor blush with arterial supply from a right atrial branch is often consistent with an angiosarcoma.

Selective coronary angiography is especially important in right atrial sarcomas because the right coronary artery is often involved and will need to be resected and reconstructed and may be helpful when planning surgical resection of an intramyocardial tumor.

The major risk of angiography is peripheral embolization due to dislodgment of tumor fragments.

24.3.3 Surgical Considerations

- Patients with malignant left-heart cardiac tumors have a dismal prognosis if untreated, due to local extension and metastatic disease. Many patients with left-heart malignant tumors die of hypotension, congestive heart failure, stroke, heart block, and tumor embolization. These tumors present a surgical challenge, because incomplete resection is followed by rapid local tumor recurrence [14].
- The primary goal of surgery is to achieve a complete and possibly en bloc resection of the tumor, encompassing the mass and about 1 cm of the surrounding healthy cardiac tissue.
- Cardiopulmonary bypass (CPB) and good surgical exposure are mandatory.

- A median sternotomy approach with aortic and bi-caval cannulation (the direct cannulation of the superior vena cava allows it to be transected, if necessary, to improve exposure) is almost always utilized.
- Deep hypothermia and occasionally circulatory arrest may be employed to improve exposure. Myocardial protection throughout the procedure is crucial.
- At the beginning of the operation, cardiac manipulation should be minimized in order to prevent the possible fragmentation of the tumor and its potential embolization.
- Whether blood removed from the surgical field during tumor manipulation should be discarded, in an attempt to minimize the systemic microemboli load, or returned to the pump circuit is controversial. Usually, the cardiotomy suction is used during the initial operation, but the wall suction is preferred by the time the tumor is actually excised. The routine use of leukocyte filter in the bypass circuit with the purpose to entrap tumor microemboli to minimize their load is still debated.
- Large complex left atrial tumors may present a considerable impediment to complete resection due to the posterior location of the left atrium and difficult accessibility.
- Intraoperative transesophageal echocardiography can be very helpful during the procedure to:
  - Reconfirm the anatomical location of the mass and reevaluate any associated valvular dysfunction.
  - Monitor the integrity of the tumor through the initial surgical maneuvers.
  - After weaning from CPB, it can provide useful information on:
    Radical exeresis
    Adequacy of an associated valve procedure
    Residual shunt after any intracardiac septal reconstruction

Surgical Approaches

The surgical approach varies according to the location of the tumor and is therefore based on a correct preoperative diagnostic evaluation:

- Left atrial tumors can be approached by:
  - A single right atrial incision allows easy removal of tumor attached to the fossa ovalis with full-thickness excision at the site of attachment and easy patch closure of the atrial septum if necessary.
  - Single incision of the interatrial groove through the anterior wall of the left atrium, anterior to the right pulmonary veins, that can be extended behind both venae cavae for greater exposure. This approach is also adequate for most benign left atrial tumors but is usually inadequate for malignant left atrial tumors, due to the posterior and inaccessible location of the chamber and to the proximity of vital cardiac structures.
  - Biatrial incision allows easy removal of huge tumors attached to the fossa ovalis, improving exposure and allowing full-thickness excision at the site of attachment and easy patch closure of the atrial septum if necessary.
- Ventricular tumors are usually approached through the atrioventricular (AV) valve (occasionally by detaching the valve to improve exposure and resection). Semilunar valve approach is also contemplated for resection of a ventricular outflow tract mass, but might be insufficient for larger malignant tumors. Ventriculotomy, although possible, is not attractive in an attempt to preserve chamber integrity and function.

Complex Tumor Resection

- Complex tumor resection is possible provided the mass is confined to the heart and, if malignant, is limited to a portion of the atrial wall, interatrial septum, and heart valve or to a limited region of the interventricular septum. In any case cardiac anatomic and functional integrity must be restored, even with the use of prosthetic material and/or biological substitution.
- Indeed, radical surgery may be technical demanding, and the necessity of securing negative margins may entail further interventions such as coronary artery bypass, valve replacement, reconstructive procedures, pacemaker implantation, pericardial repairs, and VAD support [17].
- Additional procedures may contribute to an increased risk of postoperative complication and overall mortality.
- To overcome the technical challenges of complete resection with accurate cardiac reconstruction, particularly of left-sided tumors with posterior extension, a technique of cardiac explantation, ex vivo tumor resection with cardiac reconstruction, and cardiac reimplantation—*cardiac autotransplantation*—has been utilized.
  - Surgical outcomes with cardiac autotransplantation are excellent in patients who do not require concurrent pneumonectomy.
  - More in detail, a 15 % 30-day mortality after cardiac autotransplantation has been recently reported.
  - Thirty-day mortality of patients who had concomitant pneumonectomy was 43 % compared with 11 % for those who had isolated cardiac autotransplantation [14, 16, 17].

Orthotopic cardiac transplantation in the management of locally advanced nonmetastatic cardiac tumors appears to have a limited role:
- It has been shown that more than 60 % of the treated patients die of local recurrence or distant metastases within a year.
- The overall poor availability of organ donors represents another important limitation.
- Nevertheless, about 25 % of the patients managed by orthotopic cardiac transplantation have a mean survival of more than 2 years without recurrent disease [18].

24.3.4 Survival Outcome

- For malignant tumors of the heart, the prognosis is very poor. The stated duration of survival from the time of diagnosis varies from 7 months to a maximum of 2 years.
- At follow-up, the majority of patients die of underlying disease or its complications or both [20].
- Patients rejected to surgery had a lower survival compared with operation receivers [19].
- In some studies, there were no significant differences in survival in patients rejected to surgery than in the patients who had positive surgical margins [19].
- In the study of French Sarcoma Group, surgery resulted as a major prognostic factor for survival, regardless of the quality of resection and metastatic status. This may indicate a particular paradigm as even incomplete resection appears worthwhile for immediate vital reasons and tumor control. Noteworthy, however, safe margins yielded better survival [13].

- The median survival was significantly longer when a complete surgical resection was possible (R0 vs R1/R2).
- The 1-year and 2-year survival of patients with primary sarcoma treated with cardiac autotransplantation was 46 % and 28 %, respectively (median survival 302 days). The 2-year survival of patients with and without pneumonectomy was 14 % and 32 %, respectively. The 2-year survival of sarcoma patients with positive and negative surgical margins was similar (40 % and 38 %, respectively) [14].
- The poor results with surgical resection have led to occasional attempts to treat patients with cardiac transplantation, if extracardiac disease is not present. In the largest series, results of cardiac transplantation in patients with malignant tumors (most of which were sarcomas) were evaluated in a review of 21 cases. Although mean survival was only 12 months, seven patients were free of recurrent malignancy at a mean follow-up of 27 months [21].

References

1. Oliveira GH, Al-Kindi SG, Hoimes C, Park SJ. Characteristics and survival of malignant cardiac tumors: a 40-year analysis of >500 patients. Circulation. 2015;132:2395–402.
2. Shapiro L. Cardiac tumors: diagnosis and management. Heart. 2001;85:218–22.
3. Castello J, Silvay G. Characterization and management of cardiac tumors. Semin Cardiothorac Vasc Anesth. 2010;14:6–20.
4. Randhawa JS, Budd GT, Randhawa M, et al. Primary cardiac sarcoma: 25-year Cleveland clinic experience. Am J Clin Oncol. 2014 Jul 17.
5. Ramlawi B, Leja MJ, Abu Saleh WK, et al. Surgical treatment of primary cardiac sarcomas: review of a single-institution experience. Ann Thorac Surg. 2016;101:698–702.
6. Barreiro M, Renilla A, Jimenez JM, et al. Primary cardiac tumors: 32 years of experience from a Spanish tertiary surgical center. Cardiovasc Pathol. 2013;22:424–7.
7. Hoffmeier A, Sindermann JR, Scheld HH, et al. Cardiac tumors—diagnosis and surgical treatment. Dtsch Arztebl Int. 2014;111:205–11.
8. Mayer F, Aebert H, Rudert M, et al. Primary malignant sarcomas of the heart and great vessels in adult patients: a single-center experience. Oncologist. 2007;12:1134–42.
9. O'Donnell DH, Abbara S, Chaithiraphan V, et al. Cardiac tumors: optimal cardiac MR sequences and spectrum of imaging appearances. AJR Am J Roentgenol. 2009;193:377–87.
10. Grebenc ML, Rosado de Christenson ML, Burke AP, et al. Primary cardiac and pericardial neoplasms: radiologic-pathologic correlation. Radiographics. 2000;20:1073–103.
11. Parissis H, Akbar MT, Young V. Primary leiomyosarcoma of the right atrium: a case report and literature update. J Cardiothorac Surg. 2010;5:80.
12. Burke A, Jeudy Jr J, Virmani R. Cardiac tumors: an update. Heart. 2008;94:117–23.
13. Isambert N, Ray-Coquard I, Italiano A, et al. Primary cardiac sarcomas: a retrospective study of the French Sarcoma Group. Eur J Cancer. 2014;50:128–36.
14. Blackmon SH, Patel AR, Bruckner BA, et al. Cardiac autotransplantation for malignant or complex primary left-heart tumors. Tex Heart Inst J. 2008;35:296–300.
15. Motwani M, Kidambi A, Herzog BA, et al. MR imaging of cardiac tumors and masses: a review of methods and clinical applications. Radiology. 2013;268:26–43.
16. Blackmon SH, Reardon MJ. Cardiac autotransplantation. Oper Tech Thorac Cardiovasc Surg. 2010;15: 147–61.
17. Ramlawi B, Al-Jabbari O, Blau LN. Autotransplantation for the resection of complex left heart tumors. Ann Thorac Surg. 2014;98:863–8.
18. Basso C, Valente M, Thiene G. Cardiac tumor pathology. New York: Springer; 2013.
19. Yu L, Gu T, Shi E, et al. Primary malignant cardiac tumors. J Cancer Res Clin Oncol. 2014;140:1047–55.
20. Hoffmeier A, Schmid C, Deiters S, et al. Neoplastic heart disease —the Muenster experience with 108 patients. Thorac Cardiovasc Surg. 2005;53:1–8.
21. Gowdamarajan A, Michler RE. Therapy for primary cardiac tumors: is there a role for heart transplantation? Curr Opin Cardiol. 2000;15:121–5.

Cardiac Tumors: Multimodality Approach, Follow-Up, and Prognosis

Antonino De Paoli, Gian Maria Miolo, and Angela Buonadonna

C. Lestuzzi et al. (eds.), *Manual of Cardio-oncology*, DOI 10.1007/978-3-319-40236-9_25

25.1 Primary Cardiac Lymphomas

Primary cardiac lymphomas are usually treated with chemotherapy (CT), with a good rate of success at least at short-medium term, even if survival is worse than in noncardiac lymphomas [1–4]. Surgery may be indicated in selected cases in the presence of life-threatening hemodynamic impairment [5]. Medical therapy is based on chemotherapy, steroids, and – in HIV-related lymphomas – antiretroviral therapy [6]. Radiation therapy may be considered for palliation in nonresponsive or progressive disease after CT:

- The cyclophosphamide, doxorubicin, vincristine, and prednisone with the monoclonal antibody rituximab (R-CHOP) regimen are the commonly used first-line therapy even in elderly patients [7].
- Chemotherapy, however, must be planned according to the histological diagnosis, which may be obtained through a tumor biopsy or a biopsy of other masses if multiple localizations are detected.
- Aggressive lymphomas may show a significant improvement even with steroids alone [6].

> **Since pathologic diagnosis may require some days to be defined, in the presence of large cardiac masses, steroid therapy should be started immediately. However, a prompt collaboration with an experienced oncologist/hematologist is necessary to plan further diagnostic examinations and prevent dangerous side effects as the tumor lysis syndrome [8, 9].**

25.2 Primary Cardiac Sarcomas

The mainstay of treatment is surgery, but CT and radiotherapy (RT) may play a relevant role, since in most cases it is difficult to achieve a radical resection with negative margins (R0) [10]:

- In the case of tumors with metastases at the time of diagnosis, surgery is not indicated. The first approach is CT.
- Neoadjuvant (preoperative) CT should be considered [11]:
  - In large, unresectable tumors in order to assess tumor response and thus modulate treatment
  - In borderline resectable tumors, to increase the probability of a wide resection with negative margins
- Postoperative CT should be considered [12]:
  - After resection with infiltrated margin or macroscopic residual disease [13]. However chemotherapy should never be intended to rescue inadequate surgery.
  - As adjuvant treatment in tumors at high risk of local and distant relapse (angiosarcoma and other high-grade, deep, >5 cm sarcomas).
- Postoperative RT may be considered as integrated approach after CT in resected tumors and right heart locations, with positive margins or macroscopic residual disease.
- Combined CT and RT may be considered, mainly in right heart sarcomas, to reduce the tumor burden and prolong the progression-free survival in unresectable or in relapsing tumors.
- *The first-line CT* is based on:
  - Anthracyclines and ifosfamide [14]. However there is no formal demonstration that multiagent chemotherapy is superior in terms of overall survival to single-

agent chemotherapy with doxorubicin alone although a longer response rate can be expected.
  - Taxanes may be considered an alternative option in angiosarcomas [15, 16].
- *Second-line CT* (for relapse or progression) includes several drugs, to be used alone or – more often – in combination: high-dose ifosfamide, gemcitabine, trabectedin, dacarbazine, and a number of tyrosine kinase inhibitors. Since there is a wide variety of sarcoma histotypes and – among each histotype – different aberrant pathways in tumor cells, the choice of the most appropriate chemotherapy should take into account the characteristics of the single tumor, to achieve a targeted therapy [17, 18].

Chemotherapy must be planned by a medical oncologist with experience in the management of sarcomas, which are rare tumors.

25.2.1 Radiotherapy

Radiotherapy of cardiac sarcomas is challenging:
- The target lesion is close to structures (ventricular myocardium, coronary arteries, cardiac valves) that can be irreversibly damaged by radiation [19, 20].
- Due to the heart movements, a treatment planning which includes the tumor with adequate margins but excludes the adjacent structures is nearly impossible to make if the tumor involves the ventricles or the atrioventricular junction [21].
- To optimize the curative effect of radiotherapy minimizing the cardiac risk, the following strategies should be used [22]:
  - Careful *assessment of anatomic and dynamic aspects* of the target lesion using several imaging techniques (MRI, high-definition CT, transesophageal echocardiography). In addition, echocardiography is particularly useful in evaluating the movement of the tumor mass during cardiac cycle to define the planned treatment volume (a close collaboration between the cardiologist and radiation oncologist for treatment planning is essential).
  - *Three-dimensional CRT* (3D-CRT) technique, to deliver radiation dose tightly limited to the tumor while sparing critical structures, is recommended.
  - *Image-guided RT* (IGRT) to localize the tumor at the time of treatment, to evaluate organ motion, and to improve knowledge of the partial volume tolerance of the hearth to radiation.
  - *Intensity-modulated RT* (IMRT) is another technological advancement that facilitates the delivery of highly conformal RT [23]. With IMRT, radiation is delivered with multiple small fields ("segments") within each beam, producing a modulated fluence pattern for each beam angle. Computer-aided, automated optimization of segment's weights (or "inverse planning") is conducted to obtain the best target coverage and sparing of dose to normal tissues.

Radiation therapy must be planned by a radiation oncologist with experience in the management of sarcomas, operating in a center with modern equipment, in collaboration of an experienced cardiologist. A regular cardiologic monitoring during the treatment should be planned.

25.3 Follow-Up and Prognosis

- The patients with unresectable sarcomas undergoing neoadjuvant CT should be reevaluated to assess the response after two or three courses:
  - Usually the response to a given therapy is based on the changes of tumor dimensions, according to the RECIST criteria [24]. However, large sarcomas may undergo necrosis or hemorrhages in response to therapy, without significant reduction or increase in global dimensions, leading to a false diagnosis of failure of therapy [25, 26].
  - New response criteria, based on density at computed tomography and on metabolic activity, have been proposed for gastrointestinal stromal tumors first and have been be applied also to other soft tissue sarcomas and to other tumors [27–29].
  - *At computed tomography*, a change in tumor density, as determined by measuring CT attenuation coefficient (Hounsfield unit [HU]), together with minor changes in tumor size that were insufficient for response by RECIST, may provide a consistent quantitative means to evaluate the tumor response.
  - At [18F]fluoro-2-deoxy-D-glucose (^{18}F-FDG), *positron emission tomography (PET)* imaging has been used to identify histopathologic treatment responders as early as after one cycle of neoadjuvant therapy [30, 31] An early and late decreases in maximum standardized 18FDG uptake (SUV_{peak}), respectively, were significant predictors of survival in a study on soft tissue sarcoma [32].
- Even with the best surgical treatment, soft tissue sarcomas may relapse, usually within the first years. Due to the objective difficulties in obtaining a radical surgery, cardiac sarcomas have even a more severe prognosis, with only a minority of patients surviving more than 3 years [33–35]. The risk of relapse is higher in the first years after treatment.

> **After treatment, patients should undergo a strict follow-up:**
> **Every 3 months in the first 2 years**
> **Every 6 month in the following 2 years**
> **Yearly thereafter**

- There are no blood neoplastic markers for sarcomas: the follow-up is based on imaging techniques:

> **Echocardiography is the cheapest and most easily available method for follow-up, but the transesophageal approach is necessary for the atrial masses.**

> **The best imaging technique is magnetic resonance imaging (MRI); its use is limited – however – by the availability of the equipments.**

> **Computed tomography and positron emission tomography are more widely available; their use is limited by the radiation exposure risk.**

> **The choice of the imaging technique(s) most frequently used should be tailored according to the primary site of the tumor, the technique with the best definition of the tumor at the time of diagnosis, and the possibility of comparing the imaging.**

> **Each kind of imaging (echocardiography, computed tomography, MRI, PET) should be obtained always in the same hospital, in order to reduce the variability of the results and to facilitate the comparison of the follow-up exams.**

References

1. Antoniades L, Eftychiou C, Petrou PM, et al. Primary cardiac lymphoma: case report and brief review of the literature. Echocardiography. 2009;26:214–9.
2. Lilje C, Thiel C, Weil J, et al. Non-surgical management of advanced cardiac lymphoma. J Pediatr. 2008;152:440.
3. Mohsen A, Najafi AH, Zhou L, et al. Massive, rapidly growing cardiac lymphoma with rare valvular involvement showing excellent response to chemotherapy. Can J Cardiol. 2013;29:1139. e3-4.
4. Oliveira GH, Al-Kindi SG, Hoimes C, Park SJ. Characteristics and survival of malignant cardiac tumors: a 40-year analysis of over 500 patients. Circulation. 2015;132:2395–402.
5. Gosev I, Sirić F, Gasparović H, et al. Surgical treatment of a primary cardiac lymphoma presenting with tamponade physiology. J Card Surg. 2006;21:414–6.
6. Lestuzzi C, Spina M, Martellotta F, Carbone A. Massive myocardial infiltration by HIV-related non-Hodgkin lymphoma: echocardiographic aspects at diagnosis and at follow-up. J Cardiovasc Med (Hagerstown). 2012;13:836–8.
7. Tilly H, Dreyling M, ESMO Guidelines Working Group. Diffuse large B-cell non-Hodgkin's lymphoma: ESMO Clinical Practice Guidelines for diagnosis, treatment and follow-up. Ann Oncol. 2010;21 Suppl 5:v172–4.
8. Howard SC, Jones DP, Pui CH. The tumor lysis syndrome. N Engl J Med. 2011;364:1844–54.
9. Pi J, Kang Y, Smith M, et al. A review in the treatment of oncologic emergencies. J Oncol Pharm Pract. 2015 Oct 6.
10. Kim MP, Correa AM, Blackmon S, et al. Outcomes after right-side heart sarcoma resection. Ann Thorac Surg. 2011;91:770–6.
11. Ramlawi B, Leja MJ, Abu Saleh WK, et al. Surgical treatment of primary cardiac sarcomas: review of a single-institution experience. Ann Thorac Surg. 2015 Oct 14.
12. Patrikidou A, Domont J, Cioffi A, Le Cesne A. Treating soft tissue sarcomas with adjuvant chemotherapy. Curr Treat Options Oncol. 2011;12:21–31.
13. Le Cesne A, Ouali M, Leahy MG, et al. Doxorubicin-based adjuvant chemotherapy in soft tissue sarcoma: pooled analysis of two STBSG-EORTC phase III clinical trials. Ann Oncol. 2014;25:2425–32.
14. Ravi V, Benjamin RS. Systemic therapy for cardiac sarcomas. MDCVJ. 2010;VI(3):57–60.
15. Schlemmer M, Reichardt P, Verweij J, et al. Paclitaxel in patients with advanced angiosarcomas of soft tissue: a retrospective study of the EORTC soft tissue and bone sarcoma group. Eur J Cancer. 2008;44:2433–6.
16. Oxenberg J, Khushalani NI, Salerno KE, et al. Neoadjuvant chemotherapy for primary cutaneous/soft tissue angiosarcoma: determining tumor behavior prior to surgical resection. J Surg Oncol. 2015;111:829–33.
17. Liebner DA. The indications and efficacy of conventional chemotherapy in primary and recurrent sarcoma. J Surg Oncol. 2015;111:622–31.
18. van der Graaf WT, Blay JY, Chawla SP, EORTC Soft Tissue and Bone Sarcoma Group, PALETTE study group, et al. Pazopanib for metastatic soft-tissue sarcoma (PALETTE): a randomised, double-blind, placebo-controlled phase 3 trial. Lancet. 2012;379:1879–86.
19. Basavaraju SR, Easterly CE. Pathophysiological effects of radiation on atherosclerosis development and progression, and the incidence of cardiovascular complications. Med Phys. 2002;29:2391–403.
20. Thariat J, Clément-Colmou K, Vogin G, et al. Radiation therapy of cardiac sarcomas. Cancer Radiother. 2014;18:125–31.
21. Ipsen S, Blanck O, Oborn B, et al. Radiotherapy beyond cancer: target localization in real-time MRI and treatment planning for cardiac radiosurgery. Med Phys. 2014;41:120702.
22. Thariat J, Clément-Colmou K, Vogin G, et al. Radiation therapy of cardiac sarcomas. Cancer Radiother. 2014;18:125–31.
23. Roeder F, Nicolay NH, Nguyen T, et al. Intensity modulated radiotherapy (IMRT) with concurrent chemotherapy as definitive treatment of locally advanced esophageal cancer. Radiat Oncol. 2014;9:191.
24. Eisenhauer EA, Therasse P, Bogaerts J, et al. New response evaluation criteria in solid tumours: revised RECIST guideline (version 1.1). Eur J Cancer. 2009;45:228–47.
25. Hollebecque A, Adenis A, Taieb S, et al. Inadequacy of size-based response criteria to assess the efficacy of trabectedin among metastatic sarcoma patients. Invest New Drugs. 2010;28:529–30.

26. Taieb S, Saada-Bouzid E, Tresch E, French Sarcoma Group, et al. Comparison of response evaluation criteria in solid tumours and Choi criteria for response evaluation in patients with advanced soft tissue sarcoma treated with trabectedin: a retrospective analysis. Eur J Cancer. 2015;51:202–9.
27. Choi H, Charnsangavej C, Faria SC, et al. Correlation of computed tomography and positron emission tomography in patients with metastatic gastrointestinal stromal tumor treated at a single institution with imatinib mesylate: proposal of new computed tomography response criteria. J Clin Oncol. 2007;25:1753–9.
28. Lencioni R, Llovet JM. Modified RECIST (mRECIST) assessment for hepatocellular carcinoma. Semin Liver Dis. 2010;30:52–60.
29. Ueda T, Morioka H, Nishida Y, et al. Objective tumor response to denosumab in patients with giant cell tumor of bone: a multicenter phase II trial. Ann Oncol. 2015;26:2149–54.
30. Evilevitch V, Weber WA, Tap WD, et al. Reduction of glucose metabolic activity is more accurate than change in size at predicting histopathologic response to neoadjuvant therapy in high-grade soft-tissue sarcomas. Clin Cancer Res. 2008;14:715–20.
31. Benz MR, Czernin J, Allen-Auerbach MS, et al. FDG-PET/CT imaging predicts histopathologic treatment responses after the initial cycle of neoadjuvant chemotherapy in high-grade soft-tissue sarcomas. Clin Cancer Res. 2009;15:2856–63.
32. Herrmann K, Benz MR, Czernin J, et al. 18F-FDG-PET/CT Imaging as an early survival predictor in patients with primary high-grade soft tissue sarcomas undergoing neoadjuvant therapy. Clin Cancer Res. 2012;18:2024–31.
33. Li H, Xu D, Chen Z, et al. Prognostic analysis for survival after resections of localized primary cardiac sarcomas: a single- institution experience. Ann Thorac Surg. 2014;97:1379–85.
34. Isambert N, Ray-Coquard I, Italiano A, et al. Primary cardiac sarcomas: a retrospective study of the French Sarcoma Group. Eur J Cancer. 2014;50:128–36.
35. Randhawa JS, Budd GT, Randhawa M, et al. Primary cardiac sarcoma: 25-Year Cleveland clinic experience. Am J Clin Oncol. 2014 Jul 17.

Improving the Cooperation Between Oncologists, Cardiologists, and General Practitioners

Contents

Understanding the Most Common Oncologic and Cardiologic Terms

Davide Santeufemia, Francesco Ferraù, and Iris Parrini

C. Lestuzzi et al. (eds.), *Manual of Cardio-oncology*, DOI 10.1007/978-3-319-40236-9_26

A rather frequent problem in cardio-oncology is the imperfect comprehension between cardiologists and oncologist. In the daily clinical practice, the use of acronyms is common, but the acronyms used in a particular field of medicine are easily understood by the specialists of that particular field only; they may be less obvious for specialists of other fields. This chapter will help in understanding the most common oncologic and cardiologic terms.

In ◻ Table 26.1, the acronyms most used in cardiology are explained. The principal classes of drugs are highlighted in *yellow*; arrhythmias in **blue**. In ◻ Table 26.1, the coronary artery tree is depicted in summary. The oncologists use many acronyms to define various

◻ Table 26.1 List of Acronyms and terms currently used by cardiologists

ACE	*Angiolensin-converting enzyme*	*Drugs used for hypertension, to prevent cardiac remoleding, cardioprotective*
ACS	Acute coronary syndrome	Acute cardiac ischemia (may evolve to a myocardial infarction)
AF	**Atrial Fibrillation**	**Atrial arrhythmia with desyncronized electric activity**
AMI	Acute myocardial infarction	Acute myocardial ischemia with evidence of myocardial necrosis
ARB	*Angiotensin receptor blocker*	*Drugs used for hypertension, to prevent cardiac remoleding. cardioprotective*
ASA	*Acetylsalicilic acide*	
AVB	**Atrio-ventricular block**	**A delay/block of the conduction of the electrical impulse from the atria to the ventricles, it is classified as 1st degree (all the impulse are conducted, with temporal delay). 2nd degree (some impulse only are conducted), 3rd degree or complete AVB (all the impulse are blocked: a ventricular rhythm emerges)**
BAV	Balloon aortic valvuloplasty	Dilatation of a stenotic aortic valve with a balloon catheter
BB	*Beta blockers*	*Drugs used for arrhythmias, hypertension, to prevent cardiac remoleding.*
BBB	**Bundle branch block**	**A delay in the conduction of the electrical impulse within die ventricles. it may involve the right (RBBB) or left (LBBB) branch. May me complete or incomplete.**
BMS	Bare metal stent	
BNP	Brain natriuretic peptide	
CABG	Coronary artery bypass grafting	Surgical coronary revasculatization with venous or arterial by-pass
CAD	Coronary artery disease	
CCS	Classification of the Canadian Cardiovascular Society	Classification of angina symptoms. Ranges from 1 to 4

Table 26.1 (continued)

CHD	Cardiovascular heart disease	
	Congenital heart disease	
CHF	Congestive heart failure	
CIEDs	cardiovascular implantable electronic devices	
CK-MB	MB isoenzymc of Creatine kinase	A marker of myocardial necrosis. CK is released by any muscular necrosis: the MB isoenzyme is released from the myocardium
CRT	Cardiac resynchronization therapy	
CVD	Cardiovascular discase	
DAPT	Dual antiplatelet therapy	Assocition of two different antiplatelet drugs (usually USA and dopidogrel or prasugrel). It is indicated after acute coronary syndromes and after stent implantation.
DES	Drug eluting stent	
EF	Ejection fraction	Percentage of change of ventricular volume from end-diastole to end-systole
ICD	Implantable cardioverter-defibrillator	
IMA	Internal mammary artery	A vessel used for CABG
LAD	Left anterior descending artery	
LMWH	*Low Molecular Weight Heparin*	
LV	Left ventricle (left ventricular)	
IE (or BE)	Infective endocarditis (or Bacterial Endocarditis)	A bacterial infection of the cardiac valves, of the endocardium (in congenital heart diseases) or of a cardiac device (pacemaker leads for instance)
INR	International Normalized Ratio	To assess the efficacy of classic oral anticoaugulants, as warfarin
NOA	*New Oral Anticoagulants*	*New generation anticoagulants (as dabigatran, rivaroxaban.apixaban)*
NSTEMI	Non-ST elevation myocardial infarction	Acute myocardial infarction without elevation of ST segment at ECG.

(continued)

Table 26.1 (continued)

NYMA class	New York Heart Associationclass	Classification of symptoms of congestive heart failure. Ranges from 1 (no symptoms) to IV (severe symptoms at rest)
PCI	Percutaneous coronary) intervention	
PM	Pacemaker	
PVE	Prosthetic valve endocarditis	A bacterial infection of a prosthetic cardiac valve. It may involve both biological and mechanical valves
QRS		Electrocardiographic complex corresponding to the electrical activation of the ventricles
QT		The interval between the onset of ventricular depolarization and the end of repolarization
RCA	Right coronaty artery	
SSS	**Sick sinus syndrome**	Arrhythmia due to a dysfunction of the sinoatrial node. May require PM
STEMI	ST elevation myocardial infarction	Acute myocardial infarction with elevation of ST segment at ECG.
Takotsubo	Takotsubo syndrome	Acute reversible heart failure syndrome -usually following a stressful trigger- which may mimick an acute coronary syndrome
TAVI	Transcatheter aortic valve implanation	
TdP	**Torsade de pointe**	**Ventricular arrhythmia with changing electric axes. It usually leads to syncope and may be transient or may evolve to ventricular fibrillation**
Tn	Troponin: I. T, High sensitivity (HS) I or T	A highly specific marker of myocardial necrosis.
TEE	Transesophageal echocardiography	
TTE	Transthoracic echocardiography	
VEB	**Ventricular ectopic beats**	
VF	**Ventricular fibrillation**	
VT	**Ventricular tachycardia**	**≥.3 consecutive VEB**

Highlighted: in bold: arrhythmias, in italic: drugs

kinds of tumors (Table 26.2). Any cardiac adverse effect due to an oncologic treatment raises the problem of interrupting the treatment. The decision is based on several variables: prognosis of the tumor, availability of alternative treatments, intent of therapy. The following paragraphs will help the cardiologist to better understand the clinical scenario.

Table 26.2 List of Acronyms and terms currently used by oncologists

		Notes
ADK	Adenocarcinoma	Refers to various tumor sites
AML	Acute myeloid leukemia	
BC	Breast carcinoma	
BCC	Basal cell carcinoma	
BM	Brain metastases	From any type of tumors
BT	Brain tumors	
CLL	Chronic lymphatic leukemia	
CML	Chronic myeloid leukemia	
CR	Carcinoma	
CRC	Colo-rectal carcinoma	
GCT	Germ cell tumor	Refers both to gonadal and extragonadal tumors
GIST	Gastrointestinal stromal tumor	Pertains to sarcomas family
HCC	Hepatocellular carcinoma	
HD (HL)	Hodgkin's disease, Hodgkin lymphoma	
H&Nscc	Head and Neck squamous cell carcinoma	
MDS	Myelodisplastic syndrome(s)	
MM	Malignant melanoma	
MO	Multiple myeloma	
NHL	Non-Hodgkin lymphoma	
NSCLC	Non-small cell lung carcinoma	
OC	esophageal carcinoma	
PC	Pancreatic carcinoma	
PEL	Primary effusion lymphoma	A rare type of NHL, localized in the serous cavities
PMM	Pleural malignant mesothelioma	
PNET	Primitive neuroectodermal tumor	Pertains to sarcomas family (similar to Ewing sarcoma)
RCC	Renal cell carcinoma	
SCLC	Small cell lung carcinoma	
SCC	Squamous cell carcinoma	Refers to various tumor sites

(continued)

Table 26.2 (continued)

		Notes
STS	Soft Tissue Sarcoma	
TCC	Transitional cell carcinoma	Refers both to vesical and extravesical tumors
Descriptive indices after instrumental evaluation of disease		
CR	Complete remission	Complete disappearing of disease after treatment
PR	Partial remission	Partial regression of disease after treatment
SD	Stable disease	No modification of disease after treatment
PD	Progressive disease	Diametric increase and/or new lesions of disease

26.1 Intents of Chemotherapy

- **Adjuvant:** Chemotherapy given to destroy microscopic cells that may be present after the tumor is removed by surgery with the aim to prevent a disease recurrence.
- **Neoadjuvant chemotherapy**: Chemotherapy given prior to the surgical procedure with the aim to shrink the tumor before surgery.
- **Induction chemotherapy**: Chemotherapy given to induce a remission.
- **Consolidation chemotherapy**: Chemotherapy given once a remission is achieved.
- **First-line chemotherapy**: Chemotherapy that has the best probability of treating a given cancer. This may also be called standard therapy.
- **Second-line chemotherapy**: Chemotherapy that is given if a disease has not responded or reoccurred after first-line chemotherapy. In some cases, this may also be referred to as salvage therapy.
- **Palliative chemotherapy**: Palliative chemotherapy is a type of chemotherapy that is given specifically with the aim to improve quality of life and to prolong (when possible) survival.

After chemotherapy, a clinical instrumental restaging is usually done to the patient in order to assess the treatment response:

- ***Complete remission (CR)*:** Disappearance of all target lesions
- ***Partial remission (PR)*:** *At least a 30 % decrease in the sum of the longest diameter (LD) of target lesions, taking as reference the baseline sum LD*
- ***Stable Disease (SD)***: Neither sufficient shrinkage to qualify for PR nor sufficient increase to qualify for PD, taking as reference the smallest sum LD since the treatment started
- ***Progressive Disease (PD)***: At least a 20 % increase in the sum of the LD of target lesions, taking as reference the smallest sum LD recorded since the treatment started or the appearance of one or more new lesions

26.2 Antineoplastic Drugs

Chemotherapeutic drugs may be administered alone or in combination using several different treatment schedules. In a chemotherapeutic regimen, these medications may be given at the same time or one after another for a time default. A specific regimen may be identified by an acronym, which is formed using the first letter (s) of the drug name, chemical abbreviation of the agents used in the regimen. However, it is important to know that selection, dosing, and administration of anti-cancer agents are complex, and both drugs' dose or schedule modifications are often necessary in the clinical practice because of expected toxicities and patient intrinsic variability.

In ◘ Table 26.3, the most used acronyms and short terms for cytotoxic anticancer treatments are summarized, together with the most common indications. Those more frequently involved in cardiac toxicity are highlighted in *yellow*.

◘ **Table 26.3** Most used acronyms and short names for oncologic drugs.

SHORT NAMES	EXPLANATION and dosage for each course	INDICATION; NOTES
AC	*Adriamcin + Cyclophosphmide*	Breast cancer
ABV	*Adriamicin + Bleomycin + Vinblastine*	Lymphomas
ABVD	*Adriamicin + Bleomycin + Vinblastine + Dacarbazine*	Lymphomas; administered 2 times in each course (day 1 and 15)
ADM	*Adriamicin (Doxorubicin)*	
BEACOPP	*Adriamicin + Bleomycin + Etoposide*	Lymphomas
BLM	Bleomycin	Lymphomas
CAF	*Adriamcin + Cyclophosphmide + Fluorouracil*	breast cancer
CBDCA	Carboplatin (same of JM8)	Lung cancer
CDDP	Cisplatin (same of DDP)	Lung cancer
CEOP	*Epi-adriamicin + Cyclophosphamide + vincristine + Prednisone*	Lymphomas
CHOPP	*Adriamicin + Cyclophosphamide + vincristine + Prednisone*	Lymphomas
CMF	Cyclophosphamide + Methothrexate + Fluorouracil	Breast cancer
COMP	*Myocet (nonpegilated liposomal doxorubicin) + Bleomycin + Vincristine*	Lymphomas
CV	*Capecitabine + Vinorelbine*	Breast cancer
DHAP	Dexamethasone + Cisplatin + Cytarabine	Lymphomas, high-dose chemotherapy

(continued)

26

Table 26.3 (continued)

SHORT NAMES	EXPLANATION and dosage for each course	INDICATION; NOTES
DCF	*Docetaxel + Cisplatin + Fluorouracil over 5 day*	Gastric cancer
EC	*Epi-adriamicin + Cyclophosphamide*	Breast cancer
ECF	*Epirubicin + Cisplatin + Fluorauracil via 21 day Continuous infusion*	Gastric cancer
EPI	*Epiadriamicin*	
ESHAP	Etoposide + Prednisolone + hioh-dose Cytarabine + Cisplatin	Lymphomas, high-dose chemotherapy
DDP	Cisplatin (same of CDDP)	
FOLFIRI	*Fluorauracil (bolus + continuous Infusion for 48 hours) + Leucovorin + Irinotecan*	Colorectal carcinoma
FOLFOX	*Fluorouracil (bolus + continuous infusion for 48 hours) + Leucovorin + Oxaliplatin*	Colorectal carcinoma
5-FU	Fluorouracil	Head/neck, gastrointestinal, liver, breast cancers
GDP	Dexamethasone + Cisplatin + Gemcitabine	Lymphomas
GP	Gemcitabine + Cisplatin	Lung Cancer, Biliary cancer, Transitional cell cancer
HER	Herceptin (trade name of Trastuzumab)	Breast cancer, Gastric cancer
ICE	ifosfamide + Carboplatin + Etoposide	Lymphomas, high-dose chemotherapy
IFO	ifosfamide	Sarcomas, high dose chemotherapy
JM8	Carboplatin (same of CBDCA)	
MOPP	Mechloretamine + Vincristine + Procarbazine + Prednisone	Hodgkin lymphoma
MVAC	*Methotrexate + Vinblastine + Adriamkin + Cisplatin*	Transitional cell carsinoma
Stanford V	*Doxorubicin + Vinblastine + Mechloretamine + Vincristine + Etoposide + Prednisone*	Hodgkin lymphoma. Widely used in the past, less Frequently nowadays
TAX	Taxal (Pacitaxel)	Breast cancer, Ovarian cancer, Angiosarcomas
TAC	*Docetaxel + Adriamicin + Cyclophospbamlde*	Breast cancer
TC	Docetaxel + Cyclophosphamide	Breast cancer

Table 26.3 (continued)

SHORT NAMES	EXPLANATION and dosage for each course	INDICATION; NOTES
TCF	*Docetaxel + Cisplatin + Fluorouracil*	Head & neck carcinomas
TCH	*Docetaxel + Cyclophosphamide + Trastuzumab*	Breast cancer
T-DM1	Ado-Trastuzumab emtansine (Trastuzumab conjugated to anticancer DM-1)	Breast cancer
TICE	Ifosfamide + Carboplatin + Etoposide + Taxel	Lymphomas, high-dose chemotherapy
TIP	*Taxol + Ifosfamide + Cisplatin*	Cervical carcinoma
TKI	Tyrosine kinase inhibitors (a class of drugs used in target therapy)	
TXT	Taxotere (Docetaxel)	breast cancer, ovarian cancer
VAC/IE	*vincristine + doxorubicin + cyclophosphamide alternating with ifosfamide + etoposide*	Sarcomas, Bone cancer
VAI	*vincristine + ifosfamide + dactinomycin + doxarubicin*	Bone cancer
VCR	Vincristine	
VEPEB	*Epi-adriamicin + Cyclophosphamide + Bleomycin + Vinorelbine*	Lymphomas
VIDE	*Vincristine + Ifosfamide + Doxorubicin + Etoposide*	
VP16	Etoposide	Lung cancer
XL	*Capecitabine + Lapatinib*	Breast cancer

Highlighted in italic, those which may be more frequently involved in cardiotoxicity
Adriamicin= doxorubicin= adriblastin; epi-adriamicin= epidoxorubicin= epirubicin

In Table 26.4, the commercial names are reported.

Targeted therapy is a newer type of cancer treatment that uses drugs or other substances to more precisely identify and attack specific receptors expressed by cancer cells. These treatments are aimed to limit the damage to normal cells. However, they may have several side effects, which may be caused by their therapeutic mechanism (on-target) or by the action on other organs or by immune reactions or toxic metabolites (off-target).

In Table 26.5, a list of the most used target therapies (including mechanism of action, indications, and possible side effects) is reported.

Table 26.4 Commercial names of the most common antineoplastic drugs

Drug	Commercial name
Actinomycin D	Cosmegen
Bleomycin	Bleomycin
Capecitabine	Xeloda
Carboplatin	Paraplatin
Cyclophosphamide	Endoxan
Cisplatin	Cisplatin (generic)
Cytarabine	Aracytin
Dacarbazine	Deticene
Docetaxel	Taxotere
Doxorubicin	Adriamycin, Adriblastina
Doxorubicin liposomal non-pegylated	Myocet
Doxorubicin liposomal pegylated	Caelyx
Epirubicin	Epirubicin
Etoposide	Vepesid
Fluorouracil	Fluorouracil (generic)
Gemcitabine	Gemzar
Ifosfamide	Holoxan
Irinotecan	Campto
Lapatinib	Tyverb
Methotrexate	Methotrexate
Paclitaxel	Taxol
Pertuzumab	Perjeta
Procarbazine	Natulan
Rituximab	Mabthera
Temozolomide	Temodal
Trabectedin	Yondelis
Trastuzumab	Herceptin (both ev and sc)
Trastuzumab emtansine	Kadcycla
Vinblastine	Velbe
Vincristine	Vincristine
Vinorelbine	Navelbine (both ev and oral)

Table 26.5 Target therapies

Drug	Target	Action	Indications	Cardiotoxicity	Nephrotoxicity	Indirect Nephrotoxicity	Chronic kidney disease patients	Dialysis patients
Imatinib	c-Kit BCR-ABL Receptors	Tyrosine kinase inhibitor	Chronic myeloid leukemia Gastrointestinal stromal tumors	**Common**: Edema Hypertension Heart Failure Pulmonary hypertension Tachycardia Pulmonary edema **Rare:** Arrhythmias Atrial fibrillation Cardiac angina/infarction Pericardial effusion	Hematuria Kidney Insufficiency Hypokalemia Hyperkalemia Hypomagnesemia	Diarrhea		
Dasatinib	BCR-ABL Receptor	Tyrosine kinase inhibitor	Chronic myeloid leukemia Gastrointestinal stromal tumors	**Common**: Edema Heart Failure Pericardial effusion Tachycardia **Rare:** Ventricular arrhythmias Increased QT interval Pulmonary hypertension Cardiac angina/infarction Ictus cerebri	Kidney Insufficiency Proteinuria	Nausea Vomiting Diarrhea Rabdomiolisis Hyperuricemia	No dose adjustment	

Table 26.5 (continued)

Drug	Target	Action	Indications	Cardiotoxicity	Nephrotoxicity	Indirect Nephrotoxicity	Chronic kidney disease patients	Dialysis patients
Trastuzumab Lapatinib	EGFR EGFR2 (HER2)	Protein kinase inhibitors	Breast cancer Metastatic gastric cancer	Hypertension Tachycardia Atrial flutter Ejection fraction reduction Heart failure Atrial arrhythmias Cardiomyopathy Pericardial effusion	Membranous nephropathy Kidney insufficiency	Nausea Vomiting Diarrhea	No dose adjustment	
Afatinib Erlotinib Gefitinib	EGFR	Receptors blockers	Lung cancer	Interaction with anticoagulant drugs and statins	Kidney insufficiency	Nausea Vomiting Diarrhea Anorexia	No dose adjustment Not recommended in patients with renal clearance <15 ml/m for Erlotinib and <30 ml/m for Afatinib	
Cetuximab Panitumumab	EGFR	Receptors blockers	Colorectal carcinoma	Deep vein thrombosis Cardiac ischemic disease and heart failure if associated with fluoropyrimidine	Hypomagnesemia Hypokalemia. Hypocalcemia (in association with cisplatin). Kidney insufficiency	Nausea Vomiting Diarrhea Anorexia	No dose adjustment	

Bevacizumab Aflibercept	VEGF	Anti-angiogenesis monoclonal antibodies	Metastatic colon–rectal carcinoma Metastatic renal carcinoma Breast cancer Lung cancer Ovarian carcinoma	Hypertension Arterial and venous thrombosis Heart failure (for bevacizumab).	Proteinuria Nephrotic Syndrome Kidney insufficiency Thrombotic microangiopathy	Nausea Vomiting Diarrhea	No dose adjustment	
Sunitinib Axitinib Pazopanib	VEGFR2	Tyrosine kinase inhibitor	Metastatic renal carcinoma Gastrointestinal stromal tumors	Hypertension Arterial and venous thrombosis Cardiomyopathya (for Sunitinib). Heart failure Increased QT interval	Chromaturia (for Sunitinib) Proteinuria Nephrotic Syndrome Acute kidney injury	Nausea Vomiting Diarrhea Rabdomiolisis	No dose adjustment	No dose adjustment
Sorafenib	VEGFR2 VEGFR-3, RET RET/PTC CRAF, BRAF BRAFV600E c-KIT FLT-3 PDGFR-β	Tyrosine kinase inhibitor	Hepatocellular carcinoma Renal carcinoma Differentiated thyroid carcinoma	Hypertension Cardiac angina/infarction Heart failure Interaction with Warfarin Prolungamento del QT Increased QT interval (rare)	Proteinuria Nephrotic Syndrome Acute kidney injury Hypocalcemia	Nausea Vomiting Diarrhea Rabdomiolisis	No dose adjustment	No data in literature
Cabozantinib	VEGFR2	Tyrosine kinase inhibitor	Medullary thyroid carcinoma not surgically treatable	Hypertension Atrial fibrillation Increased QT interval Cardiac angina Supraventricular tachycardia Thromboembolism Arterial thrombosis	Proteinuria Hematuria Dysuria Acute kidney injury	Nausea Vomiting Diarrhea Rabdomiolisis	Caution in patients with mild-moderate renal dysfunction	No data for severe chronic renal insufficiency and dialysis patients

(continued)

Table 26.5 (continued)

Drug	Target	Action	Indications	Cardiotoxicity	Nephrotoxicity	Indirect Nephrotoxicity	Chronic kidney disease patients	Dialysis patients
Everolimus Temsirolimus	mTOR	Serine threonine-protein kinase inhibitor	Breast cancer Neuroendocrine pancreatic tumors Renal carcinoma	Hypertension **Rare:** Heart failure Deep vein thrombosis	Proteinuria Mild renal dysfunction	Diarrhea Nausea High fever	No dose adjustment	No dose adjustment
Trametinib Cobimetinib	MEK	MEK inhibitor	Metastatic melanoma positive for BRAF V600	Hypertension Increased QT interval Reduced ejection fraction Retinal vein occlusion Deep vein thrombosis Pulmonary embolism	Glomerulonephritis (rare)	Nausea Vomiting Diarrhea High fever Rabdomiolisis Severe dehydration with acute kidney injury	No dose adjustment	No data in literature

c-Kit receptor overexpressed in gastrointestinal stromal tumors, *BCR-ABL R* Breakpoint cluster region Abelson receptor, *EGFR* Epithelial growth factor receptor, *VEGF* Vascular endothelial growth factor, *VEGFR* Vascular endothelial growth factor receptor, *BRAF* gene encoding for BRAF protein, *PDGFR* Platelet derived growth factor receptor, *mTOR*, Mammalian target of rapamycin, *MEK* protein kinase

26.3 Common Chemotherapeutic Regimen Adopted in the Clinical Practice According to Tumor Type

- Anal Cancer
  - 5-FU + mitomycin + radiotherapy (5-Fluorouracil + mitomycin + radiotherapy)
  - 5-FU+ cisplatin (5-Fluorouracil + cisplatin)
- Bone Cancer
  - VAC/IE (vincristine + doxorubicin + cyclophosphamide alternating with ifosfamide + etoposide)
  - VAI (vincristine + ifosfamide + dactinomycin + doxorubicin)
  - VIDE (vincristine + ifosfamide + doxorubicin + etoposide)
  - Docetaxel + gemcitabine (docetaxel + gemcitabine)
- Brain Tumors
  - Temozolomide (temozolamide)
  - Bevacizumab + irinotecan (Bevacizumab + irinotecan)
  - Combination PCV (lomustine + procarbazine + vincristine)
- Breast Cancer
  - CMF (cyclophosphamide + methotrexate + 5-Fluorouracil)
  - Dose dense AC followed by paclitaxel (doxorubicin + cyclophosphamide followed by paclitaxel)
  - EC (epirubicin + cyclophosphamide)
  - TC (docetaxel + cyclophosphamide)
  - TAC (docetaxel + doxorubicin + cyclophosphamide)
  - FEC followed by docetaxel (5-Fluorouracil + epirubicin + cyclophosphamide followed by docetaxel)
  - AC followed by paclitaxel with trastuzumab (doxorubicin + cyclophosphamide followed by paclitaxel with trastuzumab)
  - Pertuzumab Trastuzumab and docetaxel (pertuzumab + trastuzumab + docetaxel)
  - T-DM 1 (ado-Trastuzumab emtansine)
  - TCH (docetaxel + cyclophosphamide + trastuzumab)
  - Herceptin (trastuzumab)
  - Capecitabine (alone or together with lapatinib) 14 days/21 (2 weeks of therapy, 1 week off)
- Bladder Cancer
  - Gemcitabine + cisplatin (Gemcitabine + cisplatin)
  - MVAC (methotrexate + vinblastine + doxorubicin + cisplatin)
  - Cisplatin + paclitaxel (cisplatin + paclitaxel)
  - Gemcitabine + paclitaxel (gemcitabine + paclitaxel
- Gallbladder and Cholangiocarcinoma
  - Cisplatin + Gemcitabine (cisplatin + gemcitabine)
  - Capecitabine (capecitabine)
- Esophageal and Esophagogastric Junction Cancer
  - Cisplatin + 5-FU (cisplatin + 5-Fluorouracil)
  - Paclitaxel + carboplatin (paclitaxel + carboplatin)
  - ECF (epirubicin + cisplatin + 5-Fluorouracil)
- Gastric Cancer
  - ECF (epirubicin + cisplatin + 5-Fluorouracil)

  - DCF (docetaxel + cisplatin + 5-Fluorouracil)
  - Cisplatin + 5-FU + trastuzumab (cisplatin + 5-Fluorouracil + trastuzumab)
  - Xelox (capecitabine + oxaliplatin)
  - Folfox (5-Fluorouracil + Leucovorin + Oxaliplatin)
  - Folfiri (5-Fluorouracil + Oxaliplatin + Leucovorin + Irinotecan)
  - Ramucirumab + paclitaxel (ramucirumab + paclitaxel)
- Colorectal Cancer
  - Folfiri (5-Fluorouracil + Leucovorin + Irinotecan)
  - Folfiri + cetuximab (5-Fluorouracil + Leucovorin + Irinotecan + cetuximab)
  - Folfiri + bevacizumab (5-Fluorouracil + Leucovorin + Irinotecan + bevacizumab)
  - Folfox (5-Fluorouracil + Leucovorin + Oxaliplatin)
  - Folfiri + cetuximab (5-Fluorouracil + Leucovorin + Irinotecan + cetuximab)
  - Folfiri + bevacizumab (5-Fluorouracil + Leucovorin + Irinotecan + bevacizumab)
  - Folfoxiri + bevacizumab (5-Fluorouracil + Oxaliplatin + Leucovorin + Irinotecan + bevacizumab) Folfoxiri + cetuximab (5-Fluorouracil + Oxaliplatin + Leucovorin + Irinotecan + cetuximab)
  - Xelox (capecitabine + oxaliplatin)
  - Folfiri + aflibercept (5-Fluorouracil + Leucovorin + Irinotecan + aflibercept)
  - Cape Beva (capecitabine + bevacizumab)
  - 5-Fu/LVF (5-Fluorouracil + Leucovorin)
- Pancreatic Cancer
  - Folfirinox (5-Fluorouracil + Oxaliplatin + Leucovorin + Irinotecan+)
  - Albumin-bound paclitaxel + Gemcitabine (Nabpaclitaxel- Gemcitabine)
  - Gemox (Gemcitabine + oxaliplatin)
- Prostate Cancer
  - Docetaxel (Docetaxel)
  - Cabazitaxel (Cabazitaxel)
- Testicular cancer
  - PEB (Cisplatin + etoposide + Bleomicin)
  - PEI (Cisplatin + etoposide + Ifosfamide + mesna)
  - Carboplatin (carboplatin)
  - Gemox (Gemcitabine + oxaliplatin)
- Gynecologic Cancer
  - Carboplatin-paclitaxel (Carboplatin-Paclitaxel)
  - Carboplatin-paclitaxel + bevacizumab (Carboplatin-Paclitaxel + bevacizumab)
  - Caelyx-trabectedin (liposomial anthracycline-trabectedin)
  - Topotecan (topotecan)
  - Gemcitabine (gemcitabine)
  - TIP (Paclitaxel Cisplatin + Ifosfamide + mesna)
  - TAP (Paclitaxel + doxorubicin + Ifosfamide + mesna)
  - Cisplatin + doxorubicin (Cisplatin + doxorubicin)
- Head and Neck Cancer
  - All Sarraf (Cisplatin + 5-Fluorouracil)
  - Cisplatin + 5-Fluorouracil + cetuximab (Cisplatin + 5-Fluorouracil + cetuximab)

- Lung Cancer
  - PE (Cisplatin + Etoposide)
  - Cisplatin + gemcitabine (Cisplatin + Gemcitabine)
  - Cisplatin + docetaxel (Cisplatin + docetaxel)
  - Cisplatin + pemetrexed (Cisplatin + pemetrexed)
  - Carboplatin + paclitaxel (Carboplatin + paclitaxel)
  - Vinorelbine (vinorelbine)
  - Topotecan (topotecan)
  - Pemetrexed (pemetrexed)
- Sarcomas
  - Doxorubicin 90 mg/m^2 + Ifosfamide
  - Epirubicin + ifosfamide
  - Trabectedin (®Yondelis)
  - Gemcitabine
  - Taxol or Taxotere
- Lymphomas
  - CHOPP (Adriamycin 50 mg/m^2 + cyclophosphamide + vincristine + prednisone)
  - R-CHOPP: same as CHOPP + Rituximab
  - MOPP: Mustargen, vincristine, procarbazine, prednisone
  - ABVD: (Adriamycin 25 mg/m^2 + bleomycin + vinblastine + dacarbazine) given day 1 and day 15 of each course
  - Stanford V: Doxorubicin 25 mg/m^2 (days 1 and 15) + Vinblastine + Mechlorethamine + Vincristine + Etoposide + prednisone

Suggested readings and sites to visit; Fournier L, Ammari S, Thiam R, Cuénod CA. Imaging criteria for assessing tumour response: RECIST, mRECIST, Cheson. Diagn Interv Imaging. 2014;95:689–703. NCCN Clinical Practice Guidelines in Oncology at ► www.nccn.org/professionals/...gls/f_guidelines.asp ► https://www.cancer.gov/about-cancer/treatment/drugs ► http://chemocare.com/chemotherapy/acronyms/default.aspx

What the Oncologist Needs to Know: How to Ask for a Cardiology Consultation

Paolo Spallarossa and Matteo Sarocchi

C. Lestuzzi et al. (eds.), *Manual of Cardio-oncology*, DOI 10.1007/978-3-319-40236-9_27

Oncologists require the intervention of a cardiologist to prevent, identify, and treat the cardiovascular complication related to cancer and cancer treatment. In the near future, the need for a cardiologic consultation for cancer patients might increase. This could be related to epidemiological consideration:

- Thanks to the lifesaving anticancer treatment, long-term cancer survivor (either cancer-free or with cancer as a chronic disease) is an increasing population to take care of [1].
- Patients treated for malignancies are subject to an increased risk of comorbidities and complications, including the cardiovascular ones.
- Cardiotoxicity may worsen the health of cancer patients both during and after the treatment.
- Apart from cardiotoxicity, patients undergoing treatment for malignancies may exhibit a concomitant cardiovascular disease too. Risk factors overlap in cardiovascular and neoplastic diseases. Both relate to diabetes, smoking, overweight, and aging.

Before looking at what the cardiologist needs to know and how to transmit it, let us consider *when* a cardio-oncologic consultation is indicated and, especially, *why*.

27.1 When and Why to Ask for a Cardiologic Consultation

27.1.1 Timing of the Consultation

- Before initiating the anticancer treatment
- After the initiation
  - During the treatment
  - Treatment end
  - Later after treatment (possible late cardiotoxicity, additional treatment)

27.1.2 Different Situations for a Consultation

- Cardiovascular screening in patients with unknown CV disease (prevention, early diagnosis).
- Actual status evaluation (clinical, instrumental, therapy) of a previously known CV disease.
- Evaluate if a sign, symptom, or an instrumental abnormality may indicate a cardiovascular disease.
- Follow-up.

27.1.3 Asking a Consultation Before Initiating Anticancer Treatment

No definite recommendation establishes which patients require a first cardio-oncologic evaluation before undergoing anticancer therapy. The actual general trend is to ask for a consultation only for patients with high cardiovascular risk, concomitant cardiovascular disease, or undergoing significantly cardiotoxic treatments, but this limitation is questionable. In this matter, it is important to consider what is the key question.

27.1.4 What Is the Key Question?

If the question is whether to exclude contraindication to anticancer therapy, a cardiologic visit could be unnecessary for many patients. It is a fact that only a minority of pretreatment consultations end with a contraindication to anticancer therapies.

- Many patients are "low risk," and in the short to midterm only a minority of them will develop significant cardiovascular disease.
- In high-risk patients, a safety concern about the treatment very rarely overcomes the expected benefit: oncologic treatments are often lifesaving.

Otherwise, if the question is more comprehensive, pointing out the current cardiovascular status and the risk of complications over the entire pretreatment period and providing information for risk management, a cardiologic consultation may be useful for most patients.

- Even if the risk of cardiovascular adverse event is low, or not so high, compared to the treatment benefit, it may be reduced.
- Previous cardiovascular disease, even if stable, may require treatment modification optimized for cardiotoxicity prevention and side effect reduction.
- The consultation has a screening value. Any unknown preexisting cardiovascular disease discovered when anticancer treatment is already ongoing may raise concern and anxiety even if the diagnosis has mild clinical impact. Any cardiac complication occurring during cancer treatment may be harder to manage if a cardiologist has not previously forecast it.

> **A cardiologic consultation before initiating anticancer therapy is useful for most patients, including those with low risk of cardiotoxicity or predominating indication of anticancer treatment.**

27.2 How to Ask the First Cardio-oncologic Consult: What the Cardiologist Needs to Know in Evaluating the Patient for the First Time

The consultation should be tailored on the clinical circumstances. Thus, the oncologist should provide some oncologic information.

- **Malignancy and its prognosis.** A general description of the cancer should be provided, but more important is the interpretation of its severity. A cardiologist may find difficult to consider the prognostic implications of many details like stage, clinical presentation, histology, and molecular phenotype. The aim should be to let the cardiologist know the oncologic prognosis and impact of the treatment on it.
- **Antineoplastic treatment regimen**, including drugs combination, and radiotherapy. Different treatments have different risks, like heart failure, myocardial ischemia, thrombosis, arrhythmia, pericarditis, and hypertension [2]; moreover, the risk may be higher for specific combinations.
- **Previous anticancer treatment exposure.** The patient may underreport it. Whoever received a treatment with potentially cardiotoxic drugs is "HF class A" according to the AHA/ACC guidelines on heart failure. Chest radiation therapy increases the risk of valve degeneration and coronary disease many years after exposure.

- Forecast if the treatment could induce any *non-cardiovascular complication*. Dehydration, immune depression, pancytopenia, anemia, and ion imbalance must be considered as critical factors in exacerbating cardiovascular disease.
- *Patient enrolled in clinical trials*. Some of them withstand to strict rules about concomitant medications and clinical events monitoring. In addition, experimental anticancer treatments may bring unknown risk.

What the cardiologist needs to know is an exhaustive description of the malignancy, its past, actual and revised management, and the oncologic prognosis.

Obviously, in clinical practice there are some limitations. Some data are not always available or computable. Sometimes it is difficult to quantify the prognosis and to explain it. Not only clinicians will read the request but also the patient himself.

When requesting the consultation, the oncologist does not need to describe all the cardiovascular anamnesis, even if a brief anamnestic summary may be useful. It is more important to highlight if any new cardiologic fact or suspect were found. The cardiologist will collect an exhaustive cardiovascular anamnesis by himself, but he requires examining any documentation available.

The oncologist must request the patient to bring all the results of previous exams, visits, and discharge letters, with particular interest for ECG traces and imaging supports like coronary angiography, echocardiography, cardiac TC, and MRI.

Echocardiography is useful in many cases: it should be required on the basis of symptoms, signs (like cardiac murmur), or personal history or when a specific cardiotoxicity risk requires programmed screening, for example, for trastuzumab treatment [3].

27.3 Consultation for a Suspected Cardiovascular Problem

During or after anticancer treatment, the occurrence of a cardiovascular problem very often requires a consultation. With the term “cardiovascular problem,” the oncologist may refer not only to “cardiotoxicity” but to a widespread of signs, symptoms, and lab abnormalities (including atypical) that may rise even mild suspect of a cardiovascular issue.

27.3.1 When Reporting a Suspected Cardiovascular Problem the Oncologist Has to Focus on

- New symptoms: chest pain, dyspnea, dizziness, palpitation, fatigue, and syncope
- Objective signs: cardiac murmur, edema, pulmonary rales, pleural effusion, blood pressure, heart rate and rhythm, etc.
- Instrumental abnormalities: chest radiography images, CT scan pericardial effusion, and aortic dilation, raised cardiac biomarkers and D-dimer, anemia, reduced glomerular filtration, and ion imbalance

No long description of the cardiovascular anamnesis is required, but only few words to report the main previous cardiovascular diagnosis and procedures.

27.3.2 The Oncologist Should Also Report to the Cardiologist in Order to Help the Differential Diagnosis

- The chronologic relationship with treatments.
- Other noncardiac abnormalities. The oncologist could be aware of alterations that may simulate even typical cardiac symptoms that may reduce the "pretest" probability of a cardiovascular disease.

The oncologist should underline if the sign, symptom, or lab abnormality may have an alternative non-cardiovascular explanation for the specific patient.

It is useful to report whether the clinician took any clinical action (and the response to it): treatment interruption, medication, laboratory or imaging tests, and hospitalization.

27.4 Asking a Cardiovascular Follow-Up

A second visit may be made in asymptomatic, well-being patients, aimed at identifying preclinical alteration and allowing secondary prevention. Some groups of high-risk patients, as anthracycline-trastuzumab exposed, require prespecified strategies. Instead, for the single patient the course may be personalized. For specific groups of patients like those exposed to anthracycline, chest irradiation, and bone marrow transplant, the risk of late cardiotoxicity suggests a long-term cardiologic reevaluation, years after exposure.

Follow-up programs could be previously discussed in a multidisciplinary meeting.

Screening and prevention are "first-line" practices, and their practical application greatly depends on the physician who primarily takes care of the patient. Thus, oncologists should be actively involved in any cardiovascular prevention strategy for their patients, by asking for a consultation and providing some useful information:
- The time since last treatment
- The oncologic situation
- Any supportive therapy, even if not specifically "chemotherapy," including indication of cumulative blood-cell transfusion, if performed

The oncologist should be aware that for some patients (high risk or previous evidence of cardiotoxicity), the need of follow-up lasts for many years. Remember that losing a patient at follow-up is potentially harmful. When a patient is already on follow-up for malignancy, the oncologist should keep the link between the patient and the cardiologist [4].

The cardiologist needs to know when the patient is nearing to the end of oncologic course or diluting it. Thus, he will take care of the cardiovascular follow-up program.

27.5 How to Help the Cardiologist to Implement Cardiovascular Treatment

The risk of side effects of medications increases in such frail patients as those with malignancy. In addition, in patients with ongoing anticancer treatment, the impact of adverse event doubles, considering that an adverse event may lead to unwanted suspension of anticancer treatment. It is evident that a great effort is required to achieve an optimal safety when introducing a cardiovascular drug, with potentially harmful hemodynamic effects, bleeding risk, pro-arrhythmic potential, and liver or kidney injury.

The oncologist who starts any anticancer treatment or encounters any cancer and cancer treatment complication may develop concerns about other therapies including the cardiovascular ones. He could raise a fundamental question: "can I withdraw a cardiovascular drug or substitute it?"

27.6 Helping the Management of Cardiovascular Treatment: What the Cardiologist Has to Know?

- Explain if any concern with the cardiovascular drugs is actual or potential; reduced platelet count in anti-aggregated patient may serve as example: if the reduction is chronic and mild, the risk of bleeding could be managed with strict monitoring of the count if aspirin is mandatory. Conversely, a rapid reduction of the platelet may require preventive suspension of antiplatelet drug.
  - If the problem is *actually* suspected for being related with any cardiovascular medication, it is important to underline if an alternative explanation coexists.
  - If the problem is only a *potential* risk of adverse event, point out how high is the risk and related to what and whether any acceptable alternative exists or not to avoid the change in cardiovascular medication.
- Underline if the oncologic situation raising the concern could be reversible; thus, the cardiologist will consider a subsequent rechallenge of the cardiovascular medication.

That seen, oncologists may help greatly the decisional process leading to cardiovascular treatment. They can contribute to foresee and reduce the risk of side effects, providing information in the request.

27.7 Some Practical Considerations

Oncologist should consider to whom the request is addressed and write it consequently.

Ideally, the addressee of the request for cardio-oncologic consultation is "the cardio-oncologist," a cardiologist experienced in caring of patients with malignancy.

This skill goes far beyond the knowledge of cardiotoxicity: it includes an expanded sensibility for any issue complicating the patient's wellness. Concepts like prognosis, adverse events, and treatment goal may be differently experienced by Oncologist and Cardiologist.

In this era, many cardiologists are in the first period of their oncologic collaboration. On the other side, some patients may require their personal cardiologist. These figures are not expected to have the aforementioned practice of cardio-oncology. Talking about cancer patients, a cardiologist needs more details than a "cardio-oncologist." Even in the fortunate condition of writing to a dedicated physician, the oncologist should keep in mind a long learning curve. Only when speaking to a known cardio-oncologist, the oncologist will be allowed to save a couple of words.

The information included in any request gains an "educational" value beyond the single clinical case, contributing to formation of a future cardio-oncologist.

To facilitate comprehension, especially speaking to physicians with different professional background like cardiologists, the oncologist should be:

- Exhaustive. Incomplete information could be more dangerous than none (the absence induces research).
- Explicit. Tacit consideration from the oncologist may be unperceived from the cardiologist.
- Clear. We recommend avoiding abbreviations and acronyms.

To grant a minimal standard for data transfer, the development of an ultra-brief request form is advisable. This might also keep some data (like "technical" prognostic consideration) apart from the oncologic visit result.

Discussion on critical prognosis raises particular difficulties and requires direct multidisciplinary discussion, and the oncologist may favor to do it apart from the presence of the patient (even for ethical reasons). This wish should be specified when making the request.

This is not the only situation for such a request. Obviously the cardiologist wishes to visit the patient directly, and this should sound a little pleonastic. However, the patient's presence is unnecessary in some cases, for example, when discussing instrumental results. Avoiding a visit reduces discomfort to patients (and caregivers): some of them are not autonomous to reach the clinic or hospital or make long transfers.

Afterwards, the result of the consultation will be registered and communicated to the patient.

In conclusion, the request for a cardio-oncologic consultation should fit to the needs of cardiologist, oncologist, and patient too. How to write it clearly depends on when it is requested and why, to whom, and even where. A well-done request is the first step for a good consultation.

References

1. DeSantis CE, Lin CC, Mariotto AB, Siegel RL, Stein KD, Kramer JL, Alteri R, Robbins AS, Jemal A. Cancer treatment and survivorship statistics, 2014. CA Cancer J Clin. 2014 Jul-Aug;64(4):252–71.
2. Yeh ET, Bickford CL. Cardiovascular complications of cancer therapy: incidence, pathogenesis, diagnosis, and management. J Am Coll Cardiol. 2009 Jun 16;53(24):2231–47.
3. Plana JC, Galderisi M, Barac A, Ewer MS, Ky B, Scherrer-Crosbie M, Ganame J, Sebag IA, Agler DA, Badano LP, Banchs J, Cardinale D, Carver J, Cerqueira M, DeCara JM, Edvardsen T, Flamm SD, Force T, Griffin BP, Jerusalem G, Liu JE, Magalh„es A, Marwick T, Sanchez LY, Sicari R, Villarraga HR, Lancellotti P. Expert consensus for multimodality imaging evaluation of adult patients during and after cancer therapy: a report from the American Society of Echocardiography and the European Association of Cardiovascular Imaging. Eur Heart J Cardiovasc Imaging. 2014 Oct;15(10):1063-93.
4. Herrmann J, Lerman A, Sandhu NP, Villarraga HR, Mulvagh SL, Kohli M. Evaluation and management of patients with heart disease and cancer: cardio-oncology. Mayo Clin Proc. 2014 Sep;89(9):1287–306.

What the Cardiologist Needs to Know: How to Write the Consultation

Paolo Spallarossa and Matteo Sarocchi

C. Lestuzzi et al. (eds.), *Manual of Cardio-oncology*, DOI 10.1007/978-3-319-40236-9_28

The oncologist may require the help of the cardiologist for different reasons. Sometimes he suspects a cardiovascular problem, in general he wants to reduce complications of a cardio-toxic treatment, and, in most cases, he will find useful to have a "portrait" of the patient's actual cardiovascular status.

The cardiologist has to deal with a variety of cardiovascular issues, related or not to cancer and cancer treatment.

The cardiologist's opinion may be required even with no evidence of specific cardiovascular problem in the patient. He will be able to better exclude any cardiac disease and prevent cardio-toxicity.

The answer of the cardiologist should consider two points of view: the pure cardiological one and the relative perspective deriving from the oncologic treatments and the malignancy itself. It is very important to find each evaluation in the consultation report, integrated without strong dichotomy.

Apart from specific content, the cardio-oncologic visit is still similar in its framework to any cardiological one. We can summarise it in some key points:

- Reason for the consultation
- Non-cardiological anamnesis, with special attention for the oncologic one
- Cardiological anamnesis
  - Derived from documentation
  - Directly acquired from the patient
- Pharmacological anamnesis
- Symptoms
- Signs (physical examination during the visit)
- Actual instrumental results
- Conclusions: Cardiological interpretation
  - Presence/absence of cardiovascular disease
  - Severity of the disease
  - Eventual prognosis
- Conclusions: Cardio-oncologic considerations
  - Suspect of cardio-toxicity
  - Safety of purposed antineoplastic treatment
  - Prevention of cardio-toxicity
- Suggestions for management
  - Cardiovascular treatment
  - Consider antineoplastic treatment variation
  - Additional exams and invasive cardiological procedures

28.1 Background: Clinical Facts Acquired in the Visit

The first part of the report should include a summary of the clinical facts collected and evaluated, including both the cardiovascular and oncologic ones. The cardiologist should describe all the data he has worked on and that have allowed him/her to come to the conclusions. It is very important to make an adequate description of the oncologic anamnesis, even if the oncologist is supposed to know it optimally. A good reason to spend a little more time for this task is that possible misunderstandings may have occurred when the cardiologist has evaluated non-cardiological data, leading to inappropriate conclusions. If the oncologist, reading the consultation, finds that it has been based on wrong or inconsistent data, or that important oncologic facts have been missed, then he will require a re-evaluation.

Not only the cardiological data but also the oncologic ones should be adequately described, even if the oncologist, obviously, knows it. This practice ensures that the cardiological evaluation is coherent with the oncologic situation.

The main oncologic facts to report are:
- Oncologic or haematological diagnosis and indications about its severity, like stage and prognostic markers
- Antineoplastic treatments, including past, actual and expected ones
  - Pharmacological treatment
  - Radiotherapy
  - Therapeutic procedures and supportive cares (stem cell transplant, blood transfusion)
- Collateral facts
  - Side effects and their treatment
  - Procedures (biopsies, permanent catheter implantation)

After that, the cardiologist will proceed in collecting the cardiovascular anamnesis and symptoms, performing the physical examination and evaluating the recent instrumental exams. He will have to point out any news, for example, if the ECG or the physical examination is changed or the patient reports any symptom or anamnestic data that the oncologist could have missed. He will underline any suspicion that some relevant cardiovascular documentation is unavailable.

The availability of clinical documentation is very important, especially during the first cardio-oncologic visit. It helps the correct clinical evaluation and may reduce additional exams.

28.2 Conclusions: Cardiological Interpretation

The second part of the report is dedicated to the interpretation of the clinical data. Here any suspected or definite cardiovascular diagnosis should stand out and, in the absence of those, the cardiovascular risk. When the cardiologist describes the cardiovascular status of the patient, he should remember to inform the oncologist about:
- Actual severity of the cardiovascular disease or risk
- Possible future evolution and worsening (at first, independently from cancer and cancer treatment)
- Theoretical approach to the disease, as in a cancer-free patient

An initial "pure" cardiological description of the clinical status is propaedeutic to subsequent cardio-oncologic evaluation.

The oncologist needs an adequate description of the cardiovascular disease, enhanced by an expert interpretation. Any alteration in heart structure, ECG, biomarkers or the clinical presentation may have a broad spectrum of severity. Atrial fibrillation, for example, has different implications based on the coexistence of structural heart disease, heart failure, stroke or uncontrolled heart rate. Oncologist may be drawn to consider low ejection fraction as the main contraindication for cardio-toxic drugs, but the cardiologist will help him not to underestimate a minor reduction, in the presence of ventricular hypertrophy or any significant haemodynamic overload like valve regurgitation or stenosis [1].

In addition, the oncologist needs to know the probability that the clinical situation of the patient will require an invasive procedure or intervention, sooner or later.

28.3 Cardiological Suggestions in the Cancer Patient

In this paragraph we will discuss some of the typical situations that may require particular collaboration between the cardiologist and the oncologist:

- Prescription of cardiovascular drugs
- Requirement of additional exams
- Cardiological invasive procedures
- Variation of oncologic treatment

The cardiologist should submit any nonurgent decision to the oncologist, before translating it into actions, allowing a second evaluation of its compatibility with the oncologic needs. At the same time, in order to be effective, the cardiologist should point out the importance of the cardiovascular intervention, explaining the reason and the strength of the indication. A similar approach should guide the relations with the patient, who may have a reduced compliance to additional medical treatments, for understandable reasons related to physical and psychological effects of malignancy. The clinician should be willing to consider the patient's wishes. The informed consent is the prerequisite for any decision; the patient should receive adequate information on the risk related to some cardiovascular exams, medications and procedures and the risk of not pursuing them. This last information is mandatory when the patient refuses a cardiological exam or treatment.

28.3.1 Drug Prescription

Cardiovascular drugs are not free from side effects. When prescribing new medications, the cardiologist must be aware that cancer patients are prone to develop side effects, for various reasons:

- The pain and anxiety related to malignancy amplifies symptoms.
- Renal and hepatic impairment may be a problem during cancer treatment. Some cardiovascular drugs may worsen it.
- Anaemia and cancer-related fatigue may reduce beta-blockers tolerability.
- Normotensive cancer patients are more susceptible to side effects from haemodynamically active drugs like RAAS-inhibitors and beta-blockers, prescribed for primary or secondary prevention of left ventricular dysfunction.
- Patients often receive multiple drugs, to treat cancer and to control symptoms and side effects of chemotherapy. Polypharmacotherapy is prone to an exponentially higher incidence of side effects, due to interactions.

The containment of side effects is mandatory in cancer patients in order to avoid a loss of compliance and possible oncologic treatment discontinuation. Although some cardiovascular medications have a proven cardioprotective effect, their extensive use is still controversial in literature [2]. Prescribing drugs to cancer patients, the cardiologist will follow some basic principles:

- Start the cardiovascular treatment (in particular the haemodynamically active ones) at the lowest dose if a strong intervention is not mandatory.
- Titrate the drug gradually when necessary. Make the target of the treatment explicit, fitting for the specific patients (BP, HR, LDL) and suggest how to reach it. Plan a mid-term strategy of intervention whenever possible, for example, a step-by-step introduction of antihypertensive medications. This will help the oncologist and may save unnecessary visits to the patient.
- Forecast the typical side effects of the introduced drug, and suggest strategy to contain them.

28.3.2 Cardiovascular Exams and Invasive Procedures

A risk-benefit evaluation is the basis of a good clinical practice. A valid rule is to require exams when the result may have significant clinical consequences and to avoid those that probably will not lead to changes in the cardiological or oncologic management.

However, patients undergoing some high risk oncological procedures like stem cell transplant, may require cardiovascular exams or treatments that usually are not performed in non-cancer patient with the same cardiovascular situation. The "watchful-waiting" strategy is not always the best choice in patients that may develop other complications in a near future, thus reducing the possibility of a cardiovascular intervention.

The safety of the oncologic treatment itself may justify insisted diagnostics or anticipated intervention in order to avoid cardiovascular complications afterwards.

When taking care of cancer patients, the cardiologist should be even more careful to propose any diagnostic or interventional procedure.

Biomarkers and echocardiography are easily performed by a well-organised team, with minimal or no impact on the oncologic programme and virtually no risk to the patient. They provide important additional information for a cardiovascular diagnosis and risk stratification [3, 4].

Other useful low risk exams like cardiac TC or NMR may cause a postponement of oncologic treatment, especially where these exams are poorly available. Such a delay may be detrimental for the patient health.

Provocative tests and, especially, invasive procedures bring an intrinsic risk of complications for the patient. This may be even greater for cancer patients. The clinician will also consider the unfavourable effect of hospitalisation required for some procedures. In some cases, the cardiologist will consider the TC-scan as a good alternative to coronary angiography, especially if he/she needs to exclude a significant disease that may worsen with the anticancer treatment, while the opportunity of a coronary intervention is lowered by the oncologic situation. Obviously, in the case of unstable or high-risk cardiovascular disease, the oncologist should be made aware of the importance of the cardiovascular intervention, even if it induces a delay in oncologic programmes.

A good practice is to inform the oncologist about:

- The reason for the proposed exam, including the risk of not performing it.
- The implication of exam result. The cardiologist may forecast what he will consider as "good" or "not good". This helps the oncologist to understand the importance of the exam, to interpret the result and possibly to save time for re-evaluation. A brief telephonic consult is still advisable when the result is received, for confirmation.
- Advice about the best and fastest way to achieve the result. The aim is to reduce the impact on both patient life and oncologic needs.
- Whenever hospitalisation is required, clinical objectives and programmes should be specified. This will also help other colleagues implicated in the cardiological management, for example, interventional cardiologists.

28.3.3 Anticancer Treatment Discontinuation for Cardio-toxicity

The cardiologist should rarely put absolute contraindications to the optimal anticancer treatment. It is advisable to allow the oncologist to make a second evaluation about the risk-benefit of a life-saving treatment, being aware of the cardiovascular situation. When the suspension or variation of the treatment regimen is strongly advisable, it is a good practice to programme a short-term re-evaluation, leaving the possibility of a re-challenge, if feasible. The severity of the possible cardiovascular complications should be underlined, but avoiding demonization of anticancer medications, especially with the patient.

Sometimes it is possible to continue the oncologic treatment, with the caveat of an increased risk. The cardiologist should carefully inform the patient and the oncologist about the risk and how to minimise it.

- Propose a strategy for early identification of cardiological worsening.
  - Forecast if signs or symptoms are expected to be a warning, in order to speed up a clinical re-evaluation.
  - Plan a cardiological follow-up including physical examination, biomarkers and echocardiography.
- Suggest the introduction of cardioprotective agent (like carvedilol) or the use of a different formulation of the anticancer drug (like liposomal anthracycline) may be strongly recommended for a reasonably safe continuation of the treatment, but in severe conditions a suspension of the cardio-toxic drug is almost mandatory. A second-time re-challenge of a life-saving anticancer treatment should be contemplated, with explicit indication of a high cardiovascular risk.

28.4 The Equilibrium Between Cardiological and Oncologic Needs

The consultation will integrate the cardiovascular status with oncologic conditions. A definite cardiological opinion should fairly emerge in the result, with conclusive indications if possible. At the same time, the cardiologist should write these indications to the oncologist in the form of suggestions, not constrictions, always leaving him the possibility of challenging them for oncologic needs.

Since anticancer drugs are life-saving, the target is to find the best compromise in managing cardiovascular side effects without limiting the optimal anticancer treatment, thus granting most benefits to the patient. The aim of the cardiological consultation is not to avoid cardio-toxicity at any cost.

This is probably the most difficult role of the cardiologist in this setting: to be able to variate from typical cardiological behaviour, accepting the responsibilities of an increased cardiovascular risk at the service of the more comprehensive patient health [5].

28.5 Messages to the Patient

The cardiological consultation is not only part of a talk between the cardiologist and the oncologist. It is an important moment in the relation with the patient. Ethically, the cardiologist should explain any diagnosis and discuss any decision with the patient. This practice will reduce misunderstandings, fear and anxiety when the patient reads the consultation result. In addition, the oncologist's work will be easier in explaining the reason of any clinical intervention related to the cardiovascular status.

Some clinical suggestions imply the patient collaboration in monitoring blood pressure, symptoms and signs (e.g. oedema, nocturia, weight gain, haemorrhages). The cardiologist should explain how to perform those checks directly to the patient and write it understandably.

References

1. Spallarossa P, Maurea N, Cadeddu C, Madonna R, Mele D, Monte I, Novo G, Pagliaro P, Pepe A, Tocchetti CG, Zito C, Mercuro G. A recommended practical approach to the management of anthracycline-based chemotherapy cardiotoxicity: an opinion paper of the working group on drug cardiotoxicity and cardioprotection, Italian Society of Cardiology. J Cardiovasc Med (Hagerstown). 2016 May;17 Suppl 1:S84–92.
2. Plana JC, Galderisi M, Barac A, Ewer MS, Ky B, Scherrer-Crosbie M, Ganame J, Sebag IA, Agler DA, Badano LP, Banchs J, Cardinale D, Carver J, Cerqueira M, DeCara JM, Edvardsen T, Flamm SD, Force T, Griffin BP, Jerusalem G, Liu JE, Magalh„es A, Marwick T, Sanchez LY, Sicari R, Villarraga HR, Lancellotti P. Expert consensus for multimodality imaging evaluation of adult patients during and after cancer therapy: a report from the American Society of Echocardiography and the European Association of Cardiovascular Imaging. Eur Heart J Cardiovasc Imaging. 2014 Oct;15(10):1063–93.
3. Curigliano G, Cardinale D, Suter T, Plataniotis G, de Azambuja E, Sandri MT, Criscitiello C, Goldhirsch A, Cipolla C, Roila F; ESMO Guidelines Working Group. Cardiovascular toxicity induced by chemotherapy, targeted agents and radiotherapy: ESMO Clinical Practice Guidelines. Ann Oncol. 2012 Oct;23 Suppl 7:vii155–66.
4. Colombo A, Sandri MT, Salvatici M, Cipolla CM, Cardinale D. Cardiac complications of chemotherapy: role of biomarkers. Curr Treat Options Cardiovasc Med. 2014 Jun;16(6):313.
5. Suter TM, Ewer MS. Cancer drugs and the heart: importance and management. Eur Heart J. 2013 Apr;34(15):1102–11.

What the General Practitioner Needs to Know: When to Consult the Cardiologist and/or the Oncologist

Chiara Lestuzzi, Olivia Maria Thomas, Maria Agnese Caggegi, and Francesco Ferraù

C. Lestuzzi et al. (eds.), *Manual of Cardio-oncology*, DOI 10.1007/978-3-319-40236-9_29

29.1 Introduction

- Most patients undergoing antineoplastic treatments with anthracyclines and trastuzumab—well known to be potentially cardiotoxic—have a cardiology follow-up planned by the oncologists. Any obvious side effects occurring during treatments administered in hospital or in the day hospital unit will be referred to the local cardiologist.
- In an ideal world, every hospital with an oncology department has one or more cardiologists to whom they can refer patients, and routine cardiology exams may be planned to coincide with the patient's stay in the oncology ward. However, this is not possible in many hospitals.
  - In large hospitals with a crowded emergency department, a coronary intensive care unit and where cardiac surgery is performed, there are often limited resources for planning and performing a large number of routine 3–6-month echocardiograms, which are required in order to monitor the cardiac function of patients undergoing antineoplastic treatment.
  - In oncological referral centres with patients coming from far away, it may be difficult to plan all the check-up tests and investigations in 1 day. Patients undergoing chemotherapy usually go to the referring hospital every 3 or 6 weeks, and it may be difficult for these patients to come back for an additional visit in the event of new problems emerging before the planned follow-up.

The general practitioner might have to cope with cardiac problems related to the antineoplastic treatments or to the cancer itself in the following cases:

1. Patients followed by oncology departments with limited access to cardiology facilities
2. Outpatient treatments
   a. Oral treatments
   b. Long-lasting infusions with portable pumps
3. Thromboembolic events or other unpredicted side effects occurring at home
4. Delayed effects of treatments in patients who have been cured from cancer and are no longer in the care of the oncology department:
   a. Radiotherapy
   b. Hormonal treatments
   c. Platinum-based therapy for testicular cancer
5. Prescription of drugs which could interfere with the oncological treatments
6. Other acute problems common in cancer patients

29.1.1 What the General Practitioner Can Do to Solve These Problems

- The general practitioner should be aware of the antineoplastic treatments which require cardiologic screening/follow-up: drugs which can cause left ventricular dysfunction, cardiac ischaemia and thromboembolic diseases (see chapters 6–14 for more detailed information). If the follow-up has not already been done in the hospital where the oncological treatments are given, the patient should be referred to a local cardiologist.

- If the patient is receiving treatment as an outpatient, the adverse effects are usually referred to his/her general practitioner. The GP should be aware of the risk of:
  - Cardiac ischaemia during treatments with fluoropyrimidines (fluorouracil and capecitabine) and vascular endothelial growth factor inhibitors (VEGFI) (bevacizumab, sunitinib, sorafenib and other drugs mostly used in the treatment of renal cell or gastrointestinal carcinomas (see chapter…). Any new symptom potentially related to angina should be carefully assessed, and the patient should be referred as soon as possible to the cardiologist.
  - Severe hypertension during treatments with VEGFI. Blood pressure should be monitored regularly and promptly treated.
  - Some antineoplastic drugs may induce atrial fibrillation or ventricular arrhythmia. Any change in heart rhythm, or any complaint of palpitations, is worth investigating with an electrocardiogram. In case of ventricular arrhythmias, check for any electrolyte imbalance, and ask for a cardiologist's review.
- In patients at high risk of *thromboembolic disorders*, see also ▶ Chap. 5.
  - The appearance of leg oedema (with/without pain or local signs of inflammation) should raise suspicion of a *deep-vein thrombosis* (DVT).
  - The appearance of jugular vein distension and/or face oedema should raise suspicion of a superior vena cava thrombosis (more likely in presence of intrathoracic masses or central vein infusion catheters).
  - If the patient has a rapidly worsening dyspnoea, or new symptoms of dyspnoea and unexplained tachycardia, a pulmonary embolism should be suspected.
  - It is not always easy to diagnose a DVT, particularly in patients in the terminal phase of their illness, nor is the decision to treat such patients with a DVT straightforward.

29.2 Deep-Vein Thrombosis (DVT)

29.2.1 Diagnosis

There is little use in continuing with diagnostic procedures if a patient, due to the stage of their disease, is not a suitable candidate to commence anticoagulant therapy. Anticoagulant therapy is associated with risks as well as benefits; therefore, these must be weighed up in each individual case on the basis of prognosis, haemorrhagic risk, possibility of controlling symptoms and offering a good quality of life even without anticoagulants and patient compliance [1].

Colour Doppler Ultrasound:
High accuracy for proximal and distal DVT (questionable for an isolated distal DVT)
Requires sending the patient to a vascular ultrasound clinic

Compression Ultrasound:
Noninvasive, no exposure to ionising radiation, easily reproducible
Can be performed at the bedside of the patient and/or at the patient's home if a portable ultrasound machine is available and a trained member of the palliative care team or trained GP is available
High accuracy for a first presentation of a proximal DVT in symptomatic patients (patients with a history of ipsilateral DVTs retain a proximal residual incompressible vein)

D-dimer:
Its use is limited in oncological patients due to the elevated number of false positives encountered in neoplastic disease.

29.2.2 Treatment

Palliative care patients have additional risk factors:
1. Disseminated intravascular coagulation (DIC)
2. Coagulation factor deficiency
3. Platelet dysfunction/thrombocytopenia
4. Vascular tumours
5. Hepatic metastases
   - Useful General Measures
   - Elevation of the lower limbs
   - Analgesics (NSAIDs can increase haemorrhagic risk)
   - Compression stockings (if tolerated)

29.2.3 Recurrent DVTs in Cancer Patients

Patients that develop recurring DVTs despite an adequate anticoagulant therapy must be investigated to exclude disease progression.

Cancer patients have triple the risk of developing recurring DVTs and of bleeding whilst on anticoagulant therapy with vitamin K antagonists compared to non-cancer patients [2]. Patients on long-term vitamin K antagonist anticoagulant therapy who develop a DVT with a subtherapeutic INR can be treated with low molecular weight heparin (LMWH) or unfractionated heparin (UFH) until a stable INR between 2.0 and 3.0 is achieved with vitamin K antagonists. If the DVT recurs with an INR within the therapeutic range, there are two options available:
1. Switch to an alternative anticoagulation method, such as subcutaneous (sc) UFH maintaining a therapeutic range (aPTT ratio 1.5–2.5) or with a weight-adjusted dose of LMWH.
2. Increase the INR (target 3.5). This option can be dangerous due to the elevated bleeding risk in cancer patients.

Full-dose LMWH (200 U/kg once daily) can be reinstated in patients with a recurrent DVT, whilst they also receive long-term low-dose LMWH or a vitamin K antagonist. A second episode of DVT occurs in 9 % of these patients in whom this treatment strategy is well tolerated with few haemorrhagic complications [3].

In palliative care, long-term LMWH should represent the first line of treatment.

29.2.4 DVT Prevention

- Medical bedridden patients: Prophylaxis with UFH, LMWH or fondaparinux is advised in bedridden oncological patients and/or patients with an acute medical complication [4].

- Patients undergoing palliative chemotherapy for locally advanced or metastatic disease as outpatients:
  - Routine prophylaxis is not recommended in patients with advanced-stage disease who are undergoing chemotherapy as outpatients, but may be discussed and considered in patients deemed to be at high risk [5].
  - Consider LMWH or warfarin (INR ≈ 1.5) in patients affected by multiple myeloma who receive thalidomide and dexamethasone or thalidomide and chemotherapy [6].
  - Prophylaxis in oncological patients treated with adjuvant chemotherapy and/or hormonal therapy is not recommended.

29.2.5 Central Venous Catheters (CVCs)

In the 1990s, two open-label randomised clinical trials suggested using warfarin or LMWH prophylaxis in patients with CVCs [7, 8]. More recent studies assessed the incidence of CVC-related DVTs and found that the incidence is generally low, approximately 3–4 %, and that there was no statistically significant difference between patients who underwent prophylaxis and those that did not [9–12]. The risk of thrombosis depends on the size and type of the catheter and on the site of insertion (peripheral vein, femoral, subclavian or jugular) [13]. Long-term skin-tunnelled catheters have a lower incidence of thrombosis compared to peripheral catheters [14].

> **Routine prophylaxis in order to avoid CVC-related DVTs is therefore not recommended [15].**

29.3 Long-Term Side Effects

A patient with a past history of neoplasm may be at risk of delayed side effects (sometimes occurring many years later). Therefore, the GP should plan regular check-ups and screening tests for these patients:

- Patients treated with mediastinal and/or chest wall radiotherapy (RT) (see chapter):
  - Coronary artery disease
  - Valvular heart disease
  - Arrhythmias
  - Pericardial disease
  - Lung dysfunction
  - Carotid artery disease and thyroid function if RT involved the upper mediastinum and/or the neck
  - Radio-induced tumours: skin cancer, sarcomas in the irradiated area and breast cancer [16–18]
- People treated for cancer in childhood are at high risk of second tumour due to either chemo- and/or radiotherapy [19].
- Hormonal treatments. Check:
  - Metabolic function (diabetes, dyslipidemia)
  - Screen for ischaemic heart disease
- Testicular cancer:
  - Check blood lipids regularly.
  - Screen for ischaemic heart disease in patients treated with platinum

29.4 Drug Interactions

Remember that several oncological drugs (in particular the tyrosine kinase inhibitors) may interfere with some cardiovascular drugs. If the oncological and cardiac treatments are prescribed independently by specialists who do not consult each other, the risk of interaction may be undervalued. The GP is the only physician who is fully aware of all the patient's ongoing treatments.

- Check for interactions (see sites as ▶ http://www.drugs.com/drug_interactions.html).
- Ask for a cardiology check-up or advice to potentially change the therapy if the patient is taking or has been given a prescription of:
  - Verapamil, diltiazem, other calcium channel blockers
  - Amiodarone, dronedarone, propafenone, flecainide
  - Statins
  - Digoxin
  - Ranolazine
  - Warfarin, dabigatran, rivaroxaban, apixaban
  - Sotalol and any other drug which could prolong the QT interval

29.5 Most Frequent Cardiac Problems in Cancer Patients

Some cardiac problems are more frequent in cancer patients in comparison to the general population:

- **Pericardial effusion** at risk of cardiac tamponade. It should be considered as a possibility if the patient has a worsening, dyspnoea, tachycardia, low blood pressure, pulsus paradoxus and engorged jugular veins (see chapter…).
- **Atrial fibrillation** and ventricular arrhythmias may significantly worsen the patient's clinical condition and should be promptly treated. Ask for an electrocardiogram if an irregular heart rate is detected by the patient or observed during a routine visit.
- **Dyspnoea**, peripheral oedema and superficial thrombophlebitis are common problems which are worth to be analysed in details.

29.6 Dyspnoea

Dyspnoea is one of the most common symptoms in cancer patients.

- Breathlessness, 'an uncomfortably awareness of breathing', is a common symptom in cancer patients and particularly in palliative care patients (40–80 % prevalence) [20, 21].
- Breathlessness is a complicated symptom that involves physiological, psychological and environmental factors.

29.6.1 Causes of Dyspnoea [22]

- Primary lung cancer
- Mesothelioma
- Superior vena cava obstruction

- Lung metastases
- Lymphoadenopathy
- Pleural effusion
- Pulmonary embolism/lung collapse/pneumonia
- Fibrosis
- Respiratory muscle weakness
- Carcinomatous lymphangitis
- COPD/asthma
- Heart failure/arrhythmias/pericardial effusion
- Diaphragmatic weakness or pressure by ascites
- Anaemia
- Uraemia
- Anxiety

29.6.2 Assessment of Dyspnoea

- A detailed history and examination of the patient is essential:
  - Ask about timing and speed of onset of breathlessness.
  - Ask about exacerbating and relieving factors.
  - Identify co-morbidities and ask about the patient's past medical history.

Attention
Dyspnoea may not be directly caused by cancer.

29.6.3 Investigations (Personalised for Each Individual Patient)

- Full blood count (for anaemia)
- Chest X-ray (for consolidation/pleural effusion/lung collapse/heart failure)
- CT scan of the chest (for pulmonary embolus)
- ECG for arrhythmias

29.6.4 Management of Dyspnoea

General Measures

- Communication with the patient is essential: allowing the patient to talk freely about their concerns, about symptoms that they are experiencing and how these are affecting their quality of life.
- Explaining potential factors, which may be contributing to the patient's breathlessness, as well as discussing the management plan of the symptoms, helps to gain both the patient's and their carer's trust. Using a calm approach and reassuring the patient that there are different drugs that can help reduce the symptoms can go some way to alleviate the distress of the patient and their carers.

Treatment of Reversible Causes and Disease-Specific Measures [22]

Symptomatic Measures: Drugs

▪ Bronchodilators

A trial of bronchodilators can be useful if there are signs of bronchoconstriction (even without an obvious 'wheeze'):

- Beta-adrenoceptor agonists, e.g. salbutamol 2.5–5 mg via nebuliser or two puffs with an inhaler every 6 h. NB: can give anxiety, tremors or tachycardia if used frequently.
- Anticholinergic bronchodilators, e.g. ipratropium bromide 250–500 mcg via nebuliser or two puffs with an inhaler every 6 h.
- Saline chloride (0.9 %) 5 ml via nebuliser may reduce dense secretions and aid expectoration (◘ Table 29.1).

▪ Corticosteroids

Steroids can reduce tumour-associated oedema and can improve dyspnoea in lung metastases, tracheal obstruction/SVCO or lymphangitis carcinomatosa:

- Dexamethasone 4–8 mg daily (one should see an improvement within 1 week)

▪ Opioids

Morphine reduces an excessive respiratory drive and significantly reduces the respiratory response to hypoxia and hypercapnia. By reducing the rate of respiration, each breath becomes deeper and more efficient; anxiety and the sense of dyspnoea are reduced.

◘ Table 29.1 Dyspnoea: causes and disease-specific management options

Cause	Management options
Lung cancer	Chemotherapy/radiotherapy
Bronchospasm	Bronchodilators/corticosteroids
Infection	Antibiotics +/– corticosteroids if COPD
Pleural effusion	Pleural aspiration/drainage/pleurodesis
Pulmonary embolism	Anticoagulation (LMWH)
Heart failure	Diuretics/nitrates/antiarrhythmics
Anaemia	Blood transfusion/iron/erythropoietin
Lymphangitis carcinomatosa	Corticosteroids/diuretics/bronchodilators
Large airway obstruction	Radiotherapy/stenting if extrinsic compression/laser treatment/ brachytherapy/corticosteroids
SVC obstruction	Radiotherapy/chemotherapy/stent/corticosteroids

Evidence has shown that morphine is useful in treating breathlessness related to cancer, heart failure, COPD and pulmonary fibrosis [23]:

- Oral morphine 2.5–5 mg as required or at regular 4 h intervals if dyspnoea is continuous

■ Benzodiazepines

These can be useful in patients who experience symptoms of panic and hyperventilation or at night when breathlessness disturbs sleep:

- Diazepam 2–5 mg at night, twice daily or as required
- Lorazepam 0.5–2 mg as required
- Midazolam 5 mg (SC) at night

■ Oxygen [24]

Oxygen may help patients who are breathless and hypoxic at rest or on exertion. It may help relieve dyspnoea in patients (even with a normal PaO_2) due to the effect of facial cooling by the oxygen or as a placebo effect. Many cancer patients feel breathless in the absence of hypoxia; therefore, it is difficult to know which patients may benefit from additional oxygen. Intermittent or continuous domiciliary oxygen can be prescribed for the palliation of breathlessness in patients with cancer.

■ Terminal Stage of Disease

Dyspnoea can be difficult to manage despite the use of all available measures and medication, particularly in the end stages of disease. If this is the case, sedation may be required to alleviate the patient's distress.

Medications used to manage dyspnoea can include morphine and midazolam delivered in a syringe driver as a continuous subcutaneous/intravenous infusion.

Symptomatic, Non-pharmacological Measures [22]

These measures can be used in conjunction with pharmacological measures:

- A draught of air from a fan or open window
- Massaging the back of the neck during an episode of respiratory distress
- Positioning the patient appropriately:
  - Upright position to improve lung expansion and to reduce pressure from the abdomen.
  - Lying high on one side can help if the patient has copious secretions and avoids aspiration.
  - Sitting forward with arms resting on thighs helps relax the upper chest muscles and aids expansion of the diaphragm.
- Physiotherapy for breathing exercises
- Teaching relaxation techniques
- Cognitive behaviour therapy to help manage negative thoughts

  Complementary therapies such as acupuncture

29.7 Peripheral Oedema

Peripheral oedema is rather common in cancer patients, mostly in those with advanced-stage disease and/or limited physical activity. It raises the problem of differential diagnosis between:

- Cellulitis
- Lymphoedema
  (pelvic tumours, lymph node dissection, tumour infiltration or damage secondary to radiotherapy to regional lymph nodes)
- Severe hypoalbuminaemia
  (malnutrition, metabolic effects of cancer, hepatic insufficiency, third spacing, e.g. ascites)
- Rupture of a Baker's cyst
- Salt and water retention
  (NSAIDs; corticosteroids; cardiac, hepatic or renal failure; increased intra-abdominal pressure, e.g. ascites)
- Deep-vein thrombosis (DVT)

If unilateral or predominantly affecting one limb, the first step is to exclude a diagnosis of DVT (see above).

If a DVT has been excluded, it is important to distinguish between simple oedema and lymphoedema (▣ Table 29.2).

- Blood tests: serum electrolytes, urea, creatinine, liver enzymes, serum albumin

29.7.1 Treatment

1. Furosemide 25–40 mg PO OD (am). If, after 3–4 days, there is no response to the treatment, the morning dose can be doubled, and/or a second dose can be added (half the morning dose can be given at midday).
2. Spironolactone 100 mg PO OD (am).
3. Dexamethasone 8 mg PO OD (dose to be gradually reduced).

▣ **Table 29.2** Differential approach for simple oedema vs. lymphoedema

	Simple oedema	Lymphoedema
Pitting oedema	Present	Usually absent
Elevation of the affected limb	Useful	Not useful
Diuretics	Useful	Not useful
Skin	Taught, smooth	Hyperkeratotic, secretory
Affected limbs	Bilateral, lower limbs	Unilateral, can affect upper limbs
Cortisone	No	Yes, high dose

Note:

If serum albumin levels are low (<2.5 g/dl), **there are neither pathophysiological explanations nor are there trials or observational studies to justify the use of exogenous albumin in order to re-establish normal albumin levels in malnourished patients.**

Albumin should not be used in patients that require a nutritional intervention as its composition is unbalanced and lacking in particular amino acids; it can interfere both with protein synthesis and with endogenous albumin itself [25]. For these reasons as well as its capability to accelerate the breakdown of endogenous albumin, hypoalbuminaemia can rapidly be accentuated by exogenous albumin.

For nutritional purposes, albumin must be substituted with enteral or parenteral nutrition.

Rigid salt and water restriction has little sense in palliative care as such restrictions only go to reduce the patient's quality of life. However, limiting the foods with a high sodium content (e.g. sausages, jam, cheese, foods containing preservatives, canned foods) and promoting an adequate potassium intake are useful to prevent excessive water retention [26, 27].

Tip

Accurate skin care to avoid infections (in case of impetigo, start oral treatment with AM-CL, azithromycin, clarithromycin or mupirocin 2 % cream or fusidic acid 2 % cream TDS for 5–7 days)
Protection against trauma
Lymphatic drainage
Compression stockings
Exercises at the patient's bedside

29.8 Superficial Thrombophlebitis

Superficial thrombophlebitis should be suspected in presence of striae or a hot painful palpable subcutaneous cord along the course of a healthy vein, in the presence of a traumatised varicose vein and/or which has been used for an infusion, sclerotherapy or CVC insertion or in a patient with a source of infection.

29.8.1 Superficial Thrombophlebitis in a Healthy Vein

Request *colour Doppler ultrasound*:
- To assess its size, location and embolisation risk
- To follow its evolution and establish length of treatment
- To search for possible DVTs

Management

Objectives:
- To prevent its progression and possible embolisation
- To address the inflammation and clinical problem

Treatment

- Low- or medium-dose LMWH or UFH for a variable duration based on the degree of the clinical problem (on average 4 weeks) (Grade A)
- Low-dose fondaparinux (2.5 mg/die) for 45 days (Grade A)
- Alternative treatment: warfarin (target INR 2–3) for 4 weeks (Grade B)
- Graduated compression stockings (Grade B)

Note: If the superficial thrombophlebitis progresses into the deep venous system or 2–3 cm from it = treat at a DVT. Assess PE risk (if suspicious → send to A&E).

Follow-up

- Check full blood count and coagulation profile after 7 days.
- Check-up after 20 days + colour Doppler ultrasound if required.
- The decision on the LMWH or UFH dose is related to the presence of risk factors, its size, location and the severity of the clinical presentation.

29.8.2 Superficial Thrombophlebitis in a Varicose Vein

Request occasionally *colour Doppler ultrasound (based on clinical opinion).*

Management

Objectives:
- To address the inflammation and clinical problem

Treatment

- Remove the cause
- Topical of systemic NSAIDs
- Antibiotics if signs of infection
- Graduated compression stockings
- LMWH or fondaparinux in selected cases (see below)

29.8.3 Superficial Thrombophlebitis of the Great Saphenous Vein Progressing into the Deep Femoral Vein

This should be considered to all intents and purposes a DVT and therefore treated as such with anticoagulant therapy [28].

29.8.4 Superficial Thrombophlebitis of the Small and Great Saphenous Veins not Extending to the Deep Venous System

First-line therapy is LMWH (based on the patient's weight, at therapeutic doses) continued for 2–4 weeks or fondaparinux (2.5 mg in a single daily dose) for 45 days or heparin calcium (25,000 U/daily in two subcutaneous daily doses) maintaining an aPTT ratio of 1.5–2.5 [29].

29.8.5 Superficial Thrombophlebitis Affecting Other Parts of the Body

Low-dose heparin calcium or LMWH is recommended for 2 weeks in association with NSAIDs. Compression bandaging is extremely important, using bandages that have a medium–high elasticity with a low-pressure gradient between pressure during activity and pressure at rest.

References

1. Watson M, Lucas C, Hoy A, Wells J. Oxford handbook of palliative care. 2nd ed. Oxford: Oxford University Press; 2009 (Chapter 6L-Palliative Haematological Aspects).
2. Prandoni P, Lensing AW, Piccioli A, et al. Recurrent venous thromboembolism and bleeding complications during anticoagulant treatment in patients with cancer and venous thrombosis. Blood. 2002;100:3484–8.
3. Carrier M, Le Gal G, Cho R, et al. Dose escalation of low molecular weight heparin to manage recurrent venous thromboembolic events despite systemic anticoagulation in cancer patients. J Thromb Haemost. 2009;7:760–5.
4. Samama MM, Cohen AT, Darmon JY, et al. A comparison of enoxaparin with placebo for the prevention of venous thromboembolism in acutely ill medical patients: prophylaxis in medical patients with enoxaparin study group. N Engl J Med. 1999;341:793–800.
5. Agnelli G, Gussoni G, Bianchini C, et al. Nadroparin for the prevention of thromboembolic events in ambulatory patients with metastatic or locally advanced solid cancer receiving chemotherapy: a randomised, placebo-controlled, double-blind study. Lancet Oncol. 2009;10:943–9.
6. Palumbo A, Cavo M, Bringhen S, et al. Aspirin, warfarin, or enoxaparin thromboprophylaxis in patients with multiple myeloma treated with thalidomide: a phase III, open-label, randomized trial. J Clin Oncol. 2011;29:986–93.
7. Bern MM, Lokich JJ, Wallach SR, et al. Very low doses of warfarin can prevent thrombosis in central venous catheters. A randomised prospective trial. Ann Intern Med. 1990;112:423–8.
8. Monreal M, Alastrue A, Rull M, et al. Upper extremity deep venous thrombosis in cancer patients with venous access devices: prophylaxis with a low molecular weight heparin (Fragmin). Thromb Haemost. 1996;75:251–3.
9. Heaton DC, Han DY, Inder A. Minidose (1 mg) warfarin as prophylaxis for central vein catheter thrombosis. Intern Med J. 2002;32:84–8.
10. Couban S, Goodyear M, Burnell M, et al. Randomized placebo-controlled study of low-dose warfarin for the prevention of central venous catheter-associated thrombosis in patients with cancer. J Clin Oncol. 2005;23:4063–9.
11. Karthaus M, Kretzschmar A, Kroning H, et al. Dalteparin for prevention of catheter-related complications in cancer patients with central venous catheters: final results of a double-blind, placebo-controlled phase III trial. Ann Oncol. 2006;17:289–96.
12. Verso M, Agnelli G, Bertoglio S, et al. Enoxaparin for the prevention of venous thromboembolism associated with central vein catheter: a double-blind, placebo-controlled, randomized study in cancer patients. J Clin Oncol. 2005;23:4057–62.

13. Geerts W. Central venous catheter-related thrombosis. Hematology Am Soc Hematol Educ Program. 2014;2014:306–11.
14. Sriskandarajah P, Webb K, Chisholm D, et al. Retrospective cohort analysis comparing the incidence of deep vein thromboses between peripherally-inserted and long-term skin tunneled venous catheters in hemato-oncology patients. Thromb J. 2015;13:21.
15. Chaukiyal P, Nautiyal A, Radhakrishnan S, et al. Thromboprophylaxis in cancer patients with central venous catheters. A systematic review and meta-analysis. Thromb Haemost. 2008;99:38–43.
16. Travis LB, Hill DA, Dores GM, et al. Breast cancer following radiotherapy and chemotherapy among young women with Hodgkin disease. JAMA. 2003;290:465–75.
17. Travis LB, Ng AK, Allan JM, et al. Second malignant neoplasms and cardiovascular disease following radiotherapy. J Natl Cancer Inst. 2012;104:357–70.
18. Thiagarajan A, Iyer NG. Radiation-induced sarcomas of the head and neck. World J Clin Oncol. 2014;5:973–81. Review.
19. Choi DK, Helenowski I, Hijiya N. Secondary malignancies in pediatric cancer survivors: perspectives and review of the literature. Int J Cancer. 2014;135:1764–73. Review.
20. Dudgeon DJ, Lertzman M. Dyspnea in advanced cancer patient. J Pain Symptom Manage. 1998;16: 212–9.
21. Bruera E. The frequency and correlates of dyspnoea in patients with advanced cancer. J Pain Symptom Manage. 2000;19:357–62.
22. Watson M, et al. Respiratory symptoms, Oxford handbook of palliative care. 2nd ed. Oxford: Oxford University Press; 2009. p. 363–75.
23. Brown DJF. Palliation of breathlessness. Clin Med. 2006;6:133–6.
24. Goody R. Using oxygen therapy in the palliative care setting. Eur J Palliat Care. 2007;14:120–3.
25. Vermeulen LC, et al. A paradigm for consensus. The University Hospital Consortium guidelines for the use of albumin, nonprotein colloid, and crystalloid solutions. Arch Intern Med. 1995;155(16):1817.
26. Adrogué HJ, Madias NE. Sodium and potassium in the pathogenesis of hypertension. N Engl J Med. 2007;356:1966–78. Review.
27. Penton D, Czogalla J, Loffing J. Dietary potassium and the renal control of salt balance and blood pressure. Pflugers Arch. 2015;467:513–30.
28. American College of Chest Physicians. Antithrombotic therapy for venous thromboembolic disease: ACCP E-BCPG (8 th Edition). Chest. 2008;133 Suppl 6:454S–545.
29. Trentin L. Valutazione e Trattamento dei sintomi nel malato oncologico. 2015 Edition. AIOM (Associazione Italiana di Oncologia Medica) with contribution of ESMO (European Society for Medical Oncology).

MIX
Papier aus verantwortungsvollen Quellen
Paper from responsible sources
FSC® C105338

If you have any concerns about our products, you can contact us on
ProductSafety@springernature.com

In case Publisher is established outside the EU, the EU authorized representative is:
Springer Nature Customer Service Center GmbH
Europaplatz 3, 69115 Heidelberg, Germany

Printed by Libri Plureos GmbH
in Hamburg, Germany